Metabolic Syndrome

Metabolic Syndrome: From Etiology to Prevention and Clinical Management

Editors

Isabelle Lemieux
Jean-Pierre Després

MDPI • Basel • Beijing • Wuhan • Barcelona • Belgrade • Manchester • Tokyo • Cluj • Tianjin

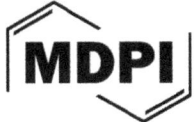

Editors
Isabelle Lemieux
Québec Heart and Lung Institute Research Centre
Canada

Jean-Pierre Després
Québec Heart and Lung Institute Research Centre
Canada

Editorial Office
MDPI
St. Alban-Anlage 66
4052 Basel, Switzerland

This is a reprint of articles from the Special Issue published online in the open access journal *Nutrients* (ISSN 2072-6643) (available at: https://www.mdpi.com/journal/nutrients/special_issues/Metabolic_syndrome_etiology_prevention_clinical_management).

For citation purposes, cite each article independently as indicated on the article page online and as indicated below:

LastName, A.A.; LastName, B.B.; LastName, C.C. Article Title. *Journal Name* **Year**, *Volume Number*, Page Range.

ISBN 978-3-03943-989-8 (Hbk)
ISBN 978-3-03943-990-4 (PDF)

Cover image courtesy of Isabelle Lemieux.

© 2020 by the authors. Articles in this book are Open Access and distributed under the Creative Commons Attribution (CC BY) license, which allows users to download, copy and build upon published articles, as long as the author and publisher are properly credited, which ensures maximum dissemination and a wider impact of our publications.

The book as a whole is distributed by MDPI under the terms and conditions of the Creative Commons license CC BY-NC-ND.

Contents

About the Editors ix

Isabelle Lemieux and Jean-Pierre Després
Metabolic Syndrome: Past, Present and Future
Reprinted from: *Nutrients* 2020, 12, 3501, doi:10.3390/nu12113501 1

Jiao Wang, Javier S. Perona, Jacqueline Schmidt-RioValle, Yajun Chen, Jin Jing and Emilio González-Jiménez
Metabolic Syndrome and Its Associated Early-Life Factors among Chinese and Spanish Adolescents: A Pilot Study
Reprinted from: *Nutrients* 2019, 11, 1568, doi:10.3390/nu11071568 9

Jacopo Troisi, Federica Belmonte, Antonella Bisogno, Luca Pierri, Angelo Colucci, Giovanni Scala, Pierpaolo Cavallo, Claudia Mandato, Antonella Di Nuzzi, Laura Di Michele, Anna Pia Delli Bovi, Salvatore Guercio Nuzio and Pietro Vajro
Metabolomic Salivary Signature of Pediatric Obesity Related Liver Disease and Metabolic Syndrome
Reprinted from: *Nutrients* 2019, 11, 274, doi:10.3390/nu11020274 23

Luigi Barrea, Giuseppe Annunziata, Giovanna Muscogiuri, Carolina Di Somma, Daniela Laudisio, Maria Maisto, Giulia de Alteriis, Gian Carlo Tenore, Annamaria Colao and Silvia Savastano
Trimethylamine-N-oxide (TMAO) as Novel Potential Biomarker of Early Predictors of Metabolic Syndrome
Reprinted from: *Nutrients* 2018, 10, 1971, doi:10.3390/nu10121971 41

Kaiser Wani, Sobhy M. Yakout, Mohammed Ghouse Ahmed Ansari, Shaun Sabico, Syed Danish Hussain, Majed S. Alokail, Eman Sheshah, Naji J. Aljohani, Yousef Al-Saleh, Jean-Yves Reginster and Nasser M. Al-Daghri
Metabolic Syndrome in Arab Adults with Low Bone Mineral Density
Reprinted from: *Nutrients* 2019, 11, 1405, doi:10.3390/nu11061405 61

Vasanti S. Malik and Frank B. Hu
Sugar-Sweetened Beverages and Cardiometabolic Health: An Update of the Evidence
Reprinted from: *Nutrients* 2019, 11, 1840, doi:10.3390/nu11081840 75

Marja-Riitta Taskinen, Chris J Packard and Jan Borén
Dietary Fructose and the Metabolic Syndrome
Reprinted from: *Nutrients* 2019, 11, 1987, doi:10.3390/nu11091987 93

Michèle Rousseau, Frédéric Guénard, Véronique Garneau, Bénédicte Allam-Ndoul, Simone Lemieux, Louis Pérusse and Marie-Claude Vohl
Associations Between Dietary Protein Sources, Plasma BCAA and Short-Chain Acylcarnitine Levels in Adults
Reprinted from: *Nutrients* 2019, 11, 173, doi:10.3390/nu11010173 109

Alicia Julibert, Maria del Mar Bibiloni, David Mateos, Escarlata Angullo and Josep A. Tur
Dietary Fat Intake and Metabolic Syndrome in Older Adults
Reprinted from: *Nutrients* 2019, 11, 1901, doi:10.3390/nu11081901 125

Stéphanie Harrison, Patrick Couture and Benoît Lamarche
Diet Quality, Saturated Fat and Metabolic Syndrome
Reprinted from: *Nutrients* **2020**, *12*, 3232, doi:10.3390/nu12113232 . . . . **141**

Anne-Laure Borel
Sleep Apnea and Sleep Habits: Relationships with Metabolic Syndrome
Reprinted from: *Nutrients* **2019**, *11*, 2628, doi:10.3390/nu11112628 . . . . **151**

Javier S. Perona, Jacqueline Schmidt-RioValle, Ángel Fernández-Aparicio, María Correa-Rodríguez, Robinson Ramírez-Vélez and Emilio González-Jiménez
Waist Circumference and Abdominal Volume Index Can Predict Metabolic Syndrome in Adolescents, but only When the Criteria of the International Diabetes Federation are Employed for the Diagnosis
Reprinted from: *Nutrients* **2019**, *11*, 1370, doi:10.3390/nu11061370 . . . . **167**

Robinson Ramírez-Vélez, MiguelÁngel Pérez-Sousa, Mikel Izquierdo, Carlos A. Cano-Gutierrez, Emilio González-Jiménez, Jacqueline Schmidt-RioValle, Katherine González-Ruíz and María Correa-Rodríguez
Validation of Surrogate Anthropometric Indices in Older Adults: What Is the Best Indicator of High Cardiometabolic Risk Factor Clustering?
Reprinted from: *Nutrients* **2019**, *11*, 1701, doi:10.3390/nu11081701 . . . . **183**

Mark D. DeBoer
Assessing and Managing the Metabolic Syndrome in Children and Adolescents
Reprinted from: *Nutrients* **2019**, *11*, 1788, doi:10.3390/nu11081788 . . . . **199**

Scott A. Lear and Danijela Gasevic
Ethnicity and Metabolic Syndrome: Implications for Assessment, Management and Prevention
Reprinted from: *Nutrients* **2020**, *12*, 15, doi:10.3390/nu12010015 . . . . **211**

Peter Clifton
Metabolic Syndrome—Role of Dietary Fat Type and Quantity
Reprinted from: *Nutrients* **2019**, *11*, 1438, doi:10.3390/nu11071438 . . . . **227**

Siti Raihanah Shafie, Stephen Wanyonyi, Sunil K. Panchal and Lindsay Brown
Linseed Components Are More Effective Than Whole Linseed in Reversing Diet-Induced Metabolic Syndrome in Rats
Reprinted from: *Nutrients* **2019**, *11*, 1677, doi:10.3390/nu11071677 . . . . **235**

Robert Ross, Simrat Soni and Sarah Houle
Negative Energy Balance Induced by Exercise or Diet: Effects on Visceral Adipose Tissue and Liver Fat
Reprinted from: *Nutrients* **2020**, *12*, 891, doi:10.3390/nu12040891 . . . . **251**

Jonathan Myers, Peter Kokkinos and Eric Nyelin
Physical Activity, Cardiorespiratory Fitness, and the Metabolic Syndrome
Reprinted from: *Nutrients* **2019**, *11*, 1652, doi:10.3390/nu11071652 . . . . **265**

Vincenzo Di Marzo and Cristoforo Silvestri
Lifestyle and Metabolic Syndrome: Contribution of the Endocannabinoidome
Reprinted from: *Nutrients* **2019**, *11*, 1956, doi:10.3390/nu11081956 . . . . **283**

Maria Garralda-Del-Villar, Silvia Carlos-Chillerón, Jesus Diaz-Gutierrez, Miguel Ruiz-Canela, Alfredo Gea, Miguel Angel Martínez-González, Maira Bes-Rastrollo, Liz Ruiz-Estigarribia, Stefanos N. Kales and Alejandro Fernández-Montero
Healthy Lifestyle and Incidence of Metabolic Syndrome in the SUN Cohort
Reprinted from: *Nutrients* **2019**, *11*, 65, doi:10.3390/nu11010065 307

Hitoshi Nishizawa and Iichiro Shimomura
Population Approaches Targeting Metabolic Syndrome Focusing on Japanese Trials
Reprinted from: *Nutrients* **2019**, *11*, 1430, doi:10.3390/nu11061430 323

About the Editors

Isabelle Lemieux is a research associate at the Centre de recherche de l'Institut universitaire de cardiologie et de pneumologie de Québec—Université Laval (Québec Heart and Lung Institute). Her scientific work has contributed to a better understanding of the links between visceral obesity and emerging risk factors for cardiometabolic diseases, from etiologic studies (association of abdominal obesity with inflammation) to the development of clinical tools (hypertriglyceridemic waist) to assess and monitor changes in visceral adiposity. Together with Dr. Jean-Pierre Després, she co-authored an invited review paper on the link between abdominal obesity and metabolic syndrome, which was published in Nature in 2006 and is considered a classic in the field. Her work has led to the production of more than 100 scientific articles and 6 book chapters (more than 19,000 Google Scholar citations; h-index: 54). As the Scientific Content Manager of the International Chair on Cardiometabolic Risk, Dr. Lemieux has also made a significant contribution to the translation of knowledge with the development of an educational website on visceral obesity (www.myhealthywaist.org).

Jean-Pierre Després is a professor in the Department of Kinesiology at Université Laval in Québec City. He established himself as a research scholar at Université Laval in 1986. He previously served as Assistant Director of the Centre for Research on Lipid Diseases at the CHUL Research Centre from 1991 to 1999, and Director of Research in Cardiology at the Québec Heart and Lung Institute from 1999 to 2018. He is currently the Scientific Director of VITAM – Centre de recherche en santé durable (Sustainable Health Research Centre) affiliated with Université Laval (appointed in 2018), and Scientific Director of the International Chair on Cardiometabolic (since 2005). He is one of the most cited researchers in the world in his field (752 scientific articles and 60 book chapters with over 145,000 Google Scholar citations; h-index: 153) and is currently the most cited active scientist at Université Laval. His research interests include obesity, adipose tissue distribution, visceral obesity, type 2 diabetes, lipids, lipoproteins, cardiovascular disease and their prevention through physical activity and healthy living. Thirty years ago, he was the first to report that an excess of fat in the abdominal cavity (visceral obesity) is particularly harmful to health. He is personally involved in major education and mobilization activities to prevent chronic societal diseases. He has received numerous prestigious awards such as "Grand Québécois" from the Québec Chamber of Commerce and Knight of the Ordre national du Québec (the highest distinction of the Québec government).

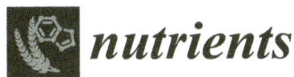

Editorial

Metabolic Syndrome: Past, Present and Future

Isabelle Lemieux [1,*] and Jean-Pierre Després [1,2,3]

1. Centre de recherche de l'Institut universitaire de cardiologie et de pneumologie de Québec—Université Laval, Québec, QC G1V 4G5, Canada; jean-pierre.despres.ciussscn@ssss.gouv.qc.ca
2. Department of Kinesiology, Faculty of Medicine, Université Laval, Québec, QC G1V 0A6, Canada
3. VITAM—Centre de recherche en santé durable, CIUSSS de la Capitale-Nationale, Québec, QC G1J 0A4, Canada
* Correspondence: isabelle.lemieux@criucpq.ulaval.ca; Tel.: +1-418-656-8711 (ext. 3603)

Received: 28 October 2020; Accepted: 29 October 2020; Published: 14 November 2020

1. Syndrome X: A Tribute to a Pioneer, Gerald M. Reaven

Most clinicians and health professionals have heard or read about metabolic syndrome. For instance, as of October 2020, entering "metabolic syndrome" in a PubMed search generated more than 57,000 publications since the introduction of the concept by Grundy and colleagues in 2001 [1]. Although many health professionals are familiar with the five criteria proposed by the National Cholesterol Education Program-Adult Treatment Panel III for its diagnosis (waist circumference, triglycerides, high-density lipoprotein (HDL) cholesterol, blood pressure and glucose), how these variables were selected and the rationale used for the identification of cut-offs remain unclear for many people. In addition, the conceptual definition of metabolic syndrome is often confused with the tools (the five criteria) that have been proposed to make its diagnosis [2,3].

In the seminal paper of his American Diabetes Association 1988 Banting award lecture, Reaven put forward the notion that insulin resistance was not only a fundamental defect increasing the risk of type 2 diabetes, but he also proposed that it was a prevalent cause of cardiovascular disease [4]. The latter point was a paradigm shift as cardiovascular medicine had, at that time, a legitimate focus on cholesterol in risk assessment and management. Reaven was therefore the first to propose that insulin resistance was a central component of a cluster of abnormalities which included hyperinsulinemia, dysglycemia, high triglycerides, low HDL cholesterol and elevated blood pressure. Under his theory, this constellation of abnormalities would not only increase the risk of type 2 diabetes but would also be a complex risk factor for cardiovascular outcomes, even in the absence of type 2 diabetes. Reaven initially referred to this condition as syndrome X. However, as there is also a syndrome X in cardiology [5,6] and because insulin resistance is a core component of Reaven's syndrome, insulin resistance syndrome was a term that then gained popularity in the literature [7,8].

As measuring insulin resistance or circulating insulin levels was not considered as feasible on a large scale in clinical practice, a group of experts then examined whether it could be possible to identify insulin-resistant individuals with common clinical tools widely used in primary care [1]. Because of the strong link between abdominal obesity and insulin resistance, the panel thus agreed on the use of waist circumference as a crude index of abdominal adiposity and then proposed sex-specific waist cut-off values [1]. However, these waist circumference thresholds were based on the relationship between waist circumference and body mass index (BMI) values defining obesity (men: 102 cm = 30 kg/m^2 and women: 88 cm = 30 kg/m^2) [9]. Thus, waist circumference thresholds were simply determined from BMI values defining obesity and, most importantly, were not based on clinical outcomes. In addition, because waist circumference and BMI are correlated [10], an elevated waist girth, observed in isolation, cannot properly assess abdominal fat accumulation [11]. For instance, a waist circumference of 104 cm in a middle-aged man with a BMI of 26 kg/m^2 is not the same adiposity phenotype as an age-matched man with the same waist girth but with a BMI of 32 kg/m^2. In this specific example, the man with a

BMI of 26 kg/m^2 is clearly abdominally obese (high-risk form of obesity) whereas the man with a BMI of 32 kg/m^2 is mostly characterized by overall obesity. This is why a recent consensus paper on the use of waist circumference in clinical practice has proposed that waist circumference should not be measured as a single adiposity index but rather interpreted along with the BMI in order to properly discriminate abdominally obese (higher risk) from overall obese (lower risk) persons [11].

Regarding simple metabolic markers of insulin resistance and other indices of metabolic syndrome, triglycerides, HDL cholesterol levels and blood glucose are easily obtained from routine clinical biochemistry laboratories, whereas blood pressure is measured in primary care. On that basis, it was proposed that individuals showing any combination of any three out of these five simple clinical criteria were likely to be characterized by insulin resistance. Prospective analyses have also shown that any combination of these factors was predictive of an increased risk of both type 2 diabetes and cardiovascular disease [12–17].

As it had also been suggested that the waist cut-offs initially proposed were probably too high, their values were thereafter lowered in harmonized criteria proposed by other organizations [18]. Studies have shown that subgroups of individuals meeting or not meeting the clinical criteria of metabolic syndrome (harmonized or not) were quite distinct from each other in terms of risk of type 2 diabetes and cardiovascular disease [12–17]. Of course, using different waist circumference cut-off values generated different prevalence values but the subgroups identified were nevertheless found to show different levels of risk.

2. From Syndrome X, Insulin Resistance/Metabolic Syndrome to Excess Visceral Adiposity

Because Reaven could find nonobese individuals with insulin resistance and individuals with obesity who were insulin sensitive, he did not include obesity in his initial definition of syndrome X. In that regard, early imaging studies measuring adiposity with the use of computed tomography initially conducted by Matsuzawa and colleagues and by ourselves suggested that there was a remarkable heterogeneity in abdominal fat accumulation (visceral vs. subcutaneous) [19,20]. Additionally, subgroup analyses revealed that there was substantial variation in glucose tolerance as well as in plasma insulin and lipoprotein levels among equally overweight or obese individuals characterized by low or high levels of visceral adipose tissue [21–24]. Since then, many large cardiometabolic imaging studies have shown that an excess accumulation of visceral adipose tissue (and not of subcutaneous fat) was a key correlate of the features of insulin resistance, explaining why Reaven could not find a robust association between total body fatness and his syndrome X: it was all about body fat distribution [2,3,25–31].

3. Liver Fat: A Key Partner in Crime in Visceral Obesity

More recently, with the availability of magnetic resonance spectroscopy, it has become possible to noninvasively measure with great accuracy liver fat accumulation. With the use of this technique, excess liver fat has been found to be associated with essentially the same clustering metabolic abnormalities as those observed in visceral obesity [32–34]. It is important, however, to point out that excess liver fat in isolation (in the absence of excess visceral adipose tissue) is a relatively rare phenomenon as its most frequent form is accompanied by high levels of visceral adipose tissue [35–37]. Thus, it has recently become obvious that the most dangerous adiposity phenotype includes excessive amounts of both visceral adipose tissue and liver fat, which is by far the most prevalent form of insulin resistance or metabolic syndrome [31]. On that basis, we have proposed that the clustering abnormalities of excess visceral adiposity/liver fat for which insulin resistance is a key feature should be called Reaven syndrome [3,38].

4. This Issue

Despite the progress made in our understanding of the constellation of atherogenic and diabetogenic abnormalities found in the subgroup of individuals with excess levels of visceral adipose tissue and liver fat, many questions remain regarding their etiology and the most efficient approaches to prevent or to manage it.

Some of these questions are examined in this special issue of *Nutrients*. The reader will find a mix of narrative reviews and communications written by well-published investigators, top international experts in the field. We are very grateful to these experts who have agreed to contribute to this issue [39–49]. Original papers that are relevant to our theme are also included [50–59].

As expected from the topics covered in *Nutrients*, this issue deals mostly with dietary factors, although some other important lifestyle features, such as physical activity/exercise and sleeping habits, are addressed. Both individual- and population-based solutions are discussed. For instance, the link between dietary fat as well as dietary fructose and sugar-sweetened beverages and some chronic diseases is reviewed. Considering the importance of physical activity/exercise and cardiorespiratory fitness in the prevention and treatment of features of metabolic syndrome, some papers review the literature relevant to these topics. Moreover, other papers deal with the assessment of metabolic syndrome in various age and ethnic groups. Finally, other highly relevant themes are explored, such as sleep habits, sleep apnea and the development of metabolic syndrome and lifestyle habits, the endocannabinoidome and features of metabolic syndrome.

5. The Future

Of course, it was not possible to cover all topics relevant to the assessment, prevention and management of such a complex modifiable risk factor which results from the interaction of genetic and environmental/lifestyle factors. The established relationship between the presence of metabolic syndrome and the development of type 2 diabetes and cardiovascular disease has been amply demonstrated, but the interest around metabolic syndrome and visceral obesity is renewed as it has also been related to other chronic diseases, such as brain health and some types of cancer [60,61]. Numerous studies are currently under way to confirm these relationships, to elucidate the underlying mechanisms or even to examine whether lifestyle intervention habits could prevent these diseases and improve their treatment. As we are going through a major epidemic of chronic lifestyle diseases, metabolic syndrome, although criticized as a concept, has been helpful as a screening approach to better identify a subgroup of high-risk individuals who would benefit from clinical and population-based approaches targeting their lifestyle habits. Finally, with the relatively new concept of precision lifestyle medicine, which consists of simultaneously taking into account the individual's genetic profile as well as his/her living environments and lifestyle habits [62], we propose that the multiplex modifiable risk factor that represents metabolic syndrome will require concerted efforts between clinical approaches and public health solutions if we want to reduce the burden associated with this condition. We hope that the content of this Special Issue will be found useful.

Author Contributions: I.L. and J.-P.D. wrote the paper together. All authors have read and agreed to the published version of the manuscript.

Funding: J.-P.D. is the Scientific Director of the International Chair on Cardiometabolic Risk supported by the Fondation de l'Université Laval. Research from J.-P.D. discussed in this editorial has been and is currently supported by the Canadian Institutes of Health Research (Foundation grant: FDN-167278) as well as by the Fondation of the Québec Heart and Lung Institute.

Conflicts of Interest: The author declares no conflict of interest.

References

1. Expert Panel on Detection, Evaluation, and Treatment of High Blood Cholesterol in Adults. Executive Summary of The Third Report of The National Cholesterol Education Program (NCEP) Expert Panel on Detection, Evaluation, and Treatment of High Blood Cholesterol in Adults (Adult Treatment Panel III). *JAMA* **2001**, *285*, 2486–2497. [CrossRef] [PubMed]
2. Després, J.P.; Lemieux, I. Abdominal obesity and metabolic syndrome. *Nature* **2006**, *444*, 881–887. [CrossRef] [PubMed]
3. Després, J.P.; Lemieux, I.; Bergeron, J.; Pibarot, P.; Mathieu, P.; Larose, E.; Rodés-Cabau, J.; Bertrand, O.F.; Poirier, P. Abdominal obesity and the metabolic syndrome: Contribution to global cardiometabolic risk. *Arterioscler. Thromb. Vasc. Biol.* **2008**, *28*, 1039–1049. [CrossRef] [PubMed]
4. Reaven, G.M. Banting lecture 1988. Role of insulin resistance in human disease. *Diabetes* **1988**, *37*, 1595–1607. [CrossRef] [PubMed]
5. Cheng, T.O. Cardiac syndrome X versus metabolic syndrome X. *Int. J. Cardiol.* **2007**, *119*, 137–138. [CrossRef]
6. Kemp, H.G., Jr. Left ventricular function in patients with the anginal syndrome and normal coronary arteriograms. *Am. J. Cardiol.* **1973**, *32*, 375–376. [CrossRef]
7. DeFronzo, R.A.; Ferrannini, E. Insulin resistance: A multifaced syndrome responsible for NIDDM, obesity, hypertension, dyslipidemia, and atherosclerotic cardiovascular disease. *Diabetes Care* **1991**, *14*, 173–194. [CrossRef]
8. Haffner, S.M.; Valdez, R.A.; Hazuda, H.P.; Mitchell, B.D.; Morales, P.A.; Stern, M.P. Prospective analysis of the insulin-resistance syndrome (syndrome X). *Diabetes* **1992**, *41*, 715–722. [CrossRef]
9. Lean, M.E.; Han, T.S.; Morrison, C.E. Waist circumference as a measure for indicating need for weight management. *BMJ* **1995**, *311*, 158–161. [CrossRef]
10. Després, J.P. Excess visceral adipose tissue/ectopic fat: The missing link in the obesity paradox? *J. Am. Coll. Cardiol.* **2011**, *57*, 1887–1889. [CrossRef]
11. Ross, R.; Neeland, I.J.; Yamashita, S.; Shai, I.; Seidell, J.; Magni, P.; Santos, R.D.; Arsenault, B.; Cuevas, A.; Hu, F.B.; et al. Waist circumference as a vital sign in clinical practice: A Consensus Statement from the IAS and ICCR Working Group on Visceral Obesity. *Nat. Rev. Endocrinol.* **2020**, *16*, 177–189. [CrossRef] [PubMed]
12. Wilson, P.W.; D'Agostino, R.B.; Parise, H.; Sullivan, L.; Meigs, J.B. Metabolic syndrome as a precursor of cardiovascular disease and type 2 diabetes mellitus. *Circulation* **2005**, *112*, 3066–3072. [CrossRef] [PubMed]
13. Ford, E.S. Risks for all-cause mortality, cardiovascular disease, and diabetes associated with the metabolic syndrome: A summary of the evidence. *Diabetes Care* **2005**, *28*, 1769–1778. [CrossRef] [PubMed]
14. Galassi, A.; Reynolds, K.; He, J. Metabolic syndrome and risk of cardiovascular disease: A meta-analysis. *Am. J. Med.* **2006**, *119*, 812–819. [CrossRef] [PubMed]
15. Gami, A.S.; Witt, B.J.; Howard, D.E.; Erwin, P.J.; Gami, L.A.; Somers, V.K.; Montori, V.M. Metabolic syndrome and risk of incident cardiovascular events and death: A systematic review and meta-analysis of longitudinal studies. *J. Am. Coll. Cardiol.* **2007**, *49*, 403–414. [CrossRef]
16. Mottillo, S.; Filion, K.B.; Genest, J.; Joseph, L.; Pilote, L.; Poirier, P.; Rinfret, S.; Schiffrin, E.L.; Eisenberg, M.J. The metabolic syndrome and cardiovascular risk: A systematic review and meta-analysis. *J. Am. Coll. Cardiol.* **2010**, *56*, 1113–1132. [CrossRef]
17. Ford, E.S.; Li, C.; Sattar, N. Metabolic syndrome and incident diabetes: Current state of the evidence. *Diabetes Care* **2008**, *31*, 1898–1904. [CrossRef]
18. Alberti, K.G.; Eckel, R.H.; Grundy, S.M.; Zimmet, P.Z.; Cleeman, J.I.; Donato, K.A.; Fruchart, J.C.; James, W.P.; Loria, C.M.; Smith, S.C., Jr. Harmonizing the metabolic syndrome: A joint interim statement of the International Diabetes Federation Task Force on Epidemiology and Prevention; National Heart, Lung, and Blood Institute; American Heart Association; World Heart Federation; International Atherosclerosis Society; and International Association for the Study of Obesity. *Circulation* **2009**, *120*, 1640–1645.
19. Ferland, M.; Després, J.P.; Tremblay, A.; Pinault, S.; Nadeau, A.; Moorjani, S.; Lupien, P.J.; Thériault, G.; Bouchard, C. Assessment of adipose tissue distribution by computed axial tomography in obese women: Association with body density and anthropometric measurements. *Br. J. Nutr.* **1989**, *61*, 139–148. [CrossRef]

20. Tokunaga, K.; Matsuzawa, Y.; Ishikawa, K.; Tarui, S. A novel technique for the determination of body fat by computed tomography. *Int. J. Obes.* **1983**, *7*, 437–445.
21. Pouliot, M.C.; Després, J.P.; Nadeau, A.; Moorjani, S.; Prud'homme, D.; Lupien, P.J.; Tremblay, A.; Bouchard, C. Visceral obesity in men. Associations with glucose tolerance, plasma insulin, and lipoprotein levels. *Diabetes* **1992**, *41*, 826–834. [CrossRef] [PubMed]
22. Després, J.P.; Moorjani, S.; Lupien, P.J.; Tremblay, A.; Nadeau, A.; Bouchard, C. Regional distribution of body fat, plasma lipoproteins, and cardiovascular disease. *Arteriosclerosis* **1990**, *10*, 497–511. [CrossRef] [PubMed]
23. Ross, R.; Aru, J.; Freeman, J.; Hudson, R.; Janssen, I. Abdominal adiposity and insulin resistance in obese men. *Am. J. Physiol. Endocrinol. Metab.* **2002**, *282*, E657–E663. [CrossRef] [PubMed]
24. Ross, R.; Freeman, J.; Hudson, R.; Janssen, I. Abdominal obesity, muscle composition, and insulin resistance in premenopausal women. *J. Clin. Endocrinol. Metab.* **2002**, *87*, 5044–5051. [CrossRef]
25. Després, J.P. Body fat distribution and risk of cardiovascular disease: An update. *Circulation* **2012**, *126*, 1301–1313. [CrossRef]
26. Neeland, I.J.; Poirier, P.; Després, J.P. Cardiovascular and metabolic heterogeneity of obesity: Clinical challenges and implications for management. *Circulation* **2018**, *137*, 1391–1406. [CrossRef]
27. Shah, R.V.; Murthy, V.L.; Abbasi, S.A.; Blankstein, R.; Kwong, R.Y.; Goldfine, A.B.; Jerosch-Herold, M.; Lima, J.A.; Ding, J.; Allison, M.A. Visceral adiposity and the risk of metabolic syndrome across body mass index: The MESA Study. *JACC Cardiovasc. Imaging* **2014**, *7*, 1221–1235. [CrossRef]
28. Smith, U. Abdominal obesity: A marker of ectopic fat accumulation. *J. Clin. Investig.* **2015**, *125*, 1790–1792. [CrossRef]
29. Matsuzawa, Y. Pathophysiology and molecular mechanisms of visceral fat syndrome: The Japanese experience. *Diabetes Metab. Rev.* **1997**, *13*, 3–13. [CrossRef]
30. Matsuzawa, Y.; Funahashi, T.; Nakamura, T. The concept of metabolic syndrome: Contribution of visceral fat accumulation and its molecular mechanism. *J. Atheroscler. Thromb.* **2011**, *18*, 629–639. [CrossRef]
31. Neeland, I.J.; Ross, R.; Després, J.P.; Matsuzawa, Y.; Yamashita, S.; Shai, I.; Seidell, J.; Magni, P.; Santos, R.D.; Arsenault, B.; et al. Visceral and ectopic fat, atherosclerosis, and cardiometabolic disease: A position statement. *Lancet Diabetes Endocrinol.* **2019**, *7*, 715–725. [CrossRef]
32. Adiels, M.; Olofsson, S.O.; Taskinen, M.R.; Boren, J. Overproduction of very low-density lipoproteins is the hallmark of the dyslipidemia in the metabolic syndrome. *Arterioscler. Thromb. Vasc. Biol.* **2008**, *28*, 1225–1236. [CrossRef] [PubMed]
33. Yki-Jarvinen, H. Non-alcoholic fatty liver disease as a cause and a consequence of metabolic syndrome. *Lancet Diabetes Endocrinol.* **2014**, *2*, 901–910. [CrossRef]
34. Stefan, N.; Schick, F.; Haring, H.U. Causes, characteristics, and consequences of metabolically unhealthy normal weight in humans. *Cell Metab.* **2017**, *26*, 292–300. [CrossRef] [PubMed]
35. Nazare, J.A.; Smith, J.D.; Borel, A.L.; Haffner, S.M.; Balkau, B.; Ross, R.; Massien, C.; Alméras, N.; Després, J.P. Ethnic influences on the relations between abdominal subcutaneous and visceral adiposity, liver fat, and cardiometabolic risk profile: The International Study of Prediction of Intra-Abdominal Adiposity and Its Relationship With Cardiometabolic Risk/Intra-Abdominal Adiposity. *Am. J. Clin. Nutr.* **2012**, *96*, 714–726. [PubMed]
36. Liu, J.; Fox, C.S.; Hickson, D.; Bidulescu, A.; Carr, J.J.; Taylor, H.A. Fatty liver, abdominal visceral fat, and cardiometabolic risk factors: The Jackson Heart Study. *Arterioscler. Thromb. Vasc. Biol.* **2011**, *31*, 2715–2722. [CrossRef] [PubMed]
37. Guerrero, R.; Vega, G.L.; Grundy, S.M.; Browning, J.D. Ethnic differences in hepatic steatosis: An insulin resistance paradox? *Hepatology* **2009**, *49*, 791–801. [CrossRef]
38. Després, J.P. The Reaven syndrome: A tribute to a giant. *Nat. Rev. Endocrinol.* **2018**, *14*, 319–320. [CrossRef]
39. Lear, S.A.; Gasevic, D. Ethnicity and metabolic syndrome: Implications for assessment, management and prevention. *Nutrients* **2019**, *12*, 15. [CrossRef]
40. Taskinen, M.R.; Packard, C.J.; Boren, J. Dietary fructose and the metabolic syndrome. *Nutrients* **2019**, *11*, 1987. [CrossRef]

41. DeBoer, M.D. Assessing and managing the metabolic syndrome in children and adolescents. *Nutrients* **2019**, *11*, 1788. [CrossRef] [PubMed]
42. Nishizawa, H.; Shimomura, I. Population approaches targeting metabolic syndrome focusing on Japanese trials. *Nutrients* **2019**, *11*, 1430. [CrossRef] [PubMed]
43. Borel, A.L. Sleep apnea and sleep habits: Relationships with metabolic syndrome. *Nutrients* **2019**, *11*, 2628. [CrossRef] [PubMed]
44. Di Marzo, V.; Silvestri, C. Lifestyle and metabolic syndrome: Contribution of the endocannabinoidome. *Nutrients* **2019**, *11*, 1956. [CrossRef] [PubMed]
45. Malik, V.S.; Hu, F.B. Sugar-sweetened beverages and cardiometabolic health: An update of the evidence. *Nutrients* **2019**, *11*, 1840. [CrossRef]
46. Myers, J.; Kokkinos, P.; Nyelin, E. Physical activity, cardiorespiratory fitness, and the metabolic syndrome. *Nutrients* **2019**, *11*, 1652. [CrossRef]
47. Clifton, P. Metabolic syndrome-role of dietary fat type and quantity. *Nutrients* **2019**, *11*, 1438. [CrossRef]
48. Ross, R.; Soni, S.; Houle, S.A. Negative energy balance induced by exercise or diet: Effects on visceral adipose tissue and liver fat. *Nutrients* **2020**, *12*, 891. [CrossRef]
49. Harrison, S.; Couture, P.; Lamarche, B. Diet quality, saturated fat and metabolic syndrome. *Nutrients* **2020**, *12*, 3232. [CrossRef]
50. Julibert, A.; Bibiloni, M.D.M.; Mateos, D.; Angullo, E.; Tur, J.A. Dietary fat intake and metabolic syndrome in older adults. *Nutrients* **2019**, *11*, 1901. [CrossRef]
51. Ramirez-Velez, R.; Perez-Sousa, M.A.; Izquierdo, M.; Cano-Gutierrez, C.A.; Gonzalez-Jimenez, E.; Schmidt-RioValle, J.; Gonzalez-Ruiz, K.; Correa-Rodriguez, M. Validation of surrogate anthropometric indices in older adults: What is the best indicator of high cardiometabolic risk factor clustering? *Nutrients* **2019**, *11*, 1701. [CrossRef] [PubMed]
52. Shafie, S.R.; Wanyonyi, S.; Panchal, S.K.; Brown, L. Linseed components are more effective than whole linseed in reversing diet-induced metabolic syndrome in rats. *Nutrients* **2019**, *11*, 1677. [CrossRef] [PubMed]
53. Wang, J.; Perona, J.S.; Schmidt-RioValle, J.; Chen, Y.; Jing, J.; Gonzalez-Jimenez, E. Metabolic syndrome and its associated early-life factors among Chinese and Spanish adolescents: A pilot study. *Nutrients* **2019**, *11*, 1568. [CrossRef] [PubMed]
54. Wani, K.; Yakout, S.M.; Ansari, M.G.A.; Sabico, S.; Hussain, S.D.; Alokail, M.S.; Sheshah, E.; Aljohani, N.J.; Al-Saleh, Y.; Reginster, J.Y.; et al. Metabolic syndrome in Arab adults with low bone mineral density. *Nutrients* **2019**, *11*, 1405. [CrossRef] [PubMed]
55. Perona, J.S.; Schmidt-RioValle, J.; Fernandez-Aparicio, A.; Correa-Rodriguez, M.; Ramirez-Velez, R.; Gonzalez-Jimenez, E. Waist circumference and abdominal volume index can predict metabolic syndrome in adolescents, but only when the criteria of the International Diabetes Federation are employed for the diagnosis. *Nutrients* **2019**, *11*, 1370. [CrossRef]
56. Troisi, J.; Belmonte, F.; Bisogno, A.; Pierri, L.; Colucci, A.; Scala, G.; Cavallo, P.; Mandato, C.; Di Nuzzi, A.; Di Michele, L.; et al. Metabolomic salivary signature of pediatric obesity related liver disease and metabolic syndrome. *Nutrients* **2019**, *11*, 274. [CrossRef]
57. Rousseau, M.; Guénard, F.; Garneau, V.; Allam-Ndoul, B.; Lemieux, S.; Pérusse, L.; Vohl, M.C. Associations between dietary protein sources, plasma BCAA and short-chain acylcarnitine levels in adults. *Nutrients* **2019**, *11*, 173. [CrossRef]
58. Garralda-Del-Villar, M.; Carlos-Chilleron, S.; Diaz-Gutierrez, J.; Ruiz-Canela, M.; Gea, A.; Martinez-Gonzalez, M.A.; Bes-Rastrollo, M.; Ruiz-Estigarribia, L.; Kales, S.N.; Fernandez-Montero, A. Healthy lifestyle and incidence of metabolic syndrome in the SUN cohort. *Nutrients* **2018**, *11*, 65. [CrossRef]
59. Barrea, L.; Annunziata, G.; Muscogiuri, G.; Di Somma, C.; Laudisio, D.; Maisto, M.; de Alteriis, G.; Tenore, G.C.; Colao, A.; Savastano, S. Trimethylamine-N-oxide (TMAO) as novel potential biomarker of early predictors of metabolic syndrome. *Nutrients* **2018**, *10*, 1971. [CrossRef]
60. Yates, K.F.; Sweat, V.; Yau, P.L.; Turchiano, M.M.; Convit, A. Impact of metabolic syndrome on cognition and brain: A selected review of the literature. *Arterioscler. Thromb. Vasc. Biol.* **2012**, *32*, 2060–2067. [CrossRef]

61. Avgerinos, K.I.; Spyrou, N.; Mantzoros, C.S.; Dalamaga, M. Obesity and cancer risk: Emerging biological mechanisms and perspectives. *Metabolism* **2019**, *92*, 121–135. [CrossRef] [PubMed]
62. Després, J.P. Predicting longevity using metabolomics: A novel tool for precision lifestyle medicine? *Nat. Rev. Cardiol.* **2020**, *17*, 67–68. [CrossRef] [PubMed]

Publisher's Note: MDPI stays neutral with regard to jurisdictional claims in published maps and institutional affiliations.

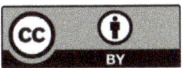

© 2020 by the authors. Licensee MDPI, Basel, Switzerland. This article is an open access article distributed under the terms and conditions of the Creative Commons Attribution (CC BY) license (http://creativecommons.org/licenses/by/4.0/).

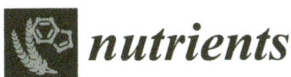

Article

Metabolic Syndrome and Its Associated Early-Life Factors among Chinese and Spanish Adolescents: A Pilot Study

Jiao Wang [1], Javier S. Perona [2], Jacqueline Schmidt-RioValle [3,*], Yajun Chen [1,*], Jin Jing [1] and Emilio González-Jiménez [3]

[1] Department of Maternal and Child Health Care, School of Public Health, Sun Yat-Sen University, Guangzhou 510080, China
[2] Instituto de la Grasa (CSIC), Campus Universidad Pablo de Olavide, Edificio 46, 41013 Seville, Spain
[3] Departamento de Enfermería, CTS-436 Adscrito al Centro de Investigación Mente, Cerebro y Comportamiento (CIMCYC), University of Granada, Av/Ilustración 60, 18016 Granada, Spain
* Correspondence: jschmidt@ugr.es (J.S.-R.V.); chenyj68@mail.sysu.edu.cn (Y.C.); Tel./Fax: +34-958-243-495 (J.S.-R.V.); Tel.:+86-20-87334627 (Y.C.); Fax: +86-20-87335498 (Y.C.)

Received: 5 June 2019; Accepted: 10 July 2019; Published: 11 July 2019

Abstract: Metabolic syndrome (MetS) is a growing problem worldwide in adolescents. This study compared two sample populations of young people in Spain and China, and analyzed the association of birth weight and breastfeeding duration with MetS. A cross-sectional study was conducted in adolescents (10–15 years old); 1150 Chinese and 976 Spanish adolescents. The variables analyzed were anthropometric characteristics, biochemical markers, and demographic characteristics using the same methodology and data collection protocol. Also, birth weight and breastfeeding were retrospectively analyzed during the first year of life. The results showed statistically significant differences between the two groups in reference to body mass index (BMI), blood pressure, triglyceride, glucose, and high-density lipoprotein cholesterol (HDL-C) levels. The MetS prevalence was higher in Spanish adolescents (2.5%) than in the Chinese group (0.5%). Breastfeeding duration was inversely associated with hypertriglyceridemia, low HDL-C, and MetS, whereas higher birth weight was associated with hyperglycemia, low HDL-C, hypertriglyceridemia, and abdominal obesity. Spanish adolescents showed more altered MetS components, and consequently, a higher MetS prevalence than the Chinese adolescents. This made them more vulnerable to cardiometabolic risk. Our results highlight the need for interventions designed by health professionals, which would encourage pregnant women to breastfeed their children.

Keywords: metabolic syndrome; adolescents; breastfeeding duration; birth weight

1. Introduction

Metabolic syndrome (MetS) involves a cluster of risk factors. Subjects with MetS typically have at least three of the following conditions; abdominal obesity, hyperglycemia, hypertension, hypertriglyceridemia, and low HDL-cholesterol (HDL-C) levels [1]. MetS has been found to be strongly associated with a higher risk of cardiovascular disease in adults [2,3]. Unfortunately, there is a lack of data regarding MetS and its associated factors in childhood and adolescence. This is particularly the case in emerging countries such as China [4].

The prevalence of MetS in adolescents is currently increasing throughout the world [5]. In a Spanish population of 976 adolescents, 10–15 years of age, González-Jiménez et al. [6] observed a MetS prevalence of 3.9% in girls and 5.4% in boys. In contrast, Xu et al. [7] obtained a prevalence of 0.8% in Chinese adolescents over 10 years old. Similarly, in a study of 1770 Chinese adolescents by Wang et al. [8], the overall prevalence was 1.1%, though boys were more affected by MetS than girls. In these three studies, MetS was defined following to the criteria proposed by the International Diabetes Federation (IDF) for children and adolescents. According to these studies carried out in China and Spain it might be expected that MetS would be less frequent in Chinese adolescents. However, to date there has been no comparative study of MetS in sample populations in Spain and China.

It is crucial to identify the risk factors leading to the development of MetS in young people so that this disorder can be rapidly detected and prevented [9]. Accordingly, it has been suggested that a higher birth weight may be associated with an early development of insulin resistance and MetS [10]. An excessively short period (or absence) of breastfeeding during the first year of childhood seems to be another risk factor for MetS [11]. In González-Jiménez et al. [6] and Wang et al. [8], a high birth weight was significantly associated with MetS, whereas breastfeeding for longer than six months was inversely associated with the syndrome. Nevertheless, there is no consensus of opinion on this issue since the absence of conclusive results in Western and Chinese populations [12] has generated a certain controversy regarding the influence of these variables [13].

The initial hypothesis of this research was that the difference in MetS prevalence in China and Spain was probably related to differences in birth weight and breastfeeding duration. To confirm this hypothesis, our objectives were to compare the prevalence of MetS in Chinese and Spanish adolescents, and then analyze the associations of MetS with birth weight and breastfeeding duration (first year of life).

2. Materials and Methods

2.1. Study Design and Participants

Accordingly, we decided to conduct a comparative analysis of two cross-sectional studies. The first study was of a sample of Chinese adolescents, and the second study was of a sample of Spanish adolescents. In China, the research was carried out in the city of Guangzhou (southern China). Four districts were randomly selected, which comprised a total of ten schools. A letter of invitation was sent to the school principals along with an information sheet and an explanation of the research methodology and objectives. All parents, tutors, and legal guardians of the minors gave their written informed consent. The study had been previously approved by the Ethics Committee of the School of Public Health in Sun Yat-sen University.

In each of the ten schools, two classes per course were randomly selected and invited to participate in the study. A total of 1150 adolescents (554 boys and 596 girls), 10–15 years of age, were finally recruited for the study. All participants had a medium socioeconomic status and the response rate was 87%.

In Spain, the study was conducted in the province of Granada (southeastern Spain), a total of eighteen schools throughout the province were randomly selected. The study had been previously approved by the Board of Education of the Andalusian Regional Government (Granada Delegation), and authorized by the school directors. It had also been approved by the Ethics Committee of the University of Granada. All parents, tutors, and guardians had explicitly authorized the participation of their children.

In each of the schools, two classes per course were randomly selected and invited to participate in the study. Finally, a total of 976 adolescents, (457 boys and 519 girls), 10–15 years of age, were recruited. All of the subjects were Spanish and had a medium socioeconomic status.

Both in the Chinese and Spanish groups, adolescents with serious physical handicaps or psychological conditions (e.g., congenital disorder and cognitive dysfunction) were excluded from the study. The flow diagram (Figure 1) describes the selection process followed in both countries.

All procedures used in this study were in accordance with the ethical standards of the institutional and/or national research committee and with the 1964 Helsinki declaration and its later amendments or comparable ethical standards.

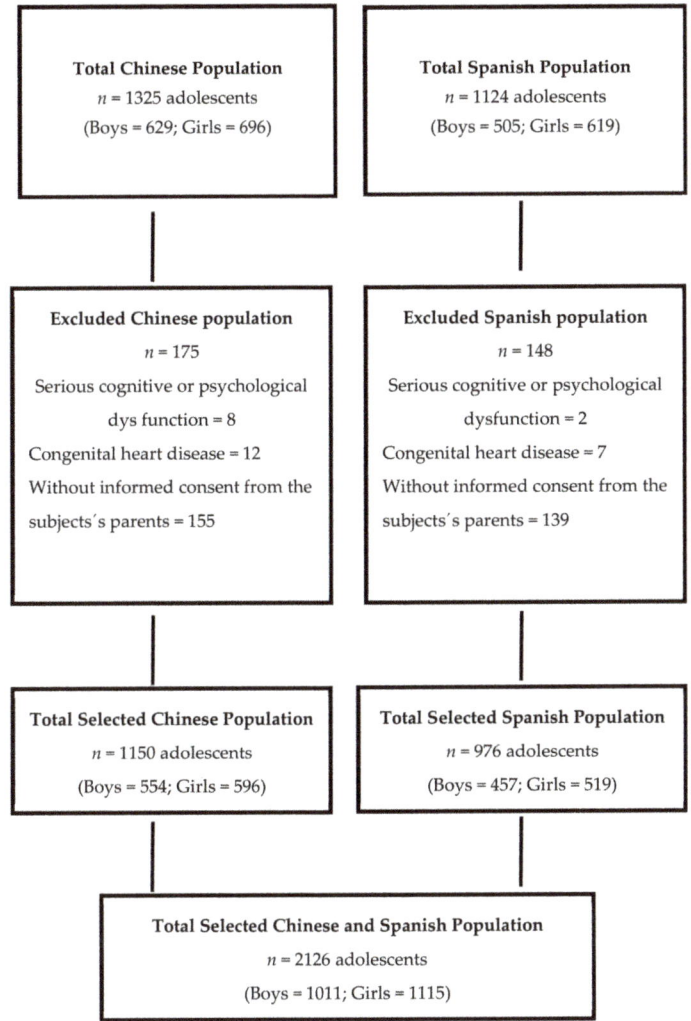

Figure 1. Flow diagram of the recruitment progress.

2.2. Data Collection and Measurements

The instrument used for data collection was a standard questionnaire elaborated ad hoc. The questionnaire was filled out during a face-to-face interview with one of the parents or guardians. The average questionnaire completion time was 20–25 min.

Questionnaire items focused on the collection of demographic data and information regarding birth weight and breastfeeding during the subjects' first year of life. All of this information was collected retrospectively. Furthermore, in order to guarantee the accuracy of the answers, parents were asked to bring the Child Health Record of their son/daughter. This document had been previously filled out by health professionals and contained accurate birth-weight and breastfeeding information. The completed questionnaires were reviewed by trained staff and uploaded into the database.

All participants underwent a complete anthropometric evaluation in accordance with the guidelines of the International Society for the Advancement of Kinanthropometry [14]. The variables assessed were weight, height, waist circumference (WC), hip circumference (HC), and BMI (weight (kg)/height (m)^2). In the Chinese sample, fasting body weight was measured to the nearest 0.1 kg on a double ruler scale (RGT-140, Wujin Hengqi Co. Ltd, Changzhou, China). During this assessment, participants were wearing light clothing and no shoes. In the Spanish sample, the subjects (also in light clothing and no shoes) were weighed on a self-calibrating Seca 861 Class (III) Digital Floor Scale (Hamburg, Germany) with a precision of up to 0.1 kg.

In the Chinese sample, height was measured to an accuracy of 1mm with a freestanding stadiometer mounted on a rigid tripod (GMCS-I; Xindong Huateng Sports Equipment Co. Ltd, Beijing, China) by trained interviewers following a standardized protocol. Participants were asked to stand erect with their back, buttocks, and heels in continuous contact with the vertical height rod of the stadiometer and their head orientated in the Frankfurt plane. The horizontal headpiece was then placed on top of their head to measure their height. The height of the Spanish children was measured with a Seca 214* portable stadiometer (seca gmbh & co., Hamburg, Germany), following the same procedure as in the Chinese study.

WC was measured with a Seca automatic roll-up measuring tape (precision of 1 mm) using the horizontal plane midway between the lowest rib and the upper border of the iliac crest at the end of a normal inspiration/expiration. HC was measured at the maximum extension of the buttocks as viewed from the right side. The average of two consecutive measurements was the value used in the analyses. In both samples, waist-to-height ratio was calculated as WC (cm) divided by height (cm), whereas waist-to-hip ratio was calculated by dividing WC by HC. The corresponding intraobserver technical error (reliability) of the measurements was 0.95%.

In the Chinese sample, blood pressure levels were calculated with a previously calibrated aneroid sphygmomanometer and a Littmann® stethoscope (3M Health Care, Saint Paul, MI, USA) after each participant had rested for at least 15 min in a sitting position, according to the BP measurement guidelines of the Subcommittee of Professional and Public Education of the American Heart Association Council on High Blood Pressure Research [15]. Diastolic pressure was defined as the point of disappearance of the Korotkoff sounds (fifth phase). Blood pressure was taken twice on the right arm with an appropriately sized cuff. The average of two readings obtained at a minimum interval of 5 min was recorded. In the Spanish sample, blood pressure levels were calculated with the same equipment and following the same procedure as the research team in China.

2.3. Serum Biochemical Examination

The biochemical variables analyzed were fasting glucose (FG), HDL-C, and triglycerides (TG). At 8 a.m., after a 12 h overnight fast, 10 mL of blood was extracted by venipuncture from the antecubital fossa of the right arm with a disposable vacuum blood collection tube. In the 4 hours after extraction, all samples were centrifuged at 3500 rpm for 15 min (Z400 K, Hermle, Wehingen, Germany). Red blood cells were separated and serum was finally frozen at −80 °C for its subsequent analysis. FG was measured with a colorimetric enzymatic method (GOD-PAP Method, Human Diagnostics, Germany). HDL-C and TG were also calculated by means of a colorimetric enzymatic method with an Olympus analyzer (GmbH company, Hamburg, Germany). The techniques and equipment employed in the biochemical analysis were the same in both samples. The precision performance of these assays was within the manufacturer's specifications. In both populations, blood samples were taken at the educational center in a classroom especially designated for this purpose and on different days in order to guarantee the fasting of the participants.

2.4. Diagnostic Criteria of Metabolic Syndrome according to the International Diabetes Federation, IDF

The definition of MetS was based on the criteria of the IDF, adapted for children and adolescents. These criteria were abdominal obesity (defined by WC adult ethnicity-specific cutoffs: ≥94 cm in men and ≥80 cm in women for the Spanish and ≥90 cm in men and ≥80 cm in women for the Chinese) and the presence of two or more clinical features, including TG ≥1.7 mmol/L, HDL-C <1.03 mmol/L, systolic blood pressure (SBP) ≥130 mmHg and/or diastolic blood pressure (DBP) ≥85 mmHg, and serum FG ≥5.6 mmol/L [16].

2.5. Statistical Analysis

Descriptive statistics were calculated for all of the variables, including continuous variables (reported as mean and standard deviation) and categorical variables (reported as number and percentage). A p-value of 0.05 and a power of 80% were used to determine sample sizes. The differences between sexes, ages, and countries for the variables studied were evaluated using Student's t-test, ANOVA, nonparametric test, or the χ^2 test, as appropriate. Pearson/Spearman's correlation coefficients between MetS components and their associated factors were also calculated. In the total sample and separated sample, multivariable logistic regression analyses (Enter method) were employed to identify the relationship between MetS and its features in the form of outcomes (abdominal obesity, low HDL-C, hyperglycemia, hypertriglyceridemia, hypertension), and associated factors. The multivariable logistic analysis in the country of origin (China), breastfeeding duration (months), and birth weight (100 g) was sex-adjusted and age-adjusted to control the influence of puberty. The prevalence odds ratios and the corresponding 95% confidence intervals were calculated as well. All statistical analyses were performed with the statistical software package SPSS version 21.0 (IBM, Armonk, NY, USA). In this study, p-values of less than 0.05 were regarded as statistically significant.

3. Results

Table 1. shows the data collected from the participants, including demographic information, anthropometry, MetS features, and early-life factors. It was observed that Spanish children had higher mean values for height, weight, BMI, WC, TG, and SBP than Chinese children. Generally speaking, the Spanish sample had also been breastfed for a longer period of time in their first year of life (9 months on average).

Table 1. Demographic and clinical characteristics of Chinese and Spanish adolescents.

Variable	Chinese Adolescents	Spanish Adolescents	p-Value
Demographic information			
n	1150	976	
Boys (%)	554 (48.2)	457 (45.7)	0.28
Age (years)	12.9 ± 1.8	13.1 ± 1.2	0.09
Anthropometry			
Height (m)	1.55 ± 0.14	1.59 ± 0.10	<0.01 **
Weight (kg)	46.28 ± 14.01	54.77 ± 12.71	<0.01 **
BMI (kg/m^2)	19.24 ± 7.25	21.22 ± 3.79	<0.01 **
HC (cm)	81.06 ± 16.91	83.82 ± 9.35	0.21
WHR	0.84 ± 0.09	0.87 ± 0.16	<0.01 **
WHtR	0.44 ± 0.07	0.45 ± 0.07	0.01 *
Metabolic syndrome features			
WC (cm)	66.7 ± 10.6	72.3 ± 10.8	<0.01 **
FG (mmol/L)	4.62 ± 0.49	4.77 ± 1.68	0.01 *
HDL-C (mmol/L)	1.4 ± 0.3	1.0 ± 0.1	<0.01 **
TG (mmol/L)	0.97 ± 0.51	1.43 ± 0.60	<0.01 **
SBP (mmHg)	99.9 ± 23.2	118.0 ± 15.5	<0.01 **
DBP (mmHg)	63.6 ± 15.7	64.1 ± 9.0	0.35
Information of early-life factors			
Breastfeeding duration (month)	4.2 ± 3.7	9.2 ± 2.7	<0.01 **
Breastfeeding duration range (month)	0~13	0~13	
Birth weight (kg)	3.23 ± 0.47	3.20 ± 0.50	0.09
Birth weight range (kg)	1.4~4.9	2.0~5.7	

Notes: BMI, body mass index; HC, hip circumference; WHR, waist-to-hip ratio; WHtR, waist-to-height ratio; WC, waist circumference; FG, fasting glucose; HDL-C, high-density lipoprotein cholesterol; TG, triglyceride; SBP, systolic blood pressure; DBP, diastolic blood pressure. Values are expressed as mean ± SD. The p-value was calculated by chi-square test for category variables and two-sample t-test for continuous variables. * $p < 0.05$, ** $p < 0.01$.

Regarding the prevalence of MetS and its components, Table 2 shows statistically significant differences between the two cohorts. As can be observed, the Spanish adolescents had a higher prevalence of abdominal obesity, hyperglycemia, and hypertension. In contrast, Chinese adolescents were more prone to hypertriglyceridemia though TG mean values were higher in the Spanish cohort. Consequently, the prevalence of MetS was 2.5% in the Spanish adolescents in comparison to 0.5% in the Chinese group.

Table 2. Prevalence of metabolic syndrome and its components in Chinese and Spanish adolescents.

Characteristics	Chinese Adolescents ($n = 1150$)	Spanish Adolescents ($n = 976$)
Abdominal obesity	65 (5.5)	128 (13.1) **
Hypertension	11 (1.0)	256 (26.2) **
Hyperglycemia	23 (2.0)	65 (6.7) **
Low HDL-C	160 (13.9)	176 (18.0) *
Hypertriglyceridemia	84 (7.3)	32 (3.3) **
Pattern of risk factors clustering		
0 Component	886 (77.0)	568 (58.2) **
1 Component	193 (16.8)	234 (24.0) **
2 Components	61 (5.6)	120 (12.3) **
≥3 Components	7 (0.6)	54 (5.5) **
MetS	6 (0.5)	24 (2.5) **

Notes: HDL-C, high-density lipoprotein cholesterol; MetS, metabolic syndrome. Values are expressed as numbers of individuals (%). p-value was calculated by chi-square; * $p < 0.05$, ** $p < 0.01$.

Generally, the correlations of breastfeeding duration or birth weight with MetS and its components (Table 3) differed in Chinese and Spanish individuals. In Chinese adolescents correlations were weak. In the case of the Spaniards, the duration of breastfeeding correlated positively with HDL-C (0.81) and negatively with FG (−0.89) and TG (−0.64). In contrast, birth weight correlated negatively with HDL-C (−0.58) and positively with FG (0.65) and TG (0.48). In the Chinese cohort, birth weight was found to be positively associated with WC (0.15), SBP (0.08), and DBP (0.07).

Table 3. The association of metabolic syndrome features and early-life factors in Chinese and Spanish adolescents.

	Chinese Adolescents ($n = 1150$)		Spanish Adolescents ($n = 976$)	
	Breastfeeding Duration	Birth Weight	Breastfeeding Duration	Birth Weight
WC	−0.04	0.15 **	0.05	0.10 **
FG	0.03	0.01	−0.89 **	0.65 **
HDL-C	−0.04	−0.01	0.81 **	−0.58 **
TG	0.09 **	−0.04	−0.64 **	0.48 **
SBP	0.03	0.08 *	−0.03	0.06
DBP	−0.02	0.07 *	−0.02	0.07 *

Notes: WC, waist circumference; FG, fasting glucose; HDL-C, high-density lipoprotein cholesterol; TG, triglyceride; SBP, systolic blood pressure; DBP, diastolic blood pressure; MetS, metabolic syndrome. Data are presented as Pearson/Spearman's correlation coefficients. * $p < 0.05$ ** $p < 0.01$.

Table 4 shows the adjusted associations of Mets features with early life factors including breastfeeding duration and birth weight in Chinese and Spanish adolescents. In the Spanish adolescents, breastfeeding duration had stronger associations with low HDL-C (OR 0.18), hyperglycemia (OR 0.17), hypertriglyceridemia (OR 0.52), and MetS (0.62) than in the Chinese adolescents. However, birth weight had closer associations with abdominal obesity (OR 1.09) in Chinese subjects and closer associations with hyperglycemia (OR 6.65) in Spanish subjects.

Table 4. Risk of MetS features based on associated factors from multivariable logistic regression in two sample.

	Chinese Adolescents (*n* = 1150)		Spanish Adolescents (*n* = 976)	
	Breastfeeding Duration (month)	Birth Weight (100 g)	Breastfeeding Duration (month)	Birth Weight (100 g)
	OR (95% CI)	OR (95% CI)	OR (95% CI)	OR (95% CI)
Abdominal obesity	0.95 (0.88, 1.02)	1.09 (1.03, 1.16)	0.98 (0.90, 1.07)	1.04 (0.99, 1.10)
Low HDL-C	1.03 (0.98, 1.08)	1.17 (0.98, 1.06)	0.18 (0.13, 0.26)	1.06 (0.93, 1.21)
Hyperglycemia	0.96 (0.86, 1.08)	0.96 (0.88, 1.05)	0.17 (0.04, 0.72)	6.65 (1.83, 24.19)
Hypertriglyceridemia	1.03 (0.97, 1.10)	0.99 (0.94, 1.04)	0.52 (0.40, 0.70)	1.09 (0.93, 1.27)
Hypertension	1.10 (0.91, 1.32)	1.07 (0.92, 1.23)	0.96 (0.90, 1.03)	1.02 (0.99, 1.07)
MetS	1.07 (0.87, 1.32)	0.93 (0.80, 1.08)	0.62 (0.51, 0.76)	0.98 (0.86, 1.12)

Note: Age and gender were adjusted in all above models.

Furthermore, the combined multivariable analysis of MetS and its components showed that girls were more likely to develop abdominal obesity than boys (Table 5). In addition, there was a strong association of MetS and its components with the participants' country of origin. In general, Spanish participants were at greater risk of MetS or of the alteration of certain MetS components. In this regard, the Spaniards had a higher risk of hypertension (OR 45.05), hyperglycemia (OR 26.85), and MetS (OR 13.6) than the Chinese adolescents. For the early-life factors, breastfeeding duration was negatively associated with hypertriglyceridemia (OR 0.87), low HDL-C (OR 0.81), hyperglycemia (OR 0.60), and MetS (OR 0.74), whereas higher birth weight was positively associated with MetS components such as hyperglycemia (OR 1.96) and abdominal obesity (OR 1.15) in the total sample. We also performed analyses to assess the interaction of breastfeeding duration and the country of origin and birth weight with the country of origin, using China as reference. When the interaction of breastfeeding duration and the country of origin was assessed, we observed that the effect was significant for low HDL-C, hyperglycemia and hypertriglyceridemia. In contrast, the interaction of birth weight with the country of origin was significant only for hyperglycemia. The results of the sensitivity analysis showed that breastfeeding duration (longer than 6 months) was a protective factor for MetS (Supplementary Table S1).

Table 5. Risk of MetS features based on associated factors from multivariable logistic regression.

Variables (Reference)	Abdominal Obesity OR (95% CI)	Low HDL-C OR (95% CI)	Hyperglycemia OR (95% CI)	Hypertriglyceridemia OR (95% CI)	Hypertension OR (95% CI)	MetS OR (95% CI)
Age	1.20 (1.09, 1.32)	1.07 (0.99, 1.15)	0.96 (0.80, 1.16)	0.92 (0.83, 1.02)	1.04 (0.93, 1.17)	1.01 (0.80, 1.28)
Gender (Boy)	2.40 (1.72, 3.35)	0.78 (0.58, 1.07)	0.30 (0.12, 0.73)	0.79 (0.53, 1.20)	0.77 (0.58, 1.02)	1.76 (0.79, 3.89)
Country (China)	12.04 (0.58, 24.23)	3.84 (2.68, 5.49)	26.85 (11.76, 61.34)	0.70 (0.43, 1.15)	45.05 (21.71, 93.45)	13.6 (4.16, 44.54)
Breastfeeding duration (month)	0.91 (0.77, 1.08)	0.81 (0.78, 0.85)	0.60 (0.53, 0.68)	0.87 (0.82, 0.92)	1.10 (0.91, 1.32)	0.74 (0.65, 0.84)
Birth weight (100 g)	1.15 (1.01, 1.31)	0.98 (0.84, 1.10)	1.96 (1.88, 3.08)	0.99 (0.95, 1.04)	1.07 (0.92, 1.23)	0.94 (0.80, 1.09)
	p value	p value	p value	p value	p value	p value
Breastfeeding duration*Country	0.504	<0.001	<0.017	<0.001	0.187	<0.001
Birth weight*Country	0.211	0.578	<0.001	0.213	0.605	0.743

Notes: HDL-C, high-density lipoprotein cholesterol; MetS, metabolic syndrome. Data are presented as prevalence odds ratio (OR) with 95% confidence intervals (CI) using logistic regression model. Bold type indicates $p < 0.05$. All the shown risk factors in this model were included in the model at the same time.

4. Discussion

The results obtained showed that there were significant differences in the Chinese and Spanish samples in regard to most of the clinical features analyzed, whether anthropometric or metabolic. More specifically, Spanish adolescents were found to have considerably higher levels of TG and SBP in comparison to Chinese adolescents. In contrast, the children in the Chinese sample had lower BMI, WHR, and WC values. Generally speaking, these results suggest that the Chinese subjects were healthier than their Spanish counterparts, who had higher values for most of the clinical features [17,18]. This may be partially explained by the ethnic difference and different living environments. This evidently placed their health at risk and made them more vulnerable to cardiometabolic disorders [19]. These results indicate the need for an in-depth study of the lifestyle, and environmental factors affecting the population in China and Spain. Any or all of these could be factors that would explain the differences found between adolescents in the two countries.

Our results also showed differences between the Chinese and Spanish samples regarding MetS components. As in previous studies of the Spanish population [20] and based on the definition of MetS used, Spanish children and adolescents had higher levels of abdominal obesity, hyperglycemia, as well as a higher rate of hypertension when compared to the Chinese group. Nevertheless, the prevalence of MetS was still lower than that reported by Holst-Schumacher et al. [21] for adolescents in Costa Rica (5.6%) or that described by Alvarez et al. [22] for adolescents in Brazil (6%). The only variable that was higher in Chinese cohort was the value for hypertriglyceridemia, which was in agreement with Liang et al. [23] who studied another population of 976 Chinese adolescents.

Breastfeeding duration and birth weight correlated closely with the components of MetS. In this regard, Spanish schoolchildren had been breastfed for a longer time. This correlated positively with HDL-C levels and negatively with other variables such as FG, TG, and MetS. These findings suggest the potentially positive effect of breastfeeding as a way to prevent the development of metabolic disorders in young subjects. These results contrasted with Yakubov et al. [24], who found no association between breastfeeding duration and the development of MetS and/or impairments of its components. However, this lack of association could be explained by factors such as the small size of the sample, a possible selection bias of the subjects or the range of breastfeeding duration.

In contrast, other studies did find a correlation between breastfeeding duration and a reduced incidence of MetS later in life [25,26]. Yet, it could be argued that since in the present study Spanish adolescents were breastfed for a longer time and had a higher prevalence of MetS compared to the Chinese group, breastfeeding would increase, rather than decrease, the risk of developing MetS. However, this assumption can not be made directly, due to the multifactorial nature of the metabolic syndrome. The inverse association between breastfeeding duration and MetS in childhood and adolescence has been observed elsewhere [12,27]. Indeed, in a previous study, we found a higher prevalence of MetS in young subjects that had not been breastfed as babies [6]. Moreover, Ekelund et al. [28] stated that the most important benefits of maternal breastfeeding in terms of MetS prevention were for those subjects who had been breastfed for more than 6 months.

In the present study, breastfeeding duration was the main factor affecting the differences observed in the risk of MetS features between Chinese and Spanish adolescents. In fact, the interaction between breastfeeding duration and country for MetS and its components resulted strongly significant. Chinese mother breastfed their infants for less than half of the time than did Spanish mothers but no differences were on served for the range (0–13 months). A survey carried out in the city of Guangzhou (the same city of origin of our study), revealed that Chinese mothers tend to stop breastfeeding early before the six months. The reasons given for breastfeeding cessation were, among others, insufficient milk supply, medical reasons, lactational factors, and return to work [29]. Regardless of their antenatal intention, women with higher BMI have a higher risk of early cessation of exclusive breastfeeding [30], which has been associated to anatomical and physiological issues, medical conditions, and sociocultural and psychological factors [31]. Unfortunately, we do not have data on the prevalence of overweight mothers at the time of pregnancy. In our study, birth weight correlated positively with FG, TG, and MetS in

Spanish subjects, as well as with WC in Chinese subjects. These findings do not coincide with those in Dos Santos et al. [32], who studied a population of 172 adolescents in Brazil and found that birth weight was not a risk factor in the development of MetS during adolescence. This result was probably conditioned by the small size of the Brazilian cohort, a possible bias in the selection of participants, or methodological differences in the evaluation of adiposity. Nonetheless, Yuan et al. [33] did find an association between birth weight and disorders such as adolescent obesity and MetS. Their population sample was much larger and was composed of 16,580 Chinese children and adolescents, 7–17 years of age, which is consistent with the Chinese sample in our study. Strikingly, the results obtained by Yuan et al. [33] were more in consonance with the Spanish results in our study than with the Chinese ones.

The results of the multivariable analysis of early MetS predictors with MetS and MetS components showed that girls had a higher risk of abdominal obesity, which agrees with previous research [34,35]. The high prevalence of central obesity in Spanish and Chinese girls is a matter of concern, since according to Lee et al. [36], it increases the risk of morbidity and mortality at early ages. Additionally, MetS and its components showed a strong association with the participants' country of origin. In other words, Spanish adolescents had a greater risk of MetS or the alteration of any of its components (e.g., hypertension or hyperglycemia) than the Chinese adolescents.

These results also contrast with those of Haldar et al. [37], who reported that Asian adults who emigrated and lived in European countries were more apt to become obese than Caucasians, regardless of the degree of adiposity. However, this may very well be due to changes in their dietary habits. To explain the discrepancies between the Chinese and Spanish populations, it could be argued that Spaniards are not typical Caucasians in regard to metabolic disorders. In comparison to young people in other European countries, children and adolescents in Spain are more prone to be overweight, which means greater metabolic risk. Accordingly, the prevalence of MetS in Spanish adolescents is higher than the MetS prevalence in other European countries, such as Finland (2.1%), Greece (0.7%) [38], Denmark, Estonia, and Portugal (1.4%) [28]. Other studies also highlight differences between ethnic groups in the distribution of body fat, which signifies that they are at greater risk of developing cardiovascular and metabolic pathologies [39,40].

Interestingly, our study found that hypertriglyceridemia was strongly affected by the duration of breastfeeding (OR 0.87), regardless of the participants' gender or country of origin. The association between breastfeeding in infancy and triglyceride concentrations later in life is still a matter of debate. The absence of an association was reported by Victoria et al. [41] in a Brazilian population of 18-year-old boys and by Lawlor et al. [42] in Estonian and Danish children and adolescents. In Lawlor et al. [42], BMI and TG values were similar to those obtained for the Chinese sample in our study, but lower than those for the Spanish group. More recently, Ramirez-Silva et al. [43] observed that children who had not been breastfed had higher TG levels at the age of 4, compared with those who had been partially or exclusively breastfed. There is a lack of consensus regarding the influence of birth weight on hyperglycemia.

This research has a number of strengths as well as certain limitations. Without a doubt, one of its strengths is its pioneering nature. Our study focused on two populations of adolescents with very different cultural backgrounds and analyzed not only the prevalence of MetS, but also the association between MetS and early predictors such as breastfeeding duration (first year of life) and birth weight. Yet another strength is the size of the sample, which enhances the validity of the results and assures comparability in future studies. Nonetheless, an evident limitation of the study is its cross-sectional nature and the lack of information about the eating habits and physical activity of both populations. Finally, no data regarding pubertal status were collected or taken into account but two subjects were excluded as outliers with extremely high triglyceride levels. This may have been a factor in the differences between the two countries. The results should thus be interpreted with caution.

5. Conclusions

In conclusion, our initial hypothesis was confirmed since Spanish adolescents showed a higher number of altered MetS components, and consequently a higher prevalence of MetS than Chinese adolescents. In addition, in the Spanish sample, breastfeeding duration and birth weight strongly correlated with MetS components in comparison to the Chinese group, where this was not the case. The Spanish adolescents also had a higher risk for hyperglycemia, hypertension, hypertriglyceridemia, and abdominal obesity.

The results of this study should have an impact on clinical practice. It is advisable for healthcare professionals to have an in-depth understanding of all of the factors associated with MetS. This knowledge and awareness are crucial to the prevention of this disease in adolescents. Likewise, as reflected in our results, it is important for healthcare professionals to encourage pregnant women to breastfeed their babies. This would improve the metabolic status of the mothers and at the same time make their children less vulnerable to obesity, diabetes mellitus type 2, and MetS. This is especially true for Spain, as we found important differences in the prevalence of MetS and its components between Chinese and Spanish adolescents, which were importantly affected by differences in breastfeeding duration in both countries. For this reason, a clear priority for health professionals should be to encourage breastfeeding.

Supplementary Materials: The following are available online at http://www.mdpi.com/2072-6643/11/7/1568/s1, Supplementary Table S1: Risk of MetS features based on associated factors from multivariable logistic regression (categorical variables).

Author Contributions: J.W. and E.G.-J. had full access to all the data in the study and takes responsibility for the integrity of the data and the accuracy of the data analysis. E.G.-J., J.S.P., and J.S.-R. drafted the manuscript, critically revised the manuscript, and agreed to be accountable for all aspects of work ensuring integrity and accuracy. E.G.J., J.S.P., Y.C., and J.J. contributed to conception and whole study design. All authors have read and approved the final manuscript.

Funding: The research conducted in Spain was funded by the Spanish Interministerial Commission of Science and Technology (CYCIT, AGL2011-23810). The research in China was funded by the National Natural Science Foundation of China (grant number 81673193) as well as by a special research grant for nonprofit public service of the Ministry of Health of China (grant number 201202010).

Acknowledgments: In China, the authors gratefully acknowledge the contribution of Yuexiu, Haizhu, Liwan and Luogang Education Bureau and ten schools. In Spain, we would like to thank the schools, parents, and guardians as well as the students for participating in this study.

Conflicts of Interest: The authors declare no conflicts of interest.

References

1. Weiss, R.; Bremer, A.A.; Lustig, R.H. What is metabolic syndrome, and why are children getting it? *Ann. N. Y. Acad. Sci.* **2013**, *1281*, 123–140. [CrossRef] [PubMed]
2. Schubert, C.M.; Sun, S.S.; Burns, T.L.; Morrison, J.A.; Huang, T.T. Predictive ability of childhood metabolic components for adult metabolic syndrome and type 2 diabetes. *J. Pediatr.* **2009**, *155*, S1–S6. [CrossRef] [PubMed]
3. Huang, T.T.; Sun, S.S.; Daniels, S.R. Understanding the nature of metabolic syndrome components in children and what they can and cannot do to predict adult disease. *J. Pediatr.* **2009**, *155*, e13–e14. [CrossRef] [PubMed]
4. Chen, F.; Wang, Y.; Shan, X.; Cheng, H.; Hou, D.; Zhao, X.; Wang, T.; Zhao, D.; Mi, J. Association between childhood obesity and metabolic syndrome: Evidence from a large sample of Chinese children and adolescents. *PLoS ONE* **2012**, *7*, e47380. [CrossRef] [PubMed]
5. Miller, J.M.; Kaylor, M.B.; Johannsson, M.; Bay, C.; Churilla, J.R. Prevalence of metabolic syndrome and individual criterion in US adolescents: 2001–2010 national health and nutrition examination survey. *Metab. Syndr. Relat. Disord.* **2014**, *12*, 527–532. [CrossRef] [PubMed]
6. Gonzalez-Jimenez, E.; Montero-Alonso, M.A.; Schmidt-RioValle, J.; Garcia-Garcia, C.J.; Padez, C. Metabolic syndrome in Spanish adolescents and its association with birth weight, breastfeeding duration, maternal smoking, and maternal obesity: A cross-sectional study. *Eur. J. Nutr.* **2015**, *54*, 589–597. [CrossRef] [PubMed]

7. Xu, H.; Li, Y.; Liu, A.; Zhang, Q.; Hu, X.; Fang, H.; Li, T.; Guo, H.; Li, Y.; Xu, G.; et al. Prevalence of the metabolic syndrome among children from six cities of China. *BMC Public Health* **2012**, *12*, 13. [CrossRef] [PubMed]
8. Wang, J.; Zhu, Y.; Cai, L.; Jing, J.; Chen, Y.; Mai, J.; Ma, L.; Ma, Y.; Ma, J. Metabolic syndrome and its associated early-life factors in children and adolescents: A cross-sectional study in Guangzhou, China. *Public Health Nutr.* **2016**, *19*, 1147–1154. [CrossRef]
9. Ahmadi, A.; Gharipour, M.; Nouri, F.; Sarrafzadegan, N. Metabolic syndrome in Iranian youths: A population-based study on junior and high schools students in rural and urban areas. *J. Diabetes Res.* **2012**, *2013*, 738485. [CrossRef]
10. Agius, R.; Savona-Ventura, C.; Vassallo, J. Transgenerational metabolic determinants of fetal birth weight. *Exp. Clin. Endocrinol. Diabetes.* **2013**, *121*, 431–435. [CrossRef]
11. Stuebe, A. The risks of not breastfeeding for mothers and infants. *Rev. Obstet. Gynecol.* **2009**, *2*, 222–231. [PubMed]
12. Yang, Z.; Huffman, S.L. Nutrition in pregnancy and early childhood and associations with obesity in developing countries. *Matern. Child. Nutr.* **2013**, *9*, 105–119. [CrossRef] [PubMed]
13. Wang, X.; Liang, L.; Junfen, F.U.; Lizhong, D.U. Metabolic syndrome in obese children born large for gestational age. *Indian J. Pediatr.* **2007**, *74*, 561–565. [CrossRef] [PubMed]
14. Marfell-Jones, M.; Olds, T.; Stewart, A. *International Standards for Anthropometric Assessment*; ISAK: Potchefstroom, South Africa, 2006.
15. Pickering, T.G.; Hall, J.E.; Appel, L.J.; Falkner, B.; Graves, J.; Hill, M.; Jones, D.W.; Kurtz, T.; Sheps, S.G.; Roccella, E.J. Subcommittee of professional and public education of the American heart association council on high blood pressure research. Recommendations for blood pressure measurement in humans and experimental animals, part 1: Blood pressure measurement in humans: A statement for professionals from the subcommittee of professional and public education of the American heart association council on high blood pressure research. *Hypertension* **2005**, *45*, 142–161. [PubMed]
16. Zimmet, P.; Alberti, K.G.; Kaufman, F.; Tajima, N.; Silink, M.; Arslanian, S.; Wong, G.; Bennett, P.; Shaw, J.; Caprio, S.; et al. The metabolic syndrome in children and adolescents—An IDF consensus report. *Pediatr. Diabetes* **2007**, *8*, 299–306. [CrossRef]
17. Kelishadi, R. Childhood overweight, obesity, and the metabolic syndrome in developing countries. *Epidemiol. Rev.* **2007**, *29*, 62–76. [CrossRef] [PubMed]
18. Gupta, N.; Shah, P.; Nayyar, S.; Misra, A. Childhood obesity and the metabolic syndrome in developing countries. *Indian J. Pediatr.* **2013**, *80*, S28–S37. [CrossRef]
19. Faienza, M.F.; Wang, D.Q.; Fruhbeck, G.; Garruti, G.; Portincasa, P. The dangerous link between childhood and adulthood predictors of obesity and metabolic syndrome. *Intern. Emerg. Med.* **2016**, *11*, 175–182. [CrossRef]
20. Alvarez, L.E.; Ribas, B.L.; Serra, M.L. Prevalence of the metabolic syndrome in the population of Canary Islands, Spain. *Med. Clin.* **2003**, *120*, 172–174.
21. Holst-Schumacher, I.; Nunez-Rivas, H.; Monge-Rojas, R.; Barrantes-Santamaria, M. Components of the metabolic syndrome among a sample of overweight and obese Costa Rican schoolchildren. *Food Nutr. Bull.* **2009**, *30*, 161–170. [CrossRef]
22. Alvarez, M.M.; Vieira, A.C.; Sichieri, R.; Veiga, G.V. Prevalence of metabolic syndrome and of its specific components among adolescents from Niteroi city, Rio de Janeiro state, Brazil. *Arq. Bras. Endocrinol. Metab.* **2011**, *55*, 164–170. [CrossRef] [PubMed]
23. Liang, J.; Fu, J.; Jiang, Y.; Dong, G.; Wang, X.; Wu, W. TriGlycerides and high-density lipoprotein cholesterol ratio compared with homeostasis model assessment insulin resistance indexes in screening for metabolic syndrome in the chinese obese children: A cross section study. *BMC Pediatr.* **2015**, *15*, 138. [CrossRef] [PubMed]
24. Yakubov, R.; Nadir, E.; Stein, R.; Klein-Kremer, A. The duration of breastfeeding and its association with metabolic syndrome among obese children. *Sci. World J.* **2015**, *2015*, 731319. [CrossRef] [PubMed]
25. Owen, C.G.; Martin, R.M.; Whincup, P.H.; Smith, G.D.; Cook, D.G. Effect of infant feeding on the risk of obesity across the life course: A quantitative review of published evidence. *Pediatrics* **2005**, *115*, 1367–1377. [CrossRef] [PubMed]

26. Harder, T.; Bergmann, R.; Kallischnigg, G.; Plagemann, A. Duration of breastfeeding and risk of overweight: A meta-analysis. *Am. J. Epidemiol.* **2005**, *162*, 397–403. [CrossRef]
27. De Armas, M.G.; Megías, S.M.; Modino, S.C.; Bolaños, P.I.; Guardiola, P.D.; Alvarez, T.M. Importance of breastfeeding in the prevalence of metabolic syndrome and degree of childhood obesity. *Endocrinol. Nutr.* **2009**, *56*, 400–403. [CrossRef]
28. Ekelund, U.; Anderssen, S.; Andersen, L.B.; Riddoch, C.J.; Sardinha, L.B.; Luan, J.; Froberg, K.; Brage, S. Prevalence and correlates of the metabolic syndrome in a population-based sample of European youth. *Am. J. Clin. Nutr.* **2009**, *89*, 90–96. [CrossRef]
29. Sun, K.; Chen, M.; Yin, Y.; Wu, L.; Gao, L. Why Chinese mothers stop breastfeeding: Mothers' self-reported reasons for stopping during the first six months. *J. Child Health Care* **2017**, *21*, 353–363. [CrossRef]
30. De Jersey, S.J.; Mallan, K.; Forster, J.; Daniels, L.A. A prospective study of breastfeeding intentions of healthy weight and overweight women as predictors of breastfeeding outcomes. *Midwifery* **2017**, *53*, 20–27. [CrossRef]
31. Amir, L.H.; Donath, S. A systematic review of maternal obesity and breastfeeding intention, initiation and duration. *BMC Pregnancy Childbirth* **2007**, *7*, 9. [CrossRef]
32. Dos Santos Alves, P.J.; Henriques, A.C.; Pinto, L.R.; Mota, R.M.; Alencar, C.H.; Alves, R.S.; Carvalho, F.H. Endothelial and metabolic disorders in adolescence: Low birth weight is not an isolated risk factor. *J. Pediatr. Endocrinol. Metab.* **2015**, *28*, 407–413. [CrossRef] [PubMed]
33. Yuan, Z.P.; Yang, M.; Liang, L.; Fu, J.F.; Xiong, F.; Liu, G.L.; Gong, C.X.; Luo, F.H.; Chen, S.K.; Zhang, D.D.; et al. Possible role of birth weight on general and central obesity in Chinese children and adolescents: A cross-sectional study. *Ann. Epidemiol.* **2015**, *25*, 748–752. [CrossRef] [PubMed]
34. Zabeen, B.; Tayyeb, S.; Naz, F.; Ahmed, F.; Rahman, M.; Nahar, J.; Nahar, N.; Azad, K. Prevalence of obesity and central obesity among adolescent girls in a district school in Bangladesh. *Indian J. Endocrinol. Metab.* **2015**, *19*, 649–652. [CrossRef] [PubMed]
35. Schroder, H.; Ribas, L.; Koebnick, C.; Funtikova, A.; Gomez, S.F.; Fíto, M.; Perez-Rodrigo, C.; Serra-Majem, L. Prevalence of abdominal obesity in Spanish children and adolescents. Do we need waist circumference measurements in pediatric practice? *PLoS ONE* **2014**, *9*, e87549. [CrossRef] [PubMed]
36. Lee, C.M.; Huxley, R.R.; Wildman, R.P.; Woodward, M. Indices of abdominal obesity are better discriminators of cardiovascular risk factors than BMI: A meta-analysis. *J. Clin. Epidemiol.* **2008**, *61*, 646–653. [CrossRef]
37. Haldar, S.; Chia, S.C.; Henry, C.J. Body composition in Asians and caucasians: Comparative analyses and influences on cardiometabolic outcomes. *Adv. Food Nutr. Res.* **2015**, *75*, 97–154. [PubMed]
38. Papoutsakis, C.; Yannakoulia, M.; Ntalla, I.; Dedoussis, G.V. Metabolic syndrome in a Mediterranean pediatric cohort: Prevalence using international diabetes federation-derived criteria and associations with adiponectin and leptin. *Metabolism* **2012**, *61*, 140–145. [CrossRef] [PubMed]
39. Tai, E.S.; Lau, T.N.; Ho, S.C.; Fok, A.C.; Tan, C.E. Body fat distribution and cardiovascular risk in normal weight women. Associations with insulin resistance, lipids and plasma leptin. *Int. J. Obes. Relat. Metab. Disord.* **2000**, *24*, 751–757. [CrossRef]
40. Park, Y.W.; Allison, D.B.; Heymsfield, S.B.; Gallagher, D. Larger amounts of visceral adipose tissue in Asian Americans. *Obes. Res.* **2001**, *9*, 381–387. [CrossRef]
41. Victora, C.G.; Horta, B.L.; Post, P.; Lima, R.C.; De Leon Elizalde, J.W.; Gerson, B.M.; Barros, F.C. Breast feeding and blood lipid concentrations in male Brazilian adolescents. *J. Epidemiol. Community Health* **2006**, *60*, 621–625. [CrossRef]
42. Lawlor, D.A.; Riddoch, C.J.; Page, A.S.; Andersen, L.B.; Wedderkopp, N.; Harro, M.; Stansbie, D.; Smith, G.D. Infant feeding and components of the metabolic syndrome: Findings from the European youth heart study. *Arch. Dis. Child.* **2005**, *90*, 582–588. [CrossRef] [PubMed]
43. Ramirez-Silva, I.; Rivera, J.A.; Trejo-Valdivia, B.; Martorell, R.; Stein, A.D.; Romieu, I.; Ramakrishnan, U. Breastfeeding status at age 3 months is associated with adiposity and cardiometabolic markers at age 4 years in Mexican children. *J. Nutr.* **2015**, *145*, 1295–1302. [CrossRef] [PubMed]

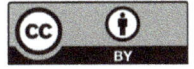 © 2019 by the authors. Licensee MDPI, Basel, Switzerland. This article is an open access article distributed under the terms and conditions of the Creative Commons Attribution (CC BY) license (http://creativecommons.org/licenses/by/4.0/).

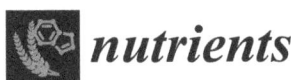

Article

Metabolomic Salivary Signature of Pediatric Obesity Related Liver Disease and Metabolic Syndrome

Jacopo Troisi [1,2,3,4,*], Federica Belmonte [1], Antonella Bisogno [1], Luca Pierri [1], Angelo Colucci [1,2], Giovanni Scala [4], Pierpaolo Cavallo [5], Claudia Mandato [6], Antonella Di Nuzzi [1], Laura Di Michele [1], Anna Pia Delli Bovi [1], Salvatore Guercio Nuzio [1] and Pietro Vajro [1,7]

1. Department of Medicine and Surgery and Dentistry, "Scuola Medica Salernitana", Pediatrics Section University of Salerno, 84081 Baronissi (Salerno), Italy; fecu91@gmail.com (F.B.); a.bisogno91@gmail.com (A.B.); luca.pierri@hotmail.com (L.P.); angelocolucci2@gmail.com (A.C.); antonelladinuzzi@gmail.com (A.D.N.); lauradimichele05091993@gmail.com (L.D.M.); delliboviannapia@gmail.com (A.P.D.B.); sguercio.nuzio@gmail.com (S.G.N.); pvajro@unisa.it (P.V.)
2. Theoreo srl, Via degli Ulivi 3, 84090 Montecorvino Pugliano (SA), Italy
3. European Biomedical Research Institute of Salerno (EBRIS), Via S. de Renzi, 3, 84125 Salerno, Italy
4. Hosmotic srl, Via R. Bosco 178, 80069 Vico Equense (NA), Italy; scala@hosmotic.com
5. Department of Physics, University of Salerno, 84084 Fisciano (Salerno), Italy; pcavallo@unisa.it
6. Department of Pediatrics, Children's Hospital Santobono-Pausilipon, 80129 Naples, Italy; cla.mandato@gmail.com
7. European Laboratory of Food Induced Intestinal Disease (ELFID), University of Naples Federico II, 80100 Naples, Italy
* Correspondence: troisi@theoreosrl.com; Tel./Fax: +39-089-0977435

Received: 24 December 2018; Accepted: 21 January 2019; Published: 26 January 2019

Abstract: Pediatric obesity-related metabolic syndrome (MetS) and nonalcoholic fatty liver disease (NAFLD) are increasingly frequent conditions with a still-elusive diagnosis and low-efficacy treatment and monitoring options. In this study, we investigated the salivary metabolomic signature, which has been uncharacterized to date. In this pilot-nested case-control study over a transversal design, 41 subjects (23 obese patients and 18 normal weight (NW) healthy controls), characterized based on medical history, clinical, anthropometric, and laboratory data, were recruited. Liver involvement, defined according to ultrasonographic liver brightness, allowed for the allocation of the patients into four groups: obese with hepatic steatosis ([St+], $n = 15$) and without hepatic steatosis ([St−], $n = 8$), and with ($n = 10$) and without ($n = 13$) MetS. A partial least squares discriminant analysis (PLS-DA) model was devised to classify the patients' classes based on their salivary metabolomic signature. Pediatric obesity and its related liver disease and metabolic syndrome appear to have distinct salivary metabolomic signatures. The difference is notable in metabolites involved in energy, amino and organic acid metabolism, as well as in intestinal bacteria metabolism, possibly reflecting diet, fatty acid synthase pathways, and the strict interaction between microbiota and intestinal mucins. This information expands the current understanding of NAFLD pathogenesis, potentially translating into better targeted monitoring and/or treatment strategies in the future.

Keywords: pediatric obesity; nonalcoholic fatty liver disease; metabolic syndrome; saliva; metabolomics; gas-chromatography mass spectrometry

1. Introduction

The incidence of obesity and its related conditions, including metabolic syndrome (MetS) and non-alcoholic fatty liver disease (NAFLD), has dramatically increased worldwide in all age groups including pediatrics [1]. Pediatric obesity definitely is an early risk factor for adult morbidity and mortality [2,3]. Due to the existence of a well-established tracking phenomenon, the early detection and treatment of MetS and fatty liver in childhood represents a valuable tool to prevent further health complications and to minimize the global socioeconomic burden of hepato-metabolic and cardiovascular obesity-associated complications in adulthood [4]. Although the exact definition of MetS is still debated regarding the pediatric population, most researchers agree (a) that it includes hypertension, hyperglycemia, dyslipidemia together with visceral obesity, and (b) that NAFLD has to be considered its hepatic component.

Metabolomics has recently started to pave the way to a better pathomechanistic understanding of these hepatometabolic complications, leading to a more efficient diagnosis and better therapeutic approaches. In this regard, studies have shown that high urinary/blood levels of aromatic (AAA) ± branched chain (BCAA) amino acids are known to be associated with insulin resistance (IR) and the risk of obesity-related MetS [5–8].

Lipid metabolism, tyrosine [9], alanine and the urea cycle [5], acylcarnitine catabolism ± changes in nucleotides, lysolipids, and inflammation markers [10], and several other components [11–13] also appear to be implicated in obesity and its related disorders.

We have recently shown a complex network of urinary molecules prevalently represented by intestinally-derived bacterial products [14] which are correlated with the clinical phenotype and can differentiate between normal weight and obese children, distinguishing between those with and without liver involvement, based also on the characteristics of their gut-liver axis (GLA) function [15].

To identify an even more easily accessible and readily obtained biofluid for possible minimally invasive disease recognition [16], few studies have shown saliva suitability for investigations of individual metabolites of oxidative stress in obesity [17] and obesity-related MetS/NAFLD [4,18]. We showed that salivary testing of uric acid, glucose, insulin and HOMA together with selected anthropometric parameters may help to identify noninvasively obese children with hepatic steatosis and/or having MetS components [4]. However, salivary metabolomics studies in this respect are lacking.

Based on these and a few other urine-and/or plasma-based metabolomic studies of pediatric obesity and MetS [15,19–21], we hypothesized that differences in the metabolite profiling of lean and obese children with and without NAFLD/MetS might also be evident in saliva, which might be ideal to screen noninvasively obese children at a higher risk of hepatometabolic complications. Prospectively, better delineation of individual or clusters of specific metabolites could serve as diagnostic biomarkers to be further investigated in future studies appraising even early stages of these comorbidities.

2. Materials and Methods

2.1. Population and Study Design

Among 46 consecutive subjects (aged 7–15 years) seen at our obesity clinic or planned for only minor surgery, 41 with verified good oral health and not taking medications were enrolled in a nested case-control study over a transversal design. Eighteen had a normal weight (NW; body mass index (BMI) < 85th percentile) and 23 were obese (BMI > 95th percentile). The patients were characterized based on clinical, anthropometric (blood pressure, BMI, waist circumference (WC), and neck circumference (NC)), laboratory (serum alanine aminotransferase (ALT), aspartate aminotransferase (AST), total and high-density lipoprotein (HDL) cholesterol, triglycerides, uric acid (UA), glucose, and insulin) parameters. An ultrasound (US) was used to determine the presence [St+] or absence [St−] of hepatic steatosis [22,23]. Blood tests were performed using a standard laboratory analyzer (Abbott Diagnostics, Santa Clara, CA, USA).

ALT upper normal values referred either to the customary normal range cut-off value of 40 IU/L or more precise SAFETY study cut-off pediatric values of 25.8 and 22.0 IU/L for boys and girls, respectively [24].

Patients with hepatic steatosis and/or transaminases >1.5 times the upper customary normal values were screened for celiac disease, Wilson disease, autoimmune hepatitis, and major and minor hepatotropic viruses [25]. According to the International Diabetes Foundation (IDF), MetS was defined as the presence of at least three of the following parameters: WC >95th percentile; triglycerides >150 mg/dL; blood glucose >100 mg/dL; systolic blood pressure (SBP) >95th percentile; and HDL cholesterol <40 mg/dL [26].

2.2. Saliva Samples

Each subject was asked to refrain from eating, drinking and brush tooting procedures for at least 1 h before saliva collection. Then he/she underwent a morning, whole saliva sampling using a saliva cotton roll commercial collection device (Salivette®; Sarstedt, Nümbrecht, Germany). As recommended by the manufacturer, to stimulate salivation patients, patients were asked to roll and gently chew the cotton swab in their mouth for 60–90 s. Then the swab was spitted in the collection tube of the kit and centrifuged within 1 h at $2000\times g$ for 2 min. The collected clear, fluid saliva sample was aliquoted without any further processing and frozen at $-80\ °C$ until samples' analysis, as previously described [4].

2.3. Ethical Approval

The study complied with the terms of the Declaration of Helsinki of 1975 (as revised in 2013) [27] for the investigation of human subjects, with written informed consent from patients and their families. All participants agreed to participate in this study and contribute saliva samples for metabolomic analysis. All samples were collected in accordance with the ethical guidelines mandated by and approved by our institutional Health Research Ethics Board. The study protocol was approved by the Ethics Review Committee of the University Hospital S. Giovanni di Dio e Ruggi d'Aragona of Salerno (Prot. No 18.02.2013/98).

2.4. Untargeted Metabolomics Analysis

2.4.1. Metabolites Extraction and Derivatization

Metabolome extraction, purification and derivatization were carried out using the MetboPrep GC kit (Theoreo srl, Montecorvino Pugliano (SA), Italy) according to the manufacturer's instructions.

2.4.2. GC-MS Analysis

GC-MS analysis was performed on the derivatized extracted metabolome according to Troisi et al. [15] with a few minor changes. Briefly, 2 µL of the sample solution was injected into the GC-MS system (GC-2010 Plus gas chromatograph coupled to a 2010 Plus single quadrupole mass spectrometer; Shimadzu Corp., Kyoto, Japan) equipped with a 30-m, 0.25-mm ID CP-Sil 8 CB fused silica capillary GC column with 1.00-µm film thickness from Agilent (Agilent, J&W Scientific, Folsom, CA, USA), using He as a carrier gas. The initial oven temperature of 100 °C was maintained for 1 min and then raised by 6 °C/min to 320 °C with a further 2.33 min of hold time. The gas flow was set to obtain a constant linear velocity of 39 cm/s, and injections were performed in the splitless mode. The mass spectrometer was operated in electron impact (70 eV) in the full-scan mode in the interval of 35–600 m/z with a scan velocity of 3333 amu/s and a solvent cut-off time of 4.5 min. The complete GC analysis duration was 40 min. Untargeted metabolites were identified by comparing the mass spectrum of each peak with the NIST library collection (NIST, Gaithersburg, MD, USA).

2.4.3. Metabolites Identification

Of the over 240 signals per sample produced by GC-MS analysis, only 222 were investigated further because they were consistently found in at least 85% of samples.

To identify metabolites under the peaks, the Kovats' index [28] difference max tolerance was set at 10, while the minimum matching for the NIST library search was set at 85%. The results were summarized in a comma-separate matrix file and loaded in the appropriate software for statistical manipulation. The chromatographic data for PLS-DA analysis were tabulated with one sample per row and one variable (metabolite) per column. The normalization procedures consisted of data transformation and scaling. Data transformation was made by generalized log transformation and data scaling by autoscaling (mean-centered and divided by standard deviation of each variable) [29]. Relevant metabolites selected using statistical analysis were further confirmed with an analytical standard purchased from Sigma-Aldrich (Milan, Italy) as indicated in the Metabolomic Standard Initiative reports [30].

2.5. Statistical Analysis

2.5.1. Demographical and Clinical Data

Statistical analysis was performed using Statistica software (StatSoft, Tulsa, OK, USA) and Minitab (Minitab Inc., State College, PA, USA). The normal distribution of data was verified using the Shapiro–Wilks test. Because the data were normally distributed, we used one-way ANOVA with Tukey's post-hoc test for intergroup comparisons. A result with $p < 0.05$ was considered statistically significant.

2.5.2. Metabolomics Univariate Data Analysis

Metabolite concentration differences among the classes (NW, OB[St+] and OB[St−]) were evaluated in terms of fold change (FC) and p-value (assessed using Student's t-test because the metabolite amount was previously normalized).

The volcano plot representation was used to encounter both criteria. Metabolites with high FC (>1 or <−1) and lower p-value (<0.05) were selected as the most relevant.

2.5.3. Metabolomic Multivariate Data Analysis

Partial least squares discriminant analysis (PLS-DA) was performed on the internal standard peak area [31] normalized chromatogram using R (Foundation for Statistical Computing, Vienna, Austria). Mean centering and unit variance scaling were applied for all analyses. Class separation was archived by PLS-DA, which is a supervised method that uses multivariate regression techniques to extract, via linear combinations of original variables (X), the information that can predict class membership (Y). PLS regression was performed using the *plsr* function included in the R pls package [32]. Classification and cross-validation were performed using the wrapper function included in the caret package [33]. A permutation test was performed to assess the significance of class discrimination. In each permutation, a PLS-DA model was built between the data (X) and permuted class labels (Y) using the optimal number of components determined by cross validation for the model based on the original class assignment. Two types of test statistics were used to measure class discrimination. The first is based on prediction accuracy during training. The second used separation distance based on the ratio of the between groups sum of the squares and the within group sum of squares (B/W-ratio). If the observed test statistics were part of the distribution based on the permuted class assignments, class discrimination cannot be considered significant from a statistical point of view [34]. Variable importance in projection (VIP) scores were calculated for each component. A VIP score is a weighted sum of squares of the PLS loadings, considering the amount of explained Y-variation in each dimension.

The metabolic pathway was constructed using the MetScape application [35] of the software Cytoscape [36].

3. Results

The demographic and clinical laboratory characteristics of the case and control subjects are reported in Table 1. None of the NW controls had either biochemical or US hepato-metabolic abnormalities.

Table 1. Characteristics of the study population.

Anthropometric and Laboratory Parameters	Controls (n = 18)	Obese with Steatosis (n = 15)	Obese without Steatosis (n = 8)	All Obese (n = 23)
Gender (M/F)	13/5	10/5	4/4	14/9
Age (years)	10.53 ± 2.57	12.48 ± 2.77 *	12.51 ± 2.79 *	12.49 ± 2.71 *
Weight (kg)	37.42 ± 11.26	79.99 ± 28.76 *	71.9 ± 17.31 *	77.18 ± 25.24 *
Height (cm)	140.17 ± 15.17	153.41 ± 19.27 *	157.45 ± 11.97 *	154.52 ± 16.88 *
BMI (kg/cm^2)	18.52 ± 2.92	32.80 ± 6.94 *	28.93 ± 5.58 *	31.45 ± 6.65 *
BMI percentile	23.75 ± 34.25	95.14 ± 0.53 *	95.67 ± 1.03 *	95.40 ± 1.05 *
Waist circumference (cm)	61.14 ± 7.11	93.27 ± 12.68 *	86.00 ± 14.53 *	90.74 ± 13.49 *
WC percentile	65.85 ± 24.58	94.98 ± 0.97 *	94.38 ± 1.77 *	94.78 ± 1.04 *
Cm WC > 95th percentile	0	21.03 ± 10.57 *	14.00 ± 10.99 *	18.59 ± 11.01 *
WtHR	0.43 ± 0.03	0.61 ± 0.05 *	0.55 ± 0.08 *	0.59 ± 0.07 *
Neck circumference (cm)	27.67 ± 2.41	36.05 ± 4.33 *	34.69 ± 4.08 *	35.58 ± 4.20 *
NC percentile	44.12 ± 33.22	95.57 ± 5.35 *	92.61 ± 3.15	94.09 ± 4.26 *
Cm NC > 95th percentile	0	3.71 ± 2.77 *	2.41 ± 2.75 *	3.26 ± 2.77 *
SBP (mmHg)	95.98 ± 11.95	127.47 ± 8.95 *	125.63 ± 20.23 *	126.83 ± 13.49 *
SBP percentile	50.00 ± 0	86.93 ± 19.36 *	83.50 ± 20.96 *	85.74 ± 19.52 *
DBP (mmHg)	55.00 ± 10.77	61.53 ± 10.42 *	60.75 ± 11.70 *	61.26 ± 10.62 *
DBP percentile	50.00 ± 0	56.00 ± 15.83 *	55.00 ± 14.14 *	55.65 ± 14.95 *
ALT (U/L)	17.33 ± 4.31	50.17 ± 28.75 *	34.50 ± 37.74 *	44.72 ± 32.21 *
AST (U/L)	24.72 ± 4.87	46.19 ± 28.58 *	19.75 ± 5.85	37.00 ± 26.39 *
Total cholesterol (mg/dL)	148.78 ± 16.38	158.17 ± 21.91 *	162.00 ± 24.20 *	159.50 ± 22.26 *
HDL (mg/dL)	56.94 ± 14.45	45.07 ± 10.21 *	48.00 ± 5.50 *	46.09 ± 8.83 *
Triglyceride (mg/dL)	Not available	90.59 ± 26.97	138.63 ± 91.90	107.30 ± 60.80
Blood glucose (mg/dL)	83.17 ± 6.61	88.59 ± 10.36 *	90.00 ± 10.34 *	89.08 ± 10.14 *
Salivary glucose (µM)	3338.36 ± 1274.73	3167.86 ± 1192.75	2647.09 ± 1227.77	2986.70 ± 1203.86
Blood insulin (U/L)	10.27 ± 5.22	24.24 ± 10.95 *	19.60 ± 6.63 *	22.62 ± 9.77 *
Salivary insulin (nM)	5.79 ± 2.85	20.89 ± 8.69 *	17.26 ± 6.37 *	19.60 ± 8.00 *
Blood HOMA-IR	2.01 ± 1.16	5.34 ± 2.60 *	4.11 ± 2.16 *	4.91 ± 2.48 *
Salivary HOMA-IR	119.7 ± 73.99	401.81 ± 231.17 *	278.79 ± 162.48 *	358.20 ± 215.35 *
Blood uric acid (mg/dL)	4.04 ± 0.76	5.06 ± 1.23 *	4.42 ± 0.92 *	4.84 ± 1.15 *
Salivary uric acid (µM)	143.46 ± 4.53	157.29 ± 13.04 *	156.45 ± 15.31 *	157.00 ± 13.53 *

Abbreviations = ALT: alanine transaminase; AST: aspartate transaminase; BMI: Body Mass Index; DBP: diastolic blood pressure; HDL: high density lipoproteins; HOMA-IR: Homeostasis Assessment Model—Insulin Resistance WC: waist circumference; NC: neck circumference; SBP: systolic blood pressure; WtHR: Waist to Height Ratio; * p value < 0.05 compared to controls.

More than 50% of obese children (n = 15) had ultrasonographic (US) signs of NAFLD and hypertransaminasemia not due to the most common causes of liver diseases, as well as significantly higher values of systolic blood pressure (127 ± 9 vs. 96 ± 11 mm Hg, p = 0.0003) and glycemia (88.6 ± 10.4 vs. 83.2 ± 6.6 mg/dL, p = 0.002) compared with NW subjects. Twenty-one patients had no component of MetS, 7 had at least one component, 10 had two or three components, and only 3 had more than three components (Table 2).

As shown in Figure 1, the PLS-DA score plots clearly differentiated between obese (OB) and normal weight (NW) children (Figure 1A1) and between OB with and without steatosis and NW controls (Figure 1B1). Twelve and 13 metabolites with a VIP-score > 2 separated NW/OB and NW/OB[St+]/OB[St−], respectively (Figure 1A2,B2). A third PLS-DA model (Figure 1C1) separated children according to MetS via five metabolites that had a VIP-score >2 (Figure 1C2).

As shown in Figure 1 and Table 3, compared with NW subjects, the saliva of obese children had higher levels of palmitic acid, myristic acid, urea, N-acetyl galactosamine, maltose, gluconic acid and isoleucine and lower levels of hydroxy butyric acid and malic acid, which were prevalent in those without steatosis and lauric acid, maltose and methyl maleic acid, which were prevalent in those with steatosis.

Table 2. Metabolic Syndrome components in obese patients with and without hepatic steatosis.

	Number (%) of Obese Patients with Hepatic Steatosis	Number (%) of Obese Patients without Hepatic Steatosis	Total (%)
Sample size	15(65%)	8(35%)	23(100%)
Waist circumference >90th percentile	15(65%)	7(30%)	22(95%)
Glucose blood levels >100 mg/dL	4(17%)	2(9%)	6(26%)
Blood pressure >95th percentile	10(43%)	4(17%)	14(60%)
HDL <40 mg/dL	3(13%)	0(0%)	3(13%)
TG >150 mg/dL	2(9%)	3(13%)	5(22%)
HOMA-IR > 3	13(57%)	5(22%)	18(79%)
Numbers of patients fulfilling MetS Criteria: (WC > 90th percentile and more than two out of four other criteria)	7(30%)	3(13%)	10(43%)

Abbreviations = HDL: high density lipoproteins; HOMA-IR: Homeostasis Assessment Model – Insulin Resistance; MetS: Metabolic Syndrome; TG: Triglycerides; WC: waist circumference

Table 3. Variables important in projection (VIP) metabolites fold changes in patients versus controls' saliva.

VIP	NW ($n = 18$) [a]	OB[St−] ($n = 15$)	OB[St+] ($n = 8$)	p-Value [b]	MetS− ($n = 38$) [a]	MetS+ ($n = 3$)	p-Value [c]
Hydroxy butyric acid	0.00697	−0.14	−0.62 *	NS	0.00622	−1.02	NS
Palmitic acid [d]	0.00088	4.46 ***	8.06 **	NS	0.00398	−0.74	NS
Myristic acid	0.00092	3.71 **	7.58 *	NS	0.00375	−0.66	NS
Lauric acid	0.00061	−7.21 **	−3.35	NS	0.00267	0.73	NS
Urea	0.00093	4.15 **	7.65 **	NS	0.00404	−0.71	NS
N-acetyl galactosamine	0.00088	3.72 **	7.60 *	NS	0.00375	−0.66	NS
Malic acid	0.17825	−0.98	−0.98	NS	0.09066	0.96	NS
Methyl maleic acid	0.01375	−0.72	−0.24	NS	0.01164	0.81	NS
Maltose	0.07047	−0.54	−0.25	NS	0.05846	0.24	NS
Xylose	0.00864	−0.62	−0.34	NS	0.00681	0.27	NS
Butanediol	0.00070	−6.16 **	−2.79	NS	0.00272	0.34	NS
Proline	0.00999	−0.56	−0.25	NS	0.00752	−1.02	NS
Tartaric acid	0.06401	0.52	0.40	NS	0.04729	−0.40	NS

* indicates a p-value < 0.05 compared to NW, ** indicates a p-value < 0.01 compared to NW, *** indicates a p-value < 0.001 compared to NW, NS indicates a p-value > 0.05. [a] Normalized chromatographic peak area; [b] p-values of OB[St+]/OB[St−] comparison; [c] p-values of MetS−/MetS+ comparison; [d] Metabolite selected by both PLS-DA models. Abbreviations: MetS−: No metabolic syndrome diagnosis; MetS+: Diagnosis of metabolic syndrome; NW: Normal Weight; OB[St+]: Obese without steatosis; OB[St+]: Obese with Steatosis; PLS-DA: Partial Least Squares Discriminant Analysis; VIP: Variable Important in Projections

The volcano plot representation and histogram of the metabolites selected using volcano plot analysis (FC > 1 or < −1, p < 0.05) of the OB patients compared with NW (Figure S1-A1) and of the OB[St+] patients compared with the OB[St−] patients (Figure S1-A2) is reported in supplementary Figure S1.

The levels of valine, mannose, acetopyruvic acid, palmitic acid, triethylene glycol, gluconic acid, citric acid, scyllo-inositol, deoxyglucose, psicopyranose, myo-inositol and cycloserine were higher in OB patients (Figure 2B1). Conversely, the levels of 1,2,3-butanetriol, 2-oxovaleric acid, 2-palmitoylglycerol, Di-n-octyl phthalate, itaconic acid, methyl galactoside, stearic acid, 2-piperidinone, maltose, 2-deoxy-D-ribose, pentane dioic acid, glycerol, pentitol, glyceric acid, methyl maleic acid, 2-deoxypentofuranose, β-hydroxy pyruvic acid, 2-hydroxy- methylcyclopentanol, and L-serine were higher in NW patients (Figure S1-B1). OB[St+] patients had higher levels of D-glucuronic acid γ-lactone, 2′-deoxyribolactone, 2-hydroxyisocaproic acid, pyroglutamic acid, and propanoic acid. Instead, OB[St−] patients had higher levels of butanoic acid, maltose, thiamine, glucopyranose, 2-hydroxybutyric acid, and mannose (Figure S1-B).

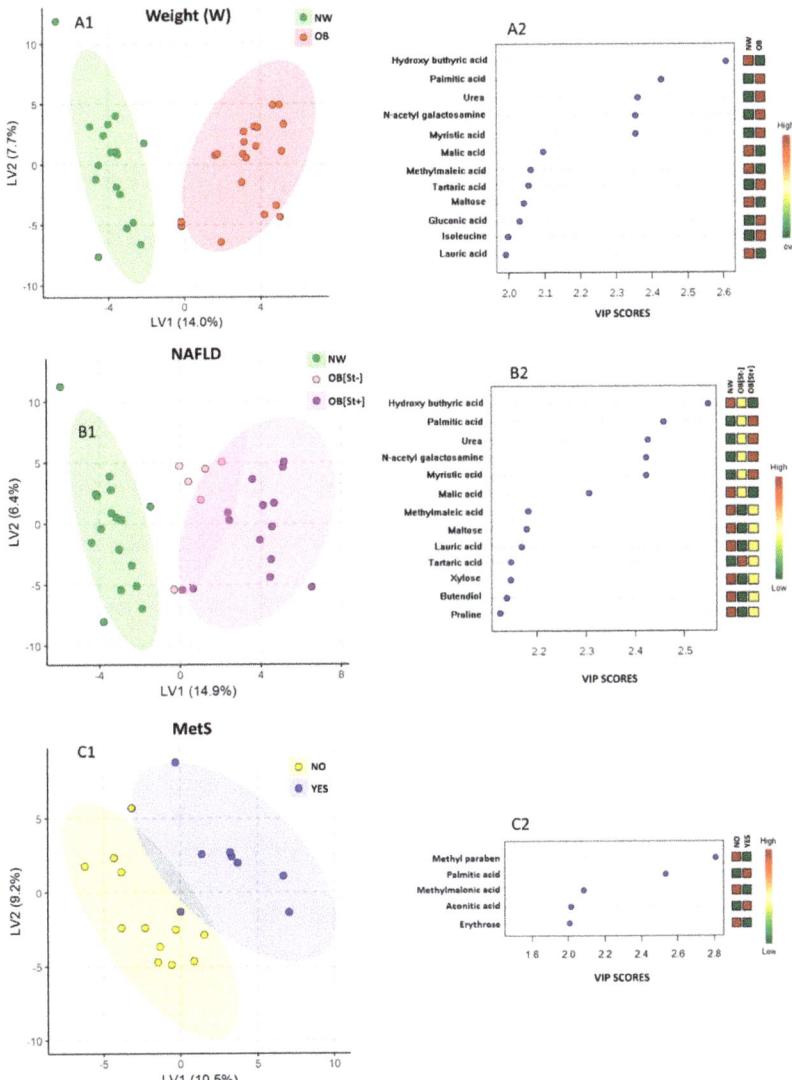

Figure 1. Partial least square discriminant analysis (PLS-DA) models to discriminate children according to Body Mass Index (BMI) (**A1**) and Non Alcoholic Fatty Liver Disease (NAFLD) (**B1**), as unique parameters investigated. The explained variance of each component is shown in parenthesis on the corresponding axis. In panel **A1**, the green ellipse contains normal weight children, while the red one contains the obese children. In panel **B1**, the purple circles represent the obese children with NAFLD (OB[St+]), the pink circles represent obese children without NAFLD (OB[St−]), while green circles represent the normal weight controls (NW). In panel **C1**, the blue circles represent the children with a diagnosis of metabolic syndrome (MetS), while the yellow ones represent the children without MetS diagnosis. The first 12, 13 and 5 variables important in projection (VIP) identified by the corresponding PLS-DA are shown in Panels **A2**, **B2** and **C2** respectively. The number of VIPs was established by setting the VIP-score ≥ 2 as a cut off value. In all cases, the colored boxes on the right indicate the relative amount of the corresponding metabolite in each group under study.

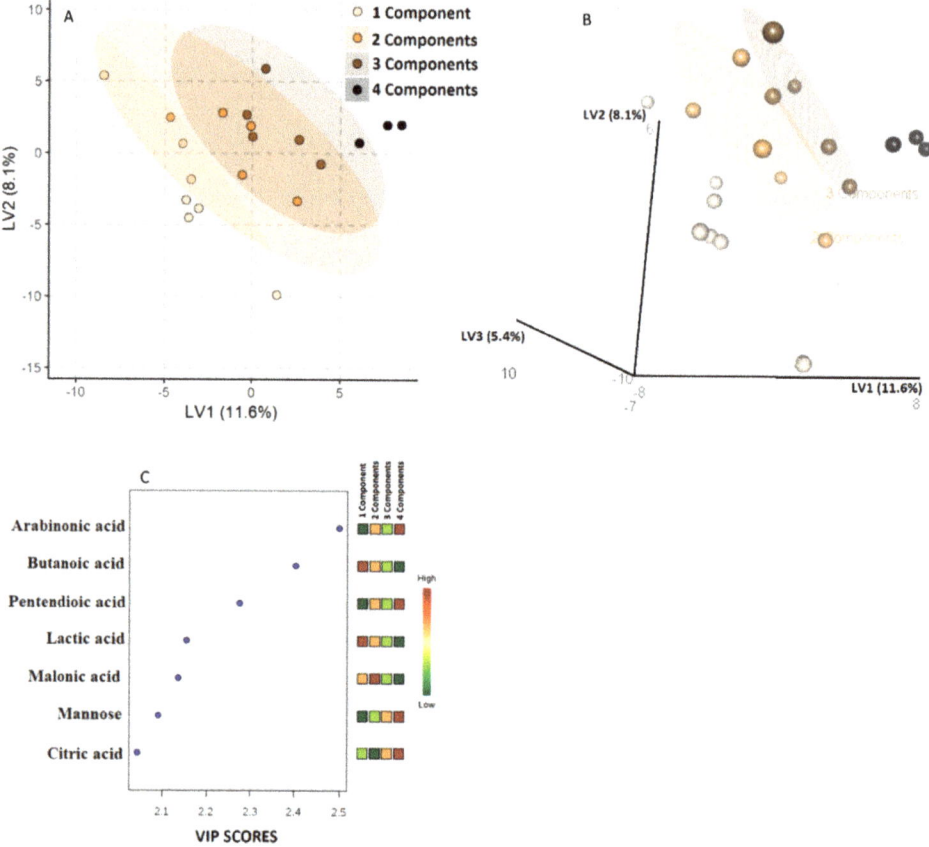

Figure 2. Partial least squares discriminant analysis (PLS-DA) model to discriminate obese children according to the number of Metabolic Syndrome (MetS) components. The explained variance of each component is shown on the corresponding axis. In panels **A** and **B**, the color darkness progression denotes the MetS components increase. The seven metabolites with a variable important in projection score (VIP-score) higher than 2 are shown in Panel **C**.

Figure 2 represents the PLS-DA model regarding the aggregation of saliva samples by the number of MetS components.

A clear-cut class separation was achieved, following the increase in the number of MetS components (Figure 2A,B). The metabolites with a VIP-score > 2 were as follows: arabinoic, butanoic, pentendioic, lactic, malonic and citric acid and mannose (Figure 2C).

Obese patients were also aggregated considering the serum ALT concentration. Figure 3A reports on the PLS-DA model when the serum ALT level higher than 40 mg/mL was considered hypertransaminasemia. Nine metabolites (butentriol, methyl valeric acid, pentanedioic acid, valine, hydroxy butanoic acid, mannose, di-n-octyl-phthalate and stearic and glyceric acid) showed a VIP-score higher than 2 (Figure 3C).

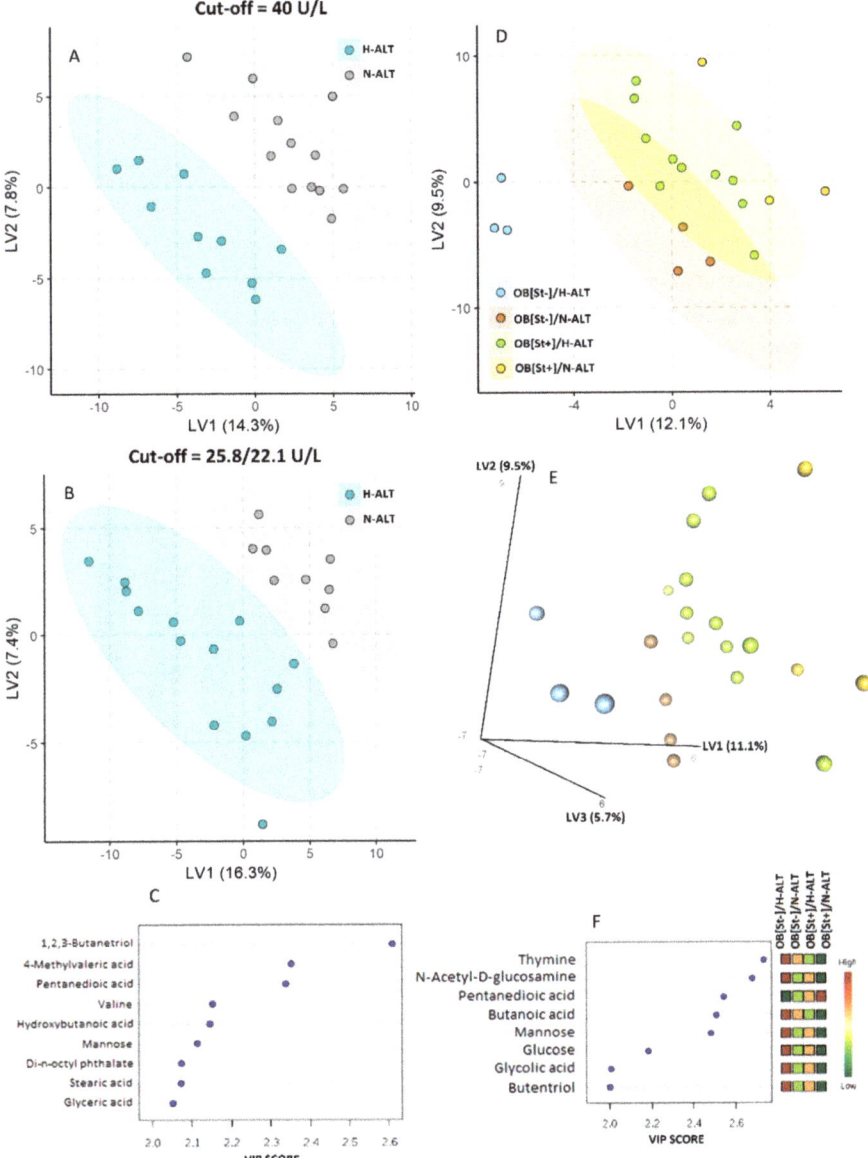

Figure 3. Partial least squares discriminant analysis (PLS-DA) model to discriminate children according to the presence/absence of hypertransaminasemia. Panel **A**: Serum Alanine transaminase (ALT) > 40 U/L was considered as hypertransaminasemia for both boys and girls. The explained variance of each component is shown on the corresponding axis. Panel **B**. Serum ALT > 25.8 U/L for boys and 22.1 U/L for girls was considered as hypertransaminasemia. In panels **A** and **B**, the cyan ellipse contains children with ALT > cut off values, while gray circles represent the children with serum ALT lower than cut off values. The nine metabolites with a VIP-score higher than 2 are shown in Panel **C**. PLS-DA shown in Panels **D/E** cumulates information on the status of both hepatic steatosis and transaminases values with respective variable important in projection scores (VIP-scores) shown in Panel **F**.

When the serum ALT level >25.8U/L for boys and 22.1 U/L for girls were considered hypertransaminasemia [24], the PLS-DA model remained discriminant (panel 3B), and the metabolites showing a VIP score >2 remained unchanged (panel 3C). PLS-DA shown in Panel 3D/E cumulates information on the status of both hepatic steatosis and transaminase values with respective VIP-scores shown in Panel F.

Figure 4 illustrates the UpSet [37] representation summarizing the selected metabolites in several classifications and the relationships between sets.

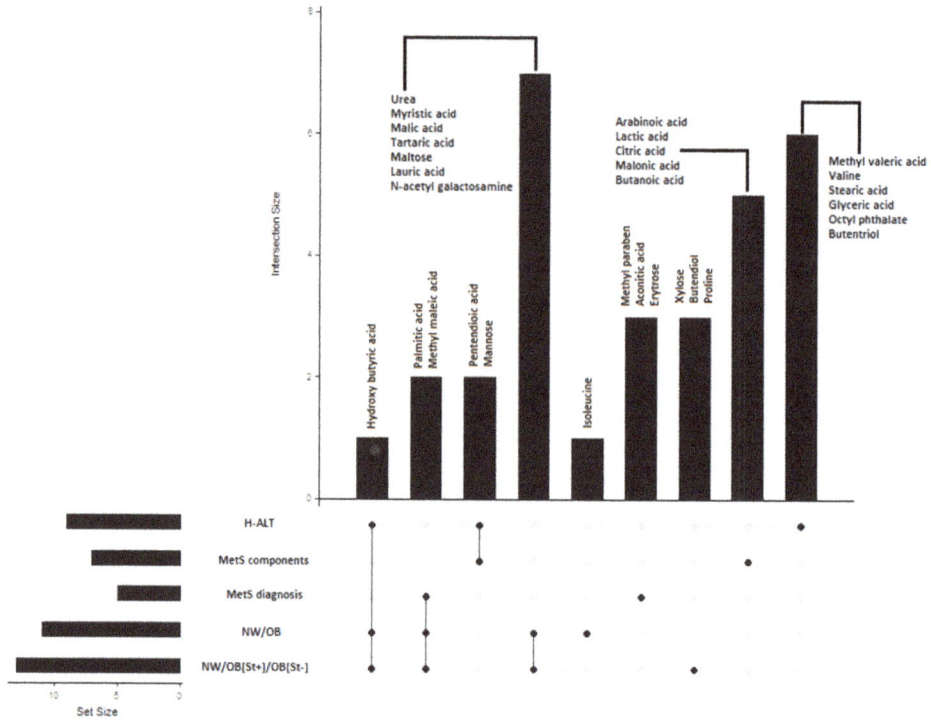

Figure 4. UpSet representation of the metabolites selected in the different classification models. H-ALT: Hypertransaminasemia; MetS: Metabolic Syndrome; NW: normal weight, OB: obese, [St]: hepatic steatosis.

Overall, as shown in the metabolic systemic map (Figure 5), there is a definite interplay of several pathways involving the following processes: de novo fatty acid biosynthesis; saturated fatty acid beta-oxidation; butanoate metabolism; glycolysis and gluconeogenesis; tricarboxylic acid cycle; urea cycle and metabolism of proline, glutamate, aspartate and asparagine; valine, leucine and isoleucine (BCCA) degradation; amino sugar metabolism; purine metabolism; and glycerophospholipid metabolism.

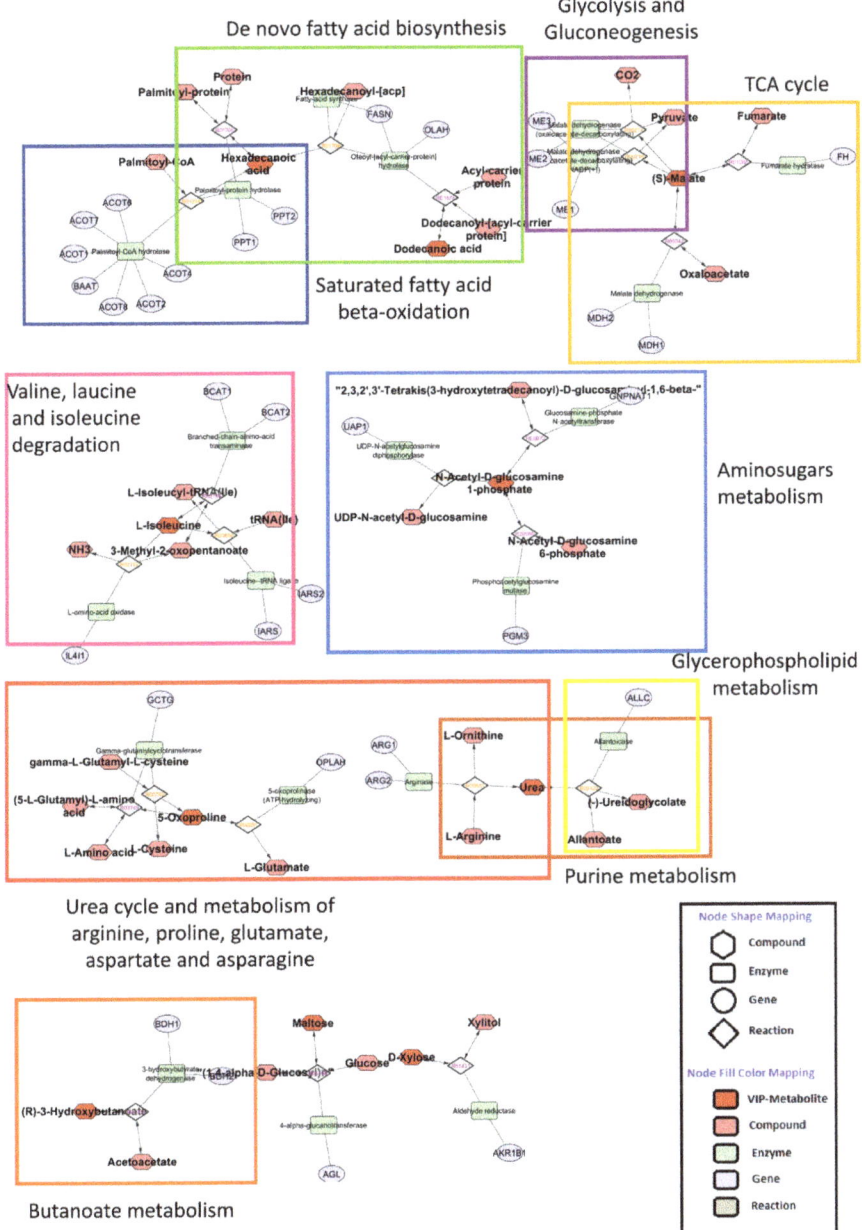

Figure 5. Metabolic systems map summarizing the shortest route that may explain the interactions among the metabolites with a variable important in projection scores higher than 2. There is a clear interplay of several pathways involving: de novo fatty acid biosynthesis; saturated fatty acid beta-oxidation; butanoate metabolism; glycolysis and gluconeogenesis; tricarboxylic acid cycle (TCA); urea cycle and metabolism of proline, glutamate, aspartate and asparagine; valine, and isoleucine (branched chain amino acids) degradation; aminosugars metabolism; purine metabolism; glycerophospholipid metabolism.

4. Discussion

As in a few other conditions (pediatric celiac disease [38], mild cognitive impairment [2], sport performance/fatigue [3,39], T2D [5,40]/T1D [41], and some neurological conditions [42]), our study shows that salivary metabolomics may represent a useful tool to obtain additional pathomechanistic information and serve as a possible clue to individuate novel disease diagnostic biomarkers data also in pediatric obesity. From our results, overall it appears that several salivary metabolites and metabolic pathways contribute to a complex metabolic fingerprint of obesity, obesity-related NAFLD and obesity-related MetS. Some of these metabolites were easily predictable based on obesity pathophysiology whereas others were not.

In line with blood and urinary metabolomic results obtained by others [43–45], the BCAAs valine and isoleucine were among the AAs more prevalently involved in the obesity-deranged pathways, but they did not appear to accurately reflect specific hepatic [43] or metabolic [44,45] involvement. The network of salivary molecules separating the lean and obese groups in obese individuals (independently from having or not MetS/NAFLD comorbidities) was also notably characterized by higher levels of two saturated fatty acids, palmitic acid and myristic acid, which tended to be prevalent in those with steatosis. Interestingly, this finding is in line with recently reported data suggesting that elevated total serum ceramide, as well as specific concentrations of myristic, palmitic, palmitoleic, stearic, oleic, behenic and lignoceric ceramide, with insulin resistance and play a potential role in the development of NAFLD in obese children [46]. The correlation of the lipid profile with glucose and insulin levels has been reported to probably mirror a still preserved ability to adapt to a caloric challenge compared with metabolically unhealthy individuals [47,48], in line with recent suggestions that propose a fatty acid profile is a useful tool to explain part of the heterogeneity between abdominal obesity and MetS [11,48,49]. Others have reported that, in addition to palmitic and stearic acid, other FAs are deranged and that increased activity of C16 Δ9-desaturase and C18 Δ9-desaturase in parallel with decreased Δ5-desaturase activity may be a causative factor in disturbed fatty acid metabolism [50]. In line with recent mouse model studies [51] where chronic oral administration of myristic acid improved hyperglycemia by decreasing insulin-responsive glucose levels and reducing body weight, myristic acid in our enrichment pathway is a fatty acid that appears to be associated with obesity but not with MetS. Finally, patients with fatty liver had higher levels of salivary pyroglutamic acid, a metabolite that has recently been proposed as a possible diagnostic biomarker for more severe liver disease [52].

Even more interestingly, as seen also by others in blood [12], PLS-DA showed that the salivary metabolic profiles could correctly identify children with a fewer number of MetS criteria than those who displayed more. This suggests that metabolic profiles can stratify MetS subpopulations, therefore, paving the way for their utilization for both early disease diagnosis and monitoring in those with MetS. This appears particularly relevant as in a recent Clinical Report, the American Academy of Pediatrics (AAP) Committee on Nutrition [53] acknowledged that although several attempts have been made to define MetS in the pediatric population, the construct at this age is difficult to define and has unclear implications for clinical care. For this reason, the Committee focused on the importance of (a) screening for and treating each individual risk factor component of MetS and (b) increasing awareness of comorbid conditions including NAFLD to be addressed and referred to specialists, as needed.

Study Limitations and Strengths

Our findings should be considered in the context of several study limitations, including a relatively small sample size, methodological flaws, and the lack of liver biopsy and prospective data during follow-up. First, our sample size was somewhat limited, and we may have had insufficient power to detect significant associations, particularly for stratified analyses. Larger series with patient follow-up are needed to confirm the preliminary results of our pilot study. Second, our findings related to VIP metabolites should be interpreted with caution given that these were obtained on only one saliva sample for each of the participant children. Although saliva was revealed to be a reliable biofluid for metabolomics studies [17], neurological disorder [42], and T1D [41], the likely risks of poor reproducibility persist. In fact, possible, differences among unstimulated, stimulated (e.g., obtained with oral movements such as gentle mastication), and pure parotid saliva exist [54,55]. Third, ultrasound may be insensitive compared with biopsy or magnetic resonance imaging (MRI). Nevertheless, it is the reference test for use in pediatric clinical practice. Furthermore, liver biopsy cannot be considered a screening procedure because it is invasive, not riskless and not exempt from possible sampling errors. As a non-invasive alternative to assess hepatic steatosis, US is repeatable because it does not require sedation or the delivery of ionizing radiation [1,56]. Although it is the less robust of the numerous imaging options [57], methodological progress has shown good diagnostic specificity and sensitivity, especially if the steatosis involves at least 20% of the hepatocytes [58]. Overall, these limitations do not allow us to draw definite conclusions but strongly suggest the viability of such an approach. These limitations, however, are balanced by several important strengths, including a full auxological and biochemical characterization of our subjects' cohort that allowed us to build several classification models on the same group of patients and delineate the metabolite/metabolic pathways. Moreover, this represents the first study to show the potential usefulness of saliva to define a metabolomic signature of pediatric obesity and related hepato-metabolic comorbidities.

5. Conclusions

Using the saliva of children affected by obesity, we showed a definite interplay of several metabolic pathways with possible specific patterns capable of sorting fatty liver and MetS. The involved metabolic processes include the following: de novo fatty acid biosynthesis; saturated fatty acid beta-oxidation; butanoate metabolism; glycolysis and gluconeogenesis; tricarboxylic acid cycle; urea cycle; metabolism of proline, glutamate, aspartate and asparagine; valine, leucine and isoleucine (BCAA) degradation; aminosugar metabolism; purine metabolism; and glycerophospholipid metabolism. Overall, this information, along with that of other recent progress regarding the study of salivary simple analytes [4], trace elements [59], major adipocytokines [60,61], and specific microRNAs [62], reinforces the idea that saliva will soon represent a useful tool for deepening pathomechanismistic aspects, noninvasive diagnosis and monitoring of pediatric and adult individuals with obesity. The early and non-invasive detection of incipient MetS/fatty liver in childhood through salivary metabolomics as described here, therefore, appears as a promising helpful tool to prevent further health hepato-metabolic and cardiovascular complications in adulthood, and ultimately serves to minimize their related global socioeconomic burden.

Supplementary Materials: The following are available online at http://www.mdpi.com/2072-6643/11/2/274/s1, Figure S1: Panels (A) show the selected metabolites with fold change (FC) values <-1 or >+1 with a simultaneous p-value < 0.05 (red dot). (A1) Normal weight (NW) versus Obese (OB) metabolite. (A2) Steatosis obese patients (OB[St+]) versus non-steatosis obese patients (OB[St−]). FC of the selected metabolites are shown in the corresponding panel (B1 and B2).

Author Contributions: J.T. and P.V. conceived and designed the experimental study, and contributed equally; F.B., A.B., L.P., C.M., A.D.N., A.G.D.A, L.D.M., A.P.D.B. and S.G.N. characterized clinical/lab features of the patients; J.T., A.C. and G.S. performed GC/MS experiments; P.C., G.S. and J.T. analyzed the data; J.T and G.S. contributed reagents/materials/analysis tools and to the development of the analytical methods; J.T. and P.V. wrote the paper which was integrated and fully agreed by all authors.

Funding: The research work was partially funded to PV by University of Salerno UNISA/FARB 2016 and 2017 and to GS by "POR FESR CAMPANIA 2014/2020-O.S. 1.1—Avviso pubblico per il sostegno alle imprese nella realizzazione di studi di fattibilità (Fase 1) e progetti di trasferimento tecnologico (Fase 2) coerenti con la RIS 3—Concessione contributo in forma di sovvenzione—Soggetto proponente: HOSMOTIC Srl—Progetto: Strumenti di supporto alla prevenzione, diagnosi e monitoraggio dell'obesità in età pediatrica—CUP:B73D18000100007".

Conflicts of Interest: The authors declare no conflict of interest.

References

1. Clemente, M.G.; Mandato, C.; Poeta, M.; Vajro, P. Pediatric non-alcoholic fatty liver disease: Recent solutions, unresolved issues, and future research directions. *World J. Gastroenterol.* **2016**, *22*, 8078–8093. [CrossRef] [PubMed]
2. Zheng, J.; Dixon, R.A.; Li, L. Development of Isotope Labeling LC-MS for Human Salivary Metabolomics and Application to Profiling Metabolome Changes Associated with Mild Cognitive Impairment. *Anal. Chem.* **2012**, *84*, 10802–10811. [CrossRef] [PubMed]
3. Ra, S.-G.; Maeda, S.; Higashino, R.; Imai, T.; Miyakawa, S. Metabolomics of salivary fatigue markers in soccer players after consecutive games. *Appl. Physiol. Nutr. Metab.* **2014**, *39*, 1120–1126. [CrossRef] [PubMed]
4. Troisi, J.; Belmonte, F.; Bisogno, A.; Lausi, O.; Marciano, F.; Cavallo, P.; Guercio Nuzio, S.; Landolfi, A.; Pierri, L.; Vajro, P. Salivary markers of hepato-metabolic comorbidities in pediatric obesity. *Dig. Liver Dis.* **2018**. [CrossRef] [PubMed]
5. Martos-Moreno, G.A.; Sackmann-Sala, L.; Barrios, V.; Berrymann, D.E.; Okada, S.; Argente, J.; Kopchick, J.J. Proteomic analysis allows for early detection of potential markers of metabolic impairment in very young obese children. *Int. J. Pediatr. Endocrinol.* **2014**, *2014*, 9. [CrossRef] [PubMed]
6. Miccheli, A.; Capuani, G.; Marini, F.; Tomassini, A.; Pratico, G.; Ceccarelli, S.; Gnani, D.; Baviera, G.; Alisi, A.; Putignani, L.; et al. Urinary (1)H-NMR-based metabolic profiling of children with NAFLD undergoing VSL#3 treatment. *Int. J. Obes.* **2015**, *39*, 1118–1125.
7. Wiklund, P.K.; Pekkala, S.; Autio, R.; Munukka, E.; Xu, L.; Saltevo, J.; Cheng, S.; Kujala, U.M.; Alen, M.; Cheng, S. Serum metabolic profiles in overweight and obese women with and without metabolic syndrome. *Diabetol. Metab. Syndr.* **2014**, *6*, 40. [CrossRef]
8. Wurtz, P.; Makinen, V.-P.; Soininen, P.; Kangas, A.J.; Tukiainen, T.; Kettunen, J.; Savolainen, M.J.; Tammelin, T.; Viikari, J.S.; Ronnemaa, T.; et al. Metabolic signatures of insulin resistance in 7098 young adults. *Diabetes* **2012**, *61*, 1372–1380. [CrossRef]
9. Jin, T.; Yu, H.; Huang, X.-F. Selective binding modes and allosteric inhibitory effects of lupane triterpenes on protein tyrosine phosphatase 1B. *Sci. Rep.* **2016**, *6*, 20766. [CrossRef]
10. Butte, N.F.; Liu, Y.; Zakeri, I.F.; Mohney, R.P.; Mehta, N.; Voruganti, V.S.; Goring, H.; Cole, S.A.; Comuzzie, A.G. Global metabolomic profiling targeting childhood obesity in the Hispanic population. *Am. J. Clin. Nutr.* **2015**, *102*, 256–267. [CrossRef]
11. Baek, S.H.; Kim, M.; Kim, M.; Kang, M.; Yoo, H.J.; Lee, N.H.; Kim, Y.H.; Song, M.; Lee, J.H. Metabolites distinguishing visceral fat obesity and atherogenic traits in individuals with overweight. *Obesity* **2017**, *25*, 323–331. [CrossRef] [PubMed]
12. Zhong, F.; Xu, M.; Bruno, R.S.; Ballard, K.D.; Zhu, J. Targeted high performance liquid chromatography tandem mass spectrometry-based metabolomics differentiates metabolic syndrome from obesity. *Exp. Biol. Med.* **2017**, *242*, 773–780. [CrossRef]
13. Pujos-Guillot, E.; Brandolini, M.; Pétéra, M.; Grissa, D.; Joly, C.; Lyan, B.; Herquelot, É.; Czernichow, S.; Zins, M.; Goldberg, M. Systems metabolomics for prediction of metabolic syndrome. *J. Proteome Res.* **2017**, *16*, 2262–2272. [CrossRef] [PubMed]
14. Pierri, L.; Saggese, P.; Guercio Nuzio, S.; Troisi, J.; Di Stasi, M.; Poeta, M.; Savastano, R.; Marchese, G.; Tarallo, R.; Massa, G.; et al. Relations of gut liver axis components and gut microbiota in obese children with fatty liver: A pilot study. *Clin. Res. Hepatol. Gastroenterol.* **2018**, *42*, 387–390. [CrossRef]
15. Troisi, J.; Pierri, L.; Landolfi, A.; Marciano, F.; Bisogno, A.; Belmonte, F.; Palladino, C.; Guercio Nuzio, S.; Campiglia, P.; Vajro, P. Urinary Metabolomics in Pediatric Obesity and NAFLD Identifies Metabolic Pathways/Metabolites Related to Dietary Habits and Gut-Liver Axis Perturbations. *Nutrients* **2017**, *9*, E485. [CrossRef] [PubMed]
16. Dame, Z.T.; Aziat, F.; Mandal, R.; Krishnamurthy, R.; Bouatra, S.; Borzouie, S.; Guo, A.C.; Sajed, T.; Deng, L.; Lin, H.; et al. The human saliva metabolome. *Metabolomics* **2015**, *11*, 1864–1883. [CrossRef]
17. Hartman, M.-L.; Goodson, J.M.; Barake, R.; Alsmadi, O.; Al-Mutawa, S.; Ariga, J.; Soparkar, P.; Behbehani, J.; Behbehani, K. Salivary Biomarkers in Pediatric Metabolic Disease Research. *Pediatr. Endocrinol. Rev.* **2016**, *13*, 602–611.

18. Belmonte, F.; Bisogno, A.; Troisi, J.; Landolfi, A.M.; Lausi, O.; Lamberti, R.; Nuzio, S.G.; Pierri, L.; Siano, M.; Viggiano, C.; et al. Salivary levels of uric acid, insulin and HOMA: A promising field of study to non-invasively identify obese children at risk of metabolic syndrome and fatty liver. *Dig. Liver Dis.* **2017**, *49*, e247. [CrossRef]
19. Cho, K.; Moon, J.S.; Kang, J.-H.; Jang, H.B.; Lee, H.-J.; Park, S.I.; Yu, K.-S.; Cho, J.-Y. Combined untargeted and targeted metabolomic profiling reveals urinary biomarkers for discriminating obese from normal-weight adolescents. *Pediatr. Obes.* **2017**, *12*, 93–101. [CrossRef]
20. Ho, J.E.; Larson, M.G.; Ghorbani, A.; Cheng, S.; Chen, M.-H.; Keyes, M.; Rhee, E.P.; Clish, C.B.; Vasan, R.S.; Gerszten, R.E.; et al. Metabolomic Profiles of Body Mass Index in the Framingham Heart Study Reveal Distinct Cardiometabolic Phenotypes. *PLoS ONE* **2016**, *11*, e0148361. [CrossRef]
21. Zheng, H.; Yde, C.C.; Arnberg, K.; Molgaard, C.; Michaelsen, K.F.; Larnkjaer, A.; Bertram, H.C. NMR-based metabolomic profiling of overweight adolescents: An elucidation of the effects of inter-/intraindividual differences, gender, and pubertal development. *Biomed. Res. Int.* **2014**, *2014*, 537157. [CrossRef] [PubMed]
22. Vajro, P.; Lenta, S.; Pignata, C.; Salerno, M.; D'Aniello, R.; De Micco, I.; Paolella, G.; Parenti, G. Therapeutic options in pediatric non alcoholic fatty liver disease: Current status and future directions. *Ital. J. Pediatr.* **2012**, *38*, 55. [CrossRef]
23. Schwenzer, N.F.; Springer, F.; Schraml, C.; Stefan, N.; Machann, J.; Schick, F. Non-invasive assessment and quantification of liver steatosis by ultrasound, computed tomography and magnetic resonance. *J. Hepatol.* **2009**, *51*, 433–445. [CrossRef] [PubMed]
24. Schwimmer, J.B.; Dunn, W.; Norman, G.J.; Pardee, P.E.; Middleton, M.S.; Kerkar, N.; Sirlin, C.B. SAFETY study: Alanine aminotransferase cutoff values are set too high for reliable detection of pediatric chronic liver disease. *Gastroenterology* **2010**, *138*, 1357–1364. [CrossRef] [PubMed]
25. Vajro, P.; Maddaluno, S.; Veropalumbo, C. Persistent hypertransaminasemia in asymptomatic children: A stepwise approach. *World J. Gastroenterol.* **2013**, *19*, 2740–2751. [CrossRef] [PubMed]
26. Zimmet, P.; Alberti, K.G.M.; Kaufman, F.; Tajima, N.; Silink, M.; Arslanian, S.; Wong, G.; Bennett, P.; Shaw, J.; Caprio, S. The metabolic syndrome in children and adolescents—An IDF consensus report. *Pediatr. Diabetes* **2007**, *8*, 299–306. [CrossRef] [PubMed]
27. World Medical Association. World medical association declaration of helsinki: Ethical principles for medical research involving human subjects. *JAMA* **2013**, *310*, 2191–2194. [CrossRef]
28. Kovats, E.S. Gas-chromatographische charakterisierung organischer verbindungen. Teil 1: Retentionsindices aliphatischer halogenide, alkohole, aldehyde und ketone. *Helv. Chim. Acta* **1958**, *41*, 1915–1932. [CrossRef]
29. van den Berg, R.A.; Hoefsloot, H.C.; Westerhuis, J.A.; Smilde, A.K.; van der Werf, M.J. Centering, scaling, and transformations: Improving the biological information content of metabolomics data. *BMC Genom.* **2006**, *7*, 142. [CrossRef]
30. Sumner, L.W.; Amberg, A.; Barrett, D.; Beale, M.H.; Beger, R.; Daykin, C.A.; Fan, T.W.-M.; Fiehn, O.; Goodacre, R.; Griffin, J.L.; et al. Proposed minimum reporting standards for chemical analysis Chemical Analysis Working Group (CAWG) Metabolomics Standards Initiative (MSI). *Metabolomics* **2007**, *3*, 211–221. [CrossRef]
31. Sysi-Aho, M.; Katajamaa, M.; Yetukuri, L.; Oresic, M. Normalization method for metabolomics data using optimal selection of multiple internal standards. *BMC Bioinformatics* **2007**, *8*, 93. [CrossRef] [PubMed]
32. Mevik, B.-H.; Wehrens, R. The pls Package: Principal Component and Partial Least Squares Regression in R. *J. Stat. Softw.* **2007**. [CrossRef]
33. Kuhn, M. Building Predictive Models in R Using the caret Package. *J. Stat. Softw.* **2008**, *28*, 1–26. [CrossRef]
34. Bijlsma, S.; Bobeldijk, I.; Verheij, E.R.; Ramaker, R.; Kochhar, S.; Macdonald, I.A.; van Ommen, B.; Smilde, A.K. Large-scale human metabolomics studies: A strategy for data (pre-) processing and validation. *Anal. Chem.* **2006**, *78*, 567–574. [CrossRef] [PubMed]
35. Karnovsky, A.; Weymouth, T.; Hull, T.; Tarcea, V.G.; Scardoni, G.; Laudanna, C.; Sartor, M.A.; Stringer, K.A.; Jagadish, H.V.; Burant, C.; et al. Metscape 2 bioinformatics tool for the analysis and visualization of metabolomics and gene expression data. *Bioinformatics* **2012**, *28*, 373–380. [CrossRef] [PubMed]
36. Nishida, K.; Ono, K.; Kanaya, S.; Takahashi, K. KEGGscape: A Cytoscape app for pathway data integration. *F1000Research* **2014**, *3*, 144. [CrossRef] [PubMed]
37. Lex, A.; Gehlenborg, N.; Strobelt, H.; Vuillemot, R.; Pfister, H. UpSet: Visualization of Intersecting Sets. *IEEE Trans. Vis. Comput. Gr.* **2014**, *20*, 1983–1992. [CrossRef] [PubMed]

38. Francavilla, R.; Ercolini, D.; Piccolo, M.; Vannini, L.; Siragusa, S.; De Filippis, F.; De Pasquale, I.; Di Cagno, R.; Di Toma, M.; Gozzi, G.; et al. Salivary microbiota and metabolome associated with celiac disease. *Appl. Environ. Microbiol.* **2014**, *80*, 3416–3425. [CrossRef]
39. Santone, C.; Dinallo, V.; Paci, M.; D'Ottavio, S.; Barbato, G.; Bernardini, S. Saliva metabolomics by NMR for the evaluation of sport performance. *J. Pharm. Biomed.* **2014**, *88*, 441–446. [CrossRef]
40. Rao, P.V.; Reddy, A.P.; Lu, X.; Dasari, S.; Krishnaprasad, A.; Biggs, E.; Roberts, C.T.; Nagalla, S.R. Proteomic identification of salivary biomarkers of type-2 diabetes. *J. Proteome Res.* **2009**, *8*, 239–245. [CrossRef]
41. Pappa, E.; Vastardis, H.; Mermelekas, G.; Gerasimidi-Vazeou, A.; Zoidakis, J.; Vougas, K. Saliva Proteomics Analysis Offers Insights on Type 1 Diabetes Pathology in a Pediatric Population. *Front. Physiol.* **2018**, *9*, 444. [CrossRef] [PubMed]
42. Walton, E.L. Saliva biomarkers in neurological disorders: A "spitting image" of brain health? *Biomed. J.* **2018**, *41*, 59–62. [CrossRef] [PubMed]
43. Goffredo, M.; Santoro, N.; Tricò, D.; Giannini, C.; D'Adamo, E.; Zhao, H.; Peng, G.; Yu, X.; Lam, T.T.; Pierpont, B. A branched-chain amino acid-related metabolic signature characterizes obese adolescents with non-alcoholic fatty liver disease. *Nutrients* **2017**, *9*, 642. [CrossRef] [PubMed]
44. Wu, N.; Wang, W.; Yi, M.; Cheng, S.; Wang, D. *Study of the Metabolomics Characteristics of Patients with Metabolic Syndrome Based on Liquid Chromatography Quadrupole Time-Of-Flight Mass Spectrometry*; Elsevier: Amsterdam, The Netherlands, 2018; Volume 79, pp. 37–44.
45. Reddy, P.; Leong, J.; Jialal, I. Amino acid levels in nascent metabolic syndrome: A contributor to the pro-inflammatory burden. *J. Diabetes Complicat.* **2018**, *32*, 465–469. [CrossRef] [PubMed]
46. Wasilewska, N.; Bobrus-Chociej, A.; Harasim-Symbor, E.; Tarasów, E.; Wojtkowska, M.; Chabowski, A.; Lebensztejn, D. Serum concentration of ceramides in obese children with nonalcoholic fatty liver disease. *J. Pediatr. Gastroenterol. Nutr.* **2018**, *66*, S2. [CrossRef] [PubMed]
47. Badoud, F.; Lam, K.P.; Perreault, M.; Zulyniak, M.A.; Britz-McKibbin, P.; Mutch, D.M. Metabolomics reveals metabolically healthy and unhealthy obese individuals differ in their response to a caloric challenge. *PLoS ONE* **2015**, *10*, e0134613. [CrossRef] [PubMed]
48. Aristizabal, J.C.; Barona, J.; Gonzalez-Zapata, L.I.; Deossa, G.C.; Estrada, A. Fatty acid content of plasma triglycerides may contribute to the heterogeneity in the relationship between abdominal obesity and the metabolic syndrome. *Metab. Syndr. Relat. Disord.* **2016**, *14*, 311–317. [CrossRef] [PubMed]
49. Aristizabal, J.C.; González-Zapata, L.I.; Estrada-Restrepo, A.; Monsalve-Alvarez, J.; Restrepo-Mesa, S.L.; Gaitán, D. Concentrations of plasma free palmitoleic and dihomo-gamma linoleic fatty acids are higher in children with abdominal obesity. *Nutrients* **2018**, *10*, 31. [CrossRef]
50. Kang, M.; Lee, A.; Yoo, H.J.; Kim, M.; Kim, M.; Shin, D.Y.; Lee, J.H. Association between increased visceral fat area and alterations in plasma fatty acid profile in overweight subjects: A cross-sectional study. *Lipids Health Dis.* **2017**, *16*, 248. [CrossRef]
51. Takato, T.; Iwata, K.; Murakami, C.; Wada, Y.; Sakane, F. Chronic administration of myristic acid improves hyperglycaemia in the Nagoya–Shibata–Yasuda mouse model of congenital type 2 diabetes. *Diabetologia* **2017**, *60*, 2076–2083. [CrossRef]
52. Qi, S.; Xu, D.; Li, Q.; Xie, N.; Xia, J.; Huo, Q.; Li, P.; Chen, Q.; Huang, S. Metabonomics screening of serum identifies pyroglutamate as a diagnostic biomarker for nonalcoholic steatohepatitis. *Clin. Chim. Acta* **2017**, *473*, 89–95. [CrossRef]
53. Magge, S.N.; Goodman, E.; Armstrong, S.C. The Metabolic Syndrome in Children and Adolescents: Shifting the Focus to Cardiometabolic Risk Factor Clustering. *Pediatrics* **2017**, *24*, e20171603. [CrossRef]
54. Denny, P.; Hagen, F.K.; Hardt, M.; Liao, L.; Yan, W.; Arellanno, M.; Bassilian, S.; Bedi, G.S.; Boontheung, P.; Cociorva, D. The proteomes of human parotid and submandibular/sublingual gland salivas collected as the ductal secretions. *J. Proteome Res.* **2008**, *7*, 1994–2006. [CrossRef]
55. Tiwari, M. Science behind human saliva. *J. Nat. Sci. Biol. Med.* **2011**, *2*, 53–58. [CrossRef]
56. Vajro, P.; Lenta, S.; Socha, P.; Dhawan, A.; McKiernan, P.; Baumann, U.; Durmaz, O.; Lacaille, F.; McLin, V.; Nobili, V. Diagnosis of nonalcoholic fatty liver disease in children and adolescents: Position paper of the ESPGHAN Hepatology Committee. *J. Pediatr. Gastroenterol. Nutr.* **2012**, *54*, 700–713. [CrossRef]

57. Vos, M.B.; Abrams, S.H.; Barlow, S.E.; Caprio, S.; Daniels, S.R.; Kohli, R.; Mouzaki, M.; Sathya, P.; Schwimmer, J.B.; Sundaram, S.S. NASPGHAN clinical practice guideline for the diagnosis and treatment of nonalcoholic fatty liver disease in children: Recommendations from the Expert Committee on NAFLD (ECON) and the North American Society of Pediatric Gastroenterology, Hepatology and Nutrition (NASPGHAN). *J. Pediatr. Gastroenterol. Nutr.* **2017**, *64*, 319–334.
58. Koot, B.G.; van der Baan-Slootweg, O.H.; Bohte, A.E.; Nederveen, A.J.; van Werven, J.R.; Tamminga-Smeulders, C.L.; Merkus, M.P.; Schaap, F.G.; Jansen, P.L.; Stoker, J. Accuracy of prediction scores and novel biomarkers for predicting nonalcoholic fatty liver disease in obese children. *Obesity* **2013**, *21*, 583–590. [CrossRef]
59. Marin Martinez, L.; Molino Pagan, D.; Lopez Jornet, P. Trace Elements in Saliva as Markers of Type 2 Diabetes Mellitus. *Biol. Trace Elem. Res.* **2018**, *186*, 354–360. [CrossRef]
60. Abdalla, M.M.I.; Soon, S.C. Salivary adiponectin concentration in healthy adult males in relation to anthropometric measures and fat distribution. *Endocr. Regul.* **2017**, *51*, 185–192. [CrossRef]
61. Ibrahim Abdalla, M.M.; Siew Choo, S. Salivary Leptin Level in Young Adult Males and its Association with Anthropometric Measurements, Fat Distribution and Muscle Mass. *Eur. Endocrinol.* **2018**, *14*, 94–98. [CrossRef]
62. Vriens, A.; Provost, E.B.; Saenen, N.D.; De Boever, P.; Vrijens, K.; De Wever, O.; Plusquin, M.; Nawrot, T.S. Children's screen time alters the expression of saliva extracellular miR-222 and miR-146a. *Sci. Rep.* **2018**, *8*, 8209. [CrossRef]

© 2019 by the authors. Licensee MDPI, Basel, Switzerland. This article is an open access article distributed under the terms and conditions of the Creative Commons Attribution (CC BY) license (http://creativecommons.org/licenses/by/4.0/).

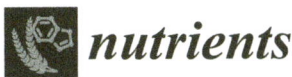

Article

Trimethylamine-N-oxide (TMAO) as Novel Potential Biomarker of Early Predictors of Metabolic Syndrome

Luigi Barrea [1,*,†], Giuseppe Annunziata [2,†], Giovanna Muscogiuri [1], Carolina Di Somma [3], Daniela Laudisio [1], Maria Maisto [2], Giulia de Alteriis [1], Gian Carlo Tenore [2], Annamaria Colao [1] and Silvia Savastano [1]

- [1] Dipartimento di Medicina Clinica e Chirurgia, Unit of Endocrinology, Federico II University Medical School of Naples, Via Sergio Pansini 5, 80131 Naples, Italy; giovanna.muscogiuri@gmail.com (G.M.); daniela.laudisio@libero.it (D.L.); dealteriisgiulia@gmail.com (G.d.A.); colao@unina.it (A.C.); sisavast@unina.it (S.S.)
- [2] Department of Pharmacy, University of Naples "Federico II", Via Domenico Montesano 49, 80131 Naples, Italy; giuseppe.annunziata@unina.it (G.A.); maria.maisto@unina.it (M.M.); giancarlo.tenore@unina.it (G.C.T.)
- [3] IRCCS SDN, Napoli Via Gianturco 113, 80143 Naples, Italy; cdisomma@unina.it
- * Correspondence: luigi.barrea@unina.it; Tel.: +39-081-746-3779
- † These Authors contributed equally to this work.

Received: 14 November 2018; Accepted: 11 December 2018; Published: 13 December 2018

Abstract: There is a mechanistic link between the gut-derived metabolite trimethylamine-N-oxide (TMAO) and obesity-related diseases, suggesting that the TMAO pathway may also be linked to the pathogenesis of obesity. The Visceral Adiposity Index (VAI), a gender-specific indicator of adipose dysfunction, and the Fatty Liver Index (FLI), a predictor of non-alcoholic fatty liver disease (NAFLD), are early predictors of metabolic syndrome (MetS). In this cross-sectional observational study, we investigated TMAO levels in adults stratified according to Body Mass Index (BMI) and the association of TMAO with VAI and FLI. One hundred and thirty-seven adult subjects (59 males; 21–56 years) were enrolled. TMAO levels were detected using HPLC/MS analysis. Homeostatic Model Assessment of Insulin Resistance (HoMA-IR), VAI and FLI were included as cardio-metabolic indices. TMAO levels increased along with BMI and were positively associated with VAI and FLI, independently, on common potential covariates. The most sensitive and specific cut-offs for circulating levels of TMAO to predict the presence of NAFLD-FLI and MetS were ≥ 8.02 µM and ≥ 8.74 µM, respectively. These findings allow us to hypothesize a role of TMAO as an early biomarker of adipose dysfunction and NAFLD-FLI in all borderline conditions in which overt MetS is not present, and suggest that a specific cut-off of TMAO might help in identifying subjects at high risk of NAFLD.

Keywords: trimethylamine N-oxide (TMAO); obesity; visceral adiposity index (VAI); fatty liver index (FLI); metabolic syndrome (MetS)

1. Introduction

TMAO is a small, organic, gut microbiota-derived metabolite, which is emerging as a new potentially important cause of increased atherosclerosis and cardiovascular risk [1–3]. Circulating levels of TMAO increase after the gut microbial metabolism of dietary L-carnitine and phosphatidylcholine-rich foods, including red meat, eggs, dairy products, which are common nutrients of the Western diet. Very recently we reported a novel association between circulating levels of TMAO and the Mediterranean diet in healthy normal-weight adults, with a clear gender difference in this association [4]. The metabolic pathway of TMAO includes the digestion of these amines from gut microbiota with the production of trimethylamine (TMA), which is then converted to TMAO via flavin-monooxygenase-3 (FMO3) in the liver [5,6]. The interplay between dietary composition, gut microbiota and microbe-generated metabolites has been intensely investigated [7,8].

Several studies have shown a mechanistic link between TMAO, inflammatory pathways [9] atherosclerosis, type 2 diabetes mellitus (T2DM), and cardiovascular diseases (CVD) [1–3,6,10,11]. Namely, circulating levels of TMAO and its metabolites (choline and betaine) are associated with atherosclerosis risks in both humans and mice [1]. Among the pro-atherosclerotic mechanisms proposed for TMAO there are the inhibition of the reverse cholesterol transport, although this effect was reported in animal studies only [6], and the enhancement of human platelet hyperresponsiveness and thrombosis potential [10]. A systematic review and meta-analysis by Schiattarella et al. [2] demonstrated that in humans there is a positive dose-dependent association between circulating levels of TMAO and increased cardiovascular risk and mortality [2]. Nevertheless, in this metanalysis, the population samples were not divided according the BMI classes. More recently, Kanitsoraphan et al. [3] reported that in patients with T2DM higher circulating levels of TMAO were significantly associated with higher overall mortality by 2.07- to 2.7-fold, also after adjustment for BMI [3]. Recently, the strong association between gut microbiota and either obesity and obesity-related diseases in humans on the one hand, and the association between the TMAO pathway and cardio-metabolic diseases on the other, suggested that the TMAO pathway may be also mechanistically linked to the pathogenesis of obesity. Schugar et al. [11] reported that plasma TMAO levels were linked to with obesity traits in the different inbred strains of mice receiving a high-fat diet and suggested that the TMAO-generating pathway is linked to obesity and energy metabolism [11], although scientific evidence to support this association in humans has not yet been provided. Only Randrianarisoa et al. [12] reported that TMAO correlated positively with BMI, insulin resistance, visceral fat mass, and liver fat content [12]. In addition, Chen et al. [13] showed positive associations of the circulating TMAO levels and two of its nutrient precursors, choline, and betaine, with the presence and severity of NAFLD, the hepatic manifestation of the MetS [14], in a large sample of hospital- and community-based Chinese adults [13].

Nevertheless, controversy remains over the exact role of TMAO in the pathogenesis of MetS, a constellation of cardio-metabolic risk factors, including central obesity, hypertriglyceridemia, low high-density lipoprotein (HDL) cholesterol, hyperglycemia, and hypertension [15], which predispose T2DM and CVD [16], according to the definition of nascent MetS [17]. Very recently, a clinical study investigating several biogenic amines in urine, including TMAO in a sample of patients with MetS showed that these subjects presented higher levels of TMAO compared with their counterparts without MetS [18]. In addition, a further study investigating unselected white patients undergoing coronary angiography for the evaluation of suspected coronary artery disease showed a positive correlation between TMAO and MetS [19]. However, this association was lost after adjusting for impaired kidney function and poor metabolic control in this population sample.

On the other hand, this association was not found in a sample of patients with nascent MetS (without CVD or T2DM), but not with the commonly used surrogate index of insulin resistance, i.e., the HoMA-IR [9]. Again, in these recent studies, the population samples were not divided according to BMI classes.

The VAI, a gender-specific indicator of adipose distribution and dysfunction [20], and the FLI, an accurate predictor of the NAFLD [21], are two surrogate indices of cardio-metabolic risk and are linked to the inflammatory pathways [22,23]. Both indices are based on simple anthropometric and metabolic parameters, and are strictly correlated with MetS, representing early predictors of MetS [20,24]. VAI has been counted as an effective marker to assess insulin resistance and metabolic disturbances that contribute to CVD in primary-care non-obese subjects, with specific cut-off values depending on the population of interest [20]. Also, FLI has been proposed as a marker of insulin resistance [21] and recently the clinical utility of FLI as a predictor of incident T2DM has been reported [25]. As three of the variables making up VAI (waist circumference (WC), plasma triglycerides (TG), and HDL cholesterol) and FLI (BMI, WC, and TG) are used as continuous variables, and while they are dichotomically expressed in the criteria for MetS, VAI and FLI might represent useful indicators of early cardio-metabolic risk in all borderline conditions in which overt MetS is not present [22].

Considering the lack of evidence in humans of a progressive increase of TMAO levels across BMI classes and to gain further insight into the levels of TMAO in the setting of obesity, in this study we aimed to investigate the circulating levels of TMAO in a sample of the adult population stratified according to BMI. In addition, considering the still controversial role of TMAO in the pathogenesis of MetS and the predictive value of VAI and FLI as easy and early indicators of MetS, we investigated the association of circulating levels of TMAO with VAI and FLI and hypothesized that this association could serve as a biological marker of early metabolic derangement in subjects with overweight and obesity.

2. Materials and Methods

2.1. Design and Setting

This is a cross-sectional observational study carried out at the Department of Clinical Medicine and Surgery, Unit of Endocrinology, University Federico II, Naples (Italy), from January 2017 to August 2018. The work has been carried out in accordance with the Code of Ethics of the World Medical Association (Declaration of Helsinki) for experiments involving humans, and it has been approved by the Ethical Committee of the University of Naples "Federico II" Medical School (n. 173/16). The purpose of the protocol was explained to all the study participants, and written informed consent was obtained. This trial was registered at http://register.clinicaltrials.gov/. Unique identifier: NCT03060811.

2.2. Population Study

Recruitment strategies included a sample of 330 adult Caucasians subjects (20–63 years) of both genders consecutively enrolled among patients of our outpatient clinic, hospital volunteers, and employees from the same geographical area around Naples, Italy). All female subjects were non-pregnant and non-lactating. A full medical history, including drug use, was collected.

To increase the homogeneity of the subject sample, we included only adults of both genders with the following criteria of exclusion:

- Impaired renal function (normal values: estimated glomerular filtration rate $\geq$ 90 mL/min/1.73 m^2 calculated by chronic kidney disease epidemiology collaboration equation; CKD EPI) (15 patients)
- Presence of T2DM (defined by criteria of the American Diabetes Association as follows: basal plasma glucose level $\geq$ 126 mg/dL on two occasions, or glycated hemoglobin (HbA1c) $\geq$ 6.5% ($\geq$48 mmol/mol) on two occasions, or both at the same time (35 patients). Participants on antidiabetic medication were considered to have T2DM [26].
- Clinical atherosclerosis (coronary artery disease, peripheral vascular disease, CVD) (41 patients)
- Current therapy with anti-inflammatory drugs, statins and other hypolipidemic agents (34 patients);
- User of antibiotics or probiotics within 2 months of recruitment (19 subjects);
- Specific nutritional regimens, including vegan or vegetarian diets (eight subjects);
- Vitamin/mineral or antioxidant supplementation (34 subjects);
- Alcohol abuse according to the Diagnostic and Statistical Manual of Mental Disorders (DSM)-V diagnostic criteria (eleven subjects);

The flow chart of the study subjects is shown in Figure 1.

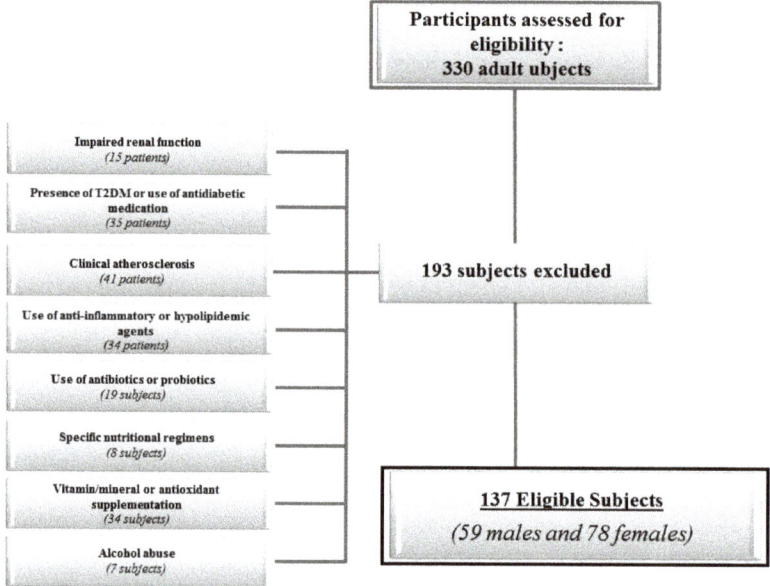

Figure 1. Flow chart of the studied subjects.

2.3. Lifestyle Habits

Lifestyle habits, including smoking and physical activity level, have been investigated as follows: subjects smoking at least one cigarette per day were considered current smokers, while former smokers were the subjects who stopped smoking at least one year before the interview. Remaining participants were defined as non-smokers. Physical activity levels were expressed according to whether the participant habitually engaged at least 30 min/day of aerobic exercise (YES/NO).

2.4. Anthropometric Measurements and Blood Pressure

Measurements were performed between 8 and 12 a.m. All subjects were measured after an overnight fast. The measurements were made in a standard way by the same operator (a nutritionist experienced in providing nutritional assessment and body composition). At the beginning of the study, all anthropometric measurements were taken with subjects wearing only light clothes and without shoes. In each subject, weight and height were measured to calculate the BMI [weight (kg) divided by height squared (m^2), kg/m^2]. Height was measured to the nearest 0.5 cm using a wall-mounted stadiometer (Seca 711; Seca, Hamburg, Germany). Body weight was determined to the nearest 0.1 kg using a calibrated balance beam scale (Seca 711; Seca, Hamburg, Germany). BMI was classified according to the World Health Organization (WHO)'s criteria with normal weight: 18.5–24.9 kg/m^2; overweight, 25.0–29.9 kg/m^2; grade I obesity, 30.0–34.9 kg/m^2; grade II obesity, 35.0–39.9 kg/m^2; grade III obesity $\geq$ 40.0 kg/m^2 [27]. WC was measured to the closest 0.1 cm using a non-stretchable measuring tape at the natural indentation or at a midway level between the lower edge of the rib cage and the iliac crest if no natural indentation was visible, as per the National Center for Health Statistics (NCHS) [28]. In all subjects Systolic Blood Pressure (SBP) and Diastolic Blood Pressure (DBP) were measured three times, two min apart, with a random zero sphygmomanometer (Gelman Hawksley Ltd., Sussex, UK) after the subject had been sitting for at least 10 min. The average of the second and third reading was recorded.

2.5. Determination of Circulating Levels of TMAO

TMAO serum levels were measured in samples stored at −80 °C. A previous study indicated that, under these conditions, TMAO is stable for several years [29]. The quantification of circulating TMAO levels has been performed using the method described by Beale and Airs [30], and reported in our previous study [4], with slight modifications. Briefly, serum proteins were precipitated with methanol (serum:methanol, 1:2, v/v); samples were vortex-mixed for 2 min, centrifuged at 14,000 g for 10 min (4 °C) [31] and supernatants were collected and analyzed by High-Performance Liquid Chromatography-Mass Spectrometry (HPLC-MS) method. Both HPLC-MS conditions and method optimization were performed in accordance with Beale and Airs [30]. The HPLC system Jasco Extrema LC-4000 system (Jasco Inc., Easton, MD, USA) was coupled to a single quadrupole mass spectrometer (Advion ExpressIonL CMS, Advion Inc., Ithaca, NY, USA) equipped with an Electrospray ionization (ESI) source, operating in positive ion mode. The chromatographic separation was performed with a Luna HILIC column (150 × 3 mm, 5 µm particles) in combination with a guard column (HILIC), both supplied by Phenomenex (Torrance, CA, USA).

2.6. Assay Methods

Samples were collected in the morning between 8 and 10 a.m., after an overnight fast of at least 8 h and stored at −80 °C until being processed. All biochemical analyses including fasting plasma glucose, total cholesterol, fasting plasma TG, Alanine Transaminase (ALT), Aspartate Aminotransferase (AST), and γ-Glutamyltransferase (γGT) were performed with a Roche Modular Analytics System in the Central Biochemistry Laboratory of our Institution. Low-Density Lipoprotein (LDL) cholesterol and HDL cholesterol were determined by a direct method (homogeneous enzymatic assay for the direct quantitative determination of LDL and HDL cholesterol). Fasting insulin levels were measured by a solid-phase chemiluminescent enzyme immunoassay using commercially available kits (Immunolite Diagnostic Products Co., Los Angeles, CA, USA). The intra-assay coefficients of variations (CV) was <5.5%, as already widely reported in our previous studies [32–36].

2.7. Cardio-Metabolic Indices

HoMA-IR was calculated according to Matthews et al. [37]. A value of HoMA-IR >2.5 was used as cut-off of insulin resistance. VAI score has been calculated by the following sex-specific formula, with TG levels expressed in mmol/L and HDL levels expressed in mmol/L:

$$\text{Males: VAI} = [WC/39.68 + (1.88 \times BMI)] \times (TG/1.03) \times (1.31/HDL), \tag{1}$$

$$\text{Females: VAI} = [WC/36.58 + (1.89 \times BMI)] \times (TG/0.81) \times (1.52/HDL), \tag{2}$$

Age-specific VAI cut-off values were used according to Amato et al. [22,38]. In detail, cut-offs in subjects aged ≤30, 31–42, 43–52, and 53–66 years old were 2.52, 2.23, 1.92, 1.93, respectively [22,38].

FLI was calculated with the formula:

$$[FLI = e^L/(1 + e^L) \times 100, L = 0.953 \times \log_e \text{triglycerides} + 0.139 \times BMI \\ + 0.718 \times \log_e \gamma GT + 0.053 \times WC - 15.745]. \tag{3}$$

FLI of 30 was considered as the cut-off value based on Bedogni's criterion [21].

2.8. Criteria to Define MetS

According to the National Cholesterol Education Program Adult Treatment Panel (NCEP ATP) III definition, MetS is present if three or more of the following five criteria are met: WC ≥ 102 cm (men) or 88 cm (women), blood pressure ≥ 130/85 mmHg, fasting TG level ≥ 150 mg/dL, fasting HDL cholesterol level ≤ 40 mg/dL (men) or ≤50 mg/dL (women), and fasting glucose ≥ 100 mg/dL [39].

2.9. Dietary Assessment

As has been already widely reported in the literature [34–36,40], data were obtained during a face-to-face interview between the patient and a qualified nutritionist. Specifically, the dietary interview allowed the quantification of foods and drinks by using a photographic food atlas (≈1000 photographs) of known portion sizes to ensure accurate completion of the records [41]. On day 1, the diary nutritionists were trained to standardized protocols and provided participants with instructions on how to complete the diary at the health check, and asked participants to recall the previous day's intake. Participants prospectively completed the remaining 6 days and returned the records to the nutritionist [42]. Data were processed using a commercial software (Terapia Alimentare Dietosystem® DS-Medica, http://www.dsmedica.info). Considering quantities of foods consumed, the software can calculate the total energy intake, expressed in kilocalories (kcal).

2.10. Statistical Analysis

The data distribution was evaluated by Kolmogorov-Smirnov test and the abnormal data were normalized by logarithm. Skewed variables were back-transformed for presentation in tables and figures. Results are expressed as mean ± standard deviation (SD). The chi square (χ^2) test was used to determine the significance of differences in frequency distribution of smoking habit, physical activity, and presence/absence of MetS. Differences according to gender, lifestyle habits, cardio-metabolic indices, and MetS were analyzed by Student's unpaired *t*-test, while the differences among the classes of BMI were analyzed by ANOVA followed by the Bonferroni post-hoc test. The correlations between study variables were performed using Pearson *r* correlation coefficients and were estimated after adjusting for gender, BMI, smoking, physical activity, and total energy intake. Proportional Odds Ratio (OR) models, 95% Interval Confidence (IC), and R^2 were performed to assess the association between gender, lifestyle habits, classes of BMI, cardio-metabolic indices, and MetS. In addition, two multiple linear regression analysis models (stepwise method), expressed as R^2, Beta (β), and *t*, with circulating levels of TMAO as dependent variables were used to estimate the predictive value of: (a) cardio-metabolic indices; and (b) FLI and MetS. Receiver operator characteristic (ROC) curve analysis was performed to determine sensitivity and specificity, area under the curve (AUC), and IC, as well as cut-off values of circulating levels of TMAO in detecting FLI and MetS. Test AUC for ROC analysis was also performed. We wanted to show that AUC being 0.943 for a particular test is significant from the null hypothesis value 0.5 (meaning no discriminating power), so we entered 0.943 for AUC ROC and 0.5 for null hypothesis values. For α level we selected 0.05 type I error and for β level we selected 0.20 type II error. In these analyses, we entered only those variables that had a *p*-value < 0.05 in the univariate analysis (partial correlation). To avoid multicollinearity, variables with a variance inflation factor (VIF) >10 were excluded. Values ≤0.05% were considered statistically significant. Data were stored and analyzed using the MedCalc® package (Version 12.3.0 1993–2012 MedCalc Software bvba—MedCalc Software, Mariakerke, Belgium).

3. Results

The study population consisted of 137 participants, 59 males and 78 females, aged 21–56 years. Current smokers were 49.6% (68 subjects). A moderate-intensity aerobic activity at least 5 days per week was reported in 42.3% (58 subjects). BMIs ranged from 19.6 to 58.8 kg/m². Median values of HoMA-IR, VAI and FLI were 1.95 (0.1–15.16), 1.89 (0.60–13.85) and 75.30 (3.40–100.0), respectively. In particular, 64 subjects (46.7%) had HoMA-IR values higher than the cut-off. VAI was higher than sex- and age-specific cut-offs in 43.8% (60 subjects) and 59.9% (82 subjects) presented FLI values above the cut-off. MetS was present in 53 participants (38.7%).

In Table 1 we report the lifestyle habits, anthropometric measurements, blood pressure, metabolic profile, and cardio-metabolic indices in the total population grouped based on BMI categories. As shown in Table 1, no differences were observed in age (p = 0.292), while subjects with overweight and obesity exhibited statistical differences in all parameters compared with normal-weight subjects ($p < 0.001$). In particular, circulating levels of TMAO increased with the BMI classes, with the highest TMAO values in the class III obesity.

Table 1. Lifestyle habits, anthropometric characteristics, blood pressure, metabolic profile, cardio-metabolic indices, and total energy intake of participants grouped based on BMI categories.

Parameters	Normal Weight $n = 34; 24.8\%$	Over Weight $n = 29; 21.2\%$	Grade I Obesity $n = 21; 15.3\%$	Grade II Obesity $n = 15; 10.9\%$	Grade III Obesity $n = 38; 27.7\%$	p-value
Lifestyle Habits						
Age (years)	35.71 ± 8.48	38.14 ± 7.58	38.24 ± 5.89	35.80 ± 8.20	35.00 ± 6.82	0.292
Smoking (yes)	16, 47.1%	19, 65.5%	4, 19.0%	2, 13.3%	22, 10.5%	$\chi^2 = 19.21$, $p < 0.001$
Physical activity (yes)	22, 64.7%	11, 37.9%	3, 14.3%	5, 33.3%	4, 10.5%	$\chi^2 = 27.85$, $p < 0.001$
Anthropometric measurement						
BMI (kg/m^2)	23.01 ± 1.49	27.32 ± 1.43	32.41 ± 1.37	37.48 ± 1.56	46.99 ± 5.16	**<0.001**
WC (cm)	85.12 ± 10.13	94.30 ± 12.38	109.65 ± 8.14	118.81 ± 13.40	139.47 ± 15.15	**<0.001**
Blood pressure						
SBP (mmHg)	115.44 ± 8.01	121.21 ± 10.90	129.52 ± 10.83	131.00 ± 16.38	133.68 ± 11.79	**<0.001**
DBP (mmHg)	71.33 ± 6.07	75.68 ± 7.41	81.67 ± 6.77	86.33 ± 11.25	89.61 ± 9.25	**<0.001**
Metabolic profile						
Circulating levels of TMAO (μM)	3.62 ± 2.37	8.23 ± 0.67	9.03 ± 0.97	9.89 ± 0.85	11.53 ± 0.96	**<0.001**
Fasting Glucose (mg/dL)	83.65 ± 10.25	93.17 ± 13.10	96.47 ± 12.11	97.73 ± 11.00	121.87 ± 10.91	**<0.001**
Insulin (μU/mL)	2.66 ± 1.23	7.01 ± 5.35	10.69 ± 5.83	14.85 ± 9.65	31.29 ± 8.87	**<0.001**
Total cholesterol (mg/dL)	146.8 ± 20.28	176.69 ± 29.17	170.76 ± 20.85	206.87 ± 39.57	221.37 ± 33.58	**<0.001**
HDL cholesterol (mg/dL)	57.59 ± 7.53	50.21 ± 8.19	41.95 ± 13.28	39.60 ± 10.60	37.05 ± 9.42	**<0.001**
LDL cholesterol (mg/dL)	69.92 ± 23.15	101.43 ± 30.05	103.37 ± 16.67	134.49 ± 41.49	150.17 ± 38.54	**<0.001**
Triglycerides (mg/dL)	96.71 ± 26.96	125.24 ± 28.30	155.52 ± 65.23	163.87 ± 33.78	170.74 ± 70.88	**<0.001**
ALT (U/L)	23.26 ± 6.87	24.89 ± 9.06	38.14 ± 12.16	40.73 ± 17.87	41.39 ± 22.49	**<0.001**
AST (U/L)	20.44 ± 5.57	26.58 ± 6.67	36.83 ± 18.25	39.07 ± 14.10	41.00 ± 20.12	**<0.001**
γGT (U/L)	25.64 ± 6.62	26.52 ± 12.48	42.42 ± 19.71	44.47 ± 19.65	49.53 ± 27.20	**<0.001**
Cardio-metabolic indices						
HoMA-IR	0.55 ± 0.28	1.49 ± 0.96	2.51 ± 1.32	3.55 ± 2.31	9.52 ± 3.13	**<0.001**
VAI	1.28 ± 0.54	2.09 ± 1.27	3.42 ± 2.91	3.55 ± 1.97	3.77 ± 2.18	**<0.001**
FLI	19.89 ± 12.37	43.70 ± 21.36	79.39 ± 10.26	90.98 ± 6.97	98.36 ± 2.30	**<0.001**
Metabolic Syndrome						
MetS (number parameter)	0.18 ± 0.52	1.24 ± 1.02	2.33 ± 1.06	2.67 ± 1.40	3.68 ± 1.07	**<0.001**
MetS (presence)	0, 0	4, 13.8%	9, 42.9%	9, 60%	31, 81.6%	$\chi^2 = 61.53$, $p < 0.001$
Nutritional parameters						
Total energy intake (kcal)	2084.79 ± 304.05	2249.14 ± 433.86	2423.33 ± 211.27	2658.67 ± 244.80	2966.45 ± 365.69	**<0.001**

A p-value in bold type denotes a significant difference ($p < 0.05$).

Circulating levels of TMAO according to gender, lifestyle habits, and cut-off of the cardio-metabolic indices are reported in Table 2. As reported in Table 2, circulating levels of TMAO were significantly higher in males ($p = 0.015$), among current smokers or physically inactive individuals ($p < 0.001$), and in subjects with cardio-metabolic indices higher than cut-offs ($p < 0.001$). In addition, circulating levels of TMAO were significantly higher in presence of MetS ($p < 0.001$).

Table 2. Circulating levels of TMAO in the study population according to gender, lifestyle habits, cardio-metabolic indices, and MetS.

Parameters		Circulating Levels of TMAO (µM)	p-value
Gender	Males (n 59)	9.11 ± 3.09	**0.015**
	Females (n 78)	7.70 ± 3.28	
Smoking	Yes (n 68)	9.38 ± 2.63	**<0.001**
	No (n 69)	7.24 ± 3.49	
Physical activity	Yes (n 58)	6.41 ± 3.52	**<0.001**
	No (n 79)	9.69 ± 2.21	
HoMA-IR	> cut-off (n 64)	10.53 ± 1.62	**<0.001**
	< cut-off (n 73)	6.36 ± 3.01	
VAI	> cut-off (n 60)	10.08 ± 2.13	**<0.001**
	< cut-off (n 77)	6.92 ± 3.33	
FLI	> cut-off (n 82)	10.24 ± 1.56	**<0.001**
	< cut-off (n 55)	5.42 ± 3.00	
MetS (parameters)			
WC	Yes (n 87)	9.88 ± 2.06	**<0.001**
	No (n 50)	5.56 ± 3.18	
SBP/DBP	Yes (n 37)	10.49 ± 1.72	**<0.001**
	No (n 100)	7.50 ± 3.33	
Fasting Glucose	Yes (n 43)	11.29 ± 1.22	**<0.001**
	No (n 94)	6.94 ± 2.98	
HDL cholesterol	Yes (n 59)	10.13 ± 2.09	**<0.001**
	No (n 78)	6.93 ± 3.33	
Triglycerides	Yes (n 45)	10.28 ± 2.20	**<0.001**
	No (n 92)	7.34 ± 3.27	
MetS (presence/absence)	Yes (n 53)	10.65 ± 1.62	**<0.001**
	No (n 84)	6.82 ± 3.17	

A p-value in bold type denotes a significant difference ($p < 0.05$).

Correlation Analysis

The correlations between circulating levels of TMAO, age, components of the MetS, metabolic profile, cardio-metabolic indices, are summarized in Table 3. Apart from the age, circulating levels of TMAO show significant correlations with all metabolic parameters. After adjusting for gender, BMI, smoking, physical activity, and total energy intake, correlations with almost all the components of MetS and cardio-metabolic indices were still evident, as shown in Table 3.

Table 3. Correlations among circulating levels of TMAO with age, anthropometric characteristics, blood pressure, metabolic profile, cardio-metabolic indices, and nutritional parameter.

Parameters	Circulating Levels of TMAO (µM)		Circulating Levels of TMAO (µM)	
	Simple Correlation		After Adjusting	
	r	p-value	r	p-value
Age (years)	0.103	0.232	0.169	0.054
Anthropometric measurements				
BMI (kg/m^2)	0.737	<0.001	-	-
WC (cm)	0.670	<0.001	−0.055	0.538
Blood pressure				
SBP (mmHg)	0.600	<0.001	0.273	**0.002**
DBP (mmHg)	0.532	<0.001	0.149	0.091
Metabolic profile				
Fasting Glucose (mg/dL)	0.656	<0.001	0.034	0.700
Insulin (µU/mL)	0.668	<0.001	0.202	**0.021**
Total cholesterol (mg/dL)	0.628	<0.001	0.236	**0.007**
HDL cholesterol (mg/dL)	−0.568	<0.001	−0.180	**0.041**
LDL cholesterol (mg/dL)	0.663	<0.001	0.356	**<0.001**
Triglycerides (mg/dL)	0.535	<0.001	0.224	**0.010**
ALT (U/L)	0.376	**0.001**	0.065	0.461
AST (U/L)	0.506	<0.001	0.176	**0.046**
γGT (U/L)	0.396	**0.001**	0.086	0.333
Cardio-metabolic indices				
HoMA-IR	0.699	<0.001	0.211	**0.016**
VAI	0.549	<0.001	0.255	**0.003**
FLI	0.820	<0.001	0.604	**<0.001**
Nutritional parameter				
Total energy intake (kcal)	0.592	<0.001	-	-

A p-value in bold type denotes a significant difference ($p < 0.05$).

The results of bivariate proportional OR model performed to assess the association of circulating levels of TMAO with quantitative variables are reported in Table 4. The highest circulating levels of TMAO are significantly associated with the severity of obesity (OR 9.59; $p < 0.001$), and insulin resistance (OR 2.82; $p < 0.001$). Moreover, the highest levels of TMAO are associated with the highest levels of VAI (OR 1.58; $p < 0.001$) and FLI (OR 4.31; $p < 0.001$), presence of MetS (OR 2.36; $p < 0.001$) and of all components of the MetS.

Table 4. Bivariate proportional odds ratio model to assess the association between circulating levels of TMAO and gender, lifestyle habits, cardio-metabolic indices, and MetS.

Parameters	Circulating Levels of TMAO (µM)			
	OR	p-value	95% IC	R^2
Gender	1.15	**0.015**	1.029–1.295	0.047
Smoking	1.26	**0.001**	1.110–1.423	0.108
Physical activity	0.67	**<0.001**	0.576–0.788	0.240
BMI categories				
Normal weight	0.05	**0.001**	0.009–0.297	0.604
Overweight	0.27	**<0.001**	0.011–1.121	0.209
Grade I obesity	0.18	**<0.001**	0.010–0.099	0.237
Grade II obesity	1.25	**<0.001**	0.995–1.565	0.033
Grade III obesity	9.59	**<0.001**	3.946–23.344	0.561
HoMA-IR	2.82	**<0.001**	1.937–4.116	0.458
VAI	1.58	**<0.001**	1.308–1.912	0.248
FLI	4.31	**<0.001**	2.353–7.874	0.536
MetS (single parameters)				
WC	1.88	**<0.001**	1.490–2.375	0.378
SBP/DBP	1.64	**<0.001**	1.304–2.065	0.201
Fasting Glucose	5.84	**<0.001**	3.161–10.804	0.538
HDL cholesterol	1.61	**<0.001**	1.320–1.953	0.254
Triglycerides	1.57	**0.001**	1.278–1.919	0.205
MetS (presence/absence)	2.36	**<0.001**	1.727–3.227	0.389

A p-value in bold type denotes a significant difference ($p < 0.05$).

To compare the relative predictive power of the cardio-metabolic indices associated with the circulating levels of TMAO, we performed a multiple linear regression analysis using a model that included as HoMA-IR, VAI, and FLI. Using this model, FLI entered at the first step ($p < 0.001$), while HoMA-IR, VAI were excluded. To compare the relative predictive power of FLI and number of components of MetS associated with the circulating levels of TMAO, we performed a second multiple linear regression analysis model. Using this second model, FLI entered at the first step ($p < 0.001$), while the number of components of MetS were excluded. Results were reported in Table 5.

Table 5. Multiple regression analysis models (stepwise method) with the circulating levels of TMAO as dependent variable to estimate the predictive value of: (a) cardio-metabolic indices; (b) FLI and MetS.

Parameters	Multiple Regression Analysis			
Model 1	R^2	β	t	p-value
FLI	0.672	0.820	16.63	**<0.001**
Variables excluded: HoMA-IR and VAI				
Model 2				
FLI	0.469	0.685	9.2	**<0.001**
Variables excluded: MetS				

A p-value in bold type denotes a significant difference ($p < 0.05$).

A ROC analysis was then performed to determine the cut-off values of circulating levels of TMAO predictive of MetS and FLI. In particular, circulating levels of TMAO ≥ 8.74 µM ($p < 0.001$, AUC 0.876, standard error 0.029, 95% CI 0.808 to 0.926; Figure 2a), and circulating levels of TMAO ≥ 8.02 µM ($p < 0.001$, AUC 0.943, standard error 0.018, 95% CI 0.890 to 0.975; Figure 2b), could serve as thresholds for significantly increased risk of the presence of MetS and NAFLD, respectively.

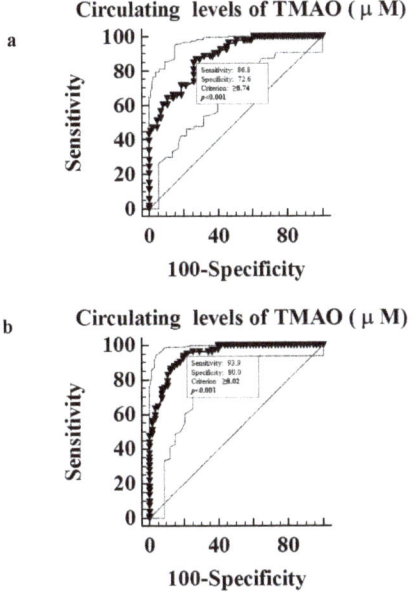

Figure 2. ROC for predictive values of circulating levels of TMAO in detecting FLI (**a**) and MetS (**b**). A *p*-value in bold type denotes a significant difference ($p < 0.05$).

4. Discussion

In this cross-sectional observational study, we evaluated the circulating levels of TMAO in a sample of adult population stratified according to categories of BMI. In addition, we investigated the association among circulating levels of TMAO and cardio-metabolic indices. The classification of the study population according to the BMI demonstrated that circulating levels of TMAO increased along with BMI. To the best of our knowledge, this is the first study that reported statistical differences in the circulating levels of TMAO across classes of BMI. Moreover, we confirmed the presence of a positive association of circulating levels of TMAO with MetS, the increasing number of its components, and HoMA-IR. Finally, a novel association was also reported among the circulating levels of TMAO and VAI and FLI, two surrogate indices of cardio-metabolic risk and early indicators of MetS, independently on common potential covariates.

There is a paucity of literature that has studied the relationship between TMAO and adiposity. A recent experimental study reported that both antisense oligonucleotide-mediated knockdown and genetic deletion of the TMAO-producing enzyme FMO3 protected mice against high-fat diet-induced obesity, thus highlighting a role of the gut microbe-driven TMA/FMO3/TMAO pathway in affecting specific transcriptional reprogramming in white adipocytes [11]. Of interest, in this study circulating levels of TMAO were positively associated with body weight, fat mass, mesenteric adiposity, and subcutaneous adiposity across the different mice-inbred strains; in addition, in cohorts of overweight or obese subjects with metabolic traits and different ethnicity the expression of FMO3 in liver biopsies was positively correlated with BMI and waist-to-hip ratio, and negatively correlated with the Matsuda Index, a measure of insulin sensitivity [11]. Consistent with these data, the findings of the present study show that there is a clear positive association of circulating TMAO levels and classes of BMI. Thus, besides its role as a risk factor for CVD and adverse event in risks subjects, emerging evidence suggests that gut microbiota-derived TMAO might represent per se a key environmental factor contributing to obesity and obesity-associated disorders.

VAI is a surrogate of adipocyte dysfunction independently correlated with insulin sensitivity, and cardio-metabolic risk in primary-care non-obese subjects [20]. In particular, VAI was proposed as a useful tool for the early detection of a condition of insulin resistance and cardio-metabolic risk before it develops into an overt MetS [38]. FLI is a surrogate marker of a fatty liver considered a screening tool to identify NAFLD, recognized as the liver manifestation of MetS, in subjects with insulin resistance and cardio-metabolic risk factors where ultrasound is unavailable [43]. In our population sample there was a positive association between circulating levels of TMAO and both indices. Of interest, the association of the circulating levels of TMAO with VAI and FLI was also shown independently on potential covariates, such as gender, BMI, smoking status, physical activity, and energy intake. In addition, among the cardio-metabolic indices included in this study, FLI, which incorporates BMI, WC, TG, and liver function, was a better predictor of TMAO variability than MetS per se. This finding was in line with the putative role of FLI as early predictor of MetS and likely reflects that the main site of expression of FMO3, the enzyme that metabolizes gut microbe-derived TMA to produce TMAO, is the liver. Based on ROC curve analysis, the most sensitive and specific cut-offs for circulating levels of TMAO to predict the presence of NAFLD-FLI and MetS were ≥ 8.02 μM and ≥ 8.74 μM, respectively. Experimental studies in mice fed with a high-fat diet showed that a high urinary excretion of TMAO was associated with insulin resistance and NAFLD in mice (129S6) prone to these diseases [44]. Miao et al. [45] found that liver insulin receptor knockout mice, characterized by a selective hepatic insulin resistance, have increased circulating TMAO levels associated with a strong up-regulation of the TMAO-producing enzyme FMO3 in the liver [45]. According to the proposed mechanism, TMAO may block the hepatic insulin signaling pathway, thereby exacerbating the impaired glucose tolerance, and promoting the development of fatty liver [46]. Turning to human studies, the above-mentioned study by Randrianarisoa et al. [12] reported a positive correlation between TMAO and liver fat content [12]. In addition, in a large sample of hospital and community-based Chinese adults, Chen et al. [13] showed positive associations of the circulating TMAO levels and two of its nutrient precursors, choline and betaine, with the presence and severity of NAFLD [13]. Choline can be oxidized to betaine, and betaine is generally regarded as safe for dietary ingestion due to its sparing effects on choline, a basic component for the synthesis of phosphatidylcholine, which in turn is necessary for promoting lipid exportation from the liver [47]. In this study, the authors suggested that TMAO may represent a possible risk factor for NAFLD due to its effect in altering the synthesis and transport of bile acids, with subsequent effects on lipid metabolism, intrahepatic triglycerides levels and glucose homeostasis [6]. More recently, Ntzouvani et al. [18] reported a strong positive association between liver function and a pattern of amino acids, which included TMAO, in a sample of Greek adult males with MetS [18].

The results of this study lend support to the evidence that circulating levels of TMAO were positively associated with body weight, thus concurring with an increased risk of developing MetS, through insulin resistance, adipocyte dysfunction, and fatty liver. In this context, it is tempting to hypothesize that circulating levels of TMAO could have a role of a biological marker of early metabolic derangement in subjects with overweight and obesity. Thus, it allows speculation on the possible beneficial and cost-effective effects to early address specific nutrition interventions aimed to reduce the excessive intake of TMAO precursors in subjects at risk of MetS and NAFLD.

Despite these very interesting results, the main limitation of this study is that the cross-sectional design does not allow identification of any causal association between the variables included. Thus, it is not possible to clearly determine the prognostic value of circulating levels of TMAO for predicting the early metabolic derangement in subjects with overweight and obesity. Second, although it is well known that the gut-derived origin of TMAO and dietary intake are important determinants of TMAO levels, we did not include in this study the gut microbiota and single-nutrient analysis. In particular, Kühn et al. [48] reported also that both dietary habits and the composition of the intestinal microbiota may be prone to changes, despite a certain stability of both factors during adulthood. On the other hand, Krüger et al. [49] reported that the large inter-individual variations TMAO levels have been mainly attributed to intestinal microbiota differences, while the influence of diet on fasting TMAO concentrations, albeit statistically significant, could be considered rather moderate. However, there is a large consensus that the study of gut microbiota is burdened by a high intra-individual variability that might hinder the interpretation of the results [48,50–52]. Third, we did not include the evaluation of markers of inflammation, such as C-reactive protein, or metabolic precursor of TMAO such as choline, betaine or carnitine, and liver expression of FMO3. However, several studies have shown that the associations between plasma TMAO and disease outcomes were independent of TMAO precursors [53–55]. In addition, the adverse effects of FMO3 on metabolic disease may be driven by factors other than TMAO, and the expression of the FMO3 or markers of inflammation encompassed the design of the present study. Fourth, we are aware that the liver biopsy is the gold-standard technique for identifying NAFLD. Liver biopsy is an invasive and costly procedure burdened with rare but potentially life-threatening complications. On the contrary, FLI has proved to represent an easy screening tool to identify NAFLD in patients with cardio-metabolic risk factors where ultrasound is unavailable [21,56,57], which is associated with reduced insulin sensitivity, and increased risk of T2DM, atherosclerosis, and cardiovascular disease [43]. Nevertheless, a major strength of this study is the good characterization of our sample population across BMI classes, with the exclusion of impaired renal function and T2DM known factors that can affect TMA metabolism, and likely with similar nutrient availability and food consumption pattern, as they were living in the same geographical area. Furthermore, we included of a variety of potential covariates, such as the total energy intake, to minimize the effect of confounding factors on the association of TMAO with adiposity. However, since complete understanding of TMAO biology is still lacking, the potential translation application of the results of this study to the clinical practice requires large-scale data investigating the beneficial and cost-effective effects of specific nutrition intervention aimed to avoid the excessive intake of TMAO precursors in subjects at risk of MetS and NAFLD. The main results of our study, compared to the results of the general literature, is reported in Table 6.

Table 6. A summary table with the main results of our study compared to the results of the general literature.

Parameters	Methodology	Participants	Effects	Hypothesis	Studies	Concordance
Nascent Metabolic Syndrome (MetS)	Case-control clinical study	30 patients 20 controls	TMAO with a trend of positive correlation	TMAO levels rise only after MetS has advanced to the later stages including T2DM and/or CVD	[9]	Yes
HoMA-IR	Case-control clinical study	30 patients 20 controls	TMAO not significantly correlated	No major role for TMAO in glucose metabolism or insulin sensitivity	[9]	No
	Intervention Program	220 subjects	A negative correlation between circulating TMAO levels insulin sensitivity	In obese, hyperglycemic humans FMO3 expression and TMAO levels are increased in hepatic insulin resistance.	[12]	Yes
NAFLD	Experimental study	Mouse strain 129S6, documented for its susceptibility to IR or NAFLD	Mice 129S6 fed with a high-fat diet showed a high urinary excretion of TMAO associated with insulin resistance and NAFLD	A high-fat diet reduces the conversion and the bioavailability of choline by microbiota, causing NAFLD	[44]	Yes
	Experimental study	Male ob/ob mice and their lean, wild-type C57BL/6J controls	Liver insulin receptor knockout mice with selective hepatic insulin resistance have increased circulating TMAO levels associated with a strong up-regulation of the TMAO-producing enzyme FMO3 in the liver	TMAO may block the hepatic insulin signaling pathway promoting the development of fatty liver	[11]	Yes
	Case-control study (CCS) and cross-sectional study (CSS)	60 adult patients and 35 controls for CCS 1.628participants for CSS	TMAO is an independent risk marker for NAFLD in humans, in both the CCS and CSS studies	TMAO decreases the total bile acid pool size and influences the hepatic triglycerides levels, as a potential risk factor for fatty liver disease	[13]	Yes
	Intervention Program	220 subjects	A positive correlation between circulating TMAO levels and liver fat content	Fasting levels of TMAO are regulated by hepatic FMO3	[12]	Yes
	Cross-sectional study	One hundred middle-aged men	A strong positive association between liver function and a pattern of amino acids, which included TMAO	A pattern of amino acids, included TMAO, are regulated by liver enzymes	[18]	Yes

Abbreviations: MetS, Metabolic Syndrome; TMAO, Trimethylamine N-oxide; T2DM, Type 2 Diabetes Mellitus; CVD, Cardiovascular Diseases; HoMA-IR, Homeostatic Model Assessment Insulin Resistance; FMO3, Flavin-containing Monooxygenases; NAFLD, non-alcoholic fatty liver disease; IR, insulin Resistance; CCS, Case-control Study; CSS, Cross-sectional Study.

5. Conclusions

In conclusion, this study in a sample of adult subjects stratified according to their BMI: (i) reported a positive association between adiposity and circulating levels of TMAO; (ii) confirmed the positive association between circulating levels of TMAO and MetS; and (iii) further expanded the knowledge of the relationship of TMAO and MetS, as we reported novel associations between circulating levels of TMAO and two early indicators of MetS. In particular, in this study we demonstrated that FLI is more tightly associated with TMAO levels than the presence of MetS per se. These associations let us to hypothesize a role of TMAO as an early biomarker of NAFLD-FLI in all borderline conditions in which overt MetS is not present. Moreover, given the current performance of therapies for MetS, we suggest that a specific cut-off of TMAO might help in identifying subjects at high risk of NAFLD, who will require specific nutrition intervention strategies. Appropriate cross-validation studies in larger patient population samples are mandatory to validate the cut-off of TMAO for the identification of subjects at high risk of NAFLD-FLI.

Author Contributions: Conceptualization, L.B. and S.S.; Data curation, G.M.; Formal analysis, L.B., G.M., C.D.S. and S.S.; Funding acquisition, L.B. and G.C.T.; Investigation, L.B., G.A., C.D.S., D.L., G.d.A. and S.S.; Methodology, L.B., G.A. and C.D.S.; Project administration, L.B. and G.M.; Resources, L.B.; Software, L.B.; Supervision, L.B.; Validation, L.B.; Visualization, L.B. and M.M.; Writing—Original Draft, L.B. and S.S.; Writing—Review and Editing, L.B., G.M., A.C. and S.S.

Funding: This research received no external funding.

Acknowledgments: We would like to thank Angela Arnone for data retrieval.

Conflicts of Interest: The authors declare no conflict of interest.

Abbreviations

TMAO	Trimethylamine-N-oxide
TMA	Trimethylamine
FMO3	Flavin-monooxygenase-3
T2DM	Type 2 Diabetes Mellitus
CVD	Cardiovascular diseases
MetS	Metabolic Syndrome
HDL	High-density Lipoprotein
HoMA-IR	Homeostatic Model Assessment of Insulin Resistance
BMI	body mass index
VAI	Visceral Adiposity Index
FLI	Fatty Liver Index
NAFLD	Non-alcoholic Fatty Liver Disease
WC	Waist Circumference
TG	Triglycerides
SBP	Systolic Blood Pressure
DBP	Diastolic Blood Pressure
ALT	Alanine Transaminase
AST	Aspartate Aminotransferase
γGT	γ-Glutamyltransferase
LDL	Low-Density Lipoprotein
SD	Standard Deviation
OR	Odds Ratio
IC	Interval Confidence
ROC	Receiver Operator Characteristic
AUC	Area Under Curve.

References

1. Wang, Z.; Klipfel, E.; Bennett, B.J.; Koeth, R.; Levison, B.S.; Dugar, B.; Feldstein, A.E.; Britt, E.B.; Fu, X.; Chung, Y.M.; et al. Gut flora metabolism of phosphatidylcholine promotes cardiovascular disease. *Nature* **2011**, *472*, 57–63. [CrossRef] [PubMed]
2. Schiattarella, G.G.; Sannino, A.; Toscano, E.; Giugliano, G.; Gargiulo, G.; Franzone, A.; Trimarco, B.; Esposito, G.; Perrino, C. Gut microbe-generated metabolite trimethylamine-N-oxide as cardiovascular risk biomarker: A systematic review and dose-response meta-analysis. *Eur. Heart J.* **2017**, *38*, 2948–2956. [CrossRef] [PubMed]
3. Kanitsoraphan, C.; Rattanawong, P.; Charoensri, S.; Senthong, V. Trimethylamine N-Oxide and Risk of Cardiovascular Disease and Mortality. *Curr. Nutr. Rep.* **2018**. [CrossRef] [PubMed]
4. Barrea, L.; Annunziata, G.; Muscogiuri, G.; Ludisio, D.; Di Somma, C.; Maisto, M.; Tenore, G.C.; Colao, A.; Savastano, S. Trimethylamine N-oxide (TMAO), Mediterranean Diet and Nutrition in Healthy, Normal-weight Subjects: Is It Also A Matter Of Gender? *Nutrition* **2018**, in press. [CrossRef]
5. Zeisel, S.H.; Wishnok, J.S.; Blusztajn, J.K. Formation of methylamines from ingested choline and lecithin. *J. Pharmacol. Exp. Ther.* **1983**, *225*, 320–324.
6. Koeth, R.A.; Wang, Z.; Levison, B.S.; Buffa, J.A.; Org, E.; Sheehy, B.T.; Britt, E.B.; Fu, X.; Wu, Y.; Li, L.; et al. Intestinal microbiota metabolism of L-carnitine, a nutrient in red meat, promotes atherosclerosis. *Nat. Med.* **2013**, *19*, 576–585. [CrossRef] [PubMed]
7. Tang, W.H.; Hazen, S.L. The contributory role of gut microbiota in cardiovascular disease. *J. Clin. Investig.* **2014**, *124*, 4204–4211. [CrossRef] [PubMed]
8. Ufnal, M.; Zadlo, A.; Ostaszewski, R. TMAO: A small molecule of great expectations. *Nutrition* **2015**, *31*, 1317–1323. [CrossRef] [PubMed]
9. Lent-Schochet, D.; Silva, R.; McLaughlin, M.; Huet, B.; Jialal, I. Changes to trimethylamine-N-oxide and its precursors in nascent metabolic syndrome. *Horm. Mol. Biol. Clin. Investig.* **2018**, *35*. [CrossRef]
10. Zhu, W.; Gregory, J.C.; Org, E.; Buffa, J.A.; Gupta, N.; Wang, Z.; Li, L.; Fu, X.; Wu, Y.; Mehrabian, M.; et al. Gut Microbial Metabolite TMAO Enhances Platelet Hyperreactivity and Thrombosis Risk. *Cell* **2016**, *165*, 111–124. [CrossRef]
11. Schugar, R.C.; Shih, D.M.; Warrier, M.; Helsley, R.N.; Burrows, A.; Ferguson, D.; Brown, A.L.; Gromovsky, A.D.; Heine, M.; Chatterjee, A.; et al. The TMAO-Producing Enzyme Flavin-Containing Monooxygenase 3 Regulates Obesity and the Beiging of White Adipose Tissue. *Cell Rep.* **2017**, *19*, 2451–2461. [CrossRef] [PubMed]
12. Randrianarisoa, E.; Lehn-Stefan, A.; Wang, X.; Hoene, M.; Peter, A.; Heinzmann, S.S.; Zhao, X.; Königsrainer, I.; Königsrainer, A.; Balletshofer, B.; et al. Relationship of Serum Trimethylamine N-Oxide (TMAO) Levels with early Atherosclerosis in Humans. *Sci. Rep.* **2016**, *6*, 26745. [CrossRef] [PubMed]
13. Chen, Y.M.; Liu, Y.; Zhou, R.F.; Chen, X.L.; Wang, C.; Tan, X.Y.; Wang, L.J.; Zheng, R.D.; Zhang, H.W.; Ling, W.H.; et al. Associations of gut-flora-dependent metabolite trimethylamine-N-oxide, betaine and choline with non-alcoholic fatty liver disease in adults. *Sci. Rep.* **2016**, *6*, 19076. [CrossRef] [PubMed]
14. Marchesini, G.; Brizi, M.; Bianchi, G.; Tomassetti, S.; Bugianesi, E.; Lenzi, M.; McCullough, A.J.; Natale, S.; Forlani, G.; Melchionda, N. Nonalcoholic fatty liver disease: A feature of the metabolic syndrome. *Diabetes* **2001**, *50*, 1844–1850. [CrossRef]
15. Grundy, S.M.; Cleeman, J.I.; Daniels, S.R.; Donato, K.A.; Eckel, R.H.; Franklin, B.A.; Gordon, D.J.; Krauss, R.M.; Savage, P.J.; Smith, S.C., Jr.; et al. National Heart, Lung, and Blood Institute. Diagnosis and management of the metabolic syndrome: An American Heart Association/National Heart, Lung, and Blood Institute Scientific Statement. *Circulation* **2005**, *112*, 2735–2752. [CrossRef] [PubMed]
16. Lorenzo, C.; Williams, K.; Hunt, K.J.; Haffner, S.M. The National Cholesterol Education Program–Adult Treatment Panel III, International Diabetes Federation, and World Health Organization definitions of the metabolic syndrome as predictors of incident cardiovascular disease and diabetes. *Diabetes Care* **2007**, *30*, 8–13. [CrossRef] [PubMed]
17. Jialal, I.; Devaraj, S.; Adams-Huet, B.; Chen, X.; Kaur, H. Increased cellular and circulating biomarkers of oxidative stress in nascent metabolic syndrome. *J. Clin. Endocrinol. Metab.* **2012**, *97*, E1844–E1850. [CrossRef]

18. Ntzouvani, A.; Nomikos, T.; Panagiotakos, D.; Fragopoulou, E.; Pitsavos, C.; McCann, A.; Ueland, P.M.; Antonopoulou, S. Amino acid profile and metabolic syndrome in a male Mediterranean population: A cross-sectional study. *Nutr. Metab. Cardiovasc. Dis.* **2017**, *27*, 1021–1030. [CrossRef]
19. Mueller, D.M.; Allenspach, M.; Othman, A.; Saely, C.H.; Muendlein, A.; Vonbank, A.; Drexel, H.; von Eckardstein, A. Plasma levels of trimethylamine-N-oxide are confounded by impaired kidney function and poor metabolic control. *Atherosclerosis* **2015**, *243*, 638–644. [CrossRef]
20. Amato, M.C.; Giordano, C.; Galia, M.; Criscimanna, A.; Vitabile, S.; Midiri, M.; Galluzzo, A.; AlkaMeSy Study Group. Visceral Adiposity Index: A reliable indicator of visceral fat function associated with cardiometabolic risk. *Diabetes Care* **2010**, *33*, 920–922. [CrossRef]
21. Bedogni, G.; Bellentani, S.; Miglioli, L.; Masutti, F.; Passalacqua, M.; Castiglione, A.; Tiribelli, C. The Fatty Liver Index: A simple and accurate predictor of hepatic steatosis in the general population. *BMC Gastroenterol.* **2006**, *6*, 33. [CrossRef] [PubMed]
22. Amato, M.C.; Giordano, C. Visceral adiposity index: An indicator of adipose tissue dysfunction. *Int. J. Endocrinol.* **2014**, *2014*, 730827. [CrossRef] [PubMed]
23. Klisic, A.; Isakovic, A.; Kocic, G.; Kavaric, N.; Jovanovic, M.; Zvrko, E.; Skerovic, V.; Ninic, A. Relationship between Oxidative Stress, Inflammation and Dyslipidemia with Fatty Liver Index in Patients with Type 2 Diabetes Mellitus. *Exp. Clin. Endocrinol. Diabetes* **2018**, *126*, 371–378. [CrossRef] [PubMed]
24. Rogulj, D.; Konjevoda, P.; Milić, M.; Mladinić, M.; Domijan, A.M. Fatty liver index as an indicator of metabolic syndrome. *Clin. Biochem.* **2012**, *45*, 68–71. [CrossRef] [PubMed]
25. Yadav, D.; Choi, E.; Ahn, S.V.; Koh, S.B.; Sung, K.C.; Kim, J.Y.; Huh, J.H. Fatty liver index as a simple predictor of incident diabetes from the KoGES-ARIRANG study. *Medicine* **2016**, *95*, E4447. [CrossRef] [PubMed]
26. American Diabetes Association. Standards of Medical Care in Diabetes-2017: Summary of Revisions. *Diabetes Care* **2017**, *40*, S4–S5. [CrossRef] [PubMed]
27. World Health Organization (WHO). Waist Circumference and Waist-Hip Ratio. Report of WHO Expert Consultation, Geneva. 8–11 December 2008. Available online: http://apps.who.int/iris/bitstream/10665/44583/1/9789241501491_eng.pdf (accessed on 10 November 2018).
28. National Center for Health Statistics. Anthropometry Procedures Manual—National Health and Nutrition Examination Survey (NHANES). Available online: http://www.cdc.gov/nchs/data/nhanes/nhanes_11_12/Anthropometry_Procedures_Manual.pdf (accessed on 10 November 2018).
29. Wang, Z.; Levison, B.S.; Hazen, J.E.; Donahue, L.; Li, X.M.; Hazen, S.L. Measurement of trimethylamine-N-oxide by stable isotope dilution liquid chromatography tandem mass spectrometry. *Anal. Biochem.* **2014**, *455*, 35–40. [CrossRef] [PubMed]
30. Beale, R.; Airs, R. Quantification of glycine betaine, choline and trimethylamine N-oxide in seawater particulates: Minimisation of seawater associated ion suppression. *Anal. Chim. Acta.* **2016**, *938*, 114–122. [CrossRef]
31. Yu, W.; Xu, C.; Li, G.; Hong, W.; Zhou, Z.; Xiao, C.; Zhao, Y.; Cai, Y.; Huang, M.; Jin, J. Simultaneous determination of trimethylamine N-oxide, choline, betaine by UPLC-MS/MS in human plasma: An application in acute stroke patients. *J. Pharm. Biomed. Anal.* **2018**, *152*, 179–187. [CrossRef]
32. Savastano, S.; Barbato, A.; Di Somma, C.; Guida, B.; Pizza, G.; Barrea, L.; Avallone, S.; Schiano di Cola, M.; Strazzullo, P.; Colao, A. Beyond waist circumference in an adult male population of Southern Italy: Is there any role for subscapular skinfold thickness in the relationship between insulin-like growth factor-I system and metabolic parameters? *J. Endocrinol. Investig.* **2012**, *35*, 925–929. [CrossRef]
33. Savastano, S.; Di Somma, C.; Colao, A.; Barrea, L.; Orio, F.; Finelli, C.; Pasanisi, F.; Contaldo, F.; Tarantino, G. Preliminary data on the relationship between circulating levels of Sirtuin 4, anthropometric and metabolic parameters in obese subjects according to growth hormone/insulin-like growth factor-1 status. *Growth Horm. IGF Res.* **2015**, *25*, 28–33. [CrossRef]
34. Barrea, L.; Tarantino, G.; Di Somma, C.; Muscogiuri, G.; Macchia, P.E.; Falco, A.; Colao, A.; Savastano, S. Adherence to the Mediterranean Diet and Circulating Levels of Sirtuin 4 in Obese Patients: A Novel Association. *Oxid. Med. Cell Longev.* **2017**, *2017*, 6101254. [CrossRef] [PubMed]
35. Barrea, L.; Di Somma, C.; Macchia, P.E.; Falco, A.; Savanelli, M.C.; Orio, F.; Colao, A.; Savastano, S. Influence of nutrition on somatotropic axis: Milk consumption in adult individuals with moderate-severe obesity. *Clin. Nutr.* **2017**, *36*, 293–301. [CrossRef] [PubMed]

36. Barrea, L.; Macchia, P.E.; Tarantino, G.; Di Somma, C.; Pane, E.; Balato, N.; Napolitano, M.; Colao, A.; Savastano, S. Nutrition: A key environmental dietary factor in clinical severity and cardio-metabolic risk in psoriatic male patients evaluated by 7-day food-frequency questionnaire. *J. Transl. Med.* **2015**, *13*, 303. [CrossRef] [PubMed]
37. Matthews, D.R.; Hosker, J.P.; Rudenski, A.S.; Naylor, B.A.; Treacher, D.F.; Turner, R.C. Homeostasis model assessment: Insulin resistance and beta-cell function from fasting plasma glucose and insulin concentrations in man. *Diabetologia* **1985**, *28*, 412–419. [CrossRef]
38. Amato, M.C.; Giordano, C.; Pitrone, M.; Galluzzo, A. Cut-off points of the visceral adiposity index (VAI) identifying a visceral adipose dysfunction associated with cardiometabolic risk in a Caucasian Sicilian population. *Lipids Health Dis.* **2011**, *10*, 183. [CrossRef] [PubMed]
39. Expert Panel on Detection, Evaluation, and Treatment of High Blood Cholesterol in Adults. Executive Summary of The Third Report of The National Cholesterol Education Program (NCEP) Expert Panel on Detection, Evaluation, And Treatment of High Blood Cholesterol in Adults (Adult Treatment Panel III). *JAMA* **2001**, *285*, 2486–2497. [CrossRef]
40. Barrea, L.; Muscogiuri, G.; Di Somma, C.; Annunziata, G.; Megna, M.; Falco, A.; Balato, A.; Colao, A.; Savastano, S. Coffee consumption, metabolic syndrome and clinical severity of psoriasis: Good or bad stuff? *Arch. Toxicol.* **2018**, *92*, 1831–1845. [CrossRef]
41. Turconi, G.; Guarcello, M.; Berzolari, F.G.; Carolei, A.; Bazzano, R.; Roggi, C. An evaluation of a colour food photography atlas as a tool for quantifying food portion size in epidemiological dietary surveys. *Eur. J. Clin. Nutr.* **2005**, *59*, 923–931. [CrossRef]
42. Lentjes, M.A.; McTaggart, A.; Mulligan, A.A.; Powell, N.A.; Parry-Smith, D.; Luben, R.N.; Bhaniani, A.; Welch, A.A.; Khaw, K.T. Dietary intake measurement using 7 d diet diaries in British men and women in the European Prospective Investigation into Cancer-Norfolk study: A focus on methodological issues. *Br. J. Nutr.* **2014**, *111*, 516–526. [CrossRef]
43. Yang, K.C.; Hung, H.F.; Lu, C.W.; Chang, H.H.; Lee, L.T.; Huang, K.C. Association of Non-alcoholic Fatty Liver Disease with Metabolic Syndrome Independently of Central Obesity and Insulin Resistance. *Sci. Rep.* **2016**, *6*, 27034. [CrossRef] [PubMed]
44. Dumas, M.E.; Barton, R.H.; Toye, A.; Cloarec, O.; Blancher, C.; Rothwell, A.; Fearnside, J.; Tatoud, R.; Blanc, V.; Lindon, J.C.; et al. Metabolic profiling reveals a contribution of gut microbiota to fatty liver phenotype in insulin-resistant mice. *Proc. Natl. Acad. Sci. USA* **2006**, *103*, 12511–12516. [CrossRef] [PubMed]
45. Miao, J.; Ling, A.V.; Manthena, P.V.; Gearing, M.E.; Graham, M.J.; Crooke, R.M.; Croce, K.J.; Esquejo, R.M.; Clish, C.B.; Torrecilla, E.; et al. Flavin-containing monooxygenase 3 as a potential player in diabetes-associated atherosclerosis. *Nat. Commun.* **2015**, *6*, 6498. [CrossRef]
46. Gao, X.; Liu, X.; Xu, J.; Xue, C.; Xue, Y.; Wang, Y. Dietary trimethylamine N-oxide exacerbates impaired glucose tolerance in mice fed a high fat diet. *J. Biosci. Bioeng.* **2014**, *118*, 476–481. [CrossRef] [PubMed]
47. Noga, A.A.; Vance, D.E. A gender-specific role for phosphatidylethanolamine N-methyltransferase-derived phosphatidylcholine in the regulation of plasma high density and very low density lipoproteins in mice. *J. Biol. Chem.* **2003**, *278*, 21851–21859. [CrossRef] [PubMed]
48. Kühn, T.; Rohrmann, S.; Sookthai, D.; Johnson, T.; Katzke, V.; Kaaks, R.; von Eckardstein, A.; Müller, D. Intra-individual variation of plasma trimethylamine-N-oxide (TMAO), betaine and choline over 1 year. *Clin. Chem. Lab. Med.* **2017**, *55*, 261–268. [CrossRef] [PubMed]
49. Krüger, R.; Merz, B.; Rist, M.J.; Ferrario, P.G.; Bub, A.; Kulling, S.E.; Watzl, B. Associations of current diet with plasma and urine TMAO in the KarMeN study: Direct and indirect contributions. *Mol. Nutr. Food Res.* **2017**, *61*. [CrossRef]
50. Rohrmann, S.; Linseisen, J.; Allenspach, M.; von Eckardstein, A.; Müller, D. Plasma Concentrations of Trimethylamine-N-oxide Are Directly Associated with Dairy Food Consumption and Low-Grade Inflammation in a German Adult Population. *J. Nutr.* **2016**, *146*, 283–289. [CrossRef]
51. Zhernakova, A.; Kurilshikov, A.; Bonder, M.J.; Tigchelaar, E.F.; Schirmer, M.; Vatanen, T.; Mujagic, Z.; Vila, A.V.; Falony, G.; Vieira-Silva, S.; et al. Population-based metagenomics analysis reveals markers for gut microbiome composition and diversity. *Science* **2016**, *352*, 565–569. [CrossRef]
52. Cho, C.E.; Caudill, M.A. Trimethylamine-N-Oxide: Friend, Foe, or Simply Caught in the Cross-Fire? *Trends Endocrinol. Metab.* **2017**, *28*, 121–130. [CrossRef] [PubMed]

53. Senthong, V.; Li, X.S.; Hudec, T.; Coughlin, J.; Wu, Y.; Levison, B.; Wang, Z.; Hazen, S.L.; Tang, W.H. Plasma Trimethylamine N-Oxide, a Gut Microbe-Generated Phosphatidylcholine Metabolite, Is Associated With Atherosclerotic Burden. *J. Am. Coll. Cardiol.* **2016**, *67*, 2620–2628. [CrossRef]
54. Tang, W.H.; Wang, Z.; Fan, Y.; Levison, B.; Hazen, J.E.; Donahue, L.M.; Wu, Y.; Hazen, S.L. Prognostic value of elevated levels of intestinal microbe-generated metabolite trimethylamine-N-oxide in patients with heart failure: Refining the gut hypothesis. *J. Am. Coll. Cardiol.* **2014**, *64*, 1908–1914. [CrossRef] [PubMed]
55. Wang, Z.; Tang, W.H.; Buffa, J.A.; Fu, X.; Britt, E.B.; Koeth, R.A.; Levison, B.S.; Fan, Y.; Wu, Y.; Hazen, S.L. Prognostic value of choline and betaine depends on intestinal microbiota-generated metabolite trimethylamine-N-oxide. *Eur. Heart J.* **2014**, *35*, 904–910. [CrossRef] [PubMed]
56. Silaghi, C.A.; Silaghi, H.; Colosi, H.A.; Craciun, A.E.; Farcas, A.; Cosma, D.T.; Hancu, N.; Pais, R.; Georgescu, C.E. Prevalence and predictors of non-alcoholic fatty liver disease as defined by the fatty liver index in a type 2 diabetes population. *Clujul. Med.* **2016**, *89*, 82–88. [CrossRef] [PubMed]
57. Fedchuk, L.; Nascimbeni, F.; Pais, R.; Charlotte, F.; Housset, C.; Ratziu, V.; LIDO Study Group. Performance and limitations of steatosis biomarkers in patients with nonalcoholic fatty liver disease. *Aliment Pharmacol. Ther.* **2014**, *40*, 1209–1222. [CrossRef] [PubMed]

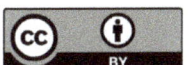 © 2018 by the authors. Licensee MDPI, Basel, Switzerland. This article is an open access article distributed under the terms and conditions of the Creative Commons Attribution (CC BY) license (http://creativecommons.org/licenses/by/4.0/).

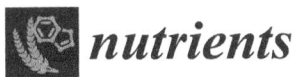

Article

Metabolic Syndrome in Arab Adults with Low Bone Mineral Density

Kaiser Wani [1], Sobhy M. Yakout [1], Mohammed Ghouse Ahmed Ansari [1], Shaun Sabico [1], Syed Danish Hussain [1], Majed S. Alokail [1], Eman Sheshah [2], Naji J. Aljohani [3], Yousef Al-Saleh [1,4,5,6], Jean-Yves Reginster [1,7] and Nasser M. Al-Daghri [1,*]

1. Chair for Biomarkers of Chronic Diseases, Department of Biochemistry, College of Science, King Saud University, Riyadh 11451, Saudi Arabia; wani.kaiser@gmail.com (K.W.); sobhy.yakout@gmail.com (S.M.Y.); ansari.bio1@gmail.com (M.G.A.A.); eaglescout01@yahoo.com (S.S.); danishhussain121@gmail.com (S.D.H.); msa85@yahoo.co.uk (M.S.A.); alaslawi@hotmail.com (Y.A.-S.); jyr.ch@bluewin.ch (J.-Y.R.)
2. Diabetes Care Center, King Salman Bin Abdulaziz Hospital, Riyadh 12769, Saudi Arabia; eman_shesha@hotmail.com
3. Specialized Diabetes and Endocrine Center, King Fahad Medical City, Riyadh 12231, Saudi Arabia; najij@hotmail.com
4. College of Medicine, King Saud bin Abdulaziz University for Health Sciences, Riyadh 22490, Saudi Arabia
5. King Abdullah International Medical Research Center, Riyadh 11481, Saudi Arabia
6. Department of Medicine, Ministry of the National Guard—Health Affairs, Riyadh 14611, Saudi Arabia
7. Department of Public Health, Epidemiology and Health Economics, University of Liège, 4000 Liège, Belgium
* Correspondence: aldaghri2011@gmail.com; Tel.: +009-661-467-5939; Fax: +009-661-467-5931

Received: 16 May 2019; Accepted: 20 June 2019; Published: 21 June 2019

Abstract: There are discrepancies in the reports on the association of metabolic syndrome (MetS) and its components with bone mineral density (BMD) and hence more population-based studies on this subject are needed. In this context, this observational study was aimed to investigate the association between T-scores of BMD at lumbar L1–L4 and full MetS and its individual components. A total of 1587 participants (84.7% females), >35 years and with risk factors associated with bone loss were recruited from February 2013 to August 2016. BMD was done at L1–L4 using dual-energy X-ray absorptiometry (DXA). T-Scores were calculated. Fasting blood samples and anthropometrics were done at recruitment. Fasting lipid profile and glucose were measured. Screening for full MetS and its components was done according to the National Cholesterol Education Programme Adult Treatment Panel III (NCEP ATP III) criteria. Logistic regression analysis revealed that the odds of having full MetS increased significantly from the lowest T-score tertile to the highest one in both sexes (OR, odd ratio (95% CI, confidence interval) of tertile 2 and 3 at 1.49 (0.8 to 2.8) and 2.46 (1.3 to 4.7), $p = 0.02$ in males and 1.35 (1.0 to 1.7) and 1.45 (1.1 to1.9), $p < 0.01$ in females). The odds remained significant even after adjustments with age, body mass index (BMI), and other risk factors associated with bone loss. Among the components of MetS, only central obesity showed a significant positive association with T-score. The study suggests a significant positive association of T-score (spine) with full MetS irrespective of sex, and among the components of MetS this positive association was seen specifically with central obesity.

Keywords: metabolic syndrome; bone mineral density; obesity; insulin resistance; bone health; osteoporosis

1. Introduction

Metabolic syndrome (MetS), a syndrome consisting of several disorders like abdominal obesity, dyslipidemia, increased blood pressure and impaired glucose regulation, represents characteristics such as low-grade inflammation and increased oxidative stress [1,2]. The increased prevalence of MetS in Saudi Arabia in recent years is blamed on rapid economic growth and Westernization of lifestyle [3,4]. The clinical impact of MetS is immense, considering its vascular harm and its predisposition to the progression of cardiovascular diseases and metabolic complications like type 2 diabetes mellitus (T2DM) [5,6].

The National Cholesterol Education Programme Adult Treatment Panel III (NCEP ATP III) [7] definition for full MetS requires the presence of at least three out of five components namely central obesity, hyperglycemia, low high-density cholesterol, hypertriglyceridemia and hypertension. The NCEP-ATPIII definition of MetS is the most commonly used definition for epidemiologic studies in the region since it does not require a pre-requisite risk factor (e.g., obesity for the International Diabetes Federation (IDF), hyperglycemia for the World Health Organization (WHO)) to reach a diagnosis. Interestingly, these components of MetS may also affect the bone mineral density (BMD) and bone metabolism through several mechanisms, one of which is the reduced blood flow to bone mass due to micro-vascular complications associated with impaired glucose regulation [8]. The other proposed mechanism is hypercalciuria induced by higher glucose levels and elevated blood pressure [9]. In spite of the associations, the overall relationship of MetS components, bone health and BMD remains blurred. For instance, although individuals with T2DM are at an increased risk for fractures [10], higher BMDs are seen in T2DM individuals [11,12]. However, a recent meta-analysis conducted on eight epidemiologic studies involving 39,938 participants suggested no explicit effect of MetS on bone fractures [13]. Apart from this, there are discrepancies in the reports on the association of MetS components and bone health in different sexes [14,15].

Clearly, more population-based studies are needed to decipher the relationship between MetS and its components on bone health. The authors' hypothesize a statistically significant association between different components of MetS and full MetS with the BMD at lumbar L1–L4 bone site. In this context, this observational study was aimed to investigate the association between T-scores of BMD at lumbar L1–L4 and full MetS and its individual components in Saudi Arab adults with risk factors associated with bone loss. Both sexes were included in this study to investigate the sexual disparity, if any, in these associations.

2. Materials and Methods

This observation study is part of a larger study dedicated to finding the biomarkers associated with bone health (titled: Osteoporosis Disease Registry); it was approved by the Ethics Committee at College of Science, King Saud University (KSU), Saudi Arabia (# H-01-R-012).

2.1. Study Design and Participants

The study was conducted in several hospitals around Riyadh city; the most prominent of them being King Fahad Medical City (KFMC), King Khalid University Hospital (KKUH) and King Salman Hospital (KSH), where the bulk of the recruitment was done. The study began in early 2013 and the recruitment ended in August 2016. The inclusion criteria were consenting males and females, >35 years old, who in their general physician visits had been advised of a bone mineral density (BMD) scan owing to their being at a risk associated with bone loss. There were no specific exclusion criteria except being ≤35 years of age or participants with malignancy, cardiac or lung diseases, etc. that required immediate medical attention. A total of 1587 participants (84.7% females and 15.3% males) were recruited during the period.

2.2. Bone Mineral Density (BMD) Scan and T-Score

A dual-energy X-ray absorptiometry (DXA) machine (Hologic Inc., Marlborough, MA, USA) was utilized to measure the bone mineral density (BMD) at lumbar vertebrae L1–L4 and the average scores were used to calculate sex-specific T-scores by the software installed in the machine which shows how much the measured bone density is higher or lower than the bone density of a healthy 30-year-old same sex individual. The machine was calibrated using a standard phantom provided by the manufacturer and the test was performed by a certified bone densitometry technologist. The results of the bone density scan were printed and transported to the Chair for Biomarkers in Chronic Diseases (CBCD) at KSU for data entry.

2.3. Anthropometry, Blood Collection and Sample Analysis

The study participants were invited for a fasting blood withdrawal procedure and administration of a standard questionnaire on the risk factors associated with the bone loss. Anthropometry measurements included height, weight, waist and hip circumference, and systolic/diastolic blood pressure, measured by trained nurses using standard procedures. Weight (Kg) was recorded using an international standard scale (Digital Pearson scale, ADAM Equipment Inc., Oxford, CT, USA). Height and waist and hip circumference (to the nearest 0.5 cm) were measured utilizing a standardized measuring tape. Body mass index (BMI) was calculated as weight in Kgs divided by height in square meters. Blood pressure (mmHG) was recorded by a trained nurse twice after 10 minutes rest using a conventional mercurial sphygmomanometer and the average was noted. A one-on-one interview was conducted by trained research associates where the participants were informed about the study and reported risk factors associated with bone loss through a 12-point questionnaire. The risk factors included whether or not the subject had T2DM, thyroid dysfunction, family history of diabetes, osteoporosis, arthritis, etc., whether they had a barium test, presence of scoliosis or kyphosis, loss of height in the last two years and history of fractures in the last five years.

Collected fasting blood samples were transported to CBCD laboratory for biochemical analysis which included lipid profile as well as glucose, calcium and albumin analysis quantified using an automated biochemical analyzer (Konelab 20, Thermo-Fischer Scientific, Espoo, Finland). The reagents were purchased from Thermo Fischer (catalogue# 981379 for glucose, 981812 for total cholesterol, 981823 for high density lipoprotein (HDL)-cholesterol, 981301 for triglyceride, 981367 for calcium and 981766 for albumin). Glucose kit employed the routine glucose-oxidase, peroxidase method; total cholesterol test employed cholesterol-esterase, oxidase method; HDL-cholesterol test employed the two-step polyethylene glycol modified cholesterol esterase and oxidase methodology; triglyceride kit employed enzymes like lipoprotein lipase and oxidase; calcium kit employed Arsenazo III methodology while albumin kit employed bromocresol purple method. The imprecision calculated as the total coefficient of variation (CV) was ≤5%, ≤3.5%, ≤4%, ≤4%, ≤4.5% and ≤3% for these tests, respectively. Insulin was also measured in these samples using Luminex multiplex (Luminexcorp, Austin, TX, USA) with fluorescent microbead technology.

2.4. T-Score Tertiles and MetS Components

Data for both males and females were divided into T-score tertiles with tertile 1 having the lowest T-score (spine) and tertile 3 having the highest T-score. The status of full MetS and its five components was assessed as present/absent (dichotomous data) using the criteria set in the National Cholesterol Education Programme Adult Treatment Panel III (NCEP-ATP III) [16] which states MetS being present if at least three of the following five components are present.

1. Central obesity: waist circumference >102 cm (males), >88 cm (females).
2. Hyperglycemia: fasting glucose >5.6 mmol/l or pharmacologic treatment for hyperglycemia (both sexes).
3. Hypertriglyceridemia: serum triglycerides ≥1.7 mmol/l (both sexes).
4. Low HDL-cholesterol: serum HDL-cholesterol <1.03 mmol/l (males), <1.30 mmol/l (females).
5. Hypertension: systolic blood pressure >130 mmHg and/or diastolic blood pressure >85 mmHg or current use of antihypertensive medications.

2.5. Data Analysis

SPSS (Version 23.0, SPSS Inc., Chicago, IL, USA) was used to analyze the data. Kolmogorov–Smirnov test was employed to assess the normal distribution of the preliminary data. Continuous normally distributed variables were presented as mean ± standard deviation while median (25th and 75th percentile) was used for continuous non-normal variables. Categorical variables like status of full MetS and its individual components; and data obtained from the bone loss risk factor questionnaires were presented as percentages. Chi-squared test (3 × 2 contingency table) was used for checking the differences in prevalence of MetS and its components in the three tertiles of T-scores. Multinomial logistic regression was performed using the T-score tertile as a dependent variable (with lowest tertile as reference) and full MetS or its individual components (present vs. absent) as independent variables. Data was presented as odds ratio 95% confidence interval (OR (95% CI)) and respective p-values represented odds of having different components of MetS at higher tertiles of T-score compared to the lowest. Different models were employed with model "a" as univariate, and all other models were adjusted accordingly for + age (model "b"), + BMI (model "c"), + other components of MetS (model "d") and + risk factors associated with bone loss like T2DM, thyroid dysfunction, etc.; family history of diabetes, osteoporosis, arthritis, etc.; barium test done previously; scoliosis or kyphosis of spine; loss of height reported; history of broken bones (model "e"). The analysis was conducted at 95% confidence level and a p-value < 0.05 was considered statistically significant. MS excel 2010 was used to prepare figures.

3. Results

3.1. General and Biochemical Characteristics of the Study Participants

Table 1 show the general and biochemical characteristics of the study participants. A total of 1587 participants were recruited for the study, out of which 84.7% (N = 1344) were females. Participants who were older than 35 years with risk factors associated with bone loss were recruited. The mean age for females and males were 56 and 58 years, respectively. It was determined that 87.3% of females and 79.4% of males were either overweight or obese (BMI >25 kg/m^2) with an average BMI in females at 32.93 kg/m^2 and males at 29.86 kg/m^2. Among the risk factors associated with bone loss, the most prominent in the participants were age greater than 50 years (77% in females and 79.8% in males); family history of diabetes (58.6% in females and 74.5% in males); and those diagnosed with T2DM (51.4% in females and 70.8% in males). The other risk factors like family history of osteoporosis and arthritis were moderately found in both males and females. The percentage of females who reported having thyroid disease, done a barium test (last two weeks of recruitment), and had scoliosis of the spine was 9.2%, 10.7% and 8.9%, respectively, while these risk factors were negligibly found in males. Additionally, 10% and 11.7% of the females reported loss of height in the last two years and a history of broken bones in the last five years of recruitment, respectively. The median (Q1, Q3) values for T-score at spine (L1–L4) for females and males were −1.70 (−2.5, −0.8) and −0.91 (−1.7, 0.1), respectively. The table also shows the biochemical characteristics of the participants, like lipid profile and fasting glucose, that were analyzed to assess different components of MetS.

3.2. Prevalence of Different MetS Components in T-Score Tertiles

Table 2 shows the prevalence of the five components of MetS and full MetS in participants with tertiles according to the T-score (L1-L4 spine). The lowest T-score (least BMD) in both groups represents the tertile 1 and the highest T-score represents the tertile 3. Among the five components of MetS, the prevalence of central obesity was significantly different in the three T-score tertiles in all participants as well as in males and females. It increased from 66.9% in tertile 1 to 82.7% in tertile 3 (p < 0.01). A similar trend was followed in males where it increased from 38.3% in tertile 1 to 71.6% in tertile 3 (p < 0.01), and in females where it increased from 72.1% in tertile 1 to 84.7% in tertile 3 (p < 0.01). The prevalence of other four components (hyperglycemia, low HDL-cholesterol, hypertriglyceridemia and hypertension) was more or less similar in different tertiles of T-score and this was seen in both males and females except for hypertriglyceridemia in all participants where it increased from 40.3% in tertile 1 to 47.7% in tertile 3 ($p = 0.04$). The prevalence of full MetS, however, increased significantly from the lowest T-score tertile to the highest and this was seen in all participants as well as when data was divided according to sexes (56.1% in tertile 1 to 67.7% in tertile 3, $p < 0.01$ in all participants as well as in males where full Mets was 50.6% in tertile 1 and 71.6% in tertile 3, $p = 0.02$; and females where it increased from 57.1% to 65.8%, $p = 0.003$).

Table 1. General and biochemical characteristics of participants.

	Overall	Males	Females
N	1587	243	1344
Anthropometrics			
Age (years)	56.7 ± 8.2	58.1 ± 9.4	56.4 ± 7.9
BMI (kg/m^2)	32.4 ± 6.4	29.9 ± 5.2	32.93 ± 6.4
Waist (cm)	100.3 ± 14.1	103.7 ± 14.2	99.7 ± 14
Hips (cm)	107.9 ± 12.9	104.4 ± 12	108.6 ± 13
Systolic BP (mmHg)	126.2 ± 16.4	131.1 ± 13.1	125.4 ± 16.8
Diastolic BP (mmHg)	76.8 ± 9.9	79.5 ± 8.2	76.3 ± 10.1
Risk Factors			
Age (>50 years) $	77.4	79.8	77.0
Family History			
Diabetes Mellitus $	61.0	74.5	58.6
Osteoporosis $	9.8	9.9	9.7
Arthritis $	6.2	4.9	6.5
Subject History			
Diabetes Mellitus $	54.4	70.8	51.4
Thyroid Disease $	8.1	2.5	9.2
Barium Test (last 2 weeks) $	9.4	2.1	10.7
Scoliosis of Spine $	7.8	1.6	8.9
Kyphosis $	3.5	0.8	4.0
Lost Height (2 years) $	8.8	1.6	10.0
Fracture (last 5 years) $	10.7	5.3	11.7
T-Score (L1–L4 Spine)	−1.49 ± 1.3	−0.84 ± 1.3	−1.60 ± 1.3
Biochemical Characteristics			
Glucose (mmol/l) #	6.7 (5.5, 9.9)	9.2 (6.5–14.1)	6.5 (5.4–9.3)
Insulin (μU/ml) #	10.4 (5.9, 18.4)	21.6 (10.7, 33.6)	9.4 (5.4, 15.6)
Total Cholesterol (mmol/l)	5.0 ± 1.1	4.9 ± 1.3	5.08 ± 1.1
Triglycerides (mmol/l) #	1.6 (1.2, 2.2)	1.9 (1.4, 2.8)	1.55 (1.1, 2.2)
HDL-Cholesterol (mol/l)	1.2 ± 0.4	1.1 ± 0.3	1.17 ± 0.4
Calcium (mmol/l)	2.3 ± 0.3	2.3 ± 0.2	2.3 ± 0.3
Albumin (g/l)	38.7 ± 6.7	40.2 ± 5.8	38.4 ± 6.8

Note: Data presented as mean ± standard deviation for normal variables; median (Q1, Q3) for non-normal variables (#) and as frequency (%) for categorical variables ($). BMI, body mass index; BP, blood pressure.

Table 2. Prevalence of metabolic syndrome (MetS) components in tertiles of T-score (spine) according to sex.

	All (N = 1587)				Males (N = 243)				Females (N = 1344)			
T-Score (L1–L4 Spine)	T1	T2	T3	p	T1	T2	T3	p	T1	T2	T3	p
Central Obesity	66.9	79.8	82.7	<0.01	38.3	60.5	71.6	<0.01	72.1	83.4	84.7	<0.01
Hyperglycemia	69.9	73.8	74.0	0.25	86.4	80.2	91.4	0.12	66.9	72.7	70.8	0.16
Low HDL-Cholesterol	63.0	64.6	68.5	0.17	40.7	45.7	42.0	0.80	67.1	68.1	73.3	0.09
Hypertriglyceridemia	40.3	46.2	47.7	0.04	54.3	58.0	64.2	0.43	37.7	44.0	44.6	0.07
Hypertension	29.3	32.5	34.4	0.20	38.3	35.8	39.5	0.88	27.6	31.9	33.5	0.15
Full MetS	56.1	63.3	67.6	<0.01	50.6	60.5	71.6	0.02	57.1	64.4	65.8	0.003

Note: Data presented as frequency (%) for the components of MetS and full MetS. T1, T2 and T3 are the three tertiles of T-score (spine) whose respective values as median (Q1, Q3) are −2.70 (−3.1, −2.4), −1.65 (−1.9, −1.3) and −0.30 (−0.7, 0.4) for all participants; −2.20 (−2.7, −1.7), 0.80 (−1.2, −0.5) and 0.55 (0.1, 1.1) for males; −2.80 (−3.2, −2.5), −1.70 (−2.0, −1.5) and −0.40 (−0.8, 0.2) for females. Chi-squared test was used to check the differences of frequencies in different tertiles of T-score. $p < 0.05$ was considered significant. HDL, high density lipoprotein.

Figure 1 shows the average T-score (spine) in individuals with one or more MetS components in males and females. A statistically significant trend was observed in both sexes with average T-score values increasing with increasing MetS components and this remained so even after multiple adjustments.

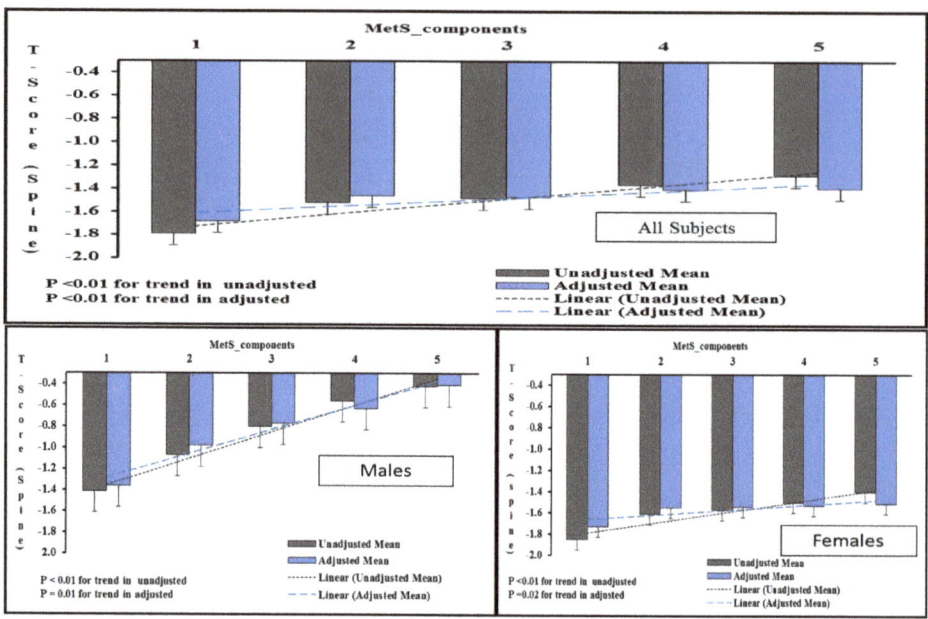

Figure 1. Increasing T-score (spine) values with increasing MetS components according to sex. Note: The figure shows the average T-score (spine) in participants with 1 or more MetS components. The data was generated by univariate analysis by taking T-score (spine) values as dependent variables and "number of components" as factors. The values were adjusted for age, BMI and other risk factors associated with bone loss. $p < 0.05$ was considered as significant.

3.3. Association of T-score with Different Components of MetS and Full MetS.

Table 3 shows the results of a multinomial regression analysis done using T-score (spine) tertiles as dependent variables (with lowest tertile as reference) and different components of MetS as factors. The results are shown as odds ratio (95% confidence interval) and respective *p*-values representing odds of having different components of metabolic syndrome with different tertiles of T-score. The odds of having full MetS increased significantly from lowest tertile to the highest tertile of T-score in all participants (OR (95% CI) of tertile 2 and 3 at 1.55 (1.2 to 2.0) and 1.57 (1.2 to 2.0), *p* (trend) < 0.01 as well as in both males and females (1.49 (0.8 to 2.8) and 2.46 (1.3 to 4.7), *p* (trend) = 0.02 in males and 1.35 (1.0 to 1.7) and 1.45 (1.1 to 1.9), *p* < 0.01 in females) and the odds ratio remained statistically significant even after multiple adjustments with age, BMI and other risk factors associated with bone loss. Among the components of MetS, the odds of hyperglycemia and hypertriglyceridemia increased significantly with T-score tertiles when unadjusted only in all participants, however, the association lost significance after adjusting with confounders. This association was not significant when the data was divided according to sexes. Only the odds of central obesity as a component of MetS increased significantly with T-score tertiles in univariate as well as adjusted models, and this trend was seen when investigated in all participants as well as when the data were divided into different sexes.

Table 3. Odds ratio of full metabolic syndrome and its components at different tertile of T-score (spine) according to sex.

MODEL	ALL				MALES				FEMALES			
	TERTILE			p	TERTILE			p	TERTILE			p
	1	2	3		1	2	3		1	2	3	
CENTRAL OBESITY												
a	1	1.96 (1.5–2.6)	2.37 (1.8–3.2)	<0.01	1	2.47 (1.3–4.6)	4.07 (2.1–7.9)	<0.01	1.0	1.94 (1.4–2.7)	2.14 (1.5–2.9)	<0.01
b	1	1.95 (1.5–2.6)	2.44 (1.8–2.3)	<0.01	1	2.58 (1.4–4.9)	4.23 (2.2–8.3)	<0.01	1.0	1.95 (1.4–2.7)	2.21 (1.6–3.1)	<0.01
c	1	1.98 (1.4–2.6)	2.24 (1.6–3.1)	<0.01	1	1.94 (0.8–4.6)	3.06 (1.3–7.4)	0.04	1.0	2.01 (1.4–2.8)	2.27 (1.6–3.3)	<0.01
d	1	1.88 (1.4–2.5)	2.21 (1.6–3.0)	<0.01	1	1.97 (0.8–4.7)	2.95 (1.2–7.1)	0.04	1.0	1.82 (1.3–2.5)	1.98 (1.4–2.8)	<0.01
e	1	1.90 (1.4–2.5)	2.20 (1.6–3.0)	<0.01	1	2.00 (0.8–4.8)	3.07 (1.2–7.5)	0.04	1.0	1.83 (1.3–2.6)	1.97 (1.4–2.8)	<0.01
HYPERGLYCEMIA												
a	1	1.21 (0.9–1.6)	1.23 (0.9–1.6)	0.25	1	0.64 (0.3–1.5)	1.66 (0.6–4.5)	0.12	1.0	1.32 (1.0–1.8)	1.20 (0.9–1.6)	0.16
b	1	1.32 (1.0–1.7)	1.54 (1.2–2.1)	0.01	1	0.82 (0.3–1.9)	2.25 (0.8–6.4)	0.10	1.0	1.40 (1.0–1.9)	1.47 (1.1–2.0)	0.02
c	1	1.28 (1.0–1.8)	1.34 (1.2–2.2)	0.04	1	0.71 (0.3–1.8)	1.71 (0.6–5.1)	0.21	1.0	1.32 (1.0–1.8)	1.44 (1.1–2.0)	0.05
d	1	1.18 (0.9–1.6)	1.29 (0.9–1.7)	0.23	1	0.66 (0.3–1.7)	1.59 (0.5–4.8)	0.24	1.0	1.25 (0.9–1.7)	1.26 (0.9–1.7)	0.29
e	1	1.17 (0.9–1.6)	1.15 (0.8–1.6)	0.57	1	0.62 (0.2–1.7)	1.58 (0.5–5.1)	0.26	1.0	1.25 (0.9–1.7)	1.21 (0.8–1.6)	0.41
LOW HDL-CHOLESTEROL												
a	1	1.07 (0.8–1.4)	1.28 (1.0–1.6)	0.16	1	1.22 (0.6–2.3)	1.05 (0.6–1.9)	0.80	1.0	1.05 (0.8–1.4)	1.35 (1.0–1.8)	0.09
b	1	1.08 (0.8–1.4)	1.32 (1.0–1.7)	0.11	1	1.43 (0.8–2.7)	1.20 (0.6–2.3)	0.55	1.0	1.05 (0.8–1.4)	1.38 (1.0–1.9)	0.08
c	1	1.05 (0.9–1.6)	1.30 (1.0–1.9)	0.32	1	1.19 (0.6–2.3)	1.01 (0.5–1.9)	0.84	1.0	1.02 (0.8–1.4)	1.29 (0.9–1.8)	0.21
d	1	0.96 (0.7–1.2)	1.13 (0.9–1.5)	0.46	1	1.20 (0.6–2.4)	0.90 (0.4–1.8)	0.69	1.0	0.94 (0.7–1.3)	1.30 (0.9–1.7)	0.21
e	1	0.96 (0.7–1.3)	1.15 (0.9–1.5)	0.39	1	1.17 (0.6–2.4)	0.82 (0.4–1.7)	0.59	1.0	0.94 (0.7–1.3)	1.24 (0.9–1.7)	0.18
HYPERTRIGLYCERIDEMIA												
a	1	1.27 (1.0–1.6)	1.35 (1.1–1.7)	0.04	1	1.16 (0.6–2.2)	1.51 (0.8–2.8)	0.43	1.0	1.30 (1.0–1.7)	1.34 (1.0–1.7)	0.06
b	1	1.29 (1.0–1.7)	1.42 (1.1–1.8)	0.02	1	1.25 (0.7–2.4)	1.62 (0.8–3.1)	0.34	1.0	1.30 (1.0–1.7)	1.34 (1.0–1.8)	0.07
c	1	1.25 (1.0–1.7)	1.29 (1.2–1.9)	0.04	1	1.18 (0.6–2.3)	1.47 (0.8–2.9)	0.51	1.0	1.20 (0.9–1.6)	1.24 (0.9–1.7)	0.29
d	1	1.18 (0.9–1.5)	1.22 (0.9–1.6)	0.30	1	1.24 (0.6–2.4)	1.38 (0.7–2.7)	0.64	1.0	1.16 (0.9–1.5)	1.13 (0.8–1.5)	0.56
e	1	1.17 (0.9–1.7)	1.15 (0.9–1.5)	0.46	1	1.16 (0.6–2.3)	1.47 (0.7–2.9)	0.56	1.0	1.16 (0.9–1.5)	1.07 (0.8–1.5)	0.61
HYPERTENSION												
a	1	1.16 (0.9–1.5)	1.27 (1.0–1.6)	0.20	1	0.90 (0.5–1.7)	1.05 (0.6–1.9)	0.88	1.0	1.23 (0.9–1.6)	1.32 (1.0–1.8)	0.15
b	1	1.12 (0.9–1.6)	1.45 (0.9–1.9)	0.06	1	1.07 (0.5–2.1)	1.25 (0.6–2.4)	0.80	1.0	1.27 (0.9–1.7)	1.45 (1.1–1.9)	0.05
c	1	1.20 (0.9–1.7)	1.32 (1.0–1.9)	0.21	1	0.95 (0.5–1.9)	1.10 (0.6–2.2)	0.91	1.0	1.24 (0.9–1.7)	1.37 (1.0–1.9)	0.13
d	1	1.10 (0.8–1.4)	1.24 (0.9–1.6)	0.33	1	0.93 (0.5–1.8)	1.16 (0.6–2.3)	0.79	1.0	1.11 (0.8–1.5)	1.24 (0.9–1.7)	0.40
e	1	1.10 (0.8–1.4)	1.20 (0.9–1.6)	0.50	1	0.90 (0.4–1.8)	1.16 (0.6–2.4)	0.77	1.0	1.11 (0.8–1.5)	1.19 (0.9–1.6)	0.56
FULL METS												
a	1	1.55 (1.2–2.0)	1.57 (1.2–2.0)	<0.01	1	1.49 (0.8–2.8)	2.46 (1.3–4.7)	0.02	1.0	1.35 (1.0–1.7)	1.45 (1.1–1.9)	<0.01
b	1	1.61 (1.2–2.1)	1.74 (1.3–2.3)	<0.01	1	1.82 (0.9–3.5)	3.05 (1.5–6.0)	<0.01	1.0	1.53 (1.2–2.0)	1.59 (1.2–2.1)	<0.01
c	1	1.54 (1.1–2.0)	1.62 (1.2–2.2)	<0.01	1	1.31 (0.6–2.7)	2.10 (1.1–4.4)	0.03	1.0	1.48 (1.1–2.0)	1.48 (1.1–2.0)	<0.01
e	1	1.59 (1.2–2.1)	1.63 (1.2–2.2)	<0.01	1	1.29 (0.6–2.5)	2.12 (1.1–4.6)	0.03	1.0	1.46 (1.1–2.0)	1.47 (1.1–2.0)	<0.01

Note: Data presented as odds ratio (95% confidence interval) (OR (95% CI)) and respective p-values representing odds of having different components of metabolic syndrome at higher tertiles of T-score (spine) compared to the lowest tertile. MetS is full metabolic syndrome; Ref is reference; Ter1, 2 and 3 are different tertiles of T-score. The data was generated by multinomial regression taking T-score tertiles as dependent variables and MetS and its components (present versus absent) as factors. Model "a" is univariate. All other models are additionally adjusted for age (model "b"), BMI (model "c"), all other MetS components (model "d") and risk factors associated with bone loss like family history of diabetes, osteoporosis, arthritis, whether or not suffering from T2DM, thyroid disease, history of broken bones, etc. (model "e"). For full MetS, model "d" is excluded as it is a combination of these five components. $p < 0.05$ is considered significant.

Figure 2 shows the odds ratio and its associated 95% confidence interval of different components of MetS in higher tertiles of T-score (spine) compared with the lowest tertile.

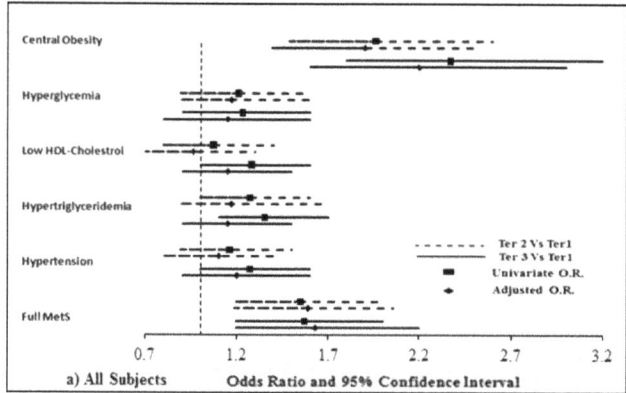
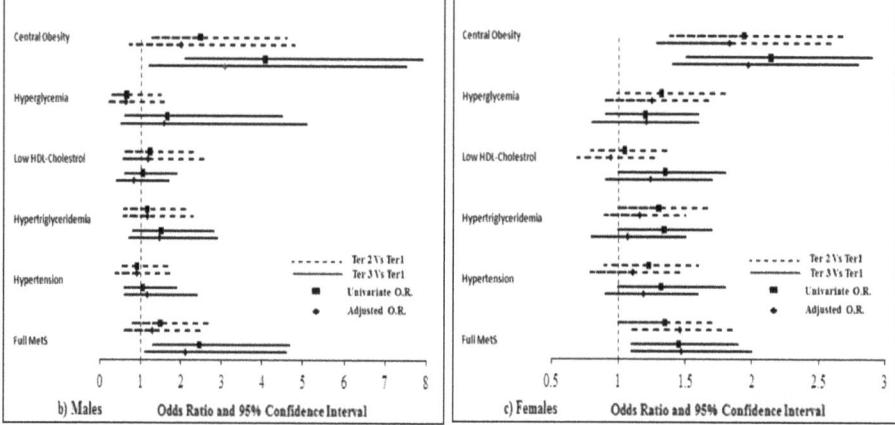

Figure 2. Odds of having full MetS and its components in individuals with higher tertiles of T-score (spine) compared with lowest tertile. Note: The figure shows the odds ratio (OR) and 95% confidence interval representing odds of having different components of metabolic syndrome at higher tertiles of T-score (spine) compared to the lowest tertile. The data was generated by multinomial regression taking T-score tertiles as dependent variables and MetS and its components (present versus absent) as factors. Unadjusted OR; and OR adjusted for age, BMI and risk factors associated with bone loss like family history of diabetes, osteoporosis, arthritis, whether or not suffering from T2DM, thyroid disease, history of broken bones, etc., are represented here.

4. Discussion

The current population-based study aimed to investigate the relationship between MetS and its components with the BMD of the spine. The main novelty of the study is that it is the first large-scale investigation on the association of MetS and BMD in a homogenous Arab ethnic group. This is clinically relevant since it is well established that bone health and risk for certain chronic conditions are influenced by genetics and environment. Several inconsistencies in associations have been found in other studies and one of the main reasons is the differences in population. The study fills this gap as it has never been investigated in this region; a well-structured logistic regression model with multiple adjustments for risk factors associated with bone loss differentiates this study from others on a similar topic. In this study, the authors found a significant positive association of full MetS with BMD spine and this association was independent of sex. The odds ratio of having full MetS, as revealed by logistic regression analysis, increased significantly from the lowest T-score tertile to the highest one and the odds remained significant even after adjustment with multiple confounders and the trend revealed similar association across both sexes. This significant positive association of MetS with BMD seemed to be driven by central obesity as all other components of MetS showed little or no association with increasing tertiles of T-score.

Many recent studies in varied populations were conducted to investigate the associations between MetS, BMD, osteoporosis and fractures. In these studies, the difference in MetS selection criteria, difference in the bone site used to calculate BMD like femoral neck, lumbar spine etc., or the difference in osteoporotic fractures and non-vertebral fractures, played a role in these associations, yet the overall picture of the relationship remains blurred. In one of the earliest studies by Muhlen et al. [17], significantly lower BMD at total hip was associated with MetS in age-adjusted models. Also, in a report by Hwang et al. [18], vertebral BMD was found to be significantly lower in women with MetS compared to non-MetS. Similarly, Jeon et al. [19] suggested higher BMD at the lumbar spine and femoral neck in post-menopausal women with MetS. The results from these studies are in conflict with the present study where a significant positive association was seen between MetS and lumbar BMD. The difference might be because of the lower prevalence of MetS in these studies [17–19] (20.9%, 20.7% and 9.0%, respectively) than the present study (62.3%), suggesting that the participants recruited in these studies were healthier than the current study group. Also, the study participants used by Muhlen et al. were much older than our study (mean age of 74.2 and 74.4 years in men and women, respectively, compared to 58.1 and 56.4 years in this study). The results in the current study are in line with some of the earlier reports [20–22] which suggest women with MetS have a significantly higher BMD than those without MetS. A meta-analysis of a total of 11 studies including 13,122 participants [23] revealed a significant overall association between MetS and increased BMD of spine, in concordance with the present study results.

The present study results of the positive association of full MetS with BMD spine seem to be driven by the component of central obesity as only this component predominantly follows the same pattern in its relationship with BMD spine as the full MetS (Table 3). A positive association of central obesity with BMD at all sites was reported first by Edelstein et al. [24] and since then BMI has been reported as a protective factor against bone loss as concluded by a meta-analysis of 12 studies including 60,000 participants [9]. However, as a flipside to this story, some studies advocate that increased obesity is correlated to low bone mass [25,26]. This paradox in the nature of this relationship of obesity with bone health may be explained by the heterogeneous role of obesity. On one hand higher waist circumference used to calculate central obesity as a component of MetS is associated with higher 17 beta-estradiol levels which may protect bone [27], while on the other hand, intra-abdominal fat or visceral fat may lead to increased bone resorption and hence lower BMD because of its association with pro-inflammatory cytokines [28,29]. Heavy weight is indeed one of the consequences since it is well-established that increased mechanical loading conferred by body weight (e.g., increased BMI or being overweight/obese) has a positive effect on bone formation, regardless of other consequences such as increased risk for other chronic health disorders [30].

The association of other components of MetS with BMD, like full MetS, as reported by many studies in the recent past is also inconclusive. In our study, in all participants, hyperglycemia increased significantly with increasing tertiles of T-score in an unadjusted model but lost significance after adjustment with multiple confounders (Table 3). This observation is supported by some of the earlier reports [31,32] which suggest an indirect effect of hyperglycemia through associated hyperinsulinemia on bone formation, as interaction between insulin, insulin like growth factor-1 and parathyroid hormone has been proposed to have an anabolic effect on bone cells [33]. At the same time, however, long-term diabetes has consistently been shown to be detrimental for bone health and associated fractures [10,34]. A direct effect of hyperglycemia and hyperinsulinemia on bone health and associated fractures would be interesting to investigate. Also, hypertriglyceridemia in our study increased, in all participants, with increased tertiles of T-score in an unadjusted model but lost significance after adjustment. Elevated triglycerides have been suggested to contribute to the overall improvement of qualitative properties of bone by forming a layer between collagen fibers and mineral crystals [35]. We did not observe a significant relationship between other components of MetS and T-score spine, but the results of some other studies present a conflicting picture [36,37].

In our study, no sexual disparity was observed as far as the relationship of MetS and T-score spine was concerned. In both sexes, a positive correlation was found in this relationship and the odds of having MetS increased significantly with higher tertiles of T-score spine even after multiple adjustments. This relationship seems to be driven by the central obesity component in both sexes. Similar to our observations, a meta-analysis conducted on participants showed no gender differences [23]. In contrast, some studies suggest gender disparity in the relationship between MetS and BMI-adjusted BMD, showing a less beneficial effect in men than women [15]. It is difficult to explain this disparity in different studies; however, an explanation might be in the age group of the study participants (e.g., the study that suggests gender differences in the relationship between MetS and BMD was conducted in much younger participants than ours (mean age 56.7 years) and it has been shown that BMD overall decreases as age progresses and the rate of decline in the BMD differs according to sex) [38].

The heterogeneity of the complex relationship between MetS and BMD as seen in various studies before may be explained on the basis of various study-level variables like ethnicity, DXA scanner manufacturer and MetS definition [23]. MetS in Asians may be more influenced by visceral adiposity as compared to Caucasians [39] and hence may explain the positive relationship of MetS and BMD seen in Caucasians rather than Asians. The choice of the DXA scanner used may also play a role in the relationship as the absolute values of BMD differ between instruments from different manufacturers [40]. Also, the differences in the definition of the MetS used in various such studies add to the heterogeneous relationship between MetS and BMD. Abdominal obesity is a necessary factor for the International Diabetes Federation (IDF) criteria of MetS whereas NCEP-ATP III criteria categorizes MetS by having any three of the five components. This difference in MetS definition may dictate the observable positive association of MetS defined by NCEP-ATP III as seen in many studies before including ours rather than when MetS was defined by IDF criteria.

Higher waist circumference (central obesity), is associated with higher 17 β-estradiol levels which is known to improve bone density by inhibiting bone resorption and stimulating bone formation [27]. On the other hand, triglycerides affect osteoblast and osteoclast differentiation, with lower levels associated with osteoporotic bone tissue [41]. Lastly, hyperglycemia and hyperinsulinemia have been demonstrated to exert an anabolic effect on bone cells by interacting insulin-growth factor (IGF)-1 receptors which are known to increase BMD by promoting osteoblast differentiation [42]. It is worthy to note that higher BMD alone cannot account for improved fracture risk since patients with T2DM and those who are obese are still at an increased risk for fragility fractures and associated mortality [43,44]. MetS being a constellation of interconnected physiological, biochemical, clinical and metabolic factors has in itself two contrasting factors: one of which is abdominal obesity known to be protective against osteoporosis and may lead to higher BMD levels [45,46] while at the same time intra-abdominal obesity, hyperglycemia and insulin resistance leads to a low-grade inflammatory state that activates bone resorption [28,47]. This might explain this heterogeneous complex relationship, however, more such studies need to be conducted in different populations to fully elucidate the pathophysiology behind this complexity.

There are several strengths of the current study. First, the sizable study sample of 1587 participants gives this study an edge over many other studies with fewer participants. Secondly, the multi-center recruitment of the study participants used in this study provides a proper representation of a population. Thirdly, this is the first study to report the relationship of MetS with BMD spine in a population with high prevalence of MetS as well as osteoporosis. Apart from these, the use of the most recent definition of MetS, well-calibrated DXA scans performed by a certified bone densitometry technologist and a well-structured logistic regression model analysis adjusted by multiple confounders gave reliable results. The authors, however, acknowledge certain limitations. The cross-sectional nature of this study limits its applicability outside cause and effect of the proposed relationship. A longitudinal study in this population would be interesting to investigate. Some of the biochemical markers that may influence BMD like 25(OH) vitamin D, serum estradiol, follicle stimulating hormone, etc. were not measured in this study. Also, the BMD was measured only at lumbar L–L4 site and hence the proposed relationship with MetS may not hold true for other anatomic sites like femoral neck, total hip, etc.

5. Conclusions

The results of the logistic regression analysis with multiple adjustments conducted in this study suggest a sex-irrespective positive association between MetS and lumbar BMD. The results also suggest that the positive relationship between MetS and lumbar BMD is predominantly driven by the central obesity component of MetS as the rest of the components show little or no association with lumbar BMD, irrespective of sex.

Author Contributions: Conceptualization: K.W., N.M.A.-D., M.S.A., N.J.A.; study execution: K.W., S.M.Y., S.S., Y.A.-S.; sample analysis: K.W., M.G.A.A., E.S.; statistical analysis: K.W., S.D.H.; manuscript writing: K.W.; Manuscript review: N.M.A.-D., S.M.Y., M.G.A.A., S.S., S.D.H., M.S.A., E.S., N.J.A., Y.A.-S., J.-Y.R.

Funding: The authors extend their appreciation to the International Scientific Partnership Program (ISPP) at King Saud University for funding this research through ISPP #0111.

Acknowledgments: The authors would like to thank the research coordinators and nurses at the recruitment centers especially KFMC, KKUH and KSH for their support and technical expertise. Also, the authors thank the CBCD biobank staff, especially Hamza Saber who deserves credit for his meticulous efforts in storing/retrieval of the study samples.

Conflicts of Interest: The authors declare no conflicts of interest. The funders had no role in the design of the study; in the collection, analyses, or interpretation of data; in the writing of the manuscript, or in the decision to publish the results.

References

1. Maiorino, M.; Bellastella, G.; Giugliano, D.; Esposito, K. From inflammation to sexual dysfunctions: A journey through diabetes, obesity, and metabolic syndrome. *J. Endocrinol. Investig.* **2018**, *41*, 1249–12580. [CrossRef] [PubMed]
2. Darroudi, S.; Fereydouni, N.; Tayefi, M.; Ahmadnezhad, M.; Zamani, P.; Tayefi, B.; Kharazmi, J.; Tavalaie, S.; Heidari-Bakavoli, A.; Azarpajouh, M.R. Oxidative stress and inflammation, two features associated with a high percentage body fat, and that may lead to diabetes mellitus and metabolic syndrome. *BioFactors* **2018**, *45*, 35–42. [CrossRef] [PubMed]
3. Al-Nozha, M.; Al-Khadra, A.; Arafah, M.R.; Al-Maatouq, M.A.; Khalil, M.Z.; Khan, N.B.; Al-Mazrou, Y.Y.; Al-Marzouki, K.; Al-Harthi, S.S.; Abdullah, M.; et al. Metabolic syndrome in saudi arabia. *Saudi Med. J.* **2005**, *26*, 1918–1925. [PubMed]
4. Al-Qahtani, D.A.; Imtiaz, M.L. Prevalence of metabolic syndrome in saudi adult soldiers. *Saudi Med. J.* **2005**, *26*, 1360–1366. [PubMed]
5. Prasad, H.; Ryan, D.A.; Celzo, M.F.; Stapleton, D. Metabolic syndrome: Definition and therapeutic implications. *Postgrad. Med.* **2012**, *124*, 21–30. [CrossRef] [PubMed]
6. Kaur, J. A comprehensive review on metabolic syndrome. *Cardiol. Res. Pract.* **2014**, *2014*, 943162. [CrossRef]
7. Huang, P.L. A comprehensive definition for metabolic syndrome. *Dis. Model. Mech.* **2009**, *2*, 231–237. [CrossRef]
8. Wong, S.; Chin, K.-Y.; Suhaimi, F.; Ahmad, F.; Ima-Nirwana, S. The relationship between metabolic syndrome and osteoporosis: A review. *Nutrients* **2016**, *8*, 347. [CrossRef]
9. De Laet, C.; Kanis, J.; Odén, A.; Johansen, H.; Johnell, O.; Delmas, P.; Eisman, J.; Kroger, H.; Fujiwara, S.; Garnero, P. Body mass index as a predictor of fracture risk: A meta-analysis. *Osteoporos. Int.* **2005**, *16*, 1330–1338. [CrossRef]
10. Janghorbani, M.; Van Dam, R.M.; Willett, W.C.; Hu, F.B. Systematic review of type 1 and type 2 diabetes mellitus and risk of fracture. *Am. J. Epidemiol.* **2007**, *166*, 495–505. [CrossRef]

11. Schwartz, A.V.; Vittinghoff, E.; Bauer, D.C.; Hillier, T.A.; Strotmeyer, E.S.; Ensrud, K.E.; Donaldson, M.G.; Cauley, J.A.; Harris, T.B.; Koster, A. Association of bmd and frax score with risk of fracture in older adults with type 2 diabetes. *JAMA* **2011**, *305*, 2184–2192. [CrossRef] [PubMed]
12. Oei, L.; Zillikens, M.C.; Dehghan, A.; Buitendijk, G.H.; Castaño-Betancourt, M.C.; Estrada, K.; Stolk, L.; Oei, E.H.; van Meurs, J.B.; Janssen, J.A. High bone mineral density and fracture risk in type 2 diabetes as skeletal complications of inadequate glucose control: The rotterdam study. *Diabetes Care* **2013**, *36*, 1619–1628. [CrossRef] [PubMed]
13. Sun, K.; Liu, J.; Lu, N.; Sun, H.; Ning, G. Association between metabolic syndrome and bone fractures: A meta-analysis of observational studies. *BMC Endocr. Disord.* **2014**, *14*, 13. [CrossRef] [PubMed]
14. Yamaguchi, T.; Kanazawa, I.; Yamamoto, M.; Kurioka, S.; Yamauchi, M.; Yano, S.; Sugimoto, T. Associations between components of the metabolic syndrome versus bone mineral density and vertebral fractures in patients with type 2 diabetes. *Bone* **2009**, *45*, 174–179. [CrossRef] [PubMed]
15. Kim, H.; Oh, H.J.; Choi, H.; Choi, W.H.; Lim, S.-K.; Kim, J.G. The association between bone mineral density and metabolic syndrome: A Korean population-based study. *J. Bone Miner. Metab.* **2013**, *31*, 571–578. [CrossRef]
16. Al-Daghri, N.M.; Al-Attas, O.S.; Wani, K.; Sabico, S.; Alokail, M.S. Serum uric acid to creatinine ratio and risk of metabolic syndrome in saudi type 2 diabetic patients. *Sci. Rep.* **2017**, *7*, 12104. [CrossRef] [PubMed]
17. Von Muhlen, D.; Safii, S.; Jassal, S.; Svartberg, J.; Barrett-Connor, E. Associations between the metabolic syndrome and bone health in older men and women: The rancho bernardo study. *Osteoporos. Int.* **2007**, *18*, 1337–1344. [CrossRef]
18. Hwang, D.-K.; Choi, H.-J. The relationship between low bone mass and metabolic syndrome in korean women. *Osteoporos. Int.* **2010**, *21*, 425–431. [CrossRef]
19. Jeon, Y.K.; Lee, J.G.; Kim, S.S.; Kim, B.H.; Kim, S.-J.; Kim, Y.K.; Kim, I.J. Association between bone mineral density and metabolic syndrome in pre- and postmenopausal women. *Endocr. J.* **2011**, *58*, 87–93. [CrossRef]
20. Hernández, J.L.; Olmos, J.M.; Pariente, E.; Martínez, J.; Valero, C.; García-Velasco, P.; Nan, D.; Llorca, J.; González-Macías, J. Metabolic syndrome and bone metabolism: The camargo cohort study. *Menopause* **2010**, *17*, 955–961. [CrossRef]
21. El Maghraoui, A.; Rezqi, A.; El Mrahi, S.; Sadni, S.; Ghozlani, I.; Mounach, A. Osteoporosis, vertebral fractures and metabolic syndrome in postmenopausal women. *BMC Endocr. Disord.* **2014**, *14*, 93. [CrossRef] [PubMed]
22. Muka, T.; Trajanoska, K.; Kiefte-de Jong, J.C.; Oei, L.; Uitterlinden, A.G.; Hofman, A.; Dehghan, A.; Zillikens, M.C.; Franco, O.H.; Rivadeneira, F. The association between metabolic syndrome, bone mineral density, hip bone geometry and fracture risk: The Rotterdam study. *PLoS ONE* **2015**, *10*, e0129116. [CrossRef] [PubMed]
23. Xue, P.; Gao, P.; Li, Y. The association between metabolic syndrome and bone mineral density: A meta-analysis. *Endocrine* **2012**, *42*, 546–554. [CrossRef] [PubMed]
24. Edelstein, S.L.; Barrett-Connor, E. Relation between body size and bone mineral density in elderly men and women. *Am. J. Epidemiol.* **1993**, *138*, 160–169. [CrossRef] [PubMed]
25. Jankowska, E.; Rogucka, E.; Mędraś, M. Are general obesity and visceral adiposity in men linked to reduced bone mineral content resulting from normal ageing? A population-based study. *Andrologia* **2001**, *33*, 384–389. [CrossRef] [PubMed]
26. Moon, S.-S.; Lee, Y.-S.; Kim, S.W. Association of nonalcoholic fatty liver disease with low bone mass in postmenopausal women. *Endocrine* **2012**, *42*, 423–429. [CrossRef] [PubMed]
27. Nelson, L.R.; Bulun, S.E. Estrogen production and action. *J. Am. Acad. Dermatol.* **2001**, *45*, S116–S124. [CrossRef]
28. Hofbauer, L.C.; Schoppet, M. Clinical implications of the osteoprotegerin/rankl/rank system for bone and vascular diseases. *JAMA* **2004**, *292*, 490–495. [CrossRef]
29. Campos, R.M.; de Piano, A.; da Silva, P.L.; Carnier, J.; Sanches, P.L.; Corgosinho, F.C.; Masquio, D.C.; Lazaretti-Castro, M.; Oyama, L.M.; Nascimento, C.M. The role of pro/anti-inflammatory adipokines on bone metabolism in nafld obese adolescents: Effects of long-term interdisciplinary therapy. *Endocrine* **2012**, *42*, 146–156. [CrossRef]
30. Cao, J.J. Effects of obesity on bone metabolism. *J. Orthop. Surg. Res.* **2011**, *6*, 30. [CrossRef]

31. Kinjo, M.; Setoguchi, S.; Solomon, D.H. Bone mineral density in adults with the metabolic syndrome: Analysis in a population-based US sample. *J. Clin. Endocrinol. Metab.* **2007**, *92*, 4161–4164. [CrossRef] [PubMed]
32. Holmberg, A.H.; Nilsson, P.; Nilsson, J.-A.; Akesson, K. The association between hyperglycemia and fracture risk in middle age. A prospective, population-based study of 22,444 men and 10,902 women. *J. Clin. Endocrinol. Metab.* **2008**, *93*, 815–822. [CrossRef] [PubMed]
33. Thrailkill, K.M.; Lumpkin, C.K., Jr.; Bunn, R.C.; Kemp, S.F.; Fowlkes, J.L. Is insulin an anabolic agent in bone? Dissecting the diabetic bone for clues. *Am. J. Physiol. -Endocrinol. Metab.* **2005**, *289*, E735–E745. [CrossRef] [PubMed]
34. Ivers, R.Q.; Cumming, R.G.; Mitchell, P.; Peduto, A.J. Diabetes and risk of fracture: The blue mountains eye study. *Diabetes Care* **2001**, *24*, 1198–1203. [CrossRef] [PubMed]
35. Xu, S.; Jianqing, J.Y. Beneath the minerals, a layer of round lipid particles was identified to mediate collagen calcification in compact bone formation. *Biophys. J.* **2006**, *91*, 4221–4229. [CrossRef]
36. Hanley, D.; Brown, J.; Tenenhouse, A.; Olszynski, W.; Ioannidis, G.; Berger, C.; Prior, J.; Pickard, L.; Murray, T.; Anastassiades, T. Associations among disease conditions, bone mineral density, and prevalent vertebral deformities in men and women 50 years of age and older: Cross-sectional results from the canadian multicentre osteoporosis study. *J. Bone Miner. Res.* **2003**, *18*, 784–790. [CrossRef] [PubMed]
37. Mussolino, M.E.; Gillum, R. Bone mineral density and hypertension prevalence in postmenopausal women: Results from the third national health and nutrition examination survey. *Ann. Epidemiol.* **2006**, *16*, 395–399. [CrossRef]
38. Krall, E.A.; Dawson-Hughes, B.; Hirst, K.; Gallagher, J.; Sherman, S.S.; Dalsky, G. Bone mineral density and biochemical markers of bone turnover in healthy elderly men and women. *J. Gerontol. A Biol. Sci. Med. Sci.* **1997**, *52*, M61–M67. [CrossRef]
39. Abate, N.; Chandalia, M. The impact of ethnicity on type 2 diabetes. *J. Diabetes Complicat.* **2003**, *17*, 39–58. [CrossRef]
40. Pocock, N.A.; Noakes, K.A.; Griffiths, M.; Bhalerao, N.; Sambrook, P.N.; Eisman, J.A.; Freund, J. A comparison of longitudinal measurements in the spine and proximal femur using lunar and hologic instruments. *J. Bone Miner. Res.* **1997**, *12*, 2113–2118. [CrossRef]
41. Dragojevič, J.; Zupan, J.; Haring, G.; Herman, S.; Komadina, R.; Marc, J. Triglyceride metabolism in bone tissue is associated with osteoblast and osteoclast differentiation: a gene expression study. *J. Bone Miner. Metab.* **2013**, *31*, 512–519. [CrossRef] [PubMed]
42. Sundararaghavan, V.; Mazur, M.M.; Evans, B.; Liu, J.; Ebraheim, N.A. Diabetes and bone health: Latest evidence and clinical implications. *Ther. Adv. Musculoskelet. Dis.* **2017**, *9*, 67–74. [CrossRef] [PubMed]
43. Komorita, Y.; Iwase, M.; Idewaki, Y.; Fujii, H.; Ohkuma, T.; Ide, H.; Jodai, K.T.; Yoshinari, M.; Murao, K.A.; Oku, Y. Impact of hip fracture on all-cause mortality in Japanese patients with type 2 diabetes mellitus: The Fukuoka Diabetes Registry. *J. Diabetes Investig.* **2019**. [CrossRef] [PubMed]
44. Tencerova, M.; Frost, M.; Figeac, F.; Nielsen, T.K.; Ali, D.; Lauterlein, J.-J.L.; Andersen, T.L.; Haakonsson, A.K.; Rauch, A.; Madsen, J.S. Obesity-Associated Hypermetabolism and Accelerated Senescence of Bone Marrow Stromal Stem Cells Suggest a Potential Mechanism for Bone Fragility. *Cell Rep.* **2019**, *27*, 2050–2062. [CrossRef] [PubMed]
45. Guh, D.P.; Zhang, W.; Bansback, N.; Amarsi, Z.; Birmingham, C.L.; Anis, A.H. The incidence of co-morbidities related to obesity and overweight: A systematic review and meta-analysis. *BMC Public Health* **2009**, *9*, 88. [CrossRef] [PubMed]
46. Salamat, M.R.; Salamat, A.H.; Janghorbani, M. Association between obesity and bone mineral density by gender and menopausal status. *Endocrinol. Metab.* **2016**, *31*, 547–558. [CrossRef] [PubMed]
47. Smith, B.; Lerner, M.; Bu, S.; Lucas, E.; Hanas, J.; Lightfoot, S.; Postier, R.; Bronze, M.; Brackett, D. Systemic bone loss and induction of coronary vessel disease in a rat model of chronic inflammation. *Bone* **2006**, *38*, 378–386. [CrossRef] [PubMed]

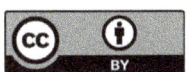

© 2019 by the authors. Licensee MDPI, Basel, Switzerland. This article is an open access article distributed under the terms and conditions of the Creative Commons Attribution (CC BY) license (http://creativecommons.org/licenses/by/4.0/).

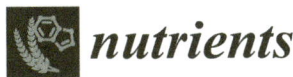

Review

Sugar-Sweetened Beverages and Cardiometabolic Health: An Update of the Evidence

Vasanti S. Malik [1,2,*] and Frank B. Hu [2,3,4]

1. Department of Nutritional Sciences, Faculty of Medicine, University of Toronto, 1 King's College Circle, Toronto, ON M5S 1A8, Canada
2. Department of Nutrition, Harvard T.H. Chan School of Public Health, 665 Huntington Avenue, Boston, MA 02115, USA
3. Department of Epidemiology, Harvard T.H. School of Public Health, Boston, MA 02115, USA
4. Channing Division of Network Medicine, Brigham and Women's Hospital and Harvard Medical School, Boston, MA 02115, USA
* Correspondence: vasanti.malik@utoronto.ca; Tel.: +416-978-5556; Fax: +416-978-5882

Received: 8 July 2019; Accepted: 6 August 2019; Published: 8 August 2019

Abstract: Sugar-sweetened beverages (SSBs) have little nutritional value and a robust body of evidence has linked the intake of SSBs to weight gain and risk of type 2 diabetes (T2D), cardiovascular disease (CVD), and some cancers. Metabolic Syndrome (MetSyn) is a clustering of risk factors that precedes the development of T2D and CVD; however, evidence linking SSBs to MetSyn is not clear. To make informed recommendations about SSBs, new evidence needs to be considered against existing literature. This review provides an update on the evidence linking SSBs and cardiometabolic outcomes including MetSyn. Findings from prospective cohort studies support a strong positive association between SSBs and weight gain and risk of T2D and coronary heart disease (CHD), independent of adiposity. Associations with MetSyn are less consistent, and there appears to be a sex difference with stroke with greater risk in women. Findings from short-term trials on metabolic risk factors provide mechanistic support for associations with T2D and CHD. Conclusive evidence from cohort studies and trials on risk factors support an etiologic role of SSB in relation to weight gain and risk of T2D and CHD. Continued efforts to reduce intake of SSB should be encouraged to improve the cardiometabolic health of individuals and populations.

Keywords: sugar-sweetened beverages; metabolic syndrome; weight gain; type 2 diabetes; cardiovascular disease; cardiometabolic risk

1. Introduction

Metabolic syndrome (MetSyn) is known as a clustering of interrelated risk factors for type 2 diabetes (T2D) and cardiovascular disease (CVD) that occur together more often than by chance alone. Although there is some confusion regarding the clinical definition of MetSyn and whether it is a unique syndrome or a mixture of unrelated phenotypes, the most widespread consensus for a diagnosis is the presence of at least three of five risk factors including hyperglycemia, raised blood pressure, elevated triglyceride levels, low high-density lipoprotein cholesterol levels, and central adiposity [1]. Given the complexity of the definition, the prevalence of MetSyn is difficult to estimate; however, data on individual risk factors suggest that MetSyn is rising across the globe in parallel with obesity trends. It was estimated that 23% of adults in the United States (US) (~50 million) have MetSyn [2,3]. This figure was relatively constant over recent years despite population-level increases in hyperglycemia and waist circumference because of decreases in hypertriglyceridemia and elevated blood pressure corresponding to medication use [4]. However, the burden of MetSyn remains high in the US and is rising in low- and middle-income countries (LMICs) [3]. This is of great concern, since individuals with MetSyn are at twice the risk of developing CVD and have a five-fold higher risk of developing T2D over the next 5–10 years [1]. Preventing or reversing MetSyn could, therefore, be an effective way to stem the rising tide of T2D and CVD.

Sugar-sweetened beverages (SSBs) are the largest source of added sugar in the diet. They include carbonated and non-carbonated soft drinks, fruit drinks, and sports drinks that contain added caloric sweeteners, and they are low in nutritional quality. To date, a large body of evidence supports a strong link between intake of SSBs and weight gain [5] and risk of T2D [6], which is the basis of many dietary guidelines and policies targeting SSBs [7]. Emerging evidence suggests that SSBs are also an important risk factor for cardiovascular diseases and related risk factors [8–12]. However, evidence linking SSBs to MetSyn is not clear. For clinicians and policy-makers to make informed recommendations about SSBs and cardiometabolic health, new evidence needs to be considered alongside existing literature. In this review, we provide an overview of global SSB intake trends and an updated summary on the evidence from prospective cohort studies and trials linking SSBs to weight gain and related cardiometabolic conditions including MetSyn. Findings from cross-sectional or case-control studies were not considered since these designs are more prone to confounding and other biases. Biological mechanisms, alternative beverage options, and policy strategies to limit SSB consumption are also discussed.

2. SSB Intake Trends

Consumption of SSBs has decreased modestly in the US since around 2002 [13]; however, intake levels are still high and, in some groups, nearly exceed the Dietary Guidelines for Americans' [14] and World Health Organization's (WHO) [7] recommendation for no more than 10% of daily calories from all added sugar. National Health and Nutrition Examination Survey (NHANES) data show that US adults consumed an average of 145 kcal/day from SSB, corresponding to 6.5% of total calories, between 2011 and 2014 with higher intake levels reported among younger age groups and among non-Hispanic black and Hispanic men and women [15].

In contrast to the US and other high-income countries where consumption of SSBs is either declining or plateauing, intake of SSBs is increasing in many LMICs as a consequence of widespread urbanization and beverage marketing. A report based on survey data from adults in 187 countries found that SSB consumption was higher in upper–middle-income countries and lower–middle-income countries compared to high-income or low-income countries [16]. Of the 21 world regions evaluated, SSB consumption was highest in the Caribbean and lowest in East Asia [16]. Another study among adolescents in 53 LMICs found that soda intake was most frequent in Central and South America, and least frequent in Southeast Asia. Across all populations surveyed, 54% consumed soda at least once a day, and one in five adolescents in Central and South America consumed soda three or more times per day [17]. These trends are supported by another study that reported that per capita sales of SSB (in daily calories per person) increased in most LMICs, while sales declined in some high-income regions, indicative of consumption patterns [18]. Chile was identified as having the highest per capita sales of SSB in 2014, followed by Mexico, the US, Argentina, and Saudi Arabia [18]. The fastest growth in sales of SSB between 2009 and 2014 was seen in Chile, along with China, Thailand, and Brazil [18] (Figure 1). For some regions, disparities in SSB intake tend to track with disparities in obesity and T2D prevalence. For example, in the US, lower socioeconomic status (SES) groups tend to have higher SSB intake levels, and these groups also tend to have a higher risk for developing obesity and T2D.

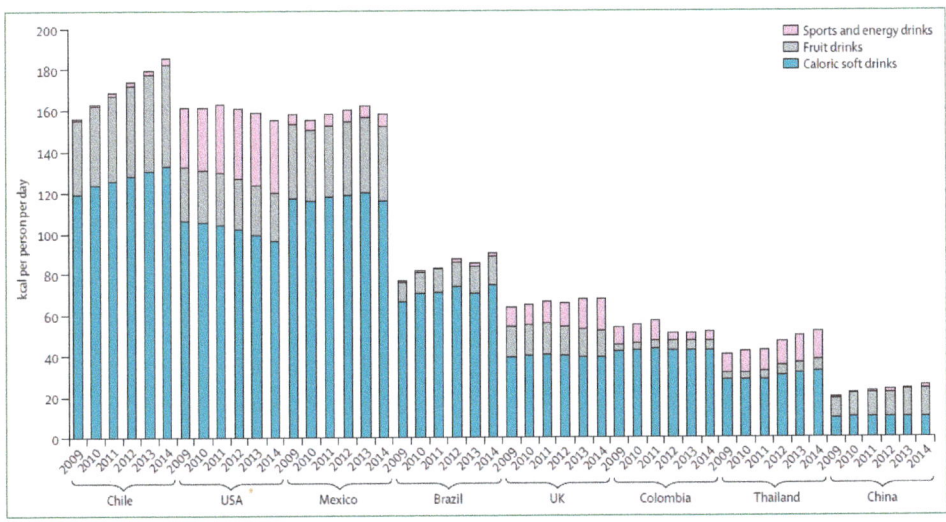

Figure 1. Sales of sugar-sweetened beverages (SSBs) in kcal per person per day by beverage type in 2009–2014 in selected countries. Data from Euromonitor Passport International, which were obtained from nutrition fact panels and websites of sugar-sweetened beverage companies; kcal = kilocalories [18].

3. Weight Gain and Obesity

Many observational studies have evaluated the relationship between consumption of SSBs and weight gain or obesity. The majority [5,19–23] of systematic reviews and meta-analyses on this topic found positive associations between SSBs and weight gain or risk of overweight or obesity. However, others reported null associations [24]. Our previous meta-analysis, the most comprehensive to date, found that a one-serving-per-day increase in SSB was associated with an additional weight gain of 0.12 kg over one year [5]. In this analysis, we included estimates that were not adjusted for total energy intake since the association between SSBs and weight gain is likely mediated through calories. In addition, all of the studies included in the meta-analysis had repeated measurements of diet and weight, and evaluated weight change in relation to change in SSB intake. This type of analysis strategy has some of the features of a quasi-experimental design, although it lacks the element of randomization. An advantage of this design is the generalizability to a real-world setting, because participants are able to change their diet and lifestyle without investigator-driven intervention. Although the results of the meta-analysis seem modest, adult weight gain in the general population is a gradual process, occurring over decades and averaging about one pound (0.45 kg) per year [25]; thus, small gains in weight from SSBs could be substantial over many years.

The association between SSBs and obesity is strengthened by our previous analysis of gene–SSB interactions [26]. Based on data from three large cohorts, we found that individuals who consumed one or more servings of SSB per day had genetic effects on body mass index (BMI) and obesity risk that were twice as large as those who consumed SSBs less than once per month. These data suggest that regular consumers of SSB may be more susceptible to genetic effects on obesity, or that persons with a greater genetic predisposition to obesity may be more susceptible to the deleterious effects of SSBs on BMI.

Compared to observational studies, most trials have evaluated short-term effects on weight change rather than long-term patterns. In our previous meta-analysis of five trials, we found that adding SSBs to the diet significantly increased body weight [5]. Another meta-analysis of seven randomized controlled trials (RCTs) also found a significant increase in body weight when SSBs were added to the diet [24]. However, in their meta-analysis of eight trials attempting to reduce SSB intake, no overall effect on BMI was observed, but a significant benefit on weight loss/less weight gain was observed among individuals who were overweight at baseline [24]. Of note, this meta-analysis included two of the largest and most rigorously conducted RCTs in children and adolescents [27,28] to date.

Another meta-analysis evaluating the effects of dietary sugars on body weight found that, in trials of adults with ad libitum diets, reducing intake of free sugar or SSB was associated with a decrease in body weight, while increasing intake was associated with a comparable weight increase [23]. Because isoenergetic exchange of dietary sugars with other carbohydrates showed no change in body weight, it seems likely that the change in body weight that occurs with modifying intakes of SSBs is mediated via changes in calories [23]. The majority of studies on SSBs and body weight focused on prevention of weight gain rather than weight loss, which is an important distinguishing factor. From a public health point of view, identifying determinants of weight gain is more impactful than short-term weight loss in reducing obesity prevalence [29]. This is because, once an individual develops obesity, it is difficult to achieve and maintain weight loss. For this reason, fewer studies have evaluated the impact of SSB restriction on weight loss.

4. Metabolic Syndrome and Risk Factors

Few prospective studies have examined intake of SSBs in relation to the development of MetSyn, most likely due to challenges in outcome assessment. However, these along with studies of individual risk factors generally show adverse associations that are consistent with studies linking SSBs to weight gain and risk of T2D. Our previous meta-analysis of three cohort studies found a higher risk of about 20% (relative risk (RR), 1.20; 95% confidence interval (CI), 1.02–1.42) comparing highest to lowest categories of SSB intake [6]. However, a recent meta-analysis of three cohort studies by Narain et al. found a marginal positive association between intake of SSB and risk of MetSyn [30]. The discrepancy may be due to inclusion of different studies. The more recent meta-analysis included a new study among children and adolescents [31], which was combined with studies in adults and excluded a study from the Multi-Ethnic Study of Atherosclerosis (MESA) cohort [32], which we included. We also included the cohort-wide estimate from the Framingham Heart study that combined diet and regular soft drinks, while Narain et al. used an estimate from a sub-group with regular soft drink consumption but limited power [33]. Recent studies not included in these meta-analyses have also found positive associations. A study in the Prevención con Dieta Mediterránea (PREDIMED) trial found a positive association between SSBs and fruit juice with MetSyn among participants at high risk for CVD, but cautioned that associations should be interpreted conservatively due to low intake levels [34]. In a cohort of healthy Korean adults, a positive association between SSB and MetSyn was observed in women but not men [35]. According to the authors, the sex difference could be due to the action of sex hormones. Some studies of MetSyn found marginal associations with SSBs; however, because they adjusted for total energy intake, the results may have been underestimated [32,36].

Studies examining individual risk factors rather than MetSyn tend to be more consistent. In the Coronary Artery Risk Development in Young Adults (CARDIA) study, higher SSB consumption was associated with a number of cardiometabolic outcomes: high waist circumference (RR: 1.09; 95% CI 1.04, 1.14), high low-density lipoprotein (LDL) cholesterol (RR: 1.18; 95% CI 1.02, 1.35), high triglycerides (RR: 1.06; 95% CI 1.01, 1.13), and hypertension (RR: 1.06; 95% CI 1.01, 1.12) [37]. Although central adiposity is a risk factor for CVD independent of body weight, few cohort studies have examined this relationship with SSBs, likely due to challenges in measurement. In the Mexican Teacher's cohort, compared to no change, increasing soda consumption by one serving per day was associated with a ~1-cm increase in waist circumference (0.9 cm; 95% CI = 0.5, 1.4) over two years [38]. Similar findings were observed in a Spanish cohort [39]. Both of these studies used waist circumference as a proxy for central adiposity. However, waist circumference does not distinguish between different types of abdominal fat accumulation, e.g., visceral vs. subcutaneous adipose tissues, which may be differently associated with cardiometabolic risk. In the Framingham Third Generation cohort, Ma and colleagues found that SSB intake was associated with a long-term adverse change in visceral adiposity as measured by abdominal computed tomography scan (i.e., increased visceral adipose tissue (VAT) volume and decrease in VAT attenuation), independent of weight gain [40].

In a systematic review including five prospective cohort studies examining SSB intake in relation to vascular risk factors, positive associations were observed for blood pressure, triglycerides, LDL cholesterol, and blood glucose, and an inverse association was observed for high-density lipoprotein (HDL) cholesterol [12]. These findings were supported by cross-sectional analyses in the Health Professionals Follow-up Study (HPFS) and Nurses' Health Study (NHS) cohorts that found associations between SSB and higher plasma triglycerides, along with inflammatory cytokines and other cardiometabolic risk factors [9,41]. Accumulating evidence also suggests a role of SSBs in the development of hypertension [42–44]. A meta-analysis of six cohort studies found that a one serving/day increase in SSB intake was associated with ~8% higher risk of hypertension (RR: 1.08, 95% CI: 1.06, 1.11) [42]. Similar results were reported in two previous meta-analyses [43,44]. Regular consumption of SSBs was also associated with hyperuricemia and with gout [45,46].

Findings from short-term trials and experimental studies also provide important evidence linking SSBs with cardiometabolic risk factors, and they provide mechanistic support for the epidemiologic evidence linking intake of SSBs to higher risk of T2D and coronary heart disease (CHD). Many of these studies explored the effects of sugars used to flavor SSBs such as high-fructose corn syrup (HFCS) (~42–55% fructose, glucose and water) or sucrose (50% fructose and glucose) in liquid form. A meta-analysis of 39 RCTs found that higher compared to lower intakes of dietary sugars or SSB significantly raised triglyceride concentrations (mean difference (MD): 0.11 mmol/L; 95% CI: 0.07, 0.15), total cholesterol (MD: 0.16 mmol/L; 95% CI: 0.10, 0.24), LDL cholesterol (MD: 0.12 mmol/L; 95% CI: 0.05, 0.19), and HDL cholesterol (MD: 0.02 mmol/L; 95% CI: 0.00, 0.03) [47]. The most pronounced effects were noted in studies that ensured energy balance and when no difference in weight change was reported, suggesting that the effects of SSBs on lipids are independent of body weight [47]. This meta-analysis also found a significant blood-pressure-raising effect of sugars, particularly in studies ≥8 weeks in duration (MD 6.9 mm Hg (95% CI: 3.4, 10.3) for systolic blood pressure, and 5.6 mm Hg (95% CI: 2.5, 8.8) for diastolic blood pressure) [47].

In a two-week parallel-arm trial, Stanhope and colleagues showed that consuming beverages containing 10%, 17.5%, or 25% of energy requirements from HFCS produced a significant linear dose–response increase in postprandial triglycerides, fasting LDL cholesterol, and 24-h mean uric acid concentrations [48]. In another study, uric acid was found to increase after six months of consuming 1 L/day of sucrose-sweetened cola compared to isocaloric consumption of milk, water, or diet beverages [49]. The change in uric acid correlated with changes in liver fat ($p = 0.005$), triglycerides ($p = 0.02$), and insulin ($p = 0.002$) [49] In a 10-week trial among overweight healthy participants, consuming a sucrose-rich diet compared to a diet rich in artificial sweeteners, significant increases in postprandial glycemia, insulinemia, and lipidemia were observed [50]. A randomized crossover trial among normal-weight healthy men found that, after three weeks, SSBs consumed in small to moderate quantities resulted in impaired glucose and lipid metabolism and promoted inflammation [51]. Other trials have found inconsistent results on markers of inflammation, which may be due to differences in study duration. [52,53].

5. Diabetes and CVD

Although experimental evidence from RCTs is lacking due to high cost and other feasibility considerations, findings from prospective cohort studies have shown strong and consistent associations in well-powered studies. A meta-analysis of 17 prospective cohort studies evaluating SSB consumption and risk of T2D found that a one-serving-per-day increment in SSB was associated with an 18% higher risk of T2D (95% CI: 9% to 28%) among studies that did not adjust for adiposity [54] (Figure 2). Among studies that adjusted for adiposity, the estimate was attenuated to 13% (6% to 21%), suggesting a partial mediating role of adiposity in this association. Positive yet weaker associations were also noted for juice and artificially sweetened beverages (ASB). This study also estimated the population attributable fraction for T2D from consumption of SSB in the US and United Kingdom (UK). Based on their estimates, 8.7% (95% CI, 3.9% to 12.9%) of T2D cases in the US and 3.6% (95% CI, 1.7% to 5.6%) in the UK would be attributable to the consumption of SSBs [54]. These results, which are consistent with previous meta-analyses [6,55,56], confirm that the consumption of SSBs is associated with increased risk of T2D independently of adiposity and suggests that the consumption of SSBs over many years could be related to a substantial number of new cases. Recent studies in the Mexican Teacher's cohort [57] and Northern Manhattan study [58], a multi ethnic urban cohort in New York City, provide additional support linking intake of SSBs to risk of T2D, and have expanded the generalizability of the findings across different populations.

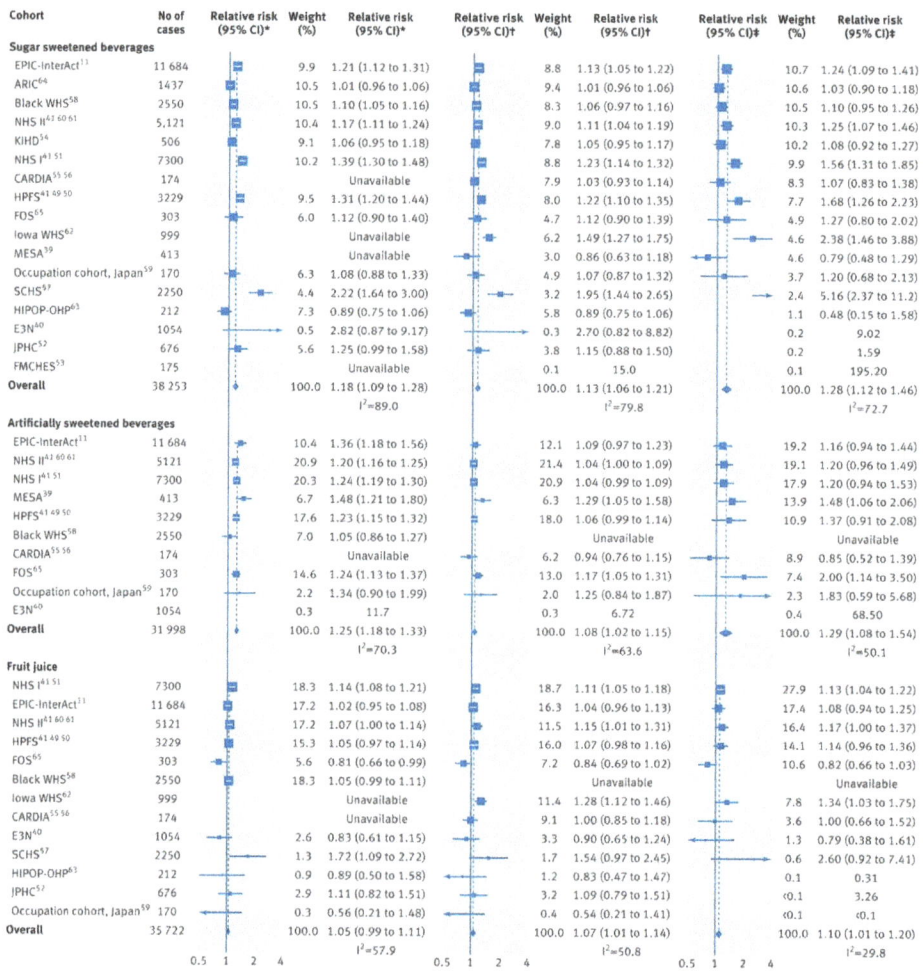

Figure 2. Prospective associations for an incremental increase in beverage consumption with incident type 2 diabetes (T2D): random effects meta-analysis. * Unadjusted for adiposity; † adjusted for adiposity; ‡ adjusted for adiposity and within person variation [54].

Emerging evidence linking intake of SSBs to CVD is strengthened by consistent associations of SSBs with cardiometabolic risk factors, in addition to weight gain and risk of T2D. A meta-analysis of nine prospective cohort studies found that a one-serving-per-day increase in SSB was associated with a 13% higher risk of stroke (RR: 1.13, 95% CI: 1.02, 1.24) based on one study, and 22% higher risk of myocardial infarction (MI) (RR: 1.22, 95% CI: 1.14, 1.30) based on two studies [10]. In the categorical analysis comparing high vs. low SSB intake, there was a 19% higher risk of MI (RR: 1.19, 95% CI: 1.09, 1.31) based on three studies, but no significant association was observed for stroke (three studies) [10]. For the association with stroke, moderate heterogeneity was evident. After stratification by sex and stroke type, the pooled results suggested that women who consume SSBs have a higher risk of ischemic stroke (RR: 1.33, 95% CI: 1.07, 1.66), while no differences were noted for men or for men and women with hemorrhagic stroke [10]. These findings are consistent with a previous meta-analysis of four prospective cohort studies, which found a 17% higher risk of CHD (95% CI: 7% to 28%) comparing extreme SSB intake categories and a 16% higher risk of CHD per one-serving-per-day increment (10% to 23%) [11]. Similar to studies of T2D, when estimates that did not adjust for BMI or energy intake were included in the meta-analysis, the magnitude of the association increased (RR: 1.26, 95% CI: 1.16, 1.37), suggesting these factors as partial mediators of the association. A systematic review by Keller et al. also reported positive associations between SSB and CHD but noted that associations were only apparent in large studies with long durations of follow-up [12]. This review also found that, among studies that evaluated SSB intake in relation to risk of stroke, positive associations were observed only among women.

Building on the clinical evidence, a few studies have also shown a link between SSB intake and risk of all-cause or CVD mortality. We recently found that, among over 118,000 women and men from the NHS and HPFS, intake of SSBs was positively associated with risk of death from any cause in a dose-dependent manner [59]. Compared with drinking SSBs less than once per month, drinking one to four per month was linked with a 1% higher risk, two to six per week with a 6% higher risk, one to two per day with a 14% higher risk, and two or more per day with a 21% higher risk [59]. The higher risk of death associated with SSBs was more pronounced among women than men and was driven by CVD mortality. Compared with infrequent SSB consumers, those who consumed two or more per day had a 31% higher risk of death from CVD [59]. These findings are consistent with a previous study conducted in a prospective analysis of NHANES, which found a 29% higher risk of CVD mortality (RR: 1.29, 95% CI: 1.04, 1.60) comparing participants who consumed seven or more servings of SSBs per week to those who consumed one serving per week or less [60]. It was also estimated in NHANES that 7.4% of all cardiometabolic deaths in the US could be attributed to intake of SSBs in 2012 [61]. More recently, in the US-based Reasons for Geographic and Racial Differences in Stroke (REGARDS) study, each additional 12-oz serving/day of SSBs was associated with an 11% higher risk of all-cause mortality [62]. However, no association was observed for risk of death from CHD, which may have been due to a limited number of cases. In contrast, results from a cohort of Chinese adults in Singapore [63] and an elderly population in the US [64], both with very low intake levels, found no significant association between SSBs and mortality.

6. Biological Mechanisms

SSBs contribute to weight gain through decreased satiety and an incomplete compensatory reduction in energy intake at subsequent meals following ingestion of liquid calories [20]. A typical 12-oz (360 mL) serving of soda contains ~140–150 calories and ~35–37.5 g of sugar. If these calories are added to the diet without compensating for the additional calories, one can of soda per day could in theory lead to a weight gain of five pounds in one year [65]. Short-term feeding trials that show greater energy intake [66] and weight gain [50,66–69] from consuming SSBs compared to ASBs indirectly illustrate this point. While few studies have evaluated this mechanism, some evidence supporting incomplete compensation for liquid calories has been provided by studies showing greater energy intake and weight gain after isocaloric consumption of beverages compared to solid food [70–72]. These studies suggest that calories from sugar in liquid beverages may not suppress intake of solid foods to the level needed to maintain energy balance; however, the mechanisms responsible for this response are largely unknown.

SSBs contribute to the development of T2D and cardiometabolic risk in part through their ability to induce weight gain, but also independently through metabolic effects of constituent sugars (Figure 3). Consumption of SSBs has been shown to induce rapid spikes in blood glucose and insulin levels [73,74]. As such, these beverages have moderate-to-high glycemic index (GI) values [75], which, in combination with the large quantities consumed, contribute to a high dietary glycemic load (GL). High-GL diets can promote insulin resistance [76], exacerbate inflammatory biomarkers [77], and are associated with higher risk of T2D [78,79] and CHD [80]. Consuming fructose from SSBs as a component of sucrose or HFCS may further impact cardiometabolic risk. Fructose alone is poorly absorbed but is enhanced by glucose in the gut, thus accounting for the rapid and complete absorption of both fructose and glucose when ingested as sucrose or HFCS. Fructose, when consumed in moderate amounts, is metabolized in the liver where it is converted to glucose, lactate, and fatty acids to serve as metabolic substrates for other cells in the body [81]. When consumed in excess, this can lead to increased hepatic de novo lipogenesis, atherogenic dyslipidemia, and insulin resistance. The increase in hepatic lipid promotes production and secretion of very-low-density lipoproteins (VLDLs) leading to increased concentrations of postprandial triglycerides. Consumption of fructose-containing sugars is associated with production of small dense LDL cholesterol, which may be due to increased levels of VLDL-induced lipoprotein remodeling [48,82]. Fructose was also shown to promote the accumulation of VAT and the deposition of ectopic fat [83–86], processes indicative of cardiometabolic risk. Accumulating evidence suggests that the metabolic effects of fructose may be modified by physical activity level with more adverse effects observed under conditions of high fructose intake and low levels of physical activity [87]. According to this model, the adverse metabolic effects of fructose would occur when fructose intake chronically exceeds the capacity of the liver to release lactate and glucose for muscle, i.e., when there is a mismatch between fructose intake and energy output in the muscle. Fructose is the only sugar known to increase production of uric acid [87]. The production of uric acid in the liver has been shown to reduce endothelial nitric oxide, which may be implicated in the association between SSBs and CHD [88]. Hyperuricemia often precedes development of obesity and T2D, and clinical evidence suggests that hyperuricemia may mediate the association between SSB consumption and hypertension through the development of renal disease, endothelial dysfunction, and activation of the renin–angiotensin system [88]. In addition, hyperuricemia is associated with the development of gout [45,46], and gout and hyperuricemia are associated with hypertension, T2D, MetSyn, kidney disease, and CVD [88,89].

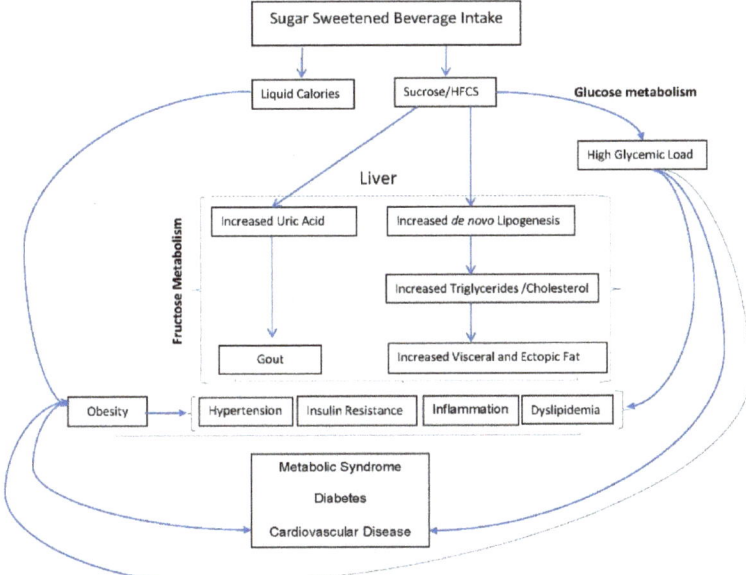

Figure 3. Biological mechanisms linking intake of sugar-sweetened beverages (SSB) to the development of obesity, metabolic syndrome (Met Syn), diabetes, and cardiovascular disease (CVD). Incomplete compensation for liquid calories leads to obesity, which is a risk factor for cardiometabolic outcomes. Increased diabetes, MetSyn, and CVD risk also occur independent of weight through development of risk factors precipitated by adverse glycemic effects and increased fructose metabolism in the liver. Excess fructose ingestion promotes hepatic uric acid production, de novo lipogenesis, and accumulation of visceral and ectopic fat, and also leads to gout. HFCS = high-fructose corn syrup.

7. Alternative Beverages

Several beverages have been suggested as alternatives to SSBs including water, 100% fruit juice, coffee, tea, and ASBs. Unlike SSBs, water does not contain liquid calories and, for most people with access to safe drinking water, it is the optimal calorie-free beverage. We found that replacement of one serving per day of SSBs with one serving of water was associated with less weight gain [90] and a lower risk of T2D [91]. With more consumers opting for water, several types of sparkling and flavored waters have emerged on the market, which may make switching to water more feasible for habitual SSB consumers.

Although 100% fruit juice might be perceived as a healthy choice since juice contains some vitamins and nutrients, they also contain a relatively high number of calories from natural sugars. Previous cohort studies have found positive associations between consumption of fruit juice and weight gain [92] and T2D [93], while the opposite has been shown for whole fruit [25,94]. Sugars in juice are absorbed more quickly than those in fruit and vegetables, which are absorbed more slowly due in part to their fiber content [95,96]. The rapid absorption of liquid fructose (from juice) compared to solid forms is more likely to result in higher concentrations of fructose in the liver and increase the rate of hepatic extraction of fructose, de novo lipogenesis, and production of lipids [97,98]. A recent study in the REGARDS cohort found that fruit juice intake was associated with a higher risk of all-cause mortality [62]. However, other studies have shown benefits of juice on cardiometabolic markers [92,99]. This suggests a need for further research that can evaluate different types of juice, since the nutrient profile and sugar content across various juices may differ. Nonetheless, based on the current evidence, it is recommended that daily intake of fruit juice be limited to 8 oz for adults.

Numerous studies have shown that regular consumption of coffee (decaffeinated or regular) and tea can have favorable effects on T2D and CVD risk [100,101], possibly due to their high polyphenol content. These beverages can thus be considered healthful alternatives to SSBs for individuals without contraindications, provided that caloric sweeteners and creamers are used sparingly, and that intake does not exceed the guidelines for caffeine. We found that substituting one serving per day of SSBs with one cup of coffee was associated with a 17% lower risk of T2D [102].

ASBs provide few to no calories but retain a sweet flavor, making them an attractive alternative to SSBs. Paradoxically, some cohort studies have reported positive associations between ASB consumption and weight gain and risk of T2D and CVD [32,36]. These findings may be due in part to residual confounding by unmeasured or poorly measured lifestyle factors or reverse causation, since individuals with obesity or metabolic risk may switch to ASBs for health reasons, which can result in spurious associations between ASBs and cardiometabolic outcomes. Studies with repeated measurements of diet, which are less prone to reverse causation, have shown only marginal nonsignificant associations with ASBs [8,9,25,59,102]. Cohort-based substitution analysis has also shown inverse associations with weight gain, T2D and mortality with replacement of SSBs with ASBs [59,90,91]. In addition, short-term trials that assessed ASBs as a replacement for SSBs reported modest benefits on body weight and metabolic risk factors [5,103]. On the other hand, some mechanisms have been proposed linking ASBs to adverse cardiometabolic health such as the intense sweetness of artificial sweeteners conditioning toward a preference for sweets or stimulating a cephalic insulin response, and more recently through alterations in gut microflora linked to insulin resistance [104]. However, these mechanisms are not well understood, and different types of artificial sweeteners may have different metabolic effects.

Consumption of ASBs in place of SSBs could be a helpful strategy to reduce cardiometabolic risk among heavy SSB consumers with the ultimate goal of switching to water or other healthful beverages. Further studies are needed to evaluate potential metabolic consequences of consuming ASBs over the life course and better understand underlying biological mechanisms. Understanding potential health impacts of ASB consumption is especially important in the context of sugar reduction policies such as taxation and labeling, which may lead to product reformulation and more ASBs in the food supply.

8. Policy Considerations

In response to the strong evidence linking consumption of SSBs to weight gain and risk of T2D and CVD, national and international organizations are already calling for reductions in intake of these beverages to help curb obesity and improve cardiometabolic health [105]. Both the WHO and 2015–2020 US Dietary Guidelines recommend an upper limit of 10% of total energy from added sugar, and numerous associations specifically recommend limiting intake of SSBs. In addition to widespread public health recommendations, public policies are needed to change consumption pattern at the population level (Box 1). The most common actions implemented to reduce SSB consumption include taxation, reduction of availability in schools, restrictions on marketing to children, public awareness campaigns, and front-of-package labelling [18,106]. Several cities in the US and globally have implemented excise taxes on SSBs as a strategy to reduce intake levels and generate revenue to support various public efforts. The most rigorously evaluated SSB tax to date is in Mexico, where a nationwide excise tax of 10% (one peso per liter) was implemented in 2014. Two years after the tax was implemented, a net decrease of 7.6% in sales of sugary drinks was observed, while sales of untaxed beverages such as water increased by 2.1% [107]. It was estimated that, between 2013 to 2022, the tax alone will prevent nearly 200,000 cases of obesity and save $980 million in direct healthcare costs, with the majority of benefits in young adults [108]. In Berkeley, California, the first US city to levy a penny-per-ounce excise tax on SSBs, sales of SSBs fell 9.6%, while sales of untaxed beverages, such as water and milk, increased 3.5%, comparing pre-tax to one-year-post-implementation trends [109]. Whether these early benefits of the tax will continue over the long term and translate into improvements in health will be important factors to monitor over time. In the US, the recently revised nutrition facts label will now require manufacturers (compliance by 1 January2020 to 1 July

2021, depending on annual food sales) to disclose the added sugar content of products, and will be accompanied by a percent daily value, with a goal of helping consumers make healthier choices. To achieve meaningful changes in beverage consumption patterns, a combination of multiple strategies will be needed, together with consumer education, and will serve as important steps in changing social norms surrounding beverage habits. Implementing and evaluating these policy actions in relation to behavior changes in the short term and clinical outcomes in the long term should remain a priority for scientists and policy-makers.

Box 1. Policy strategies to reduce consumption of sugar-sweetened beverages (SSBs).

- Governments should impose financial incentives such as taxation of SSBs of at least a 10% price increase, and implement limits for use of Supplemental Nutrition Assistance Program (SNAP) benefits for SSBs or subsidizing SNAP purchases of healthier foods, to encourage healthier beverages choices.
- Regulations are needed to reduce exposure to marketing of unhealthy foods and beverages in the media and at sports events or other activities, particularly in relation to children.
- Front-of-package labelling or other nutrition labeling strategies should be implemented to help guide consumers to make healthy food and beverage choices. These changes should be accompanied by concurrent public health awareness campaigns.
- Policies should be adopted to reduce the availability of SSBs in the workplace, healthcare facilities, government institutions, and other public spaces, and ensure access to safe water and healthy alternatives. Policies that make healthful beverages the default choice should also be adopted.
- Educational campaigns about the health risks associated with overconsumption of SSBs should be aimed at healthcare professionals and clinical populations.
- National and international campaigns targeting obesity and chronic disease prevention should include the health risks associated with overconsumption of SSBs.
- National and international dietary recommendations should include specific guidelines for healthy beverage consumption.

9. Conclusions

Intake of SSBs remains high in the US and is rising in many parts of the world. Based on findings from prospective cohort studies and short-term experimental trials of cardiometabolic risk factors, there is strong evidence for an etiological relationship between intake of SSBs and weight gain and risk of T2D and CHD. The evidence for a link with stroke is less clear and warrants further research, including the potential sex difference. Few studies have investigated intake of SSBs in relation to MetSyn, and this may be due to challenges in assessment and controversy about its clinical utility. However, findings on individual risk factors suggest a link. Since development of MetSyn often precedes onset of T2D and CHD, preventing or reversing MetSyn could be an effective way to curtail rising T2D and CHD rates.

SSBs are thought to promote weight gain through incomplete compensation for liquid calories at subsequent meals. These beverages may increase T2D and CHD in part through weight gain and independently through metabolic effects of constituent sugars. A mechanistic area that warrants future research is exploring the health effects of sugar consumed in solid form compared to SSB, and further elucidating compensatory effects of liquid vs. solid sugars. With the strength of evidence sufficient to call for reductions in intake of SSB for optimal cardiometabolic health, important research gaps exist regarding suitable alternative beverages, including the long-term health effects of consuming ASBs. Continued evaluation of SSB policies that are already in place is needed, as are more and higher-quality RCTs to identify effective strategies to reduce intake of SSBs at the individual and population level. SSBs present a clear target for health policy; however, chronic disease prevention should focus on improving overall diet quality by consuming more healthful foods and limiting unhealthy ones. Given the high levels of intake across the globe, reducing consumption of SSBs is an important step in improving diet quality that could have a measurable impact on weight control and improving cardiometabolic health.

Author Contributions: Original draft preparation, V.S.M.; critical review and editing, F.B.H. Both authors approved the submitted version and take responsibility for the accuracy and integrity of the work.

Funding: This research received no external funding.

Acknowledgments: This research was supported by NIH grants P30 DK46200 and HL607.

Conflicts of Interest: V.S.M. is on a pro bono retainer for expert support for the Center for Science in the Public Interest in litigation related to sugar-sweetened beverages, and served as a consultant for the City of San Francisco for a case related to health warning labels on soda. There are no other financial or personal conflicts of interest to disclose that are related to the contents of this paper.

References

1. Alberti, K.G.; Eckel, R.H.; Grundy, S.M.; Zimmet, P.Z.; Cleeman, J.I.; Donato, K.A.; Fruchart, J.C.; James, W.P.; Loria, C.M.; Smith, S.C., Jr.; et al. Harmonizing the metabolic syndrome: A joint interim statement of the International Diabetes Federation Task Force on Epidemiology and Prevention; National Heart, Lung, and Blood Institute; American Heart Association; World Heart Federation; International Atherosclerosis Society; and International Association for the Study of Obesity. *Circulation* **2009**, *120*, 1640–1645. [PubMed]
2. Beltran-Sanchez, H.; Harhay, M.O.; Harhay, M.M.; McElligott, S. Prevalence and trends of metabolic syndrome in the adult U.S. population, 1999–2010. *J. Am. Coll. Cardiol.* **2013**, *62*, 697–703. [CrossRef] [PubMed]
3. Saklayen, M.G. The Global Epidemic of the Metabolic Syndrome. *Curr. Hypertens. Rep.* **2018**, *20*, 12. [CrossRef] [PubMed]
4. Palmer, M.K.; Toth, P.P. Trends in Lipids, Obesity, Metabolic Syndrome, and Diabetes Mellitus in the United States: An NHANES Analysis (2003–2004 to 2013–2014). *Obesity* **2019**, *27*, 309–314. [CrossRef] [PubMed]
5. Malik, V.S.; Pan, A.; Willett, W.C.; Hu, F.B. Sugar-sweetened beverages and weight gain in children and adults: A systematic review and meta-analysis. *Am. J. Clin. Nutr.* **2013**, *98*, 1084–1102. [CrossRef] [PubMed]
6. Malik, V.S.; Popkin, B.M.; Bray, G.A.; Despres, J.P.; Willett, W.C.; Hu, F.B. Sugar-sweetened beverages and risk of metabolic syndrome and type 2 diabetes: A meta-analysis. *Diabetes Care* **2010**, *33*, 2477–2483. [CrossRef] [PubMed]
7. *Guideline: Sugar Intake for Adults and Children*; World Health Organization: Geneva, Switzerland, 2015.
8. Fung, T.T.; Malik, V.; Rexrode, K.M.; Manson, J.E.; Willett, W.C.; Hu, F.B. Sweetened beverage consumption and risk of coronary heart disease in women. *Am. J. Clin. Nutr.* **2009**, *89*, 1037–1042. [CrossRef]
9. De Koning, L.; Malik, V.S.; Kellogg, M.D.; Rimm, E.B.; Willett, W.C.; Hu, F.B. Sweetened beverage consumption, incident coronary heart disease, and biomarkers of risk in men. *Circulation* **2012**, *125*, 1735–1741. [CrossRef]
10. Narain, A.; Kwok, C.S.; Mamas, M.A. Soft drinks and sweetened beverages and the risk of cardiovascular disease and mortality: A systematic review and meta-analysis. *Int. J. Clin. Pract.* **2016**, *70*, 791–805. [CrossRef]
11. Huang, C.; Huang, J.; Tian, Y.; Yang, X.; Gu, D. Sugar sweetened beverages consumption and risk of coronary heart disease: A meta-analysis of prospective studies. *Atherosclerosis* **2014**, *234*, 11–16. [CrossRef]
12. Keller, A.; Heitmann, B.L.; Olsen, N. Sugar-sweetened beverages, vascular risk factors and events: A systematic literature review. *Public Health Nutr.* **2015**, *18*, 1145–1154. [CrossRef] [PubMed]
13. Welsh, J.A.; Sharma, A.J.; Grellinger, L.; Vos, M.B. Consumption of added sugars is decreasing in the United States. *Am. J. Clin. Nutr.* **2011**, *94*, 726–734. [CrossRef] [PubMed]
14. Dietary Guidelines for Americans 2015–2020. Available online: http://health.gov/dietaryguidelines/2015/guidelines/ (accessed on 7 August 2019).
15. Rosinger, A.; Herrick, K.; Gahche, J.; Park, S. Sugar-sweetened Beverage Consumption Among U.S. Adults, 2011–2014. *NCHS Data Brief* **2017**, *270*, 1–8.
16. Singh, G.M.; Micha, R.; Khatibzadeh, S.; Shi, P.; Lim, S.; Andrews, K.G.; Engell, R.E.; Ezzati, M.; Mozaffarian, D.; Global Burden of Diseases Nutrition and Chronic Diseases Expert Group (NutriCoDE). Global, Regional, and National Consumption of Sugar-Sweetened Beverages, Fruit Juices, and Milk: A Systematic Assessment of Beverage Intake in 187 Countries. *PLoS ONE* **2015**, *10*, e0124845. [CrossRef] [PubMed]
17. Yang, L.; Bovet, P.; Liu, Y.; Zhao, M.; Ma, C.; Liang, Y.; Xi, B. Consumption of Carbonated Soft Drinks Among Young Adolescents Aged 12 to 15 Years in 53 Low- and Middle-Income Countries. *Am. J. Public Health* **2017**, *107*, 1095–1100. [CrossRef] [PubMed]

18. Popkin, B.M.; Hawkes, C. Sweetening of the global diet, particularly beverages: Patterns, trends, and policy responses. *Lancet Diabetes Endocrinol.* **2016**, *4*, 174–186. [CrossRef]
19. Hu, F.B.; Malik, V.S. Sugar-sweetened beverages and risk of obesity and type 2 diabetes: Epidemiologic evidence. *Physiol. Behav.* **2010**, *100*, 47–54. [CrossRef]
20. Malik, V.S.; Popkin, B.M.; Bray, G.A.; Despres, J.P.; Hu, F.B. Sugar-sweetened beverages, obesity, type 2 diabetes mellitus, and cardiovascular disease risk. *Circulation* **2010**, *121*, 1356–1364. [CrossRef]
21. Malik, V.S.; Schulze, M.B.; Hu, F.B. Intake of sugar-sweetened beverages and weight gain: A systematic review. *Am. J. Clin. Nutr.* **2006**, *84*, 274–288. [CrossRef]
22. Vartanian, L.R.; Schwartz, M.B.; Brownell, K.D. Effects of soft drink consumption on nutrition and health: A systematic review and meta-analysis. *Am. J. Public Health* **2007**, *97*, 667–675. [CrossRef]
23. Te Morenga, L.; Mallard, S.; Mann, J. Dietary sugars and body weight: Systematic review and meta-analyses of randomised controlled trials and cohort studies. *BMJ* **2013**, *346*, e7492. [CrossRef] [PubMed]
24. Kaiser, K.A.; Shikany, J.M.; Keating, K.D.; Allison, D.B. Will reducing sugar-sweetened beverage consumption reduce obesity? Evidence supporting conjecture is strong, but evidence when testing effect is weak. *Obes. Rev.* **2013**, *14*, 620–633. [CrossRef] [PubMed]
25. Mozaffarian, D.; Hao, T.; Rimm, E.B.; Willett, W.C.; Hu, F.B. Changes in diet and lifestyle and long-term weight gain in women and men. *N. Engl. J. Med.* **2011**, *364*, 2392–2404. [CrossRef] [PubMed]
26. Qi, Q.; Chu, A.Y.; Kang, J.H.; Jensen, M.K.; Curhan, G.C.; Pasquale, L.R.; Ridker, P.M.; Hunter, D.J.; Willett, W.C.; Rimm, E.B.; et al. Sugar-sweetened beverages and genetic risk of obesity. *N. Engl. J. Med.* **2012**, *367*, 1387–1396. [CrossRef] [PubMed]
27. Ebbeling, C.B.; Feldman, H.A.; Chomitz, V.R.; Antonelli, T.A.; Gortmaker, S.L.; Osganian, S.K.; Ludwig, D. A randomized trial of sugar-sweetened beverages and adolescent body weight. *N. Engl. J. Med.* **2012**, *367*, 1407–1416. [CrossRef] [PubMed]
28. De Ruyter, J.C.; Olthof, M.R.; Seidell, J.C.; Katan, M.B. A trial of sugar-free or sugar-sweetened beverages and body weight in children. *N. Engl. J. Med.* **2012**, *367*, 1397–1406. [CrossRef] [PubMed]
29. Hu, F.B. Resolved: There is sufficient scientific evidence that decreasing sugar-sweetened beverage consumption will reduce the prevalence of obesity and obesity-related diseases. *Obes. Rev.* **2013**, *14*, 606–619. [CrossRef]
30. Narain, A.; Kwok, C.S.; Mamas, M.A. Soft drink intake and the risk of metabolic syndrome: A systematic review and meta-analysis. *Int. J. Clin. Pract.* **2017**, *71*, e12927. [CrossRef]
31. Mirmiran, P.; Yuzbashian, E.; Asghari, G.; Hosseinpour-Niazi, S.; Azizi, F. Consumption of sugar sweetened beverage is associated with incidence of metabolic syndrome in Tehranian children and adolescents. *Nutr. Metab.* **2015**, *12*, 25. [CrossRef]
32. Nettleton, J.A.; Lutsey, P.L.; Wang, Y.; Lima, J.A.; Michos, E.D.; Jacobs, D.R., Jr. Diet soda intake and risk of incident metabolic syndrome and type 2 diabetes in the Multi-Ethnic Study of Atherosclerosis (MESA). *Diabetes Care* **2009**, *32*, 688–694. [CrossRef]
33. Dhingra, R.; Sullivan, L.; Jacques, P.F.; Wang, T.J.; Fox, C.S.; Meigs, J.B.; D'Agostino, R.B.; Gaziano, J.M.; Vasan, R.S. Soft drink consumption and risk of developing cardiometabolic risk factors and the metabolic syndrome in middle-aged adults in the community. *Circulation* **2007**, *116*, 480–488. [CrossRef] [PubMed]
34. Ferreira-Pego, C.; Babio, N.; Bes-Rastrollo, M.; Corella, D.; Estruch, R.; Ros, E.; Fitó, M.; Serra-Majem, L.; Arós, F.; Fiol, M.; et al. Frequent Consumption of Sugar- and Artificially Sweetened Beverages and Natural and Bottled Fruit Juices Is Associated with an Increased Risk of Metabolic Syndrome in a Mediterranean Population at High Cardiovascular Disease Risk. *J. Nutr.* **2016**, *146*, 1528–1536. [PubMed]
35. Kang, Y.; Kim, J. Soft drink consumption is associated with increased incidence of the metabolic syndrome only in women. *Br. J. Nutr.* **2017**, *117*, 315–324. [CrossRef] [PubMed]
36. Lutsey, P.L.; Steffen, L.M.; Stevens, J. Dietary intake and the development of the metabolic syndrome: The Atherosclerosis Risk in Communities study. *Circulation* **2008**, *117*, 754–761. [CrossRef] [PubMed]
37. Duffey, K.J.; Gordon-Larsen, P.; Steffen, L.M.; Jacobs, D.R., Jr.; Popkin, B.M. Drinking caloric beverages increases the risk of adverse cardiometabolic outcomes in the Coronary Artery Risk Development in Young Adults (CARDIA) Study. *Am. J. Clin. Nutr.* **2010**, *92*, 954–959. [CrossRef] [PubMed]
38. Stern, D.; Middaugh, N.; Rice, M.S.; Laden, F.; Lopez-Ridaura, R.; Rosner, B.; Willett, W.; Lajous, M. Changes in Sugar-Sweetened Soda Consumption, Weight, and Waist Circumference: 2-Year Cohort of Mexican Women. *Am. J. Public Health* **2017**, *107*, 1801–1808. [CrossRef]

39. Funtikova, A.N.; Subirana, I.; Gomez, S.F.; Fito, M.; Elosua, R.; Benitez-Arciniega, A.A.; Schröder, H. Soft drink consumption is positively associated with increased waist circumference and 10-year incidence of abdominal obesity in Spanish adults. *J. Nutr.* **2015**, *145*, 328–334. [CrossRef]
40. Ma, J.; McKeown, N.M.; Hwang, S.J.; Hoffmann, U.; Jacques, P.F.; Fox, C.S. Sugar-Sweetened Beverage Consumption Is Associated With Change of Visceral Adipose Tissue Over 6 Years of Follow-Up. *Circulation* **2016**, *133*, 370–377. [CrossRef]
41. Yu, Z.; Ley, S.H.; Sun, Q.; Hu, F.B.; Malik, V.S. Cross-sectional association between sugar-sweetened beverage intake and cardiometabolic biomarkers in US women. *Br. J. Nutr.* **2018**, *119*, 570–580. [CrossRef]
42. Kim, Y.; Je, Y. Prospective association of sugar-sweetened and artificially sweetened beverage intake with risk of hypertension. *Arch. Cardiovasc. Dis.* **2016**, *109*, 242–253. [CrossRef]
43. Jayalath, V.H.; de Souza, R.J.; Ha, V.; Mirrahimi, A.; Blanco-Mejia, S.; Di Buono, M.; Jenkins, A.L.; Leiter, L.A.; Wolever, T.; Beyene, J.; et al. Sugar-sweetened beverage consumption and incident hypertension: A systematic review and meta-analysis of prospective cohorts. *Am. J. Clin. Nutr.* **2015**, *102*, 914–921. [CrossRef] [PubMed]
44. Xi, B.; Huang, Y.; Reilly, K.H.; Li, S.; Zheng, R.; Barrio-Lopez, M.T.; Martinez-Gonzalez, M.A.; Zhou, D. Sugar-sweetened beverages and risk of hypertension and CVD: A dose-response meta-analysis. *Br. J. Nutr.* **2015**, *113*, 709–717. [CrossRef] [PubMed]
45. Choi, H.K.; Curhan, G. Soft drinks, fructose consumption, and the risk of gout in men: Prospective cohort study. *BMJ* **2008**, *336*, 309–312. [CrossRef] [PubMed]
46. Choi, H.K.; Willett, W.; Curhan, G. Fructose-rich beverages and risk of gout in women. *JAMA* **2010**, *304*, 2270–2278. [CrossRef] [PubMed]
47. Te Morenga, L.A.; Howatson, A.J.; Jones, R.M.; Mann, J. Dietary sugars and cardiometabolic risk: Systematic review and meta-analyses of randomized controlled trials of the effects on blood pressure and lipids. *Am. J. Clin. Nutr.* **2014**, *100*, 65–79. [CrossRef] [PubMed]
48. Stanhope, K.L.; Medici, V.; Bremer, A.A.; Lee, V.; Lam, H.D.; Nunez, M.V.; Chen, G.X.; Keim, N.L.; Havel, P.J. A dose-response study of consuming high-fructose corn syrup-sweetened beverages on lipid/lipoprotein risk factors for cardiovascular disease in young adults. *Am. J. Clin. Nutr.* **2015**, *101*, 1144–1154. [CrossRef]
49. Bruun, J.M.; Maersk, M.; Belza, A.; Astrup, A.; Richelsen, B. Consumption of sucrose-sweetened soft drinks increases plasma levels of uric acid in overweight and obese subjects: A 6-month randomised controlled trial. *Eur. J. Clin. Nutr.* **2015**, *69*, 949–953. [CrossRef]
50. Raben, A.; Moller, B.K.; Flint, A.; Vasilaris, T.H.; Christina Moller, A.; Juul Holst, J.; Astrup, A. Increased postprandial glycaemia, insulinemia, and lipidemia after 10 weeks' sucrose-rich diet compared to an artificially sweetened diet: A Randomised controlled trial. *Food Nutr. Res.* **2011**, *55*, 5961. [CrossRef]
51. Aeberli, I.; Gerber, P.A.; Hochuli, M.; Kohler, S.; Haile, S.R.; Gouni-Berthold, I.; Berthold, H.K.; Spinas, G.A.; Berneis, K. Low to moderate sugar-sweetened beverage consumption impairs glucose and lipid metabolism and promotes inflammation in healthy young men: A randomized controlled trial. *Am. J. Clin. Nutr.* **2011**, *94*, 479–485. [CrossRef]
52. Sorensen, L.B.; Raben, A.; Stender, S.; Astrup, A. Effect of sucrose on inflammatory markers in overweight humans. *Am. J. Clin. Nutr.* **2005**, *82*, 421–427. [CrossRef]
53. Kuzma, J.N.; Cromer, G.; Hagman, D.K.; Breymeyer, K.L.; Roth, C.L.; Foster-Schubert, K.E.; Holte, S.E.; Weigle, D.S.; Kratz, M. No differential effect of beverages sweetened with fructose, high-fructose corn syrup, or glucose on systemic or adipose tissue inflammation in normal-weight to obese adults: A randomized controlled trial. *Am. J. Clin. Nutr.* **2016**, *104*, 306–314. [CrossRef] [PubMed]
54. Imamura, F.; O'Connor, L.; Ye, Z.; Mursu, J.; Hayashino, Y.; Bhupathiraju, S.N.; Forouhi, N.G. Consumption of sugar sweetened beverages, artificially sweetened beverages, and fruit juice and incidence of type 2 diabetes: Systematic review, meta-analysis, and estimation of population attributable fraction. *Br. J. Sports Med.* **2016**, *50*, 496–504. [CrossRef] [PubMed]
55. Fagherazzi, G.; Vilier, A.; Saes Sartorelli, D.; Lajous, M.; Balkau, B.; Clavel-Chapelon, F. Consumption of artificially and sugar-sweetened beverages and incident type 2 diabetes in the Etude Epidemiologique aupres des femmes de la Mutuelle Generale de l'Education Nationale-European Prospective Investigation into Cancer and Nutrition cohort. *Am. J. Clin. Nutr.* **2013**, *97*, 517–523. [PubMed]
56. Consumption of sweet beverages and type 2 diabetes incidence in European adults: Results from EPIC-InterAct. *Diabetologia* **2013**, *56*, 1520–1530. [CrossRef] [PubMed]
57. Stern, D.; Mazariegos, M.; Ortiz-Panozo, E.; Campos, H.; Malik, V.S.; Lajous, M.; López-Ridaura, R. Sugar-Sweetened Soda Consumption Increases Diabetes Risk Among Mexican Women. *J. Nutr.* **2019**, *149*, 795–803. [CrossRef] [PubMed]

58. Gardener, H.; Moon, Y.P.; Rundek, T.; Elkind, M.S.V.; Sacco, R.L. Diet Soda and Sugar-Sweetened Soda Consumption in Relation to Incident Diabetes in the Northern Manhattan Study. *Curr. Dev. Nutr.* **2018**, *2*, nzy008. [CrossRef] [PubMed]
59. Malik, V.S.; Li, Y.; Pan, A.; De Koning, L.; Schernhammer, E.; Willett, W.C.; Hu, F.B. Long-Term Consumption of Sugar-Sweetened and Artificially Sweetened Beverages and Risk of Mortality in US Adults. *Circulation* **2019**, *139*, 2113–2125. [CrossRef] [PubMed]
60. Yang, Q.; Zhang, Z.; Gregg, E.W.; Flanders, W.D.; Merritt, R.; Hu, F.B. Added Sugar Intake and Cardiovascular Diseases Mortality Among US Adults. *JAMA Intern Med.* **2014**, *174*, 516–524. [CrossRef] [PubMed]
61. Micha, R.; Penalvo, J.L.; Cudhea, F.; Imamura, F.; Rehm, C.D.; Mozaffarian, D. Association Between Dietary Factors and Mortality From Heart Disease, Stroke, and Type 2 Diabetes in the United States. *JAMA* **2017**, *317*, 912–924. [CrossRef] [PubMed]
62. Collin, L.J.; Judd, S.; Safford, M.; Vaccarino, V.; Welsh, J.A. Association of Sugary Beverage Consumption With Mortality Risk in US Adults: A Secondary Analysis of Data from the REGARDS Study. *JAMA Netw. Open* **2019**, *2*, e193121. [CrossRef] [PubMed]
63. Odegaard, A.O.; Koh, W.P.; Yuan, J.M.; Pereira, M.A. Beverage habits and mortality in Chinese adults. *J. Nutr.* **2015**, *145*, 595–604. [CrossRef] [PubMed]
64. Paganini-Hill, A.; Kawas, C.H.; Corrada, M.M. Non-alcoholic beverage and caffeine consumption and mortality: The Leisure World Cohort Study. *Prev. Med.* **2007**, *44*, 305–310. [CrossRef] [PubMed]
65. Malik, V.S.; Hu, F.B. Sweeteners and Risk of Obesity and Type 2 Diabetes: The Role of Sugar-Sweetened Beverages. *Curr. Diab. Rep.* **2012**, *12*, 195–203. [CrossRef] [PubMed]
66. DellaValle, D.M.; Roe, L.S.; Rolls, B.J. Does the consumption of caloric and non-caloric beverages with a meal affect energy intake? *Appetite* **2005**, *44*, 187–193. [CrossRef] [PubMed]
67. Raben, A.; Vasilaras, T.H.; Moller, A.C.; Astrup, A. Sucrose compared with artificial sweeteners: Different effects on ad libitum food intake and body weight after 10 wk of supplementation in overweight subjects. *Am. J. Clin. Nutr.* **2002**, *76*, 721–729. [CrossRef] [PubMed]
68. Tordoff, M.G.; Alleva, A.M. Effect of drinking soda sweetened with aspartame or high-fructose corn syrup on food intake and body weight. *Am. J. Clin. Nutr.* **1990**, *51*, 963–969. [CrossRef] [PubMed]
69. Reid, M.; Hammersley, R.; Hill, A.J.; Skidmore, P. Long-term dietary compensation for added sugar: Effects of supplementary sucrose drinks over a 4-week period. *Br. J. Nutr.* **2007**, *97*, 193–203. [CrossRef]
70. DiMeglio, D.P.; Mattes, R.D. Liquid versus solid carbohydrate: Effects on food intake and body weight. *Int. J. Obes. Relat. Metab. Disord.* **2000**, *24*, 794–800. [CrossRef]
71. Pan, A.; Hu, F.B. Effects of carbohydrates on satiety: Differences between liquid and solid food. *Curr. Opin. Clin. Nutr. Metab. Care* **2011**, *14*, 385–390. [CrossRef]
72. Mourao, D.M.; Bressan, J.; Campbell, W.W.; Mattes, R.D. Effects of food form on appetite and energy intake in lean and obese young adults. *Int. J. Obes.* **2007**, *31*, 1688–1695. [CrossRef]
73. Tey, S.L.; Salleh, N.B.; Henry, J.; Forde, C.G. Effects of aspartame-, monk fruit-, stevia- and sucrose-sweetened beverages on postprandial glucose, insulin and energy intake. *Int. J. Obes.* **2017**, *41*, 450–457. [CrossRef] [PubMed]
74. Solomi, L.; Rees, G.A.; Redfern, K.M. The acute effects of the non-nutritive sweeteners aspartame and acesulfame-K in UK diet cola on glycaemic response. *Int. J. Food Sci. Nutr.* **2019**, 1–7. [CrossRef] [PubMed]
75. Atkinson, F.S.; Foster-Powell, K.; Brand-Miller, J.C. International tables of glycemic index and glycemic load values: 2008. *Diabetes Care* **2008**, *31*, 2281–2283. [CrossRef] [PubMed]
76. Ludwig, D.S. The glycemic index: Physiological mechanisms relating to obesity, diabetes, and cardiovascular disease. *JAMA* **2002**, *287*, 2414–2423. [CrossRef] [PubMed]
77. Liu, S.; Manson, J.E.; Buring, J.E.; Stampfer, M.J.; Willett, W.C.; Ridker, P.M. Relation between a diet with a high glycemic load and plasma concentrations of high-sensitivity C-reactive protein in middle-aged women. *Am. J. Clin. Nutr.* **2002**, *75*, 492–498. [CrossRef] [PubMed]
78. Bhupathiraju, S.N.; Tobias, D.K.; Malik, V.S.; Pan, A.; Hruby, A.; Manson, J.E.; Willett, W.C.; Hu, F.B. Glycemic index, glycemic load, and risk of type 2 diabetes: Results from 3 large US cohorts and an updated meta-analysis. *Am. J. Clin. Nutr.* **2014**, *100*, 218–232. [CrossRef] [PubMed]

79. Livesey, G.; Taylor, R.; Livesey, H.F.; Buyken, A.E.; Jenkins, D.J.A.; Augustin, L.S.A.; Sievenpiper, J.L.; Barclay, A.W.; Liu, S.; Wolever, T.M.S.; et al. Dietary Glycemic Index and Load and the Risk of Type 2 Diabetes: A Systematic Review and Updated Meta-Analyses of Prospective Cohort Studies. *Nutrients* **2019**, *11*, 1280. [CrossRef]
80. Livesey, G.; Livesey, H. Coronary Heart Disease and Dietary Carbohydrate, Glycemic Index, and Glycemic Load: Dose-Response Meta-analyses of Prospective Cohort Studies. *Mayo Clin. Proc. Innov. Qual. Outcomes* **2019**, *3*, 52–69. [CrossRef]
81. Sun, S.Z.; Empie, M.W. Fructose metabolism in humans—What isotopic tracer studies tell us. *Nutr. Metab. (London)* **2012**, *9*, 89. [CrossRef]
82. Goran, M.I.; Tappy, L.; Lê, K.A. *Dietary Sugars and Health*; CRC Press, Taylor & Francis Group: Boca Raton, FL, USA, 2015.
83. Teff, K.L.; Grudziak, J.; Townsend, R.R.; Dunn, T.N.; Grant, R.W.; Adams, S.H.; Keim, N.L.; Cummings, B.P.; Stanhope, K.L.; Havel, P.J. Endocrine and metabolic effects of consuming fructose- and glucose-sweetened beverages with meals in obese men and women: Influence of insulin resistance on plasma triglyceride responses. *J. Clin. Endocrinol. Metab.* **2009**, *94*, 1562–1569. [CrossRef]
84. Stanhope, K.L.; Schwarz, J.M.; Keim, N.L.; Griffen, S.C.; Bremer, A.A.; Graham, J.L.; Hatcher, B.; Cox, C.L.; Dyachenko, A.; Zhang, W.; et al. Consuming fructose-sweetened, not glucose-sweetened, beverages increases visceral adiposity and lipids and decreases insulin sensitivity in overweight/obese humans. *J. Clin. Investig.* **2009**, *119*, 1322–1334. [CrossRef] [PubMed]
85. Stanhope, K.L.; Griffen, S.C.; Bair, B.R.; Swarbrick, M.M.; Keim, N.L.; Havel, P.J. Twenty-four-hour endocrine and metabolic profiles following consumption of high-fructose corn syrup-, sucrose-, fructose-, and glucose-sweetened beverages with meals. *Am. J. Clin. Nutr.* **2008**, *87*, 1194–1203. [CrossRef] [PubMed]
86. Stanhope, K.L.; Havel, P.J. Endocrine and metabolic effects of consuming beverages sweetened with fructose, glucose, sucrose, or high-fructose corn syrup. *Am. J. Clin. Nutr.* **2008**, *88*, 1733S–1737S. [CrossRef] [PubMed]
87. Tappy, L.; Rosset, R. Health outcomes of a high fructose intake: The importance of physical activity. *J. Physiol.* **2019**, *597*, 3561–3571. [CrossRef] [PubMed]
88. Richette, P.; Bardin, T. Gout. *Lancet* **2009**. [CrossRef]
89. Nakagawa, T.; Tuttle, K.R.; Short, R.A.; Johnson, R.J. Hypothesis: Fructose-induced hyperuricemia as a causal mechanism for the epidemic of the metabolic syndrome. *Nat. Clin. Pract. Nephrol.* **2005**, *1*, 80–86. [CrossRef] [PubMed]
90. Pan, A.; Malik, V.S.; Hao, T.; Willett, W.C.; Mozaffarian, D.; Hu, F.B. Changes in water and beverage intake and long-term weight changes: Results from three prospective cohort studies. *Int. J. Obes.* **2013**, *37*, 1378. [CrossRef] [PubMed]
91. Pan, A.; Malik, V.S.; Schulze, M.B.; Manson, J.E.; Willett, W.C.; Hu, F.B. Plain-water intake and risk of type 2 diabetes in young and middle-aged women. *Am. J. Clin. Nutr.* **2012**, *95*, 1454–1460. [CrossRef] [PubMed]
92. Schulze, M.B.; Manson, J.E.; Ludwig, D.S.; Colditz, G.A.; Stampfer, M.J.; Willett, W.C.; Hu, F.B. Sugar-sweetened beverages, weight gain, and incidence of type 2 diabetes in young and middle-aged women. *JAMA* **2004**, *292*, 927–934. [CrossRef]
93. Bazzano, L.A.; Li, T.Y.; Joshipura, K.J.; Hu, F.B. Intake of fruit, vegetables, and fruit juices and risk of diabetes in women. *Diabetes Care* **2008**, *31*, 1311–1317. [CrossRef]
94. Muraki, I.; Imamura, F.; Manson, J.E.; Hu, F.B.; Willett, W.C.; van Dam, R.M.; Sun, Q. Fruit consumption and risk of type 2 diabetes: Results from three prospective longitudinal cohort studies. *BMJ* **2013**, *347*, f5001. [CrossRef] [PubMed]
95. Ravn-Haren, G.; Dragsted, L.O.; Buch-Andersen, T.; Jensen, E.N.; Jensen, R.I.; Nemeth-Balogh, M.; Paulovicsová, B.; Bergström, A.; Wilcks, A.; Licht, T.R.; et al. Intake of whole apples or clear apple juice has contrasting effects on plasma lipids in healthy volunteers. *Eur. J. Nutr.* **2013**, *52*, 1875–1889. [CrossRef] [PubMed]
96. Pepin, A.; Stanhope, K.L.; Imbeault, P. Are Fruit Juices Healthier Than Sugar-Sweetened Beverages? A Review. *Nutrients* **2019**, *11*, 1006. [CrossRef] [PubMed]
97. Sundborn, G.; Thornley, S.; Merriman, T.R.; Lang, B.; King, C.; Lanaspa, M.A.; Johnson, R.J. Are Liquid Sugars Different from Solid Sugar in Their Ability to Cause Metabolic Syndrome? *Obesity* **2019**, *27*, 879–887. [CrossRef] [PubMed]

98. Lanaspa, M.A.; Sanchez-Lozada, L.G.; Choi, Y.J.; Cicerchi, C.; Kanbay, M.; Roncal-Jimenez, C.A.; Schreiner, G. Uric acid induces hepatic steatosis by generation of mitochondrial oxidative stress: Potential role in fructose-dependent and -independent fatty liver. *J. Biol. Chem.* **2012**, *287*, 40732–40744. [CrossRef] [PubMed]
99. Ghanim, H.; Mohanty, P.; Pathak, R.; Chaudhuri, A.; Sia, C.L.; Dandona, P. Orange juice or fructose intake does not induce oxidative and inflammatory response. *Diabetes Care* **2007**, *30*, 1406–1411. [CrossRef] [PubMed]
100. Van Dam, R.M. Coffee consumption and risk of type 2 diabetes, cardiovascular diseases, and cancer. *Appl. Physiol. Nutr. Metab.* **2008**, *33*, 1269–1283. [CrossRef]
101. Bhupathiraju, S.N.; Pan, A.; Malik, V.S.; Manson, J.E.; Willett, W.C.; van Dam, R.M.; Hu, F.B. Caffeinated and caffeine-free beverages and risk of type 2 diabetes. *Am. J. Clin. Nutr.* **2013**, *97*, 155–166. [CrossRef]
102. De Koning, L.; Malik, V.S.; Rimm, E.B.; Willett, W.C.; Hu, F.B. Sugar-sweetened and artificially sweetened beverage consumption and risk of type 2 diabetes in men. *Am. J. Clin. Nutr.* **2011**, *93*, 1321–1327. [CrossRef]
103. Malik, V.S. Non-sugar sweeteners and health. *BMJ* **2019**, *364*, k5005. [CrossRef]
104. Swithers, S.E. Not so Sweet Revenge: Unanticipated Consequences of High-Intensity Sweeteners. *Behav. Anal.* **2015**, *38*, 1–17. [CrossRef] [PubMed]
105. Yale Rudd Center for Food Policy and Obesity. SUgar-Sweetened Beverage Taxes and Sugar Intake: Policy Statements, Endorsements, and Recommendations. Available online: http://www.yaleruddcenter.org/resources/upload/docs/what/policy/SSBtaxes/SSBTaxStatements.pdf (accessed on 10 January 2013).
106. Muth, N.D.; Dietz, W.H.; Magge, S.N.; Johnson, R.K.; American Academy Of Pediatrics; Section On Obesity; Committee On Nutrition; American Heart Association. Public Policies to Reduce Sugary Drink Consumption in Children and Adolescents. *Pediatrics* **2019**, *143*, e20190282. [CrossRef] [PubMed]
107. Colchero, M.A.; Rivera-Dommarco, J.; Popkin, B.M.; Ng, S.W. In Mexico, Evidence Of Sustained Consumer Response Two Years After Implementing A Sugar-Sweetened Beverage Tax. *Health Aff.* **2017**, *36*, 564–571. [CrossRef] [PubMed]
108. Sanchez-Romero, L.M.; Penko, J.; Coxson, P.G.; Fernandez, A.; Mason, A.; Moran, A.E.; Ávila-Burgos, L.; Odden, M.; Barquera, S.; Bibbins-Domingo, K. Projected Impact of Mexico's Sugar-Sweetened Beverage Tax Policy on Diabetes and Cardiovascular Disease: A Modeling Study. *PLoS Med.* **2016**, *13*, e1002158. [CrossRef] [PubMed]
109. Silver, L.D.; Ng, S.W.; Ryan-Ibarra, S.; Taillie, L.S.; Induni, M.; Miles, D.R.; Poti, J.M.; Popkin, B.M. Changes in prices, sales, consumer spending, and beverage consumption one year after a tax on sugar-sweetened beverages in Berkeley, California, US: A before-and-after study. *PLoS Med.* **2017**, *14*, e1002283. [CrossRef] [PubMed]

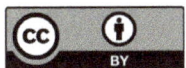 © 2019 by the authors. Licensee MDPI, Basel, Switzerland. This article is an open access article distributed under the terms and conditions of the Creative Commons Attribution (CC BY) license (http://creativecommons.org/licenses/by/4.0/).

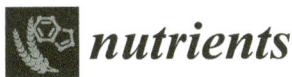

Communication

Dietary Fructose and the Metabolic Syndrome

Marja-Riitta Taskinen [1], Chris J Packard [2] and Jan Borén [3,*]

1. Research Program for Clinical and Molecular Medicine Unit, Diabetes and Obesity, University of Helsinki, 00029 Helsinki, Finland
2. Institute of Cardiovascular and Medical Sciences, University of Glasgow, Glasgow G12 8QQ, UK
3. Department of Molecular and Clinical Medicine, University of Gothenburg and Sahlgrenska University Hospital, 41345 Gothenburg, Sweden
* Correspondence: jan.boren@wlab.gu.se; Tel.: +46-733-764264

Received: 4 July 2019; Accepted: 8 August 2019; Published: 22 August 2019

Abstract: Consumption of fructose, the sweetest of all naturally occurring carbohydrates, has increased dramatically in the last 40 years and is today commonly used commercially in soft drinks, juice, and baked goods. These products comprise a large proportion of the modern diet, in particular in children, adolescents, and young adults. A large body of evidence associate consumption of fructose and other sugar-sweetened beverages with insulin resistance, intrahepatic lipid accumulation, and hypertriglyceridemia. In the long term, these risk factors may contribute to the development of type 2 diabetes and cardiovascular diseases. Fructose is absorbed in the small intestine and metabolized in the liver where it stimulates fructolysis, glycolysis, lipogenesis, and glucose production. This may result in hypertriglyceridemia and fatty liver. Therefore, understanding the mechanisms underlying intestinal and hepatic fructose metabolism is important. Here we review recent evidence linking excessive fructose consumption to health risk markers and development of components of the Metabolic Syndrome.

Keywords: fructose; metabolic syndrome; hypertriglyceridemia; metabolism

---

1. Introduction

Food patterns and diet have greatly changed during the last decades in both industrialized and developing countries together with sedentary lifestyle resulting in dramatic increases of obesity, Metabolic Syndrome (MetS), non-alcoholic fatty liver disease (NAFLD), and type 2 diabetes [1–4]. Importantly, the rapid increase in pediatric NAFLD has become the major concern globally [5,6]. As obesity is a driving force for NAFLD and type 2 diabetes, it is not surprising that the prevalence of the MetS is high in both disorders.

The main component of dietary changes is not only lack of physical activity in face of extra calories, but in particular increases of added sugar mainly in sugar sweetened beverages (SSBs). The common sweeteners are sucrose (containing 50% saccharose and 50% fructose) and high fructose corn syrup (containing up to 55% fructose). The consumption of SSBs, comprising fruit-flavored drinks and sport and energy drinks, is the main source of added sugar. It accounts for about 15–17% of the total daily energy intake in Western diets. Thus, it exceeds the recommended limit of 5% of added sugar (World Health Organization's guidelines 2018) [7]. Consequently, excess sugar consumption has become a major public health problem particularly in children and teen-age populations globally. This menace has initiated the call for the restriction of sugar consumptions [8].

There is substantial and consistent data evidence that exposure to excess fructose intake has detrimental effects on multiple cardiometabolic risk factors [9–13]. In fact, fructose consumption is considered to be a culprit in the MetS as a lipogenic compound that associates with excess ectopic fat accumulation, particularly in the liver. This review will focus on the links between fructose consumption and the MetS, highlighting specifically effects of fructose on hepatic lipid homeostasis and metabolism.

2. Metabolic Effects of Fructose Consumption

2.1. Fructose Metabolism in Enterocytes

Although fructose and glucose are both monosaccharides with closely similar formulas, their metabolism pathways are divergent in both enterocytes and in hepatocytes [14–17]. Fructose absorption is mainly mediated by glucose transporter 5 (GLUT-5), a fructose transporter expressed on the apical border of enterocytes in the small intestine across the lumen in enterocytes (Figure 1) [17,18]. Fructose trafficking from the enterocytes into the portal vein is partly also mediated by GLUT-2. Notably, a part of fructose is metabolized in the cytosol by fructokinase, an enzyme that catalyzes the transfer of a high-energy phosphate group to d-fructose. Notably, high flux of fructose into enterocytes induces GLUT-5 expression. This mechanism may respond to excess chronic fructose intake by increasing the capacity of the intestine for fructose absorption and transport to the liver. Thus, GLUT-5 activity is the key regulator of fructose concentration in the portal vein.

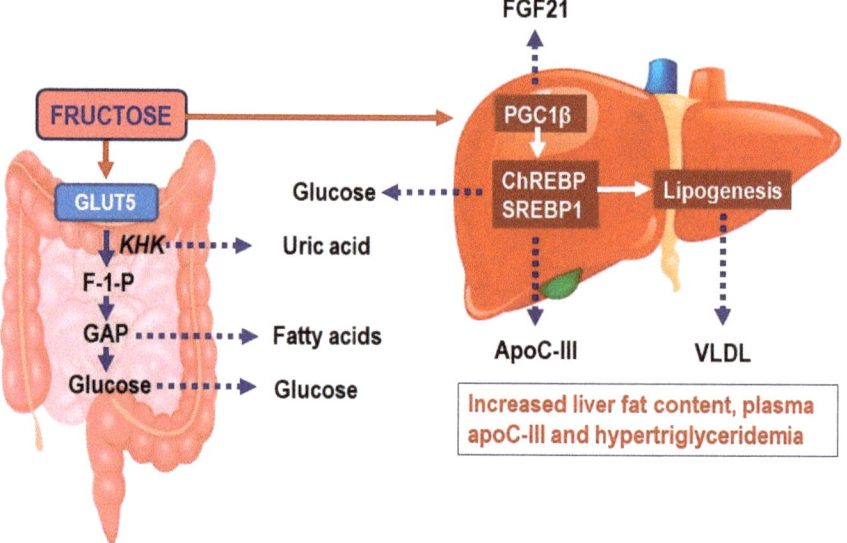

Figure 1. Metabolism of fructose in the intestine and liver. Fructose is in the small intestine metabolized by ketohexokinase (KHK) into fructose-1-phosphate (F-1-P) [19]. F-1-P is then cleaved by aldolase B into dihydroxyacetone phosphate and glyceraldehyde. Glyceraldehyde is phosphorylated by triokinase generating glyceraldehyde 3-phosphate (GAP). GAP and other triose phosphates are resynthesized into glucose via gluconeogenesis or metabolized into lactate or acetyl-CoA, which are oxidized or used for lipogenesis. In the liver, fructose activates the transcription factors carbohydrate-responsive element-binding protein (ChREBP) and sterol regulatory element-binding transcription factor 1c (SREBP1c) and their coactivator peroxisome proliferator-activated receptor-β (PGC1β) [16]. This results in upregulation of pathways that stimulate fructolysis, glycolysis, lipogenesis, and glucose production. Collectively, this results in increased hepatic glucose production, generation of lipid intermediates that may affect hepatic insulin sensitivity, increased expression of APOC3 and increased secretion of triglyceride-rich very-low density lipoproteins (VLDL). The increased APOC3 expression induces increased plasma apoC-III, an inhibitor of lipoprotein lipase and hepatic clearance of lipoprotein remnants [20]. This results in hypertriglyceridemia and accumulation of atherogenic triglyceride-rich lipoprotein (TRL) remnants.

Carbohydrate response element binding protein (ChREBP), a transcription factor responding to sugar intake, is recognized to be a key regulator of hepatic carbohydrate and lipid metabolism [21,22]. Recent data highlight the role of ChREBP in enterocytes as a regulator of intestinal GLUT-5 expression [19,23]. Interestingly, chronic fructose feeding in hamsters enhances lipid synthesis in enterocytes, resulting in increased synthesis of apoB48 and release of intestinal-derived chylomicrons, likely by activation of ChREBP and GLUT-5 [24]. In contrast, ChREBP-deficient mice fed a high fructose diet are reported to be fructose intolerant due to impaired fructose absorption and decreased expression of GLUT-5 [19]. These data highlight the role of intestinal ChREBP for fructose-induced impaired metabolism.

The liver is considered to be the major organ for fructose metabolism [16,25–27]. Plasma concentration of fructose are increased only trivially after fructose intake in humans as first pass metabolism by liver covers about 80–90% of the fructose load. Recently, this concept has been challenged by studies in mice utilizing isotope tracers and mass spectrometry [28]. The key finding suggests that the small intestine may be the major site for dietary fructose metabolism instead of the liver. Notably, the intestinal fructose metabolism seems to be a saturable process that allows high doses of dietary fructose to pass to the liver. The handling of dietary fructose in humans may be different due to the relatively smaller gut in humans than in mice [29]. This is supported by studies in healthy volunteers with stable isotope-labelled fructose to study the initial metabolism of ingested fructose [30]. The amount of dietary fructose escaping the splanchnic extraction averaged only about 14.5% and the first-pass extraction was 85.5%.

A study in healthy males ($n = 7$) demonstrated that fructose combined with Intralipid infusion (consisting of 10% soybean oil, 1.2% egg yolk phospholipids, 2.25% glycerin, and water) resulted in increased apoB48 production rate without any altered catabolism of chylomicrons [31]. Recently, we reported that in abdominally obese men, fructose consumption (75 g/per day served as fructose sweetened beverage) for 12 weeks increased postprandial responses of both plasma triglycerides and apoB48 to a fat rich meal [32]. How changes in fructose absorption and metabolism in enterocyte influence intestinal lipogenesis, reflected in handling of dietary fats and postprandial lipemia, remains to be established in future kinetic studies in humans as direct extrapolation from animal studies may be misleading.

2.2. Fructose Metabolism in the Liver

Hepatic fructose and glucose metabolism occurs via divergent pathways with consequences on hepatic lipid handling and insulin sensitivity reflected in metabolic diseases [15,27,33]. Fructose uptake from portal circulation into liver is mediated by GLUT2 via first pass metabolism by phosphorylation of fructose to fructose-1-phosphate, that is further metabolized to dihydroxyacetone phosphate and glyceraldehyde 3-phosphate. Notably only a small part of ingested fructose ends up in the circulation in contrast to glucose. These initial steps in fructose metabolism seem to be unregulated and bypass the hormonal control in contrast to the strictly regulated glucose uptake and glycolysis in the liver where insulin plays a central role. Glyceraldehyde 3-phosphate and other triose phosphate compounds derived from fructolysis are directed to the formation of pyruvate and acetyl-CoA and to lipogenesis. Consequently, fructose has effects on both glucose homeostasis and lipogenesis the partitioning depending on cellular energy needs [34].

2.3. Evidence Linking Fructose Intake to Non-Alcoholic Fatty Liver Disease (NAFLD) and to Increased Cardiometabolic Risk

The heterogeneity of obesity and its consequences on cardiometabolic risk has been addressed in several outstanding recent reviews that have recognized the importance of body fat distribution, in particular the ectopic fat in the liver as the critical link to cardiometabolic health [25,35–40]. The central role of non-alcoholic fatty liver disease (NAFLD) as the source for multiple cardiometabolic risk factors has raised the questions how the liver can handle extra influx of lipids and the consequences on lipoprotein metabolism and ultimately vascular health [9,10,13,41].

2.4. Effects of Fructose on Hepatic De Novo Lipogenesis

The hallmark of NAFLD is hepatic triglyceride accumulation. The disease develops when the influx of lipid into the liver (from circulating non-esterified fatty acids, diet-derived chylomicrons, and hepatic *de novo* lipogenesis(DNL)) exceeds hepatic lipid disposal (via β-oxidation in mitochondria and triglyceride secretion as lipoprotein particles) [42]. In the past decade, we have seen a remarkable increase in NAFLD [43–45]. It is already the most common cause of chronic liver disease in Western countries and may soon achieve this status in the rest of the world.

Accumulating evidence indicates that increased hepatic DNL is a significant pathway contributing to the development of NAFLD [6,46]. Dietary carbohydrates, in particular, fructose, have been shown to stimulate DNL and increase liver fat, although it is still debated whether this is due to excess energy or fructose per se [46]. Studies in humans are lacking but a comparison between fructose and glucose supplementation in rats for two months showed that, although total caloric consumption was higher in glucose-supplemented rats, fructose caused worse metabolic responses [47].

DNL is a highly regulated pathway, dependent upon several steps, in which key enzymes involved are upregulated in NAFLD [48–50]. Importantly, dietary fructose further increases levels of enzymes involved in DNL as fructose is absorbed via portal vein and delivered to the liver in much higher concentrations as compared to other tissues. Interestingly, in contrast to metabolism of glucose, the breakdown of fructose leads to the generation of metabolites that stimulate hepatic DNL [51–53].

Fructose drives lipogenesis in the setting of insulin resistance as fructose does not require insulin for its metabolism, and it directly stimulates sterol regulatory element-binding protein 1 (SREBP-1c), a major transcriptional regulator of DNL (Figure 1) [54]. Fructose also promotes hepatic DNL and lipid accumulation by suppressing hepatic β-oxidation and by inducing promotes ER stress and uric acid formation (see below). High-fructose feeding has also been shown to increase hepatic expression of ChREBP, a lipogenic transcription factor of carbohydrate metabolism and DNL. ChREBP regulates fructose-induced glucose production independently of insulin signaling [22], and the fructose-induced increases in circulating fibroblast growth factor 21 (FGF21) [55]. The fructose-induced FGF21 feeds back on the liver to enhance further ChREBP activity and hepatic DNL and VLDL secretion [55]. Consequently, circulating FGF21 levels correlate with rates of de novo lipogenesis in human subjects [55]. FGF21 has also been implemented in a signaling axis regulating carbohydrate consumption [11,16,27,33,46,56].

Despite convincing evidence in animals, whether fructose consumption increases DNL in humans to the extent that it induces metabolic disturbances has been more controversial [57]. However, Stanhope et al. reported that 10 weeks overfeeding of fructose (but not glucose), increased DNL (from 11% to 17%) [58]. Other studies have reported that a high fructose diet increased fasting DNL from 2% to 9% [59], and that fructose (75 g/day), served with their habitual diet over 12 weeks to abdominally obese men resulted in significant increases in DNL in both the fasting state (12.3% to 16.5%) and 4 to 8 h postprandially [32,60]. In line, 9 days of isocaloric fructose restriction in the context of an otherwise normal diet led to significant decreased DNL in 37 out of 40 children with obesity [61].

2.5. Clinical Evidence That Fructose Consumption Is Leading to Non-Alcoholic Fatty Liver Disease (NAFLD)

As fructose is recognized to be a lipogenic sugar, its contribution to the pathogenesis of NAFLD has been the focus of intensive research for more than a decade [16,27,33,54,58,62]. The ongoing interest is stimulated by the huge global burden of NAFLD as the potential driver of CVD and its clinical manifestations [11,15,16,63–65].

Although accumulated evidence has demonstrated a strong link between fructose consumption and NAFLD it is still unclear if the association is caused by fructose consumption per se, or by the increased energy intake [66]. An important reason for this is the technological problems associated with measuring liver fat content. Accurate non-invasively measurements of liver fat content require advanced equipment like magnetic resonance imaging and spectroscopy [66–69]. Notably, these technologies allow both quantitation and characterization of hepatic lipids [69,70]. NAFLD is commonly define as >5.5% hepatic fat fraction as determined by MRI [71].

Mot studies focusing on the association between fructose or saccharose overfeeding and liver fat steatosis (quantitated by MRI), have been performed in healthy or obese men [58,72–79]. Many of these studies have been positive [58,72–79]. For example, daily intake of one liter regular cola for 6 months in overweight subjects ($n = 10$) was shown to associate with significant increases of liver fat measured by MRI, but without significant changes of BMI or total fat mass [80]. However, many studies have also been negative [81–83].

Reasons for the different outcome from these earlier studies are the relatively smaller study cohorts, variable and short-duration less than 7 days) study designs, and differing doses of fructose. Despite these weaknesses, many studies seem to indicate that hypercaloric fructose feeding increases liver fat content and that this response is aggravated in obese subjects. For example, Ma et al. reported that the regular consumption of SSBs in overweight and obese subjects from the Framingham cohort ($n = 2634$) was associated with increases of liver fat content quantitated by computed tomography [84].

In line, we recently reported that fructose consumption (75 g/day as fructose sweetened beverage) for 12 weeks in abdominally obese men with cardiometabolic risk factors, significantly increased liver fat content measured by MRI despite relative low increases in weight and waist circumferences [32]. The study subjects were served their habitual diet with add on fructose feeding resulting in hypercaloric set up that also occurs in the real world with SSB intake [32].

Despite this study design, the average increase of liver fat content was modest (10%) in face of no significant change in visceral or subcutaneous fat depots and there was high variation in the response liver fat content. To better understand this variation, we genotyped all individuals for carrier status of the major risk alleles for hepatic steatosis; PNPLA3, TN6SF2, and MBOAT7. Results showed that the number of risk alleles associated with increased liver fat at the baseline. However, individuals without and with risk allele did not have differences in the response of liver fat during fructose feeding. In line with this, two other studies have confirmed increases of liver fat content during carbohydrate (simple sugars) overfeeding on hypercaloric diet for 3 weeks in overweight and obese subjects [85,86].

The key metabolic and mechanistic issues of fructose consumption has been studied during a nine days isocaloric feeding study (fructose restriction to less than 4% of calories) in obese children ($n = 40$) with MetS and a high habitual sugar consumption (>50 g/day) [61,87,88]. The metabolic assessment was extensive utilizing magnetic resonance imaging and stable isotope technology for DNL in addition to extensive biomarker platform. The first important message is that the dietary fructose restriction was associated with significant reductions of liver (from 7.2% to 3.8%, $p < 0.001$) and visceral fat content (from 123 cm^3 to 110 cm^3, $p < 0.001$). Notably, the reduction of liver fat content was not related to the baseline liver fat content. The diet intervention was also associated with a significant decrease of DNL and an improved lipoprotein profile. In addition, significant improvements were observed in biomarkers of insulin resistance and glucose metabolism. The authors also elucidated the impact of the diet intervention on the methylglyoxal (MG) pathway [15,63,89–91], and surprisingly found that fructose restriction associated with marked reduction of D-lactate, a biomarker of MG metabolism. This change of D-lactate correlated with reduction of liver fat content and DNL [88]. These observations open a new perspective of the adverse metabolic effects of excess fructose intake.

Thus, accumulating evidence supports the fact that fructose is an important mediator for the development of NAFLD and a main driver for DNL [64]. Indeed, this concept is supported by a recent meta-analysis including 6326 participants and 1361 cases with NAFLD [92]. However, it is still debated whether fructose, when consumed in isocaloric amounts, causes more liver fat accumulation than other energy-dense nutrients [93].

Kirk et al. investigated the effects of acute and chronic calorie restriction with either a low-fat, high-carbohydrate (>180 g/day) diet or a low-carbohydrate (<50 g/day) diet on hepatic and skeletal muscle insulin sensitivity in 22 obese subjects [94]. Interestingly, the low-carbohydrate diet lowered the hepatic lipids within 48 h by 30% (compared to ~10% in the low-fat, high-carbohydrate group). The mechanism for the rapid clearance of liver fat was not elucidated. After approximately 11 weeks (7% weight loss) a similar marked reduction of liver fat content was seen in both groups (38% vs. 44%). These results show that liver fat content is highly dynamic in response to energy balance and sugar intake. However, it is still debated whether a low-carbohydrate hypocaloric diet is more efficient than a low-fat hypocaloric diet in reducing intrahepatic lipid accumulation.

Haufe et al. compared the 6 months responses of a low-carbohydrate hypocaloric or a low-fat hypocaloric diet on intrahepatic lipid accumulation in overweight/obese subjects (n = 84 to 86 in each group) [95]. Results showed that both diets had the same beneficial effects on intrahepatic lipid accumulation, weight loss and insulin resistance. The decrease in intrahepatic fat was independent of visceral fat loss and not associated with changes in whole body insulin sensitivity. Interestingly, subjects with high baseline intrahepatic lipids (>5.6%) lost ≈ 7-fold more liver fat compared with those with low baseline values irrespective of the prolonged hypocaloric diet.

2.6. Effects of Fructose on Uric Acid Metabolism and MG (Methyl Glyoxal) Pathways

The role of fructose as a potential source of uric acid was recognized decades ago [96]. The rapid phosphorylation of fructose to fructose-1-phospate not only increases the fluxes of trioses for lipogenesis, but also depletes ATP stores leading to the degradation of AMP, resulting in increased generation of uric acid via purine pathway. Importantly, fructose seems to be the only carbohydrate that can generate uric acid. Cellular depletion of ATP has several adverse consequences on energy metabolism including increased ER stress and mitochondrial dysfunction [64]. ER stress has been linked to many metabolic diseases including NAFLD [97] and can be induced by a range of condition such as high protein demand, viral infection, mutant protein expression, hypoxia, energy deprivation, or exposure to excessive oxidative stress including ATP depletion [97–99]. The ER stress triggers an adaptive signaling pathway known as the Unfolded Protein Response (UPR) to restore normal ER function. If the UPR fail to restore normal ER function, the UPR aims towards apoptosis [97–99]. A sustained chronic UPR response may worsen the pathophysiological condition by inducing lipotoxicity, insulin resistance, inflammation, and apoptotic cell death [97–99].

ER stress activates the transcription factor X-box binding protein 1 (XBP1s), a key regulator of the unfolded protein response. Interestingly, XBP1 also regulates hepatic fatty acid synthesis [100]. Mitochondrial oxidative stress results in enhanced generation of citrate and acetyl coenzyme A AcCoA [101–103], two metabolites that stimulate lipogenesis. This may explain why fructose is lipogenic [16,104]. An additional nexus is that increased triose flux enhance the generation of methyl glyoxal (MG) and dicarbonyl stress. A key crossroad step is the inactivation of AMPK by MG and consequences on energy metabolism. This is a novel pathway linked to excess fructose intake and its metabolic relevance remains to be clarified [15]. In summary, fructose seems to influence multiple metabolic pathways in the liver that results in enhanced lipogenesis, generation of uric acid, ER stress, and inflammation. The association between uric acid and insulin resistance [105], raised the interest of uric acid as a potential biomarker in the Metabolic Syndrome [105]. Indeed, several studies have established that serum uric acid is a risk factor for the Metabolic Syndrome [106–113].

Substantial evidence suggest that uric acid also associates with NAFLD [114–117]. Several studies have reported that serum uric acid levels are higher in subjects with NAFLD than in those without NAFLD [64,118,119]. Importantly, hyperuricemia seems to associate with NAFLD independently of other features of the MetS and these associations are independent on body weight [120]. Thus, uric acid belongs to the cluster of biomarkers in Metabolic Syndrome and NAFLD.

Can excess intake of fructose and SSBs result in the elevation of plasma uric acid concentrations? Indeed, numerous studies have found an association between fructose/SSBs intake and uric acid levels [27,54,64,118,121,122]. For example, two large prospective cohort studies including American men (n = 46,393) or American women (n = 78,906) showed strong associations between consumption of SBBs and hyperuricemia [123,124]. Similar positive associations between SSBs intake and serum uric acid concentrations have been observed in Korean, Mexican, and Brazilian populations [125–127]. Likewise, in an adolescents cohort (n = 4867 aged 12 to 18 years) consumption of SSBs associated with higher serum uric acid and also higher systolic blood pressure [128].

So far, data from RCTs on fructose feeding trials have remained limited. Fructose feeding associated with increased uric acid in three smaller intervention studies [72,129,130]. Weaknesses of the study protocol are that the design and duration of feeding trials, as well as study cohorts, are highly variable. Unfortunately, data from available meta-analyses are not consistent. One meta-analysis reported that fructose intake as an apart of isocaloric diet did not raise uric acid levels but signaled that the hypercaloric intake of fructose may raise uric acid [131]. Although hyperuricemia is highly prevalent in patients with NAFLD and Met Syndrome, its clinical relevance remains debated. Recent French recommendations for sugar intake concluded that long-term consequences of potential small increases of uric acid by fructose/sugar intake remain insufficient [132], likewise critical analysis of the available data left open the casual link between fructose intake and hyperuricemia [133,134].

2.7. Consequences of Increased Lipid Synthesis to Very Low-Density Lipoproteins (VLDL) Metabolism and Release—Effects on Plasma Lipids, Lipoproteins, and Apolipoproteins

The association of blood lipid levels and consumption of added sugars was studied in the adult population in the National Health and Nutrition Examination Survey (NHANES) (n = 6113) [135]. In this American cross-sectional study higher fructose consumers had more unfavorable lipid levels, namely significantly lower HDL cholesterol, higher triglycerides, and a high ratio of triglycerides to high density lipoproteins (HDL), whereas women also had higher low-density lipoprotein (LDL) cholesterol levels. Likewise, in the Framingham study, daily soft drink consumers had higher incidence of elevated triglycerides and low HDL cholesterol than non-consumers (relative risk: 1.22 and 1.22, respectively) [136].

Several studies have consistently reported increased responses of fasting and postprandial triglyceride levels and 24 h. profiles to short term feeding of fructose as compared to glucose in both lean and obese subjects [8,53]. These perturbations directly lead to other lipid abnormalities including elevation of apoB levels, accumulation of small dense LDL, and increased remnant lipoproteins, combined with reduced HDL cholesterol which all are components of the atherogenic lipid triad, a strong risk factor for CVD. Interestingly, the deleterious effect of fructose on lipid metabolism is directly linked to the daily intake; a fructose intake >50 g/day is associated with postprandial hyperlipemia whereas intake above 100 g/day also results in elevation of fasting serum triglycerides [137]. Collectively, these results clearly show that fructose intake is directly linked to an atherogenic dyslipidemia.

The recent increased focus on plasma triglycerides and postprandial hyperlipidemia not only as markers but also as causal drivers of CVD has partly been driven by improved understanding of the biology and genetics of triglyceride heritability. Of particular interest is *APOC3*, which has emerged as a novel therapeutic target to reduce dyslipidemia and CVD risk [20,138–140]. Interestingly, fructose feeding is linked to a significant rise of plasma apoC-III levels (Figure 1) [32,141].

2.8. Interactions between Fructose Consumption and Changes in Gut Microbiota

High consumption of fructose, artificial sweeteners, and sugar alcohols have been shown to affect host-gastrointestinal microbe interactions and possibly contribute to the development of metabolic disorders and obesity. Multiple studies have also reported fructose as a critical factor contributing to NAFLD progression by modulating intestinal microbiota (see review [142]). Gut microbiota interacts with its host, and influences both the energy homeostasis and the immunity of the host [142]. Shifts in this composition can result in alterations of the symbiotic relationship, which can promote metabolic diseases [143]. Indeed, the microbial composition have been shown to differ between healthy individuals and NAFLD patients [144], and a diet enriched in fructose not only induced NAFLD but also negatively affected the gut barrier and the microbiota composition, leading to impaired microbiota [145]. The underlying mechanisms are complex and still unclear, but Oh et al. recently showed that dietary fructose activates the Ack-pathway, involved in generating acetic acid, which in turn triggers the bacterial stress response that promotes phage production [146]. Thus, prophages in a gut symbiont can be induced by diet and metabolites affected by diet, which provides a potential mechanistic explanation for the effects of diet on the intestinal phage community [147].

The complex interaction between dietary carbohydrates and gut microbiota was recently demonstrated in a two-week intervention with an isocaloric low-carbohydrate diet in obese subjects with NAFLD [148]. The authors observed rapid and marked reductions of liver fat paralleled by marked decreases in hepatic DNL and increases in hepatic β-oxidation. Interestingly, the marked reduction in cardiometabolic risk factors paralleled with rapid increases in the folate-producing gut microbiota Streptococcus, serum folate concentrations, and hepatic one-carbon metabolism.

3. Conclusions

Consistent data evidence that excess fructose intake as a central component of unhealthy lifestyle has detrimental effects on multiple cardiovascular risk factors. Consequently, it is not surprising that links between fructose consumption with MetS and NAFLD are strong. Fructose is a lipogenic sugar as it increases hepatic *de novo* lipogenesis in the liver through several metabolic pathways resulting in a vicious circle that further aggravates DNL. Increased DNL favors excess fat accumulation in the liver, being a driving force for increased secretion of VLDL particles leading to the atherogenic lipid profile and other metabolic derangements associated with CVD risk. The global health burden of MetS together with NAFLD is growing rapidly, sweeping across the world. It is clear that added sugars have become a threat to cardiometabolic health. These facts call for the restriction of dietary sugars, especially SSB consumption to limit fructose intake to achieve better cardiometabolic health.

Funding: This research received no external funding.

Conflicts of Interest: The authors declare no conflict of interest.

References

1. GBD 2015 Obesity Collaborators; Afshin, A.; Forouzanfar, M.H.; Reitsma, M.B.; Sur, P.; Estep, K.; Lee, A.; Marczak, L.; Mokdad, A.H.; Moradi-Lakeh, M.; et al. Health Effects of Overweight and Obesity in 195 Countries over 25 Years. *N. Engl. J. Med.* **2017**, *377*, 13–27. [CrossRef] [PubMed]
2. Bluher, M. Obesity: Global epidemiology and pathogenesis. *Nat. Rev. Endocrinol.* **2019**, *15*, 288–298. [CrossRef] [PubMed]
3. Malik, V.S.; Li, Y.; Pan, A.; De Koning, L.; Schernhammer, E.; Willett, W.C.; Hu, F.B. Long-Term Consumption of Sugar-Sweetened and Artificially Sweetened Beverages and Risk of Mortality in US Adults. *Circulation* **2019**. [CrossRef] [PubMed]
4. Younossi, Z.M. Non-alcoholic fatty liver disease—A global public health perspective. *J. Hepatol.* **2019**, *70*, 531–544. [CrossRef] [PubMed]
5. Vos, M.B.; Abrams, S.H.; Barlow, S.E.; Caprio, S.; Daniels, S.R.; Kohli, R.; Mouzaki, M.; Sathya, P.; Schwimmer, J.B.; Sundaram, S.S.; et al. NASPGHAN Clinical Practice Guideline for the Diagnosis and Treatment of Nonalcoholic Fatty Liver Disease in Children: Recommendations from the Expert Committee on NAFLD (ECON) and the North American Society of Pediatric Gastroenterology, Hepatology and Nutrition (NASPGHAN). *J. Pediatr. Gastroenterol. Nutr.* **2017**, *64*, 319–334. [CrossRef] [PubMed]
6. Younossi, Z.; Tacke, F.; Arrese, M.; Chander Sharma, B.; Mostafa, I.; Bugianesi, E.; Wai-Sun Wong, V.; Yilmaz, Y.; George, J.; Fan, J.; et al. Global Perspectives on Nonalcoholic Fatty Liver Disease and Nonalcoholic Steatohepatitis. *Hepatology* **2019**, *69*, 2672–2682. [CrossRef] [PubMed]
7. Powell, E.S.; Smith-Taillie, L.P.; Popkin, B.M. Added Sugars Intake Across the Distribution of US Children and Adult Consumers: 1977–2012. *J. Acad. Nutr. Diet.* **2016**, *116*, 1543–1550. [CrossRef] [PubMed]
8. Johnson, R.K.; Lichtenstein, A.H.; Anderson, C.A.M.; Carson, J.A.; Despres, J.P.; Hu, F.B.; Kris-Etherton, P.M.; Otten, J.J.; Towfighi, A.; Wylie-Rosett, J.; et al. Low-Calorie Sweetened Beverages and Cardiometabolic Health: A Science Advisory From the American Heart Association. *Circulation* **2018**, *138*, e126–e140. [CrossRef] [PubMed]

9. Lim, S.; Taskinen, M.R.; Boren, J. Crosstalk between nonalcoholic fatty liver disease and cardiometabolic syndrome. *Obes. Rev.* **2019**, *20*, 599–611. [CrossRef]
10. Santos, R.D.; Valenti, L.; Romeo, S. Does nonalcoholic fatty liver disease cause cardiovascular disease? Current knowledge and gaps. *Atherosclerosis* **2019**, *282*, 110–120. [CrossRef]
11. Mirtschink, P.; Jang, C.; Arany, Z.; Krek, W. Fructose metabolism, cardiometabolic risk, and the epidemic of coronary artery disease. *Eur. Heart J.* **2018**, *39*, 2497–2505. [CrossRef] [PubMed]
12. Stanhope, K.L.; Goran, M.I.; Bosy-Westphal, A.; King, J.C.; Schmidt, L.A.; Schwarz, J.M.; Stice, E.; Sylvetsky, A.C.; Turnbaugh, P.J.; Bray, G.A.; et al. Pathways and mechanisms linking dietary components to cardiometabolic disease: Thinking beyond calories. *Obes. Rev.* **2018**, *19*, 1205–1235. [CrossRef] [PubMed]
13. Stahl, E.P.; Dhindsa, D.S.; Lee, S.K.; Sandesara, P.B.; Chalasani, N.P.; Sperling, L.S. Nonalcoholic Fatty Liver Disease and the Heart: JACC State-of-the-Art Review. *J. Am. Coll. Cardiol.* **2019**, *73*, 948–963. [CrossRef] [PubMed]
14. Ferraris, R.P.; Choe, J.Y.; Patel, C.R. Intestinal Absorption of Fructose. *Annu. Rev. Nutr.* **2018**, *38*, 41–67. [CrossRef] [PubMed]
15. Mortera, R.R.; Bains, Y.; Gugliucci, A. Fructose at the crossroads of the metabolic syndrome and obesity epidemics. *Front. Biosci. (Landmark Ed.)* **2019**, *24*, 186–211.
16. Hannou, S.A.; Haslam, D.E.; McKeown, N.M.; Herman, M.A. Fructose metabolism and metabolic disease. *J. Clin. Investig.* **2018**, *128*, 545–555. [CrossRef]
17. Hoffman, S.; Alvares, D.; Adeli, K. Intestinal lipogenesis: How carbs turn on triglyceride production in the gut. *Curr. Opin. Clin. Nutr. Metab. Care* **2019**, *22*, 284–288. [CrossRef]
18. Patel, C.; Douard, V.; Yu, S.; Gao, N.; Ferraris, R.P. Transport, metabolism, and endosomal trafficking-dependent regulation of intestinal fructose absorption. *FASEB J.* **2015**, *29*, 4046–4058. [CrossRef]
19. Lee, H.J.; Cha, J.Y. Recent insights into the role of ChREBP in intestinal fructose absorption and metabolism. *BMB Rep.* **2018**, *51*, 429–436. [CrossRef]
20. Taskinen, M.R.; Packard, C.J.; Boren, J. Emerging Evidence that ApoC-III Inhibitors Provide Novel Options to Reduce the Residual CVD. *Curr. Atheroscler. Rep.* **2019**, *21*, 27. [CrossRef]
21. Abdul-Wahed, A.; Guilmeau, S.; Postic, C. Sweet Sixteenth for ChREBP: Established Roles and Future Goals. *Cell Metab.* **2017**, *26*, 324–341. [CrossRef] [PubMed]
22. Kim, M.S.; Krawczyk, S.A.; Doridot, L.; Fowler, A.J.; Wang, J.X.; Trauger, S.A.; Noh, H.L.; Kang, H.J.; Meissen, J.K.; Blatnik, M.; et al. ChREBP regulates fructose-induced glucose production independently of insulin signaling. *J. Clin. Investig.* **2016**, *126*, 4372–4386. [CrossRef] [PubMed]
23. Kim, M.; Astapova, I.I.; Flier, S.N.; Hannou, S.A.; Doridot, L.; Sargsyan, A.; Kou, H.H.; Fowler, A.J.; Liang, G.; Herman, M.A. Intestinal, but not hepatic, ChREBP is required for fructose tolerance. *JCI Insight* **2017**, *2*. [CrossRef] [PubMed]
24. Haidari, M.; Leung, N.; Mahbub, F.; Uffelman, K.D.; Kohen-Avramoglu, R.; Lewis, G.F.; Adeli, K. Fasting and postprandial overproduction of intestinally derived lipoproteins in an animal model of insulin resistance. Evidence that chronic fructose feeding in the hamster is accompanied by enhanced intestinal de novo lipogenesis and ApoB48-containing lipoprotein overproduction. *J. Biol. Chem.* **2002**, *277*, 31646–31655. [CrossRef] [PubMed]
25. Stanhope, K.L. Sugar consumption, metabolic disease and obesity: The state of the controversy. *Crit. Rev. Clin. Lab. Sci.* **2016**, *53*, 52–67. [CrossRef] [PubMed]
26. Sun, S.Z.; Empie, M.W. Fructose metabolism in humans—What isotopic tracer studies tell us. *Nutr. Metab. (Lond.)* **2012**, *9*, 89. [CrossRef] [PubMed]
27. Softic, S.; Cohen, D.E.; Kahn, C.R. Role of Dietary Fructose and Hepatic De Novo Lipogenesis in Fatty Liver Disease. *Dig. Dis. Sci.* **2016**, *61*, 1282–1293. [CrossRef] [PubMed]
28. Jang, C.; Hui, S.; Lu, W.; Cowan, A.J.; Morscher, R.J.; Lee, G.; Liu, W.; Tesz, G.J.; Birnbaum, M.J.; Rabinowitz, J.D. The Small Intestine Converts Dietary Fructose into Glucose and Organic Acids. *Cell Metab.* **2018**, *27*, 351–361. [CrossRef] [PubMed]
29. Gonzalez, J.T.; Betts, J.A. Dietary Fructose Metabolism By Splanchnic Organs: Size Matters. *Cell Metab.* **2018**, *27*, 483–485. [CrossRef]
30. Francey, C.; Cros, J.; Rosset, R.; Creze, C.; Rey, V.; Stefanoni, N.; Schneiter, P.; Tappy, L.; Seyssel, K. The extra-splanchnic fructose escape after ingestion of a fructose-glucose drink: An exploratory study in healthy humans using a dual fructose isotope method. *Clin. Nutr. ESPEN* **2019**, *29*, 125–132. [CrossRef]

31. Xiao, C.; Dash, S.; Morgantini, C.; Lewis, G.F. Novel role of enteral monosaccharides in intestinal lipoprotein production in healthy humans. *Arterioscler. Thromb. Vasc. Biol.* **2013**, *33*, 1056–1062. [CrossRef] [PubMed]
32. Taskinen, M.R.; Soderlund, S.; Bogl, L.H.; Hakkarainen, A.; Matikainen, N.; Pietilainen, K.H.; Rasanen, S.; Lundbom, N.; Bjornson, E.; Eliasson, B.; et al. Adverse effects of fructose on cardiometabolic risk factors and hepatic lipid metabolism in subjects with abdominal obesity. *J. Intern. Med.* **2017**, *282*, 187–201. [CrossRef] [PubMed]
33. Herman, M.A.; Samuel, V.T. The Sweet Path to Metabolic Demise: Fructose and Lipid Synthesis. *Trends Endocrinol. Metab.* **2016**, *27*, 719–730. [CrossRef] [PubMed]
34. Tappy, L. Fructose-containing caloric sweeteners as a cause of obesity and metabolic disorders. *J. Exp. Biol.* **2018**, *221*. [CrossRef] [PubMed]
35. Spalding, K.L.; Bernard, S.; Naslund, E.; Salehpour, M.; Possnert, G.; Appelsved, L.; Fu, K.Y.; Alkass, K.; Druid, H.; Thorell, A.; et al. Impact of fat mass and distribution on lipid turnover in human adipose tissue. *Nat. Commun.* **2017**, *8*, 15253. [CrossRef] [PubMed]
36. Kim, S.H.; Despres, J.P.; Koh, K.K. Obesity and cardiovascular disease: Friend or foe? *Eur. Heart J.* **2016**, *37*, 3560–3568. [CrossRef] [PubMed]
37. Karpe, F.; Pinnick, K.E. Biology of upper-body and lower-body adipose tissue—Link to whole-body phenotypes. *Nat. Rev. Endocrinol.* **2015**, *11*, 90–100. [CrossRef] [PubMed]
38. Schulze, M.B. Metabolic health in normal-weight and obese individuals. *Diabetologia* **2019**, *62*, 558–566. [CrossRef] [PubMed]
39. Neeland, I.J.; Poirier, P.; Despres, J.P. Cardiovascular and Metabolic Heterogeneity of Obesity: Clinical Challenges and Implications for Management. *Circulation* **2018**, *137*, 1391–1406. [CrossRef]
40. Piche, M.E.; Vasan, S.K.; Hodson, L.; Karpe, F. Relevance of human fat distribution on lipid and lipoprotein metabolism and cardiovascular disease risk. *Curr. Opin. Lipidol.* **2018**, *29*, 285–292. [CrossRef]
41. Stefan, N.; Haring, H.U.; Cusi, K. Non-alcoholic fatty liver disease: Causes, diagnosis, cardiometabolic consequences, and treatment strategies. *Lancet Diabetes Endocrinol.* **2019**, *7*, 313–324. [CrossRef]
42. Stefan, N.; Kantartzis, K.; Haring, H.U. Causes and metabolic consequences of Fatty liver. *Endocr. Rev.* **2008**, *29*, 939–960. [CrossRef] [PubMed]
43. Vernon, G.; Baranova, A.; Younossi, Z.M. Systematic review: The epidemiology and natural history of non-alcoholic fatty liver disease and non-alcoholic steatohepatitis in adults. *Aliment. Pharmacol. Ther.* **2011**, *34*, 274–285. [CrossRef] [PubMed]
44. Bellentani, S.; Scaglioni, F.; Marino, M.; Bedogni, G. Epidemiology of non-alcoholic fatty liver disease. *Dig. Dis.* **2010**, *28*, 155–161. [CrossRef] [PubMed]
45. Estes, C.; Anstee, Q.M.; Arias-Loste, M.T.; Bantel, H.; Bellentani, S.; Caballeria, J.; Colombo, M.; Craxi, A.; Crespo, J.; Day, C.P.; et al. Modeling NAFLD disease burden in China, France, Germany, Italy, Japan, Spain, United Kingdom, and United States for the period 2016–2030. *J. Hepatol.* **2018**, *69*, 896–904. [CrossRef]
46. Chiu, S.; Mulligan, K.; Schwarz, J.M. Dietary carbohydrates and fatty liver disease: De novo lipogenesis. *Curr. Opin. Clin. Nutr. Metab. Care* **2018**, *21*, 277–282. [CrossRef]
47. Sanguesa, G.; Shaligram, S.; Akther, F.; Roglans, N.; Laguna, J.C.; Rahimian, R.; Alegret, M. Type of supplemented simple sugar, not merely calorie intake, determines adverse effects on metabolism and aortic function in female rats. *Am. J. Physiol. Heart Circ. Physiol.* **2017**, *312*, H289–H304. [CrossRef]
48. Dorn, C.; Riener, M.O.; Kirovski, G.; Saugspier, M.; Steib, K.; Weiss, T.S.; Gabele, E.; Kristiansen, G.; Hartmann, A.; Hellerbrand, C. Expression of fatty acid synthase in nonalcoholic fatty liver disease. *Int. J. Clin. Exp. Pathol.* **2010**, *3*, 505–514.
49. Mitsuyoshi, H.; Yasui, K.; Harano, Y.; Endo, M.; Tsuji, K.; Minami, M.; Itoh, Y.; Okanoue, T.; Yoshikawa, T. Analysis of hepatic genes involved in the metabolism of fatty acids and iron in nonalcoholic fatty liver disease. *Hepatol. Res.* **2009**, *39*, 366–373. [CrossRef]
50. Paglialunga, S.; Dehn, C.A. Clinical assessment of hepatic de novo lipogenesis in non-alcoholic fatty liver disease. *Lipids Health Dis.* **2016**, *15*, 159. [CrossRef]
51. Tappy, L.; Le, K.A. Metabolic effects of fructose and the worldwide increase in obesity. *Physiol. Rev.* **2010**, *90*, 23–46. [CrossRef]
52. Rutledge, A.C.; Adeli, K. Fructose and the metabolic syndrome: Pathophysiology and molecular mechanisms. *Nutr. Rev.* **2007**, *65*, S13–S23. [CrossRef]

53. Stanhope, K.L.; Havel, P.J. Fructose consumption: recent results and their potential implications. *Ann. N. Y. Acad. Sci.* **2010**, *1190*, 15–24. [CrossRef]
54. Malik, V.S.; Hu, F.B. Fructose and Cardiometabolic Health: What the Evidence From Sugar-Sweetened Beverages Tells Us. *J. Am. Coll. Cardiol.* **2015**, *66*, 1615–1624. [CrossRef]
55. Fisher, F.M.; Kim, M.; Doridot, L.; Cunniff, J.C.; Parker, T.S.; Levine, D.M.; Hellerstein, M.K.; Hudgins, L.C.; Maratos-Flier, E.; Herman, M.A. A critical role for ChREBP-mediated FGF21 secretion in hepatic fructose metabolism. *Mol. Metab.* **2017**, *6*, 14–21. [CrossRef]
56. Solinas, G.; Boren, J.; Dulloo, A.G. De novo lipogenesis in metabolic homeostasis: More friend than foe? *Mol. Metab.* **2015**, *4*, 367–377. [CrossRef]
57. Stanhope, K.L. Role of fructose-containing sugars in the epidemics of obesity and metabolic syndrome. *Annu. Rev. Med.* **2012**, *63*, 329–343. [CrossRef]
58. Stanhope, K.L.; Schwarz, J.M.; Keim, N.L.; Griffen, S.C.; Bremer, A.A.; Graham, J.L.; Hatcher, B.; Cox, C.L.; Dyachenko, A.; Zhang, W.; et al. Consuming fructose-sweetened, not glucose-sweetened, beverages increases visceral adiposity and lipids and decreases insulin sensitivity in overweight/obese humans. *J. Clin. Investig.* **2009**, *119*, 1322–1334. [CrossRef]
59. Faeh, D.; Minehira, K.; Schwarz, J.M.; Periasamy, R.; Park, S.; Tappy, L. Effect of fructose overfeeding and fish oil administration on hepatic de novo lipogenesis and insulin sensitivity in healthy men. *Diabetes* **2005**, *54*, 1907–1913. [CrossRef]
60. Stanhope, K.L. More pieces of the fructose puzzle. *J. Intern. Med.* **2017**, *282*, 202–204. [CrossRef]
61. Schwarz, J.M.; Noworolski, S.M.; Erkin-Cakmak, A.; Korn, N.J.; Wen, M.J.; Tai, V.W.; Jones, G.M.; Palii, S.P.; Velasco-Alin, M.; Pan, K.; et al. Effects of Dietary Fructose Restriction on Liver Fat, De Novo Lipogenesis, and Insulin Kinetics in Children With Obesity. *Gastroenterology* **2017**, *153*, 743–752. [CrossRef]
62. Vos, M.B.; Lavine, J.E. Dietary fructose in nonalcoholic fatty liver disease. *Hepatology* **2013**, *57*, 2525–2531. [CrossRef]
63. Jegatheesan, P.; De Bandt, J.P. Fructose and NAFLD: The Multifaceted Aspects of Fructose Metabolism. *Nutrients* **2017**, *9*, 230. [CrossRef]
64. Jensen, T.; Abdelmalek, M.F.; Sullivan, S.; Nadeau, K.J.; Green, M.; Roncal, C.; Nakagawa, T.; Kuwabara, M.; Sato, Y.; Kang, D.H.; et al. Fructose and sugar: A major mediator of non-alcoholic fatty liver disease. *J. Hepatol.* **2018**, *68*, 1063–1075. [CrossRef]
65. Moore, J.B. From sugar to liver fat and public health: Systems biology driven studies in understanding non-alcoholic fatty liver disease pathogenesis. *Proc. Nutr. Soc.* **2019**. [CrossRef]
66. Alexander, M.; Loomis, A.K.; Fairburn-Beech, J.; van der Lei, J.; Duarte-Salles, T.; Prieto-Alhambra, D.; Ansell, D.; Pasqua, A.; Lapi, F.; Rijnbeek, P.; et al. Real-world data reveal a diagnostic gap in non-alcoholic fatty liver disease. *BMC Med.* **2018**, *16*, 130. [CrossRef]
67. Lee, S.S.; Park, S.H.; Kim, H.J.; Kim, S.Y.; Kim, M.Y.; Kim, D.Y.; Suh, D.J.; Kim, K.M.; Bae, M.H.; Lee, J.Y.; et al. Non-invasive assessment of hepatic steatosis: Prospective comparison of the accuracy of imaging examinations. *J. Hepatol.* **2010**, *52*, 579–585. [CrossRef]
68. Reeder, S.B.; Cruite, I.; Hamilton, G.; Sirlin, C.B. Quantitative assessment of liver fat with magnetic resonance imaging and spectroscopy. *J. Magn. Reson. Imaging* **2011**, *34*, 729–749. [CrossRef]
69. Szczepaniak, L.S.; Nurenberg, P.; Leonard, D.; Browning, J.D.; Reingold, J.S.; Grundy, S.; Hobbs, H.H.; Dobbins, R.L. Magnetic resonance spectroscopy to measure hepatic triglyceride content: Prevalence of hepatic steatosis in the general population. *Am. J. Physiol. Endocrinol. Metab.* **2005**, *288*, E462–E468. [CrossRef]
70. van de Weijer, T.; Schrauwen-Hinderling, V.B. Application of Magnetic Resonance Spectroscopy in metabolic research. *Biochim. Biophys. Acta Mol. Basis Dis.* **2019**, *1865*, 741–748. [CrossRef]
71. European Association for the Study of the Liver; European Association for the Study of Diabetes; European Association for the Study of Obesity. EASL-EASD-EASO Clinical Practice Guidelines for the management of non-alcoholic fatty liver disease. *Diabetologia* **2016**, *59*, 1121–1140. [CrossRef]
72. Le, K.A.; Ith, M.; Kreis, R.; Faeh, D.; Bortolotti, M.; Tran, C.; Boesch, C.; Tappy, L. Fructose overconsumption causes dyslipidemia and ectopic lipid deposition in healthy subjects with and without a family history of type 2 diabetes. *Am. J. Clin. Nutr.* **2009**, *89*, 1760–1765. [CrossRef]
73. Sobrecases, H.; Le, K.A.; Bortolotti, M.; Schneiter, P.; Ith, M.; Kreis, R.; Boesch, C.; Tappy, L. Effects of short-term overfeeding with fructose, fat and fructose plus fat on plasma and hepatic lipids in healthy men. *Diabetes Metab.* **2010**, *36*, 244–246. [CrossRef]

74. Lecoultre, V.; Egli, L.; Carrel, G.; Theytaz, F.; Kreis, R.; Schneiter, P.; Boss, A.; Zwygart, K.; Le, K.A.; Bortolotti, M.; et al. Effects of fructose and glucose overfeeding on hepatic insulin sensitivity and intrahepatic lipids in healthy humans. *Obesity (Silver Spring)* **2013**, *21*, 782–785. [CrossRef]
75. Theytaz, F.; Noguchi, Y.; Egli, L.; Campos, V.; Buehler, T.; Hodson, L.; Patterson, B.W.; Nishikata, N.; Kreis, R.; Mittendorfer, B.; et al. Effects of supplementation with essential amino acids on intrahepatic lipid concentrations during fructose overfeeding in humans. *Am. J. Clin. Nutr.* **2012**, *96*, 1008–1016. [CrossRef]
76. Johnston, R.D.; Stephenson, M.C.; Crossland, H.; Cordon, S.M.; Palcidi, E.; Cox, E.F.; Taylor, M.A.; Aithal, G.P.; Macdonald, I.A. No difference between high-fructose and high-glucose diets on liver triacylglycerol or biochemistry in healthy overweight men. *Gastroenterology* **2013**, *145*, 1016–1025. [CrossRef]
77. Surowska, A.; Jegatheesan, P.; Campos, V.; Marques, A.S.; Egli, L.; Cros, J.; Rosset, R.; Lecoultre, V.; Kreis, R.; Boesch, C.; et al. Effects of Dietary Protein and Fat Content on Intrahepatocellular and Intramyocellular Lipids during a 6-Day Hypercaloric, High Sucrose Diet: A Randomized Controlled Trial in Normal Weight Healthy Subjects. *Nutrients* **2019**, *11*, 209. [CrossRef]
78. Schwarz, J.M.; Noworolski, S.M.; Wen, M.J.; Dyachenko, A.; Prior, J.L.; Weinberg, M.E.; Herraiz, L.A.; Tai, V.W.; Bergeron, N.; Bersot, T.P.; et al. Effect of a High-Fructose Weight-Maintaining Diet on Lipogenesis and Liver Fat. *J. Clin. Endocrinol. Metab.* **2015**, *100*, 2434–2442. [CrossRef]
79. Cox, C.L.; Stanhope, K.L.; Schwarz, J.M.; Graham, J.L.; Hatcher, B.; Griffen, S.C.; Bremer, A.A.; Berglund, L.; McGahan, J.P.; Havel, P.J.; et al. Consumption of fructose-sweetened beverages for 10 weeks reduces net fat oxidation and energy expenditure in overweight/obese men and women. *Eur. J. Clin. Nutr.* **2012**, *66*, 201–208. [CrossRef]
80. Maersk, M.; Belza, A.; Stodkilde-Jorgensen, H.; Ringgaard, S.; Chabanova, E.; Thomsen, H.; Pedersen, S.B.; Astrup, A.; Richelsen, B. Sucrose-sweetened beverages increase fat storage in the liver, muscle, and visceral fat depot: A 6-mo randomized intervention study. *Am. J. Clin. Nutr.* **2012**, *95*, 283–289. [CrossRef]
81. Silbernagel, G.; Machann, J.; Unmuth, S.; Schick, F.; Stefan, N.; Haring, H.U.; Fritsche, A. Effects of 4-week very-high-fructose/glucose diets on insulin sensitivity, visceral fat and intrahepatic lipids: An exploratory trial. *Br. J. Nutr.* **2011**, *106*, 79–86. [CrossRef]
82. Chung, M.; Ma, J.; Patel, K.; Berger, S.; Lau, J.; Lichtenstein, A.H. Fructose, high-fructose corn syrup, sucrose, and nonalcoholic fatty liver disease or indexes of liver health: A systematic review and meta-analysis. *Am. J. Clin. Nutr.* **2014**, *100*, 833–849. [CrossRef]
83. Chiu, S.; Sievenpiper, J.L.; de Souza, R.J.; Cozma, A.I.; Mirrahimi, A.; Carleton, A.J.; Ha, V.; Di Buono, M.; Jenkins, A.L.; Leiter, L.A.; et al. Effect of fructose on markers of non-alcoholic fatty liver disease (NAFLD): a systematic review and meta-analysis of controlled feeding trials. *Eur. J. Clin. Nutr.* **2014**, *68*, 416–423. [CrossRef]
84. Ma, J.; Fox, C.S.; Jacques, P.F.; Speliotes, E.K.; Hoffmann, U.; Smith, C.E.; Saltzman, E.; McKeown, N.M. Sugar-sweetened beverage, diet soda, and fatty liver disease in the Framingham Heart Study cohorts. *J. Hepatol.* **2015**, *63*, 462–469. [CrossRef]
85. Sevastianova, K.; Santos, A.; Kotronen, A.; Hakkarainen, A.; Makkonen, J.; Silander, K.; Peltonen, M.; Romeo, S.; Lundbom, J.; Lundbom, N.; et al. Effect of short-term carbohydrate overfeeding and long-term weight loss on liver fat in overweight humans. *Am. J. Clin. Nutr.* **2012**, *96*, 727–734. [CrossRef]
86. Luukkonen, P.K.; Sadevirta, S.; Zhou, Y.; Kayser, B.; Ali, A.; Ahonen, L.; Lallukka, S.; Pelloux, V.; Gaggini, M.; Jian, C.; et al. Saturated Fat Is More Metabolically Harmful for the Human Liver Than Unsaturated Fat or Simple Sugars. *Diabetes Care* **2018**, *41*, 1732–1739. [CrossRef]
87. Gugliucci, A.; Lustig, R.H.; Caccavello, R.; Erkin-Cakmak, A.; Noworolski, S.M.; Tai, V.W.; Wen, M.J.; Mulligan, K.; Schwarz, J.M. Short-term isocaloric fructose restriction lowers apoC-III levels and yields less atherogenic lipoprotein profiles in children with obesity and metabolic syndrome. *Atherosclerosis* **2016**, *253*, 171–177. [CrossRef]
88. Erkin-Cakmak, A.; Bains, Y.; Caccavello, R.; Noworolski, S.M.; Schwarz, J.M.; Mulligan, K.; Lustig, R.H.; Gugliucci, A. Isocaloric Fructose Restriction Reduces Serum d-Lactate Concentration in Children With Obesity and Metabolic Syndrome. *J. Clin. Endocrinol. Metab.* **2019**, *104*, 3003–3011. [CrossRef]
89. Lee, O.; Bruce, W.R.; Dong, Q.; Bruce, J.; Mehta, R.; O'Brien, P.J. Fructose and carbonyl metabolites as endogenous toxins. *Chem. Biol. Interact.* **2009**, *178*, 332–339. [CrossRef]

90. Pickens, M.K.; Yan, J.S.; Ng, R.K.; Ogata, H.; Grenert, J.P.; Beysen, C.; Turner, S.M.; Maher, J.J. Dietary sucrose is essential to the development of liver injury in the methionine-choline-deficient model of steatohepatitis. *J. Lipid Res.* **2009**, *50*, 2072–2082. [CrossRef]
91. Masania, J.; Malczewska-Malec, M.; Razny, U.; Goralska, J.; Zdzienicka, A.; Kiec-Wilk, B.; Gruca, A.; Stancel-Mozwillo, J.; Dembinska-Kiec, A.; Rabbani, N.; et al. Dicarbonyl stress in clinical obesity. *Glycoconj. J.* **2016**, *33*, 581–589. [CrossRef] [PubMed]
92. Asgari-Taee, F.; Zerafati-Shoae, N.; Dehghani, M.; Sadeghi, M.; Baradaran, H.R.; Jazayeri, S. Association of sugar sweetened beverages consumption with non-alcoholic fatty liver disease: A systematic review and meta-analysis. *Eur. J. Nutr.* **2018**. [CrossRef] [PubMed]
93. Ter Horst, K.W.; Serlie, M.J. Fructose Consumption, Lipogenesis, and Non-Alcoholic Fatty Liver Disease. *Nutrients* **2017**, *9*, 981. [CrossRef] [PubMed]
94. Kirk, E.; Reeds, D.N.; Finck, B.N.; Mayurranjan, S.M.; Patterson, B.W.; Klein, S. Dietary fat and carbohydrates differentially alter insulin sensitivity during caloric restriction. *Gastroenterology* **2009**, *136*, 1552–1560. [CrossRef] [PubMed]
95. Haufe, S.; Engeli, S.; Kast, P.; Bohnke, J.; Utz, W.; Haas, V.; Hermsdorf, M.; Mahler, A.; Wiesner, S.; Birkenfeld, A.L.; et al. Randomized comparison of reduced fat and reduced carbohydrate hypocaloric diets on intrahepatic fat in overweight and obese human subjects. *Hepatology* **2011**, *53*, 1504–1514. [CrossRef] [PubMed]
96. Perheentupa, J.; Raivio, K. Fructose-induced hyperuricaemia. *Lancet* **1967**, *2*, 528–531. [CrossRef]
97. Sozen, E.; Ozer, N.K. Impact of high cholesterol and endoplasmic reticulum stress on metabolic diseases: An updated mini-review. *Redox Biol.* **2017**, *12*, 456–461. [CrossRef] [PubMed]
98. Lebeaupin, C.; Vallee, D.; Hazari, Y.; Hetz, C.; Chevet, E.; Bailly-Maitre, B. Endoplasmic reticulum stress signalling and the pathogenesis of non-alcoholic fatty liver disease. *J. Hepatol.* **2018**, *69*, 927–947. [CrossRef]
99. Henkel, A.; Green, R.M. The unfolded protein response in fatty liver disease. *Semin. Liver Dis.* **2013**, *33*, 321–329. [CrossRef]
100. Lee, A.H.; Scapa, E.F.; Cohen, D.E.; Glimcher, L.H. Regulation of hepatic lipogenesis by the transcription factor XBP1. *Science* **2008**, *320*, 1492–1496. [CrossRef]
101. Lanaspa, M.A.; Sanchez-Lozada, L.G.; Choi, Y.J.; Cicerchi, C.; Kanbay, M.; Roncal-Jimenez, C.A.; Ishimoto, T.; Li, N.; Marek, G.; Duranay, M.; et al. Uric acid induces hepatic steatosis by generation of mitochondrial oxidative stress: Potential role in fructose-dependent and -independent fatty liver. *J. Biol. Chem.* **2012**, *287*, 40732–40744. [CrossRef] [PubMed]
102. Abdelmalek, M.F.; Lazo, M.; Horska, A.; Bonekamp, S.; Lipkin, E.W.; Balasubramanyam, A.; Bantle, J.P.; Johnson, R.J.; Diehl, A.M.; Clark, J.M.; et al. Higher dietary fructose is associated with impaired hepatic adenosine triphosphate homeostasis in obese individuals with type 2 diabetes. *Hepatology* **2012**, *56*, 952–960. [CrossRef] [PubMed]
103. Satapati, S.; Kucejova, B.; Duarte, J.A.; Fletcher, J.A.; Reynolds, L.; Sunny, N.E.; He, T.; Nair, L.A.; Livingston, K.A.; Fu, X.; et al. Mitochondrial metabolism mediates oxidative stress and inflammation in fatty liver. *J. Clin. Investig.* **2015**, *125*, 4447–4462. [CrossRef] [PubMed]
104. Softic, S.; Gupta, M.K.; Wang, G.X.; Fujisaka, S.; O'Neill, B.T.; Rao, T.N.; Willoughby, J.; Harbison, C.; Fitzgerald, K.; Ilkayeva, O.; et al. Divergent effects of glucose and fructose on hepatic lipogenesis and insulin signaling. *J. Clin. Investig.* **2017**, *127*, 4059–4074. [CrossRef] [PubMed]
105. Facchini, F.; Chen, Y.D.; Hollenbeck, C.B.; Reaven, G.M. Relationship between resistance to insulin-mediated glucose uptake, urinary uric acid clearance, and plasma uric acid concentration. *JAMA* **1991**, *266*, 3008–3011. [CrossRef] [PubMed]
106. Choi, H.K.; Ford, E.S. Prevalence of the metabolic syndrome in individuals with hyperuricemia. *Am. J. Med.* **2007**, *120*, 442–447. [CrossRef]
107. Yu, T.Y.; Jee, J.H.; Bae, J.C.; Jin, S.M.; Baek, J.H.; Lee, M.K.; Kim, J.H. Serum uric acid: A strong and independent predictor of metabolic syndrome after adjusting for body composition. *Metabolism* **2016**, *65*, 432–440. [CrossRef]
108. Lee, Y.J.; Cho, S.; Kim, S.R. A possible role of serum uric acid as a marker of metabolic syndrome. *Intern. Med. J.* **2014**, *44*, 1210–1216. [CrossRef]
109. Sun, H.L.; Pei, D.; Lue, K.H.; Chen, Y.L. Uric Acid Levels Can Predict Metabolic Syndrome and Hypertension in Adolescents: A 10-Year Longitudinal Study. *PLoS ONE* **2015**, *10*, e0143786. [CrossRef]

110. Johnson, R.J.; Nakagawa, T.; Sanchez-Lozada, L.G.; Shafiu, M.; Sundaram, S.; Le, M.; Ishimoto, T.; Sautin, Y.Y.; Lanaspa, M.A. Sugar, uric acid, and the etiology of diabetes and obesity. *Diabetes* **2013**, *62*, 3307–3315. [CrossRef]
111. Zurlo, A.; Veronese, N.; Giantin, V.; Maselli, M.; Zambon, S.; Maggi, S.; Musacchio, E.; Toffanello, E.D.; Sartori, L.; Perissinotto, E.; et al. High serum uric acid levels increase the risk of metabolic syndrome in elderly women: The PRO.V.A study. *Nutr. Metab. Cardiovasc. Dis.* **2016**, *26*, 27–35. [CrossRef] [PubMed]
112. Babio, N.; Martinez-Gonzalez, M.A.; Estruch, R.; Warnberg, J.; Recondo, J.; Ortega-Calvo, M.; Serra-Majem, L.; Corella, D.; Fito, M.; Ros, E.; et al. Associations between serum uric acid concentrations and metabolic syndrome and its components in the PREDIMED study. *Nutr. Metab. Cardiovasc. Dis.* **2015**, *25*, 173–180. [CrossRef] [PubMed]
113. Yuan, H.; Yu, C.; Li, X.; Sun, L.; Zhu, X.; Zhao, C.; Zhang, Z.; Yang, Z. Serum Uric Acid Levels and Risk of Metabolic Syndrome: A Dose-Response Meta-Analysis of Prospective Studies. *J. Clin. Endocrinol. Metab.* **2015**, *100*, 4198–4207. [CrossRef] [PubMed]
114. Ouyang, X.; Cirillo, P.; Sautin, Y.; McCall, S.; Bruchette, J.L.; Diehl, A.M.; Johnson, R.J.; Abdelmalek, M.F. Fructose consumption as a risk factor for non-alcoholic fatty liver disease. *J. Hepatol.* **2008**, *48*, 993–999. [CrossRef] [PubMed]
115. Zhang, S.; Du, T.; Li, M.; Lu, H.; Lin, X.; Yu, X. Combined effect of obesity and uric acid on nonalcoholic fatty liver disease and hypertriglyceridemia. *Medicine (Baltimore)* **2017**, *96*, e6381. [CrossRef] [PubMed]
116. Liu, Z.; Que, S.; Zhou, L.; Zheng, S. Dose-response Relationship of Serum Uric Acid with Metabolic Syndrome and Non-alcoholic Fatty Liver Disease Incidence: A Meta-analysis of Prospective Studies. *Sci. Rep.* **2015**, *5*, 14325. [CrossRef] [PubMed]
117. Yang, C.; Yang, S.; Xu, W.; Zhang, J.; Fu, W.; Feng, C. Association between the hyperuricemia and nonalcoholic fatty liver disease risk in a Chinese population: A retrospective cohort study. *PLoS ONE* **2017**, *12*, e0177249. [CrossRef]
118. Lee, J.W.; Cho, Y.K.; Ryan, M.; Kim, H.; Lee, S.W.; Chang, E.; Joo, K.J.; Kim, J.T.; Kim, B.S.; Sung, K.C. Serum uric Acid as a predictor for the development of nonalcoholic Fatty liver disease in apparently healthy subjects: A 5-year retrospective cohort study. *Gut Liver* **2010**, *4*, 378–383. [CrossRef]
119. Lonardo, A.; Loria, P.; Leonardi, F.; Borsatti, A.; Neri, P.; Pulvirenti, M.; Verrone, A.M.; Bagni, A.; Bertolotti, M.; Ganazzi, D.; et al. Fasting insulin and uric acid levels but not indices of iron metabolism are independent predictors of non-alcoholic fatty liver disease. A case-control study. *Dig. Liver Dis.* **2002**, *34*, 204–211. [CrossRef]
120. Sirota, J.C.; McFann, K.; Targher, G.; Johnson, R.J.; Chonchol, M.; Jalal, D.I. Elevated serum uric acid levels are associated with non-alcoholic fatty liver disease independently of metabolic syndrome features in the United States: Liver ultrasound data from the National Health and Nutrition Examination Survey. *Metabolism* **2013**, *62*, 392–399. [CrossRef]
121. Li, Y.; Xu, C.; Yu, C.; Xu, L.; Miao, M. Association of serum uric acid level with non-alcoholic fatty liver disease: A cross-sectional study. *J. Hepatol.* **2009**, *50*, 1029–1034. [CrossRef] [PubMed]
122. Xu, C.; Yu, C.; Xu, L.; Miao, M.; Li, Y. High serum uric acid increases the risk for nonalcoholic Fatty liver disease: A prospective observational study. *PLoS ONE* **2010**, *5*, e11578. [CrossRef] [PubMed]
123. Choi, H.K.; Curhan, G. Soft drinks, fructose consumption, and the risk of gout in men: Prospective cohort study. *BMJ* **2008**, *336*, 309–312. [CrossRef] [PubMed]
124. Choi, H.K.; Willett, W.; Curhan, G. Fructose-rich beverages and risk of gout in women. *JAMA* **2010**, *304*, 2270–2278. [CrossRef] [PubMed]
125. Bae, J.; Chun, B.Y.; Park, P.S.; Choi, B.Y.; Kim, M.K.; Shin, M.H.; Lee, Y.H.; Shin, D.H.; Kim, S.K. Higher consumption of sugar-sweetened soft drinks increases the risk of hyperuricemia in Korean population: The Korean Multi-Rural Communities Cohort Study. *Semin. Arthritis Rheum.* **2014**, *43*, 654–661. [CrossRef] [PubMed]
126. Meneses-Leon, J.; Denova-Gutierrez, E.; Castanon-Robles, S.; Granados-Garcia, V.; Talavera, J.O.; Rivera-Paredez, B.; Huitron-Bravo, G.G.; Cervantes-Rodriguez, M.; Quiterio-Trenado, M.; Rudolph, S.E.; et al. Sweetened beverage consumption and the risk of hyperuricemia in Mexican adults: A cross-sectional study. *BMC Public Health* **2014**, *14*, 445. [CrossRef] [PubMed]
127. Siqueira, J.H.; Mill, J.G.; Velasquez-Melendez, G.; Moreira, A.D.; Barreto, S.M.; Bensenor, I.M.; Molina, M. Sugar-Sweetened Soft Drinks and Fructose Consumption Are Associated with Hyperuricemia: Cross-Sectional Analysis from the Brazilian Longitudinal Study of Adult Health (ELSA-Brasil). *Nutrients* **2018**, *10*, 981. [CrossRef]

128. Nguyen, S.; Choi, H.K.; Lustig, R.H.; Hsu, C.Y. Sugar-sweetened beverages, serum uric acid, and blood pressure in adolescents. *J. Pediatr.* **2009**, *154*, 807–813. [CrossRef]
129. Ngo Sock, E.T.; Le, K.A.; Ith, M.; Kreis, R.; Boesch, C.; Tappy, L. Effects of a short-term overfeeding with fructose or glucose in healthy young males. *Br. J. Nutr.* **2010**, *103*, 939–943. [CrossRef]
130. Cox, C.L.; Stanhope, K.L.; Schwarz, J.M.; Graham, J.L.; Hatcher, B.; Griffen, S.C.; Bremer, A.A.; Berglund, L.; McGahan, J.P.; Keim, N.L.; et al. Consumption of fructose- but not glucose-sweetened beverages for 10 weeks increases circulating concentrations of uric acid, retinol binding protein-4, and gamma-glutamyl transferase activity in overweight/obese humans. *Nutr. Metab. (Lond.)* **2012**, *9*, 68. [CrossRef]
131. Wang, D.D.; Sievenpiper, J.L.; de Souza, R.J.; Chiavaroli, L.; Ha, V.; Cozma, A.I.; Mirrahimi, A.; Yu, M.E.; Carleton, A.J.; Di Buono, M.; et al. The effects of fructose intake on serum uric acid vary among controlled dietary trials. *J. Nutr.* **2012**, *142*, 916–923. [CrossRef]
132. Tappy, L.; Morio, B.; Azzout-Marniche, D.; Champ, M.; Gerber, M.; Houdart, S.; Mas, E.; Rizkalla, S.; Slama, G.; Mariotti, F.; et al. French Recommendations for Sugar Intake in Adults: A Novel Approach Chosen by ANSES. *Nutrients* **2018**, *10*, 989. [CrossRef] [PubMed]
133. Caliceti, C.; Calabria, D.; Roda, A.; Cicero, A.F.G. Fructose Intake, Serum Uric Acid, and Cardiometabolic Disorders: A Critical Review. *Nutrients* **2017**, *9*, 395. [CrossRef] [PubMed]
134. Kanbay, M.; Jensen, T.; Solak, Y.; Le, M.; Roncal-Jimenez, C.; Rivard, C.; Lanaspa, M.A.; Nakagawa, T.; Johnson, R.J. Uric acid in metabolic syndrome: From an innocent bystander to a central player. *Eur. J. Intern. Med.* **2016**, *29*, 3–8. [CrossRef] [PubMed]
135. Welsh, J.A.; Sharma, A.; Abramson, J.L.; Vaccarino, V.; Gillespie, C.; Vos, M.B. Caloric sweetener consumption and dyslipidemia among US adults. *JAMA* **2010**, *303*, 1490–1497. [CrossRef] [PubMed]
136. Dhingra, R.; Sullivan, L.; Jacques, P.F.; Wang, T.J.; Fox, C.S.; Meigs, J.B.; D'Agostino, R.B.; Gaziano, J.M.; Vasan, R.S. Soft drink consumption and risk of developing cardiometabolic risk factors and the metabolic syndrome in middle-aged adults in the community. *Circulation* **2007**, *116*, 480–488. [CrossRef] [PubMed]
137. Livesey, G.; Taylor, R. Fructose consumption and consequences for glycation, plasma triacylglycerol, and body weight: Meta-analyses and meta-regression models of intervention studies. *Am. J. Clin. Nutr.* **2008**, *88*, 1419–1437. [CrossRef] [PubMed]
138. Adiels, M.; Taskinen, M.R.; Bjornson, E.; Andersson, L.; Matikainen, N.; Soderlund, S.; Kahri, J.; Hakkarainen, A.; Lundbom, N.; Sihlbom, C.; et al. Role of apolipoprotein C-III overproduction in diabetic dyslipidaemia. *Diabetes Obes. Metab.* **2019**. [CrossRef]
139. Taskinen, M.R.; Boren, J. Why Is Apolipoprotein CIII Emerging as a Novel Therapeutic Target to Reduce the Burden of Cardiovascular Disease? *Curr. Atheroscler. Rep.* **2016**, *18*, 59. [CrossRef]
140. Borén, J.; Watts, G.F.; Adiels, M.; Söderlund, S.; Chan, D.C.; Hakkarainen, A.; Lundbom, N.; Matikainen, N.; Kahri, J.; Vergès, B.; et al. Kinetic and Related Determinants of Plasma Triglyceride Concentration in Abdominal Obesity. Multicenter Tracer Kinetic Study. *Arterioscler. Thromb. Vasc. Biol.* **2015**, *35*, 2218–2224. [CrossRef] [PubMed]
141. Stanhope, K.L.; Medici, V.; Bremer, A.A.; Lee, V.; Lam, H.D.; Nunez, M.V.; Chen, G.X.; Keim, N.L.; Havel, P.J. A dose-response study of consuming high-fructose corn syrup-sweetened beverages on lipid/lipoprotein risk factors for cardiovascular disease in young adults. *Am. J. Clin. Nutr.* **2015**, *101*, 1144–1154. [CrossRef]
142. Lambertz, J.; Weiskirchen, S.; Landert, S.; Weiskirchen, R. Fructose: A Dietary Sugar in Crosstalk with Microbiota Contributing to the Development and Progression of Non-Alcoholic Liver Disease. *Front. Immunol.* **2017**, *8*, 1159. [CrossRef] [PubMed]
143. den Besten, G.; Lange, K.; Havinga, R.; van Dijk, T.H.; Gerding, A.; van Eunen, K.; Muller, M.; Groen, A.K.; Hooiveld, G.J.; Bakker, B.M.; et al. Gut-derived short-chain fatty acids are vividly assimilated into host carbohydrates and lipids. *Am. J. Physiol Gastrointest. Liver Physiol.* **2013**, *305*, G900–G910. [CrossRef] [PubMed]
144. Mouzaki, M.; Comelli, E.M.; Arendt, B.M.; Bonengel, J.; Fung, S.K.; Fischer, S.E.; McGilvray, I.D.; Allard, J.P. Intestinal microbiota in patients with nonalcoholic fatty liver disease. *Hepatology* **2013**, *58*, 120–127. [CrossRef] [PubMed]
145. Jegatheesan, P.; Beutheu, S.; Ventura, G.; Sarfati, G.; Nubret, E.; Kapel, N.; Waligora-Dupriet, A.J.; Bergheim, I.; Cynober, L.; De-Bandt, J.P. Effect of specific amino acids on hepatic lipid metabolism in fructose-induced non-alcoholic fatty liver disease. *Clin. Nutr.* **2016**, *35*, 175–182. [CrossRef] [PubMed]

146. Oh, J.H.; Alexander, L.M.; Pan, M.; Schueler, K.L.; Keller, M.P.; Attie, A.D.; Walter, J.; van Pijkeren, J.P. Dietary Fructose and Microbiota-Derived Short-Chain Fatty Acids Promote Bacteriophage Production in the Gut Symbiont Lactobacillus reuteri. *Cell Host Microbe* **2019**, *25*, 273–284. [CrossRef] [PubMed]
147. Chatterjee, A.; Duerkop, B.A. Sugar and Fatty Acids Ack-celerate Prophage Induction. *Cell Host Microbe* **2019**, *25*, 175–176. [CrossRef]
148. Mardinoglu, A.; Wu, H.; Bjornson, E.; Zhang, C.; Hakkarainen, A.; Rasanen, S.M.; Lee, S.; Mancina, R.M.; Bergentall, M.; Pietilainen, K.H.; et al. An Integrated Understanding of the Rapid Metabolic Benefits of a Carbohydrate-Restricted Diet on Hepatic Steatosis in Humans. *Cell Metab.* **2018**, *27*, 559–571. [CrossRef]

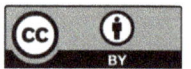

© 2019 by the authors. Licensee MDPI, Basel, Switzerland. This article is an open access article distributed under the terms and conditions of the Creative Commons Attribution (CC BY) license (http://creativecommons.org/licenses/by/4.0/).

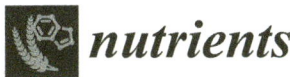

Article

Associations Between Dietary Protein Sources, Plasma BCAA and Short-Chain Acylcarnitine Levels in Adults

Michèle Rousseau [1,2], Frédéric Guénard [1,2], Véronique Garneau [1,2], Bénédicte Allam-Ndoul [1,2], Simone Lemieux [1,2], Louis Pérusse [1,3] and Marie-Claude Vohl [1,2,*]

1. Institute of Nutrition and Functional Foods (INAF), Laval University, Quebec City, QC G1V 0A6, Canada; michele.rousseau.1@ulaval.ca (M.R.); frederic.guenard@fsaa.ulaval.ca (F.G.); veronique.garneau@fsaa.ulaval.ca (V.G.); benedicte.allam-ndoul@criucpq.ulaval.ca (B.A.-N.); simone.lemieux@fsaa.ulaval.ca (S.L.); louis.perusse@kin.ulaval.ca (L.P.)
2. School of Nutrition, Laval University, Quebec City, QC G1V 0A6, Canada
3. Department of Kinesiology, Laval University, Quebec City, QC G1V 0A6, Canada
* Correspondence: marie-claude.vohl@fsaa.ulaval.ca; Tel.: +1-418-656-2131 (ext. 4676)

Received: 27 November 2018; Accepted: 11 January 2019; Published: 15 January 2019

Abstract: Elevated plasma branched-chain amino acids (BCAA) and C3 and C5 acylcarnitines (AC) levels observed in individuals with insulin resistance (IR) might be influenced by dietary protein intakes. This study explores the associations between dietary protein sources, plasma BCAA levels and C3 and C5 ACs in normal weight (NW) or overweight (OW) individuals with or without metabolic syndrome (MS). Data from 199 men and women aged 18–55 years with complete metabolite profile were analyzed. Associations between metabolic parameters, protein sources, plasma BCAA and AC levels were tested. OW/MS+ consumed significantly more animal protein ($p = 0.0388$) and had higher plasma BCAA levels ($p < 0.0001$) than OW/MS− or NW/MS− individuals. Plasma BCAA levels were not associated with BCAA intakes in the whole cohort, while there was a trend for an association between plasma BCAA levels and red meat or with animal protein in OW/MS+. These associations were of weak magnitude. In NW/MS− individuals, the protein sources associated with BCAA levels varied greatly with adjustment for confounders. Plasma C3 and C5 ACs were associated with plasma BCAA levels in the whole cohort ($p < 0.0001$) and in subgroups based on OW and MS status. These results suggest a modest association of meat or animal protein intakes and an association of C3 and C5 ACs with plasma BCAA levels, obesity and MS.

Keywords: branched-chain amino acids; acylcarnitines; dietary protein sources; meat; metabolic syndrome; metabolite profiling; diet

1. Introduction

Branched-chain amino acids (BCAA) are comprised of leucine, isoleucine and valine [1]. Their plasma levels have been positively associated with features of the metabolic syndrome (MS), such as insulin resistance (IR) and pre-diabetes [2,3], and thus with an increased risk of type 2 diabetes (T2D) and cardiovascular diseases (CVD) [4–8]. Controversies still remain on whether an increase in plasma BCAA levels is a cause or a consequence of IR. The latter is the most strongly supported hypothesis [9,10], since plasma BCAAs elevation could be the result of an impaired metabolism caused by the decreased gene expression of BCAA aminotransferase (*BCAT*) and branched-chain a-keto acid dehydrogenase (*BCKD*), as seen in mice models [11].

Most dietary BCAAs are metabolized in the skeletal muscle after passing through systemic circulation, whereas other amino acids (AA) are metabolized in the liver [12–15]. This reinforces the potential impact of BCAAs on circulating metabolites, hormones or nutrients [15]. Some studies also relate the increase of plasma BCAAs to the amount or the type (animal or vegetal) of protein ingested [16,17]. Moreover, diets high in red meat [18], animal protein or BCAAs [8,19,20] are associated with an increased risk of T2D in contrast to diets high in vegetal protein, which appears to be associated with a lower risk of T2D [19,20]. In addition, acylcarnitines (AC), a by-product of incomplete mitochondrial fatty acid oxidation, are acyl esters of carnitine that can also result from the degradation of other compounds, such as BCAAs into C3 and C5 ACs [21]. More specifically, isoleucine and leucine catabolism generate 2-methylbutyryl-CoA and isovaleryl-CoA, which will transfer their acyl group to carnitine to form C5 ACs. Isoleucine and valine catabolism will generate propionyl-CoA to be incorporated into C3 ACs [22,23]. These short-chain ACs have previously been associated with IR [21,22] along with western-type dietary habits [24], and are considered as a potential marker of animal products and meat consumption [25].

Changes in plasma BCAA levels according to dietary profiles and dietary protein intakes have been investigated. While higher BCAA intakes have been related to plasma BCAA levels in some studies [16,26], others found no or an inverse association between these two factors [27–29]. One possible explanation for this discrepancy may be related to the source of protein, either animal or vegetal [4]. Protein source might also influence the relationship between plasma BCAA levels and IR. Accordingly, red meat, poultry, fish and whole milk were reported to be the main sources of dietary BCAAs in the US [8] and UK [28] populations, two countries for which a positive association between IR and plasma BCAAs has been reported. An association between IR and plasma BCAAs have also been observed in population from Brazil where red meat, poultry, bread, rice and beans were the principal dietary sources of BCAAs [30]. In contrast, cereal, potatoes and starches, followed by fish, shellfish and finally meats were the main sources of BCAAs in a Japanese cohort where an inverse relationship between BCAA intakes and T2D risk was observed, but only in women [29]. However, up to now, no study has explored the associations between the principal dietary sources of protein and plasma BCAAs, as well as its association with C3 and C5 AC levels in one single cohort.

As such, the main objective of this study was to investigate the relationship between dietary protein source—either animal or vegetal—intakes and fasting plasma BCAA levels in adults with diverse BMI and obesity-associated metabolic perturbations. The second objective was to describe the association between plasma BCAA levels and C3 and C5 AC levels in the same subgroups according to overweight (OW) MS status. We found plasma BCAA levels to be associated with animal protein consumption, with red meat being the main source of proteins that correlates in OW/MS+ individuals. C3 and C5 plasma concentrations were also associated with plasma BCAA levels in the whole cohort, and by subgroups defined on the basis of BMI and the metabolic status.

2. Materials and Methods

2.1. Study Population

INFOGENE is a cross-sectional study investigating the familial history of obesity [31–33]. The recruitment took place in the Quebec City metropolitan area between May 2004 and March 2007 via advertisements in local newspaper and radio stations. Electronic group messages were also sent to university and hospital employees. In the first period of recruitment, only normal weight (NW) individuals were accepted while in the second phase, only OW individuals were recruited. No other criteria of exclusion were applied. After a phone interview where a trained research assistant asked the participants to report their weight and height, eligible individuals were given an appointment at the clinical investigation unit. At this appointment, anthropometric measurements were taken, and participants had to complete a food frequency questionnaire (FFQ), as well as other questionnaires assessing socio-demographic level and lifestyle habits. Individuals who were homeless (1), pregnant (1), older than 55 years (1), had acquired immune deficiency syndrome (AIDS) (1), total energy intakes greater than 4 SD (4), fibre intakes greater than 4 SD (1) or who reported unreliable data (1), were excluded. The final sample consisted of 664 adults—of which 245 men and 372 women—aged 18 to 55 years who gave their written consent to participate. Of those individuals [34], 100 men and 100 women were randomly selected for metabolic profiling of their blood samples [35]. One individual missing biochemical information was excluded from the following analyses. This study has been approved by the Université Laval Ethics Committee.

2.2. Dietary Assessment and Food Grouping

Dietary intakes over the past month were assessed using a 91-item FFQ administered by a registered dietitian. This FFQ was previously validated in French Canadian men and women, and was structured to reflect nutritional habits of the Quebec population [36]. Nutritional intakes were evaluated using the Nutrition Data System for Research (NDS-R) software version 4.03 (Nutrition Coordination Center, Minneapolis, MN, USA). For each item in the FFQ, participants were asked to report their consumption either in days, weeks or months. Many portion size examples were provided for a better estimation of the consumption. Thirty-seven food groups were made, based on the nutrient profile of each item or on its culinary usage. Some groups consisted of only one food (e.g., eggs or beer) because of their particular composition. Twelve groups typically providing most of the dietary proteins in Canada were kept for the current analysis [37]. These are red meat, processed meat, organ meat, fish and other seafood, poultry, eggs, reduced or low-fat dairy products, regular or high-fat dairy products, legumes, nuts, refined grain products and whole grains products. Total animal protein and total vegetal protein (in grams) were also available from the database by calculating the sum of each food sources and mixed dishes. Nutritional information from foods missing in the database was derived from nutritional food labels and entered manually.

2.3. Anthropometric Measurements

Participants were asked to wear light indoor clothes on the day of their appointment. All measurements were made by a trained research assistant. Weight and height were measured using a beam scale with rod graduated in centimetres (Detecto, Webb City, MO USA). Weight was measured to the nearest 0.1 kg and height was measured to the nearest 0.5 cm. Body mass index (BMI) was computed as weight in kilograms divided by height in meters squared (kg/m^2). OW was defined as having BMI over 25 kg/m^2 while individuals with a BMI below 25 kg/m^2 were defined as having a NW. Waist (WC) and hip circumferences were measured according to the procedures recommended by the Airlie Conference [38]. For the measure of systolic (SBP) and diastolic blood pressure (DBP), participants were asked to sit straight with arms and legs uncrossed. The measures were taken after a 5-minute rest.

2.4. Biochemical Parameters

Blood samples were collected from an antecubital vein into vacutainer tubes containing EDTA after a 12-h overnight fast. Blood samples were immediately centrifuged. Total cholesterol (total-C) and triglyceride (TG) concentrations were determined from plasma and lipoprotein fractions using the Olympus AU400e system (Olympus America Inc., Melville, NY, USA). A precipitation of low-density lipoprotein cholesterol (LDL-C) fraction in the infranatant with heparin-manganese chloride was used to obtain the high-density lipoprotein cholesterol (HDL-C) fraction. LDL-C concentrations were estimated using the Friedewald's equation [39]. Radioimmunoassay with polyethylene glycol separation was used to measure fasting insulin. Fasting glucose concentrations were enzymatically measured. Homeostasis model assessment of IR (HOMA-IR) was obtained using (fasting glucose × fasting insulin)/22.5. MS was defined as having three or more of the following risk factors: WC >88 cm for women and 102 cm for men, fasting plasma TG $\geq$1.7 mmol/L, HDL-C levels $\leq$1.29 mmol/L for women and 1.03 mmol/L for men, glucose levels $\geq$5.6 mmol/L and resting SBP/DBP $\geq$130/85 mmHg. Participants taking medication for lipidemia, diabetes or hypertension control were considered as having abnormal values for their respective parameters.

2.5. Metabolite Profiling

As previously described [35], the Absolute ID p180 Kit (Biocrates Life Sciences AG, Innsbruck, Australia) for mass spectrometry was used for the metabolic profiling measurements for two-hundred participants. Ninety-five metabolites were quantified. They include: 67 Glycerophospholipids (GPs), 12 AC, 10 Sphingolipids (SGs) and 6 AAs. For GPs, ACs and SGs x:y notation was used, x denoting the number of carbons in the side chain and y the number of double bonds. All metabolite concentrations are presented in µM. A metabolite would have been excluded if more than half of the values obtained were below the limit of detection or with standard out of range.

2.6. Statistical Analyses

Variables not normally distributed were transformed using $\log_{10}$ (TG, HDL-C, insulin, animal protein, processed meat, eggs, low-fat dairy), square root (legumes) or inverse transformation (nuts). Organ meat intakes were still not normally distributed after transformation and were then used as a categorical variable (eater or non-eater of organ meat). BCAA dietary intakes or plasma levels were defined as the sum of valine, leucine and isoleucine respectively calculated in FFQ or following plasma metabolite profiling. The General Linear Model (GLM) procedure with the type-III sum of squares was used to assess the association between plasma BCAA levels and age, sex, BMI, WC, BCAA intakes, energy from proteins and total energy intakes. Different models were computed to further assess the associations between plasma BCAA levels, vegetal protein and animal protein and their constituents, as well as to take into account adjustments for total daily energy intakes, age and sex. Associations between different protein sources, as well as BCAA intakes and plasma BCAA levels, were tested with and without adjustments for confounding factors. The associations between ACs levels and plasma BCAA levels were finally assessed. The same models were tested when subdividing study participants based on OW status and the absence/presence of MS (MS−/MS+). Four groups were consequently created: NW/MS−, NW/MS+, OW/MS− and OW/MS+. The NW/MS+ group was excluded from dietary, BCAAs and ACs analyses since this group was composed of only one woman and one man. The GLM procedure was also used to compare mean intakes between groups. All data analyses were performed using SAS statistical software University edition (SAS Institute Inc, Cary, NC, USA). A p-value < 0.05 was considered as statistically significant.

3. Results

3.1. Study Population

Characteristics of study participants are presented in Table 1. Mean values for the four groups are presented. Mean age of participants was 34.2 years and 49.7% of them were women. There were significant differences between groups for all anthropometric and metabolic parameters except for men/women proportions and LDL-C levels. OW individuals were older and had higher BMI, WC, total-C, TG, insulin, SBP and DBP, as well as lower HDL-C than NW/MS− subjects.

3.2. Dietary Intakes

As shown in Table 2, mean daily protein intakes were 104.2 g, which represents 16.8% of total daily energy intakes. Proteins were mainly provided by animal-based foods, with a mean intake of 70.5g versus 32.0g from plant-based sources. There were some differences between groups for total energy (p = 0.0172), total carbohydrates (p = 0.0446), % of kcal from carbohydrates (p = 0.0340), total protein (p = 0.0303), animal protein (p = 0.0086), BCAA intakes (0.0310), total fat (p = 0.0102), total SFA (p = 0.0173), total monounsaturated fatty acids (MUFA) (p = 0.0131) and total polyunsaturated fatty acids (PUFA) (p = 0.0347) intakes. These differences were no longer significant after adjustments for age, sex and energy intake except for significantly greater animal protein intakes in both OW groups (p = 0.0388). Table 3 presents mean intakes, expressed in portions/day, of the food subgroups providing most dietary proteins. OW individuals either MS- or MS+ consumed less fish (p = 0.0106) and more eggs (p = 0.0166) than NW/MS− individuals, but the difference in eggs consumption did not remain significant after adjustments for age, sex and total energy intake. OW/MS+ also consumed more red meat ($p = 0.0027$) and this was still observed, but only as a trend, after adjustments for age, sex and total energy intake ($p = 0.0899$). A detailed list of foods included in each category is provided in Supplementary Table S1.

Table 1. Characteristics of participants.

Characteristics	Total Subjects (n = 199)	NW/MS− (n = 65)	NW/MS+ (n = 2)	OW/MS− (n = 84)	OW/MS+ (n = 48)	p-Value
Women (%)	49.7	58.5	50.0	51.1	35.4	0.1130
Age (years)	34.2 ± 10.2	28.9 ± 7.4 [a]	39.1 ± 17.8 [a]	35.7 ± 10.4 [b]	38.4 ± 10.1 [b,c]	<0.0001
BMI (kg/m^2)	29.0 ± 6.2	22.2 ± 1.8 [a]	24.5 ± 0.66 [a]	31.4 ± 4.2 [b]	34.3 ± 4.8 [c]	<0.0001
WC (cm)	92.7 ± 16.5	74.7 ± 5.7 [a]	83.1 ± 0.64 [a]	97.7 ± 10.7 [b]	109.0 ± 11.8 [c]	<0.0001
Total-C (mmol)	4.49 ± 1.00	4.13 ± 0.67 [a]	3.58 ± 0.76 [a,b]	4.57 ± 1.0 [b]	4.88 ± 1.19 [b]	0.0003
TG (mmol)	1.29 ± 0.91	0.77 ± 0.31 [a]	0.88 ± 0.03 [a,b]	1.15 ± 0.56 [b,c]	2.23 ± 1.22 [d]	<0.0001 *
HDL-C (mmol)	1.33 ± 0.41	1.60 ± 0.45 [c]	1.07 ± 0.21 [a,b]	1.32 ± 0.30 [b]	0.99 ± 0.24 [a]	<0.0001 *
LDL-C (mmol)	2.76 ± 0.94	2.52 ± 0.70	2.51 ± 0.55	2.81 ± 0.91	3.00 ± 1.21	0.0545
Fasting glycemia (mmol/L)	5.65 ± 0.74	5.68 ± 0.74 [a]	6.90 ± 1.13 [b]	5.43 ± 0.52 [c]	5.94 ± 1.92 [a,b]	0.0001
Insulin (pM)	85.1 ± 60.6	48.7 ± 17.1 [a]	68.5 ± 21.9 [a,b,c]	86.1 ± 56.3 [b]	134.5 ± 72.2 [c]	<0.0001 *
SBP (mmHg)	121.3 ± 11.1	115.9 ± 9.8 [a]	130.5 ± 4.9 [b,c,d]	119.9 ± 8.9 [c]	130.5 ± 10.6 [d]	<0.0001
DBP (mmHg)	77.9 ± 9.5	74.0 ± 9.9 [a]	74.0 ± 5.7 [a,b,c]	77.7 ± 7.7 [b]	83.6 ± 9.4 [c]	<0.0001
BCAAs (μM)	455.6 ± 92.3	413.8 ± 83.5 [a]	378.8 ± 83.3 [a,b]	460.0 ± 83.2 [a,b]	507.7 ± 92.3 [b]	<0.0001
C3 ACs (μM)	0.325 ± 0.115	0.281 ± 0.104 [a]	0.181 ± 0.011 [a,b]	0.327 ± 0.100 [b]	0.387 ± 0.125 [c]	<0.0001
C5 ACs (μM)	0.137 ±0.048	0.118±0.036 [a]	0.094± 0.005 [a,b]	0.137 ± 0.045 [b]	0.163 ± 0.056 [c]	<0.0001

Values are means ± SD. Model p-values of comparisons between NW/MS−, NW/MS+, OW/MS− and MW/MS+ are shown. Between-groups comparisons were made using the LS means procedure. Results who do not share the same letter ([a,b,c,d]) are significantly different ($p < 0.05$) from each other. * indicates that the p-value was obtained with the transformed variables. Significant values ($p < 0.05$) are presented in bold. Abbreviations, NW, normal weight; OW, overweight; MS, metabolic syndrome; BMI, body mass index; WC, waist circumference; Total-C, total cholesterol; TG, triglycerides; HDL-C, high-density lipoproteins; LDL-C, low-density lipoproteins; SBP, systolic blood pressure; DBP, diastolic blood pressure; BCAAs, branched-chain amino-acids; ACs, acylcarnitines; SD, standard deviation.

Table 2. Daily dietary energy and macronutrients intakes of participants.

Nutrients	Total Subjects (n = 197)	NW/MS− (n = 65)	OW/MS− (n = 84)	OW/MS+ (n = 48)	p-Value [1]	p-Value [2]
Total energy (kcal)	2474 ± 790	2412 ± 853 [a]	2364 ± 695 [a]	2754 ± 809 [b]	0.0172	
Total carbohydrates (g)	297.5 ± 92.5	298.8 ± 95.7 [a,c]	281.7 ± 87.0 [a,b]	323.3 ± 93.5 [c]	0.0446	0.5447
Carbohydrates (%kcal)	46.7 ± 6.0	48.23 ± 6.54 [a]	45.9 ± 5.3 [b]	45.8 ± 6.1 [b]	0.0340	0.2229
Total dietary fiber (g)	23.5 ± 7.9	23.6 ± 8.7	22.8 ± 7.3	24.6 ± 7.7	0.4495	0.7690
Soluble dietary fibers (g)	7.8 ± 2.5	7.6 ± 2.6	7.5 ± 2.3	8.5 ± 2.7	0.0745	0.7736
Insoluble dietary fibers (g)	15.5 ± 5.5	15.7 ± 6.2	15.2 ± 5.2	15.9 ± 5.1	0.7463	0.5677
Total protein (g)	104.2 ± 37.1	99.9 ± 43.2 [a]	100.4 ± 29.9 [a]	116.4 ± 37.7 [b]	0.0303	0.6209
Protein (%kcal)	16.8 ± 2.4	16.4 ± 2.6	17.1 ± 2.0	17.0 ± 2.5	0.2580	0.3762
Vegetal protein (g)	32.0 ± 11.8	31.9 ± 12.5	31.0 ± 11.6	34.1 ± 11.1	0.3459	0.6093
Animal protein (g)	70.5 ± 30.3	66.2 ± 35.9 [a]	68.0 ± 23.7 [a]	80.7 ± 30.9 [b]	0.0086 *	0.0388 *
BCAA intakes (g)	18.5 ± 6.8	17.6 ± 7.8 [a]	17.9 ± 5.5 [a]	20.7 ± 7.0 [b]	0.0310	0.3789
Total fat (g)	93.4 ± 37.3	88.4 ± 39.9 [a]	89.2 ± 30.6 [a]	107.4 ± 41.3 [b]	0.0102	0.8410
Fat (%kcal)	33.6 ± 5.3	32.4 ± 5.7	33.8 ± 4.7	34.7 ± 5.6	0.0649	0.5095
Total SFA (g)	32.6 ± 14.7	30.6 ± 15.9 [a]	31.1 ± 12.3 [a]	37.8 ± 16.0 [b]	0.0173	0.8734
SFA (%kcal)	11.6 ± 2.6	11.1 ± 2.7	11.8 ± 2.6	12.1 ± 2.6	0.0902	0.4312
Total MUFA (g)	38.3 ± 15.7	36.3 ± 16.7 [a]	36.5 ± 12.5 [a]	44.0 ± 18.1 [b]	0.0131	0.9269
MUFA (%kcal)	13.8 ± 2.6	13.3 ± 2.9	13.9 ± 2.2	14.2 ± 2.8	0.2203	0.7753
Total PUFA (g)	15.2 ± 6.2	14.5 ± 6.3 [a]	14.7 ± 5.6 [a]	17.3 ± 6.9 [b]	0.0347	0.9148
PUFA (%kcal)	5.5 ± 1.4	5.4 ± 1.3	5.6 ± 1.3	5.6 ± 1.5	0.6765	0.9631
Total alcohol (g)	10.5 ± 12.1	9.8 ± 9.0	11.1 ± 13.0	10.5 ± 14.0	0.2968 *	0.1406 *
Alcohol (%kcal)	3.0 ± 2.9	2.9 ± 2.5	3.2 ± 3.2	2.5 ± 2.9	0.4770	0.3919

Values are means ± SD. %kcal from carbohydrates was calculated by difference. Model p-values of comparisons between NW/MS−, OW/MS− and MW/MS+ are shown [1] unadjusted and [2] adjusted for age, sex and total energy intakes. Between-groups comparisons were made using the LS means procedure. Results who do not share the same letter ([a,b,c]) are significantly different ($p < 0.05$) from each other. * indicates that the p-value was obtained with the transformed variables. Significant values ($p < 0.05$) are presented in bold. Abbreviations: NW, normal weight; OW, overweight; MS, metabolic syndrome; BCAA, branched-chain amino-acids; SFA, saturated fatty acids; MUFA, monounsaturated fatty acids; PUFA, polyunsaturated fatty acids.

Table 3. Mean intakes (standard portions/day) of the principal food groups contributing to protein intakes

Food Groups	Total Subjects (n = 197)	NW/MS− (n = 65)	OW/MS− (n = 84)	OW/MS+ (n = 48)	p-Value [1]	p-Value [2]
Red meat	2.25 ± 1.78	1.93 ± 1.95 [a]	2.07 ± 1.40 [a]	3.01 ± 1.94 [b]	**0.0027**	0.0899
Processed meat	0.85 ± 0.95	0.78 ± 0.83	0.72 ± 0.60	1.16 ± 1.44	0.0660 *	0.4325 *
Organ meat	0.02 ± 0.09	0.01 ± 0.04	0.03 ± 0.10	0.04 ± 0.11	0.1009 *	0.2641 *
Fish	1.21 ± 1.19	1.56 ± 1.56 [b]	1.11 ± 0.97 [a]	0.92 ± 0.81 [a]	**0.0106**	**0.0119**
Poultry	1.17 ± 0.91	1.13 ± 0.94	1.23 ± 0.89	1.12 ± 0.90	0.7332	0.1337
Eggs	0.36 ± 0.30	0.28 ± 0.23 [a]	0.38 ± 0.29 [b]	0.43 ± 0.37 [b]	**0.0166**	0.1431
Low fat dairy	1.60 ± 1.34	1.42 ± 1.08	1.59 ± 1.24	1.86 ± 1.77	0.5081 *	0.5713 *
High fat dairy	1.80 ± 1.29	1.73 ± 1.27	1.77 ± 1.17	1.95 ± 1.51	0.6389	0.7883
Legumes	0.28 ± 0.49	0.28 ± 0.41	0.31 ± 0.62	0.21 ± 0.32	0.4132 *	0.2473 *
Nuts	0.97 ± 2.99	0.75 ± 0.81	0.80 ± 1.00	1.58 ± 5.84	0.9254 *	0.9691 *
Refined grain products	2.78 ± 1.95	2.72 ± 1.65	2.54 ± 1.83	3.28 ± 2.41	0.1028	0.7890
Whole grain products	2.43 ± 1.85	2.64 ± 2.13	2.34 ± 1.63	2.29 ± 1.82	0.5212	0.1007

Values are means ± SD. [1] p-value unadjusted, [2] p-value adjusted for age, sex and total energy intakes. Results who do not share the same letter ([a,b]) are significantly different ($p < 0.05$) from each other. * indicates that the p-value was obtained with the transformed variables. Significant values ($p < 0.05$) are presented in bold. Abbreviations: NW, normal weight; OW, overweight; MS, metabolic syndrome.

3.3. Plasma BCAAs and Protein Intakes

The associations between total protein intake, total energy, BCAA intakes, age, sex and BMI with plasma BCAA levels have also been investigated. Sex and BMI or WC contributed significantly to the variance of plasma BCAA levels ($p < 0.0001$ for both), while total protein, total energy and BCAA intakes and age did not. We also investigated plasma BCAA levels according to obesity and MS status. As shown in Figure 1, there was an increase of plasma BCAA levels with obesity and the presence of MS ($p < 0.0001$) that remained significant after adjustments for age, sex and energy intake ($p < 0.0001$). A concomitant increase in BCAA intakes was also seen ($p = 0.0310$), with OW/MS+ consuming more BCAAs than the other groups (Figure 1). However, the difference in BCAA intakes was no longer significant after adjustments for confounding factors, including age, sex and energy intake ($p = 0.3789$).

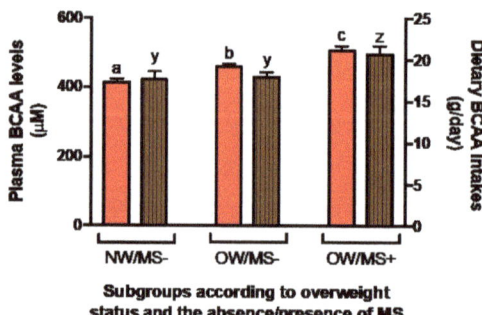

Figure 1. Mean plasma and dietary BCAA levels between subgroups of NW/OW individuals with or without MS. Plasma BCAA levels are shown in plain salmon; BCAA intakes calculated from food frequency questionnaire are shown in lined brown. Whiskers represent standard error. Results who do not share the same letter ([a,b,c] for plasma BCAA levels and [y,z] for dietary BCAA intakes) are significantly different ($p < 0.05$) from each other. Values presented are unadjusted.

The association of each of the 12 principal protein sources (red meat, processed meat, fish, poultry, eggs, legumes, nuts, high and low-fat dairy and whole and refined grain products) with plasma BCAA levels was also tested in a GLM model. Considering all 197 study participants, the only trend observed was with red meat ($p = 0.0575$). This trend was lost after adjustments for age, sex, BMI and total energy intake (data not shown).

When looking at food correlates of plasma BCAA levels in groups defined on the basis of OW and MS status (Table 4), refined and whole grain products were positively associated with plasma BCAA levels ($\beta = 16.07$, $p = 0.0338$ and $\beta = 13.04$, $p = 0.0279$, respectively) in NW/MS− subjects. Their respective contribution to the variance of plasma BCAA levels was of 5.55% and 5.97%, respectively. None of the food group was significantly associated with plasma BCAA levels in OW/MS+ subjects, but a positive trend was seen for red meat ($\beta = 15.40$, $p = 0.0713$). After adjustments for age, sex and energy intake, a negative association between red meat consumption and plasma BCAA levels ($\beta = -26.15$, $p = 0.0013$) was found in NW/MS, explaining 9.64% of its variance. When looking at men and women separately, this negative association was only found in NW/MS− men ($\beta = -49.75.16$, $p = 0.0039$) and not in NW/MS− women ($\beta = -11.81$, $p = 0.4715$). As for OW/MS+ individuals, red meat showed a trend toward a positive relationship ($\beta = 16.16$, $p = 0.0548$), and a negative association was observed with eggs ($\beta = -310.14$, $p = 0.0272$).

Finally, in a model testing the association between total animal and vegetal protein intakes and plasma BCAA levels, only animal protein intake was associated with plasma BCAA levels ($p = 0.0002$) with a weak contribution of 6.89% to the variance of the trait (not shown). After adjustments for age, sex and energy, the positive association between animal protein intakes and plasma BCAA levels remained significant ($R^2 = 0.0193$, $p = 0.0297$, not shown). When analysed by sex, this association was significant in women ($\beta = 177.16$, $p = 0.0164$), but not in men ($\beta = 98.12$, $p = 0.2908$). In subgroups, there was a positive association between total animal protein intakes and plasma BCAA levels for NW/MS− ($R^2 = 0.0675$, $p = 0.0292$), as well as a trend toward relationship for OW/MS+ ($R^2 = 0.0664$, $p = 0.0786$) individuals. After adjustments for age, sex and energy intake, the positive association between animal protein intakes and plasma BCAA levels was significant in OW/MS+ ($R^2 = 0.0422$, $p = 0.0422$), but was lost in NW/MS− individuals (not shown).

As animal protein is the main nutritional correlate of plasma BCAA levels, we further tested the association with its constituents, thus including red meat, processed and organ meats, fish, poultry, eggs and low and high fat dairy in the model. Again, red meat was the single constituent significantly and positively associated with plasma BCAA levels ($p = 0.0388$) while a positive trend was also observed with poultry ($p = 0.0801$). These associations (with respective R^2 of 0.0209 and 0.0150) were no longer significant after adjustments for age, sex and total energy intake (data not shown).

3.4. Acylcarnitines

As shown in Figure 2, plasma concentrations of both C3 and C5 ACs increased in parallel to plasma BCAA levels according to OW status and MS even after adjustments for age, sex and total energy intake ($p < 0.001$) (not shown). The associations between plasma BCAA and plasma C3 and C5 AC levels were also tested. With or without adjustments for age, sex and total energy intake, associations between plasma BCAAs and C3 and C5 ACs were significant in the whole cohort ($p < 0.0001$ for all), and in subgroups based on obesity and MS presence ($p < 0.002$ for all) (Table 5). After further adjustments for dietary BCAAs, red meat and total protein intakes, only the association between plasma BCAAs and C5 ACs in OW/MS+ was lost. The contribution of C3 and C5 ACs to the variance was weak to moderate, with R^2 values ranging from 0.0466 to 0.3817.

Table 4. Associations between all 12 principal protein sources and plasma BCAA levels in subgroups based on OW and MS status without and with adjustments for confounders.

Group	NW/MS− (n = 65)				OW/MS− (n = 84)				OW/MS+ (n = 48)			
Model	Unadjusted		Adjusted [2]		Unadjusted		Adjusted [2]		Unadjusted		Adjusted [2]	
Parameters	R^2	p-value	R^2	p-value	R^2	p-value	R^2	p-value	R^2	p-value	R^2	p-value
Red meat	0.0087	0.3910	0.0964	**0.0013**	0.0113	0.3408	0.0072	0.4330	0.0771	0.0713	0.0602	0.0548
Processed meat *	0.0088	0.3892	0.0047	0.4571	0.0004	0.8625	0.0005	0.8336	0.0025	0.7380	0.0002	0.9061
Organ meat *	0.0007	0.8112	0.0006	0.7977	0.0028	0.6313	0.0002	0.8871	0.0293	0.2591	0.0449	0.0948
Fish	0.0258	0.1429	0.0306	0.0607	0.0105	0.3589	0.0037	0.5756	0.0151	0.4160	0.0149	0.3288
Poultry	0.0197	0.1999	0.0219	0.1108	0.0046	0.5410	0.0004	0.8479	0.0397	0.1902	0.0429	0.1022
Eggs *	0.0203	0.1936	0.0214	0.1153	0.0076	0.4324	0.0074	0.4275	0.0578	0.1161	0.0812	**0.0272**
Legumes *	0.0140	0.2787	0.0003	0.8594	0.0072	0.4453	0.0066	0.4543	0.0047	0.6496	0.0424	0.1039
Nuts *	0.0164	0.2418	0.0065	0.3820	0.0045	0.5485	0.0032	0.6039	0.0049	0.6432	0.0001	0.9438
Hf dairy	0.0071	0.4395	0.0058	0.4077	0.0296	0.1248	0.0344	0.0904	0.0105	0.4973	0.0099	0.4244
Lf dairy *	0.0010	0.7721	0.0006	0.7817	0.0013	0.7469	0.0088	0.3890	0.0001	0.9434	0.0054	0.5539
Refined gp	0.0555	**0.0338**	0.0016	0.6596	0.0146	0.2785	0.0000	0.9857	0.0207	0.3415	0.0108	0.4047
Whole gp	0.0597	**0.0279**	0.0002	0.8773	0.0161	0.2552	0.0020	0.6791	0.0250	0.2963	0.0053	0.5576

Protein sources were analysed in portions/day. [2] The model is adjusted for age, sex and total energy intakes. * indicates that the values was obtained with the transformed variables. Significant values ($p < 0.05$) are presented in bold. Abbreviations: NW, normal weight; OW, overweight; MS, metabolic syndrome; Hf dairy, high fat dairy; Lf dairy, Low fat dairy; Refined gp, refined grain products; Whole gp, whole grain products.

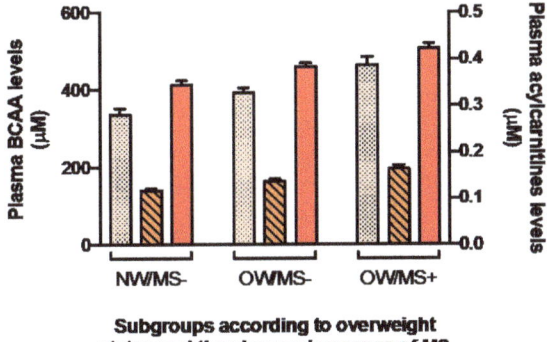

Figure 2. Mean plasma concentrations of C3 and C5 ACs in relation with mean plasma BCAA levels between subgroups of NW/OW individual with or without MS. Plasma BCAA levels are shown in salmon; C3 ACs are shown in dotted light orange; C5 ACs are shown in striped medium orange. Whiskers represent standard error. Values presented are unadjusted. All mean values are significantly different ($p < 0.05$) between groups.

Table 5. Associations between plasma BCAA and C3 and C5 ACs plasma levels in the whole cohort and by subgroups based on OW and MS status without and with adjustments for confounders. All lines were computed individually.

Parameters	Model	Total cohort ($n = 197$)		NW/MS− ($n = 65$)		OW/MS− ($n = 84$)		OW/MS+ ($n = 48$)	
		R^2	p-value	R^2	p-value	R^2	p-value	R^2	p-value
C3 ACs	Unadjusted	0.3804	**<0.0001**	0.3529	**<0.0001**	0.3069	**<0.0001**	0.2812	**0.0001**
	Adjusted [2]	0.2080	**<0.0001**	0.0909	**0.0020**	0.2356	**<0.0001**	0.2181	**0.0002**
	Adjusted [3]	0.1932	**<0.0001**	0.0775	**0.0047**	0.2140	**<0.0001**	0.1488	**0.0019**
C5 ACs	Unadjusted	0.3817	**<0.0001**	0.3608	**<0.0001**	0.3822	**<0.0001**	0.2159	**0.0009**
	Adjusted [2]	0.1614	**<0.0001**	0.0866	**0.0017**	0.2212	**<0.0001**	0.2181	**0.0002**
	Adjusted [3]	0.1504	**<0.0001**	0.0901	**0.0010**	0.2026	**<0.0001**	0.0466	0.0847

[2] Model adjusted for age, sex and total energy intakes, [3] Model adjusted for age, sex, total energy intakes and total BCAA, animal protein and red meat intakes. Significant values ($p < 0.05$) are presented in bold. Abbreviations: NW, normal weight; OW, overweight-obese; MS, metabolic syndrome; ACs, Acylcarnitines.

4. Discussion

It is not yet fully established if elevated plasma BCAA and AC levels are a cause or a consequence of IR, and if protein intakes exert an influence on their plasma concentrations. To our knowledge, we are the first to investigate the association between the individual food groups contributing the most to daily protein intakes, fasting AC and BCAA levels in normal weight and overweight/obese individuals with or without metabolic perturbations.

As expected, plasma BCAA levels were significantly greater in OW with or without MS than in NW individuals, which is consistent with the literature [22,40–43]. Worth of mention, plasma BCAAs appeared to be affected by sex, as previously reported in some studies [40–42]. However, differences in BCAA intakes between groups were not present following adjustments for age, sex and energy intake. This was expected since total protein intakes and % of energy from protein were also not different between groups after adjustments. Still, the protein's origin deserves further attention. Considering all principal protein sources, red meat seems to be driving the positive association of total animal protein intakes with plasma BCAAs since it was the only food group presenting a trend towards significance for an association with plasma BCAAs. Associations with red meat were lost in adjusted models on the whole sample, but animal protein intakes remained significant. This reflects very well the intakes of our participants: OW/MS+ consumed significantly more animal protein than

NW/MS− and OW/MS− individuals in non-adjusted and adjusted models, whereas red meat intakes were no longer different between groups after adjustments for age, sex and energy. Considering these observations, plasma BCAA levels potentially reflect the consumption of animal protein/red meat. Greater red meat intakes would have been necessary to see an effect of this food on already metabolically deteriorated individuals. These findings are concordant with recent papers reporting BCAAs consumption—correlating with animal protein and/or meat intakes—associated or correlated with plasma BCAA levels [8,17]. Still, because animal protein and red meat only explain a small portion of plasma BCAAs variance, dietary intakes might not be the main variable affecting plasma BCAA levels.

Testing the associations within the three subgroups of subjects revealed substantial differences. In OW/MS+ individuals, the association between plasma BCAAs and animal protein presented a trend toward significance that became significant after adjustments. In the model including all 12 principal protein sources, the tendency observed for red meat persisted after adjustments, but reached significance when considering animal protein sources only (not shown). Similarly to what we observed in the whole sample, red meat was the main animal protein source associated with plasma BCAA levels in metabolically disturbed individuals although the small magnitude of the relationship is probably an indicator that there are other important metabolic factors implicated in plasma BCAAs elevation in this group.

As for OW/MS−, we surprisingly did not find any association of protein intakes with plasma BCAA levels. Their intakes were more similar to NW than to OW/MS+ individuals regarding macronutrients, but were no longer significantly different after adjustments for age, sex and energy intake. Yet, compared to their MS+ counterparts, they consumed less red meat and less animal protein overall. The hypothesis that elevated plasma BCAAs is consequent to IR could explain why their levels are significantly higher than NW/MS− subjects, assuming that they are at a greater risk of developing IR. At this point, we cannot rule out the possibility that the different dietary habits of OW/MS− exert some kind of protection against elevated plasma BCAA levels. Unfortunately, the study design of the INFOGENE study does not allow the verification of this hypothesis.

What has been observed in NW/MS− individuals is quite different. All models presented different associations. In the unadjusted ones, grain products were the main protein sources positively associated with plasma BCAA levels while total animal protein, but not vegetal protein intakes, was also positively associated. This unexpected observation could rather be an indicator of a dietary pattern rich in grain products, as well as in animal protein, explaining their associations with plasma BCAAs in different models. Even more intriguing, after adjustments for confounders, red meat was negatively associated with plasma BCAA levels. Sex appeared to be a moderator of this association ($p < 0.0001$). BCAAs might be more strongly affected by sex (and other metabolic factors) than by protein sources intakes in healthy individuals. This could explain why we found very different associations depending on the model used and would corroborate with the small magnitude of the associations found with the 12 principal protein food sources intakes. Of note, a decreased predictive effect of the habitual diet on serum metabolites after sex and age adjustments was previously reported by Floegel et al [44].

Plasma AC levels were another important aspect of the present study. It appears that the association between plasma C3 and C5 ACs and plasma BCAA levels were influenced by sex but not so much by other confounders, such as age, energy intakes, animal protein, red meat or BCAA intakes, depending on the model used. Further adjustments for variables related to dietary protein intakes did not change the associations between C3 or C5 ACs and plasma BCAA levels except for the loss of the association for C5 ACs in OW/MS+. In that model, neither animal protein, red meat or BCAA intakes were significant correlates to the variance. Thus, we cannot confirm if these variables modulate the association between C5 ACs and plasma BCAA levels or if we lost the association because of a lack of statistical power, but their contribution to the variance appears to be weak. C3 and C5 ACs might be differentially associated with plasma BCAA, but literature does not report on their individual effect [25,44]. We found C3 and C5 ACs to be positively associated with plasma BCAAs as reported in a comparable study where higher levels of short-chain ACs were observed in diabetic patients compared to lean or obese individuals [45]. Since this association persisted with adjustments for confounders and animal protein, BCAA and red meat intakes in our models, there appears to be a relative independence of C3 and C5 ACs from the diet. Consequently, we propose that C3 and C5 ACs more likely represents the degree of plasma BCAAs elevation than meat consumption. For these reasons, using these short-chain ACs as a biomarker of meat consumption should be done with caution and with consideration of other metabolic markers. It would be interesting to further investigate these association in fasting and non-fasting individuals since C3 and C5 levels could be lower in fasted individuals [46].

Taken all together, these findings are in line with a study realized in a cohort of Asian Indians living in the US and at risk of CVD [47]. The investigators reported a positive association between a Western/non-vegetarian dietary pattern, characterized by higher intakes of red meat, poultry, fish, eggs and vegetables, and a metabolite signature rich in BCAAs, as well as in aromatic AAs and short-chain ACs. Participants scoring higher for that metabolite signature were also more insulin resistant, had higher fasting and 2-h insulin concentrations and had lower adiponectin levels and insulin sensitivity. Similarly, we found a metabolic signature, including BCAA leucine, C3 and C5 ACs that was associated with a Western dietary pattern in French Canadians [24]. Red meat also appeared to be an important positive loading factor for T2D risk [44]. As for our healthy volunteers, recent work found meats, sausages, meat products and eggs to be included in dietary patterns explaining variation among plasma BCAA levels in a healthy population [17]. These foods were highlighted in at least one of our models.

The mechanisms underlying the association between BCAA intakes and IR development are unclear for now and association studies reported opposite results [4,28]. The largest European prospective study found total and mostly animal protein intakes to be associated with an elevated T2D risk [48]. As observed in the present study, and in similar studies [17–20], plant-protein intakes were not inversely associated with T2D risk. Interestingly, Okekunle et al., found that a pattern rich in meat was associated with T2D risk, even if rice and wheaten foods were the main correlates of BCAAs in their study cohort [49]. These findings, alongside the higher intakes of animal protein observed in OW/MS+ individuals herein, reiterate the importance of considering the composition of the foods BCAAs are coming from. In fact, red meat does have high heme-iron content which was suggested to be associated with T2D [50–54]. Other nutrients in meats may also have an impact on IR development, including the pro-oxidant and pro-inflammatory advanced glycation end products formed by the reaction of carbonyl groups of reducing sugars with the amine groups of proteins, lipids or nucleotides [55,56]. We also cannot exclude the role of the gut microbiota (GMB) in BCAAs metabolism. Accordingly, intestinal bacteria impact AAs absorption that are used for growth or the synthesis of metabolic compounds, such as short-chain fatty acids (SCFA), including branched-chain fatty acids (BCFA), BCAA being involved in the later [57]. Finally, animal protein could have a different biodisponibility or kinetics that could predispose to IR. A small study reported that vegan, who consumed less BCAAs than omnivores at baseline, had a significant decrease in insulin sensitivity after three months of BCAA supplementation [26]. Another study found a switch to fish and plant-based protein versus meat lowered plasma BCAAs in a small sample of mainly overweight individuals [58]. Mechanisms of actions need to be the subject of future studies.

All things considered, results of the present study and a literature review lead us to two different hypotheses: First, that the protein quality has an impact on plasma BCAA levels and second, that elevated BCAAs are the consequence of a disturbed metabolism in individuals having suboptimal dietary habits. In both cases, ACs seems more likely to reflect BCAA concentrations in the plasma. If BCAA levels induce IR, the most plausible hypothesis involves the mammalian target of rapamycin (mTOR) [59,60]. BCAAs and especially leucine can activate mTORC1 through an alternative pathway ending with insulin receptor degradation. Insulin-binding to its receptor being therefore compromised, a state of insulin resistance would occur [59–66]. BCAAs could also increase the activity of p65 subunit of nuclear transcription factor Kb (NF-kβ), a pro-inflammatory pathway that could accelerate IR progression [67]. Regardless of their potential, these mechanisms might not explain the rise of plasma BCAA levels observed in our sample, granted that protein intakes and therefore amino acid pool, were not greater in OW/MS− compared to NW/MS− group. If BCAAs elevation is rather the consequence of a disturbed metabolism, it has been proposed that high fat diets, obesity, IR or insulin levels could lead to a defect in BCKD activity and expression in the liver [11]. Circulating BCAAs are transaminated into branched-chain keto acids (BCKA) by the branched-chain amino acid transferase, a reversible step, before being further oxidized by BCKD to serve as substrates in the Krebs cycle [2,11,68]. Having dysfunctional BCKD would therefore lead to BCKA and or BCAAs accumulation. BCKA being the precursors of C3 and C5 ACs, this could explain ACs elevation in conjunction with IR [2].

The present study has some limitations. As mentioned earlier, elevated BCAAs is an early predictor of IR. Individuals classified in the MS− group could be insulin resistant but without enough metabolic impairments to make it into the MS+ group and therefore dilute IR impact on our results. As previously hypothesized by Isanejad et al., the response to dietary protein might depend on metabolic health, as well as on one's degree of IR [19]. Classifying our population according to IR only could help to isolate the impact of protein intakes on BCAAs at different stages of diabetes development (healthy, insulin resistant and diabetic). Also, we considered the medication for diabetes, dyslipidemia or hypertension to define our subgroups. But taking medications artificially improve metabolic parameters, which could therefore ameliorate BCAAs metabolism and affect the associations observed. Our sample was also too small for further investigation of the effect of sex on plasma BCAA levels by subgroups based on BMI and MS presence. Finally, because we used data from a cross-sectional study, we were not able to investigate in a prospective way the associations between plasma BCAA levels and changes in consumption of plant or animal protein nor time variations in ACs. It is important to note that correction for multiple testing was not applied to data. Because of the exploratory design of this study, having applied too restrictive correction could have masked potentially interesting associations in this relatively small sample of subjects. Notwithstanding, this study has some strengths. Our decision to compare healthy and metabolically deteriorated individuals was based on the fact that plasma BCAA levels are influenced by other components of the metabolic syndrome than glycemia [2]. As such, the present work compares healthy and metabolically deteriorated individuals within a single sample allowing comparisons between groups and generalization of the results. To our knowledge, it is also the first study testing the association of BCAAs with diet between subgroups of subjects with cardiometabolic perturbations as opposed to only IR or CVD related risk factors. All measurements were standardized, including the dietary questionnaire that has been validated for our population. Finally, the detailed FFQ allowed us to explore the associations with specific subgroups of animal-derived protein sources in parallel with ACs and BCAAs, which is unique to the present study.

5. Conclusions

In summary, we found a constant tendency toward significance between plasma BCAAs and animal protein or red meat intakes in OW/MS+ individuals. In NW/MS− individuals, diverse associations were observed between models. That being said, it is likely that BCAA or animal protein/meat intakes are not the main or the sole correlate to their elevation in plasma prior to IR considering their weak contribution to the variance. Plasma ACs concentrations were also found to be associated with plasma BCAA levels. Our study cannot explain mechanisms by which plasma BCAA levels and ACs are elevated in OW/MS+ individuals, but the impact of meat, its BCAA content, the presence of other compounds in its matrix and its GMB metabolites should be further investigated.

Supplementary Materials: The following is available online at http://www.mdpi.com/2072-6643/11/1/173/s1, Table S1: Food grouping used in the dietary pattern analysis.

Author Contributions: Conceptualization and design of the experiments, L.P., S.L. and M.-C.V.; data analysis, M.R., F.G., B.A.-N. and V.G.; formal analysis and writing, M.R.; supervision, M.-C.V.; review and editing, all authors.

Funding: This research received no external funding.

Acknowledgments: The authors express gratitude to all participants for their much-appreciated collaboration. We recognize the contribution of Marie-Eve Bouchard, Steve Amireault, Diane Drolet, and Dominique Beaulieu for their involvement in the study coordination, recruitment of the subjects, and data collection. We would also like to thank Chenomx Inc. (Edmonton, AB, Canada) who performed the mass spectrometry analyses to measure plasma metabolite levels. Marie-Claude Vohl is Canada Research Chair in Genomics Applied to Nutrition and Metabolic Health. Michèle Rousseau received a studentship from the INITIA foundation.

Conflicts of Interest: The authors declare no conflict of interest.

References

1. Gannon Nicholas, P.; Schnuck Jamie, K.; Vaughan Roger, A. BCAA Metabolism and Insulin Sensitivity—Dysregulated by Metabolic Status? *Mol. Nutr. Food Res.* **2018**, *62*, 1700756. [CrossRef] [PubMed]
2. Gar, C.; Rottenkolber, M.; Prehn, C.; Adamski, J.; Seissler, J.; Lechner, A. Serum and plasma amino acids as markers of prediabetes, insulin resistance, and incident diabetes. *Crit. Rev. Clin. Lab. Sci.* **2018**, *55*, 21–32. [CrossRef]
3. Labonte, C.C.; Farsijani, S.; Marliss, E.B.; Gougeon, R.; Morais, J.A.; Pereira, S.; Bassil, M.; Winter, A.; Murphy, J.; Combs, T.P.; et al. Plasma Amino Acids vs Conventional Predictors of Insulin Resistance Measured by the Hyperinsulinemic Clamp. *J. Endocr. Soc.* **2017**, *1*, 861–873. [CrossRef] [PubMed]
4. Asghari, G.; Farhadnejad, H.; Teymoori, F.; Mirmiran, P.; Tohidi, M.; Azizi, F. High dietary intake of branched-chain amino acids is associated with an increased risk of insulin resistance in adults. *J. Diabetes* **2018**, *10*, 357–364. [CrossRef] [PubMed]
5. Ruiz-Canela, M.; Toledo, E.; Clish, C.B.; Hruby, A.; Liang, L.; Salas-Salvadó, J.; Razquin, C.; Corella, D.; Estruch, R.; Ros, E.; et al. Plasma branched-chain amino acids and incident cardiovascular disease in the PREDIMED trial. *Clin. Chem.* **2016**, *62*, 582–592. [CrossRef] [PubMed]
6. Song, M.; Fung, T.T.; Hu, F.B.; Willett, W.C.; Longo, V.; Chan, A.T.; Giovannucci, E.L. Animal and plant protein intake and all-cause and cause-specific mortality: Results from two prospective US cohort studies. *JAMA Intern. Med.* **2016**, *176*, 1453. [CrossRef]
7. Wang, T.J.; Larson, M.G.; Vasan, R.S.; Cheng, S.; Rhee, E.P.; McCabe, E.; Lewis, G.D.; Fox, C.S.; Jacques, P.F.; Fernandez, C.; et al. Metabolite profiles and the risk of developing diabetes. *Nat. Med.* **2011**, *17*, 448–453. [CrossRef] [PubMed]
8. Zheng, Y.; Li, Y.; Qi, Q.; Hruby, A.; Manson, J.E.; Willett, W.C.; Wolpin, B.M.; Hu, F.B.; Qi, L. Cumulative consumption of branched-chain amino acids and incidence of type 2 diabetes. *Int. J. Epidemiol.* **2016**, *45*, 1482–1492. [CrossRef]
9. Mahendran, Y.; Jonsson, A.; Have, C.T.; Allin, K.H.; Witte, D.R.; Jørgensen, M.E.; Grarup, N.; Pedersen, O.; Kilpeläinen, T.O.; Hansen, T. Genetic evidence of a causal effect of insulin resistance on branched-chain amino acid levels. *Diabetologia* **2017**, *60*, 873–878. [CrossRef]
10. Wang, Q.; Holmes, M.V.; Davey Smith, G.; Ala-Korpela, M. Genetic Support for a Causal Role of Insulin Resistance on Circulating Branched-Chain Amino Acids and Inflammation. *Diabetes Care* **2017**, *40*, 1779–1786. [CrossRef]
11. Shin, A.C.; Fasshauer, M.; Filatova, N.; Grundell, L.A.; Zielinski, E.; Zhou, J.-Y.; Scherer, T.; Lindtner, C.; White, P.J.; Lapworth, A.L.; et al. Brain insulin lowers circulating BCAA levels by inducing hepatic BCAA catabolism. *Cell Metab.* **2014**, *20*, 898. [CrossRef] [PubMed]
12. Lynch, C.J.; Adams, S.H. Branched-chain amino acids in metabolic signalling and insulin resistance. *Nat. Rev. Endocrinol.* **2014**, *10*, 723–736. [CrossRef] [PubMed]
13. Fernstrom, J.D. Branched-Chain Amino Acids and Brain Function. *J. Nutr.* **2005**, *135*, 1539S–1546S. [CrossRef] [PubMed]
14. Brosnan, J.T.; Brosnan, M.E. Branched-Chain Amino Acids: Enzyme and Substrate Regulation. *J. Nutr.* **2006**, *136*, 207S–211S. [CrossRef]

15. Platell, C.; Kong, S.E.; McCauley, R.; Hall, J.C. Branched-chain amino acids. *J. Gastroenterol. Hepatol.* **2001**, *15*, 706–717. [CrossRef]
16. López, A.M.; Noriega, L.G.; Diaz, M.; Torres, N.; Tovar, A.R. Plasma branched-chain and aromatic amino acid concentration after ingestion of an urban or rural diet in rural Mexican women. *BMC Obes.* **2015**, *2*, 8. [CrossRef]
17. Merz, B.; Frommherz, L.; Rist, M.J.; Kulling, S.E.; Bub, A.; Watzl, B. Dietary Pattern and Plasma BCAA-Variations in Healthy Men and Women—Results from the KarMeN Study. *Nutrients* **2018**, *10*, 623. [CrossRef] [PubMed]
18. Pan, A.; Sun, Q.; Bernstein, A.M.; Schulze, M.B.; Manson, J.E.; Willett, W.C.; Hu, F.B. Red meat consumption and risk of type 2 diabetes: 3 cohorts of US adults and an updated meta-analysis. *Am. J. Clin. Nutr.* **2011**, *94*, 1088–1096. [CrossRef]
19. Isanejad, M.; LaCroix, A.Z.; Thomson, C.A.; Tinker, L.; Larson, J.C.; Qi, Q.; Qi, L.; Cooper-DeHoff, R.M.; Phillips, L.S.; Prentice, R.L.; et al. Branched-Chain Amino Acid, Meat Intake and Risk of Type 2 Diabetes in the Women's Health Initiative. Available online: /core/journals/british-journal-of-nutrition/article/branchedchain-amino-acid-meat-intake-and-risk-of-type-2-diabetes-in-the-womens-health-initiative/2706233DCEB0422B3DCCA9D9925CCB3F (accessed on 10 April 2018).
20. Malik, V.S.; Li, Y.; Tobias, D.K.; Pan, A.; Hu, F.B. Dietary Protein Intake and Risk of Type 2 Diabetes in US Men and Women. *Am. J. Epidemiol.* **2016**, *183*, 715–728. [CrossRef] [PubMed]
21. Schooneman, M.G.; Vaz, F.M.; Houten, S.M.; Soeters, M.R. Acylcarnitines. *Diabetes* **2013**, *62*, 1–8. [CrossRef]
22. Newgard, C.B.; An, J.; Bain, J.R.; Muehlbauer, M.J.; Stevens, R.D.; Lien, L.F.; Haqq, A.M.; Shah, S.H.; Arlotto, M.; Slentz, C.A.; et al. A Branched-Chain Amino Acid-Related Metabolic Signature that Differentiates Obese and Lean Humans and Contributes to Insulin Resistance. *Cell Metab.* **2009**, *9*, 311–326. [CrossRef]
23. Roe, D.S.; Roe, C.R.; Brivet, M.; Sweetman, L. Evidence for a short-chain carnitine-acylcarnitine translocase in mitochondria specifically related to the metabolism of branched-chain amino acids. *Mol. Genet. Metab.* **2000**, *69*, 69–75. [CrossRef]
24. Bouchard-Mercier, A.; Rudkowska, I.; Lemieux, S.; Couture, P.; Vohl, M.-C. The metabolic signature associated with the Western dietary pattern: A cross-sectional study. *Nutr. J.* **2013**, *12*, 158. [CrossRef]
25. Cheung, W.; Keski-Rahkonen, P.; Assi, N.; Ferrari, P.; Freisling, H.; Rinaldi, S.; Slimani, N.; Zamora-Ros, R.; Rundle, M.; Frost, G.; et al. A metabolomic study of biomarkers of meat and fish intake. *Am. J. Clin. Nutr.* **2017**, *105*, 600–608. [CrossRef]
26. Gojda, J.; Rossmeislová, L.; Straková, R.; Tůmová, J.; Elkalaf, M.; Jaček, M.; Tůma, P.; Potočková, J.; Krauzová, E.; Waldauf, P.; et al. Chronic dietary exposure to branched chain amino acids impairs glucose disposal in vegans but not in omnivores. *Eur. J. Clin. Nutr.* **2017**, *71*, 594–601. [CrossRef]
27. Iwasaki, M. Validity of a Self-Administered Food-Frequency Questionnaire for Assessing Amino Acid Intake in Japan: Comparison with Intake From 4-Day Weighed Dietary Records and Plasma Levels. *J. Epidemiol.* **2016**, *26*, 36–44. [CrossRef]
28. Jennings, A.; MacGregor, A.; Pallister, T.; Spector, T.; Cassidy, A. Associations between branched chain amino acid intake and biomarkers of adiposity and cardiometabolic health independent of genetic factors: A twin study. *Int. J. Cardiol.* **2016**, *223*, 992–998. [CrossRef]
29. Nagata, C.; Nakamura, K.; Wada, K.; Tsuji, M.; Tamai, Y.; Kawachi, T. Branched-chain Amino Acid Intake and the Risk of Diabetes in a Japanese CommunityThe Takayama Study. *Am. J. Epidemiol.* **2013**, *178*, 1226–1232. [CrossRef]
30. Pallottini, A.C.; Sales, C.H.; Vieira, D.A.D.S.; Marchioni, D.M.; Fisberg, R.M. Dietary BCAA Intake Is Associated with Demographic, Socioeconomic and Lifestyle Factors in Residents of São Paulo, Brazil. *Nutrients* **2017**, *9*, 449. [CrossRef]
31. Paradis, A.-M.; Pérusse, L.; Godin, G.; Vohl, M.-C. Validity of a self-reported measure of familial history of obesity. *Nutr. J.* **2008**, *7*, 27. [CrossRef]
32. Paradis, A.-M.; Godin, G.; Pérusse, L.; Vohl, M.-C. Associations between dietary patterns and obesity phenotypes. *Int. J. Obes.* **2009**, *33*, 1419–1426. [CrossRef] [PubMed]
33. Paradis, A.-M.; Godin, G.; Pérusse, L.; Vohl, M.-C. Interaction between Familial History of Obesity and Fat Intakes on Obesity Phenotypes. *Lifestyle Genom.* **2009**, *2*, 37–42. [CrossRef] [PubMed]

34. Cormier, H.; Thifault, É.; Garneau, V.; Tremblay, A.; Drapeau, V.; Pérusse, L.; Vohl, M.-C. Association between yogurt consumption, dietary patterns, and cardio-metabolic risk factors. *Eur. J. Nutr.* **2016**, *55*, 577–587. [CrossRef]
35. Allam-Ndoul, B.; Guénard, F.; Garneau, V.; Cormier, H.; Barbier, O.; Pérusse, L.; Vohl, M.-C. Association between Metabolite Profiles, Metabolic Syndrome and Obesity Status. *Nutrients* **2016**, *8*, 324. [CrossRef]
36. Goulet, J.; Nadeau, G.; Lapointe, A.; Lamarche, B.; Lemieux, S. Validity and reproducibility of an interviewer-administered food frequency questionnaire for healthy French-Canadian men and women. *Nutr. J.* **2004**, *3*, 13. [CrossRef] [PubMed]
37. Johnson-Down, L.; Ritter, H.; Starkey, L.J.; Gray-Donald, K. Primary Food Sources of Nutrients In the Diet of Canadian Adults. *Can. J. Diet. Pract. Res.* **2006**, *67*, 7–13. [CrossRef]
38. Callaway, C.W.; Chumlea, W.C.; Bouchard, C.; Himes, J.H.; Lohman, T.G.; Martin, A.D.; Mitchell, C.D.; Mueller, W.H.; Roche, A.F.; Seefeldt, V.D. Standardization of Anthropometric Measurements. In *The Airlie (VA) Consensus Conference*; Human Kinetics Publisher: Champaign, IR, USA, 1988; pp. 29–80.
39. Friedewald, W.T.; Levy, R.I.; Fredrickson, D.S. Estimation of the Concentration of Low-Density Lipoprotein Cholesterol in Plasma, Without Use of the Preparative Ultracentrifuge. *Clin. Chem.* **1972**, *18*, 499–502. [PubMed]
40. Guevara-Cruz, M.; Vargas-Morales, J.M.; Méndez-García, A.L.; López-Barradas, A.M.; Granados-Portillo, O.; Ordaz-Nava, G.; Rocha-Viggiano, A.K.; Gutierrez-Leyte, C.A.; Medina-Cerda, E.; Rosado, J.L.; et al. Amino acid profiles of young adults differ by sex, body mass index and insulin resistance. *Nutr. Metab. Cardiovasc. Dis.* **2018**, *28*, 393–401. [CrossRef] [PubMed]
41. Takashina, C.; Tsujino, I.; Watanabe, T.; Sakaue, S.; Ikeda, D.; Yamada, A.; Sato, T.; Ohira, H.; Otsuka, Y.; Oyama-Manabe, N.; et al. Associations among the plasma amino acid profile, obesity, and glucose metabolism in Japanese adults with normal glucose tolerance. *Nutr. Metab.* **2016**, *13*, 5. [CrossRef]
42. Würtz, P.; Mäkinen, V.-P.; Soininen, P.; Kangas, A.J.; Tukiainen, T.; Kettunen, J.; Savolainen, M.J.; Tammelin, T.; Viikari, J.S.; Rönnemaa, T.; et al. Metabolic Signatures of Insulin Resistance in 7098 Young Adults. *Diabetes* **2012**, *61*, 1372.
43. Boulet, M.M.; Chevrier, G.; Grenier-Larouche, T.; Pelletier, M.; Nadeau, M.; Scarpa, J.; Prehn, C.; Marette, A.; Adamski, J.; Tchernof, A. Alterations of plasma metabolite profiles related to adipose tissue distribution and cardiometabolic risk. *Am. J. Physiol.-Endocrinol. Metab.* **2015**, *309*, E736–E746. [CrossRef]
44. Floegel, A.; von Ruesten, A.; Drogan, D.; Schulze, M.B.; Prehn, C.; Adamski, J.; Pischon, T.; Boeing, H. Variation of serum metabolites related to habitual diet: A targeted metabolomic approach in EPIC-Potsdam. *Eur. J. Clin. Nutr.* **2013**, *67*, 1100–1108. [CrossRef] [PubMed]
45. Mihalik, S.J.; Goodpaster, B.H.; Kelley, D.E.; Chace, D.H.; Vockley, J.; Toledo, F.G.S.; DeLany, J.P. Increased Levels of Plasma Acylcarnitines in Obesity and Type 2 Diabetes and Identification of a Marker of Glucolipotoxicity. *Obes. Silver Spring Md* **2010**, *18*, 1695. [CrossRef] [PubMed]
46. Strand, E.; Pedersen, E.R.; Svingen, G.F.T.; Olsen, T.; Bjørndal, B.; Karlsson, T.; Dierkes, J.; Njølstad, P.R.; Mellgren, G.; Tell, G.S.; et al. Serum Acylcarnitines and Risk of Cardiovascular Death and Acute Myocardial Infarction in Patients with Stable Angina Pectoris. *J. Am. Heart Assoc.* **2017**, *6*, e003620. [CrossRef]
47. Bhupathiraju, S.N.; Guasch-Ferré, M.; Gadgil, M.D.; Newgard, C.B.; Bain, J.R.; Muehlbauer, M.J.; Ilkayeva, O.R.; Scholtens, D.M.; Hu, F.B.; Kanaya, A.M.; et al. Dietary Patterns among Asian Indians Living in the United States Have Distinct Metabolomic Profiles That Are Associated with Cardiometabolic Risk. *J. Nutr.* **2018**, *148*, 1150–1159. [CrossRef] [PubMed]
48. van Nielen, M.; Feskens, E.J.M.; Mensink, M.; Sluijs, I.; Molina, E.; Amiano, P.; Ardanaz, E.; Balkau, B.; Beulens, J.W.J.; Boeing, H.; et al. Dietary Protein Intake and Incidence of Type 2 Diabetes in Europe: The EPIC-InterAct Case-Cohort Study. *Diabetes Care* **2014**, *37*, 1854–1862. [CrossRef]
49. Okekunle, A.P. Dietary Intakes of Branched-Chained Amino Acid and Risk for Type 2 Diabetes in Adults: The Harbin Cohort Study on Diet, Nutrition and Chronic Non-Communicable Diseases Study. *Can. J. Diabetes* **2018**, *42*, 484–492.e7. [CrossRef] [PubMed]
50. White, D.L.; Collinson, A. Red Meat, Dietary Heme Iron, and Risk of Type 2 Diabetes: The Involvement of Advanced Lipoxidation Endproducts. *Adv. Nutr.* **2013**, *4*, 403. [CrossRef]
51. Kunutsor Setor, K.; Apekey Tanefa, A.; Walley, J.; Kain, K. Ferritin levels and risk of type 2 diabetes mellitus: An updated systematic review and meta-analysis of prospective evidence. *Diabetes Metab. Res. Rev.* **2013**, *29*, 308–318. [CrossRef]

52. Bao, W.; Rong, Y.; Rong, S.; Liu, L. Dietary iron intake, body iron stores, and the risk of type 2 diabetes: A systematic review and meta-analysis. *BMC Med.* **2012**, *10*, 119. [CrossRef]
53. Zhao, Z.; Li, S.; Liu, G.; Yan, F.; Ma, X.; Huang, Z.; Tian, H. Body Iron Stores and Heme-Iron Intake in Relation to Risk of Type 2 Diabetes: A Systematic Review and Meta-Analysis. *PLoS ONE* **2012**, *7*, e41641. [CrossRef] [PubMed]
54. Talaei, M.; Wang, Y.-L.; Yuan, J.-M.; Pan, A.; Koh, W.-P. Meat, Dietary Heme Iron, and Risk of Type 2 Diabetes MellitusThe Singapore Chinese Health Study. *Am. J. Epidemiol.* **2017**, *186*, 824–833. [CrossRef] [PubMed]
55. O'Brien, J.; Morrissey, P.A.; Ames, J.M. Nutritional and toxicological aspects of the Maillard browning reaction in foods. *Crit. Rev. Food Sci. Nutr.* **1989**, *28*, 211–248. [CrossRef] [PubMed]
56. Calder, P.C.; Ahluwalia, N.; Brouns, F.; Buetler, T.; Clement, K.; Cunningham, K.; Esposito, K.; Jönsson, L.S.; Kolb, H.; Lansink, M.; et al. Dietary factors and low-grade inflammation in relation to overweight and obesity. *Br. J. Nutr.* **2011**, *106*, S1–S78. [CrossRef] [PubMed]
57. Neis, E.P.J.G.; Dejong, C.H.C.; Rensen, S.S. The Role of Microbial Amino Acid Metabolism in Host Metabolism. *Nutrients* **2015**, *7*, 2930–2946. [CrossRef]
58. Elshorbagy, A.; Jernerén, F.; Basta, M.; Basta, C.; Turner, C.; Khaled, M.; Refsum, H. Amino acid changes during transition to a vegan diet supplemented with fish in healthy humans. *Eur. J. Nutr.* **2017**, *56*, 1953–1962. [CrossRef]
59. Zoncu, R.; Efeyan, A.; Sabatini, D.M. mTOR: From growth signal integration to cancer, diabetes and ageing. *Nat. Rev. Mol. Cell Biol.* **2011**, *12*, 21–35. [CrossRef]
60. Jewell, J.L.; Russell, R.C.; Guan, K.-L. Amino acid signalling upstream of mTOR. *Nat. Rev. Mol. Cell Biol.* **2013**, *14*, 133–139. [CrossRef]
61. Yoon, M.-S. The Emerging Role of Branched-Chain Amino Acids in Insulin Resistance and Metabolism. *Nutrients* **2016**, *8*, 405. [CrossRef]
62. Krebs, M.; Krssak, M.; Bernroider, E.; Anderwald, C.; Brehm, A.; Meyerspeer, M.; Nowotny, P.; Roth, E.; Waldhäusl, W.; Roden, M. Mechanism of Amino Acid-Induced Skeletal Muscle Insulin Resistance in Humans. *Diabetes* **2002**, *51*, 599–605. [CrossRef]
63. Tremblay, F.; Krebs, M.; Dombrowski, L.; Brehm, A.; Bernroider, E.; Roth, E.; Nowotny, P.; Waldhäusl, W.; Marette, A.; Roden, M. Overactivation of S6 Kinase 1 as a Cause of Human Insulin Resistance During Increased Amino Acid Availability. *Diabetes* **2005**, *54*, 2674–2684. [CrossRef]
64. Laplante, M.; Sabatini, D.M. mTOR Signaling in Growth Control and Disease. *Cell* **2012**, *149*, 274–293. [CrossRef]
65. Zick, Y. Insulin resistance: A phosphorylation-based uncoupling of insulin signaling. *Trends Cell Biol.* **2001**, *11*, 437–441. [CrossRef]
66. Um, S.H.; D'Alessio, D.; Thomas, G. Nutrient overload, insulin resistance, and ribosomal protein S6 kinase 1, S6K1. *Cell Metab.* **2006**, *3*, 393–402. [CrossRef]
67. Zhenyukh, O.; Civantos, E.; Ruiz-Ortega, M.; Sanchez, M.S.; Vazquez, C.; Peiro, C.; Egido, J.; Mas, S. High concentration of branched-chain amino acids promotes oxidative stress, inflammation and migration of human peripheral blood mononuclear cells via mTORC1 activation. *Free Radic. Biol. Med.* **2017**, *104*, 165–177. [CrossRef]
68. Adeva, M.M.; Calviño, J.; Souto, G.; Donapetry, C. Insulin resistance and the metabolism of branched-chain amino acids in humans. *Amino Acids* **2012**, *43*, 171–181. [CrossRef]

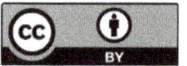

© 2019 by the authors. Licensee MDPI, Basel, Switzerland. This article is an open access article distributed under the terms and conditions of the Creative Commons Attribution (CC BY) license (http://creativecommons.org/licenses/by/4.0/).

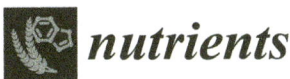

Article

Dietary Fat Intake and Metabolic Syndrome in Older Adults

Alicia Julibert [1], Maria del Mar Bibiloni [1], David Mateos [1], Escarlata Angullo [1,2] and Josep A. Tur [1,*]

[1] Research Group on Community Nutrition & Oxidative Stress, University of Balearic Islands, IDISBA & CIBEROBN, 07122 Palma de Mallorca, Spain
[2] Escola Graduada Primary Health Care Center, IBSalut, 07001 Palma de Mallorca, Spain
* Correspondence: pep.tur@uib.es; Tel.: +34-971-1731; Fax: +34-971-173184

Received: 1 July 2019; Accepted: 12 August 2019; Published: 14 August 2019

Abstract: Background: Metabolic Syndrome (MetS) is associated with higher rates of cardiovascular disease (CVD), type 2 diabetes mellitus, and cancer worldwide. Objective: To assess fat intake in older adults with or without MetS. Design: Cross-sectional nutritional survey in older adults living in the Balearic Islands (n = 477, 48% women, 55–80 years old) with no previous CVD. Methods: Assessment of fat (total fat, MUFA, PUFA, SFA, TFA, linoleic acid, α-linolenic acid, marine and non-marine ω-3 FA, animal fat and vegetable fat, cholesterol) and macronutrient intake using a validated food frequency questionnaire, and its comparison with recommendations of the US Institute of Medicine (IOM) and the Spanish Society of Community Nutrition (SENC). Results: Participants with MetS showed higher BMI, lower physical activity, higher total fat and MUFA intake, and lower intake of energy, carbohydrates, and fiber than participants without MetS. Men and women with MetS were below the Acceptable Macronutrient Distribution Range (AMDR) proposed by IOM for carbohydrates and above the AMDR for total fat and MUFAs, and women were below the AMDR proposed for α-linolenic acid (ALA) compared with participants without MetS. Conclusions: Subjects with MetS were less likely to meet IOM and SENC recommendations for fat and macronutrient intakes as compared to non-MetS subjects.

Keywords: older adults; macronutrient intake; dietary intake; fat intake; metabolic syndrome

1. Introduction

Metabolic syndrome (MetS) is a clinical condition characterized by several metabolic risk factors [1,2] associated with higher prevalence of cardiovascular disease (CVD), type 2 diabetes (T2DM), and cancer worldwide [3]. These factors involve abdominal obesity, blood pressure, glycaemia, triglyceridemia (TG), and high-density lipoprotein cholesterol (HDL-c) [1].

The prevalence of MetS has been increasing over the years and is now reaching epidemic proportions [4]. In Western countries, the prevalence of MetS is approximately one-fifth of the adult population and increases with age. However, the prevalence of MetS will vary according to the population studied, age, gender, race, and ethnicity, as well as the definition applied [5,6].

MetS is also influenced by nutrient intake, alcohol consumption, physical exercise, or smoking [3]. Unhealthy eating patterns and lifestyle, such as malnutrition and inactivity, can worsen the clinical status, with accumulation of body fat and alteration of the parameters that characterize MetS [7].

As shown in the ANIBES study, the macronutrient distribution is worsening and somewhat moving away from the recommendations and traditional Mediterranean dietary pattern, although the negative changes are less pronounced as age increases [8]. Age, sex, lower levels of education, economic status, smoking status, and alcohol intake predict lower dietary variety. There is evidence that older Spanish adults with MetS had a high risk of inadequate nutrient intake [9].

Eating patterns and their food and nutrient characteristics are the primary emphasis of the recommendations of U.S. Dietary Guidelines 2015–2020 [10]. Accordingly, therehas been a focus on the roles of macronutrients (carbohydrates, fat, and proteins) [11–17] and dietary patterns [7,18–20] on MetS.

Therefore, taking into consideration the scientific evidence on nutrients in the development of MetS, this study aimed to assess fat intake in older adults with or without MetS.

2. Materials and Methods

2.1. Design and Participants

The sample had477 participants (48% women; aged 55–80 years old)with no previously documented CVD that were engaged in social and municipal clubs, health centers, and sport clubs ofacross-sectional study conducted in the Balearic Islands. The age range was chosen since they are at high risk of suffering non communicable disease, the association of MetS with CVD, and because the increasing prevalence of MetS with age is known [21]. Exclusion criteria included being institutionalized, suffering from a physical or mental illness thatlimited their participation in physical fitness or their ability to respond to questionnaires, chronic alcoholism or drug addiction, and intake of drugs for clinical research over the past year.

The study protocols followed the Declaration of Helsinki ethical standards, and were approved by the Ethics Committee of Research of Balearic Islands (refs. CEIC-IB2251/14PI and CEIC-IB1295/09PI). All participants provided informed written consent.

2.2. Anthropometric Measurements

Anthropometric variables were measured by trained personnel to minimize the inter-observer coefficients of variation. Weight and height were measured with high-quality electronic calibrated scales and a wall-mounted stadiometer, respectively. Height was determined using a mobile anthropometer (Seca 213, SECA Deutschland, Hamburg, Germany) to the nearest millimeter, with the participant's head maintained in the Frankfort Horizontal Plane position. Body weight and body fat were determined using a Segmental Body Composition Analyzer (Tanita BC-418, Tanita, Tokyo, Japan). The participants were weighed in bare feet and light clothes (0.6 kg was subtracted for their clothing). Body mass index (BMI) was calculated as weight in kilograms divided by the square of height in meters (kg/m^2). Waist circumference (WC) was measured half-way between the last rib and the iliac crest by using an anthropometric tape. Blood pressure was measured using a validated semi-automatic oscillometer (Omron HEM-705CP, Hoofddorp, The Netherlands) after 5 min of rest inbetween measurements while the participant was in a seated position. All anthropometric variables were determined in duplicate, except for blood pressure (in triplicate).

2.3. Blood Collection and Analysis

Blood samples were collected after an overnight fast and biochemical analyses were performed on fasting plasma glucose, total cholesterol, HDL-c, and TG concentrations in local laboratories using standard enzymatic methods. Participants were classified as "with MetS" (n = 333) and "without MetS" (n = 144) according to the updated harmonized definition of the International Diabetes Federation and the American Heart Association and National Heart, Lung, and Blood Institute [2].

2.4. Dietary Intake Assessment

Licensed dieticians administered a semiquantitative, 137-item food frequency questionnaire (FFQ), repeatedly validated in Spain [22]. For each item, a typical portion size was included and consumption frequencies were registered in 9 categories that ranged from "never or almost never" to "≥6 times/day". Energy and nutrient intakes were calculated as frequency multiplied by nutrient composition of specified portion size for each food item, using a self-made computerized program based on available information in the Spanish food composition tables by Moreiras et al. [23]. When foods in the Spanish food composition tables were not available, the BEDCA food database was used in order to complete missing information [24]. Dietary intake of energy, carbohydrates (CHOs), proteins, total fat, monounsaturated fatty acids (MUFAs), polyunsaturatedfatty acids (PUFAs) and SFAs, trans-fatty acid (TFA), linoleic acid (LA), α-linolenic acid (ALA), marine and non-marine ω-3 fatty acid (ω-3 FA), animal fat and vegetable fat, cholesterol, and fiber were estimated. The vegetable fat included vegetables, fruits, nuts, legumes, total cereals, olives, oils, cookies, fritters, cocoa powder, mustard, ketchup, fried tomato, sugar, marmalade, and snacks. The animal fat included total dairy products, total meat, total fish, pizza, butter, lard, bakery goods, nougat, ready-to-eat meals, salad cream, and honey. The fat quality index (FQI) was also calculated as previously described [25]. Briefly, the FQI was calculated using the ratio (MUFA + PUFA)/(SFA + TFA) as a continuous variable.

Macronutrients and different fat intakes were compared with Institute of Medicine (IOM) and Spanish Society of Community Nutrition (SENC) recommendations. The dietary references intakes (DRIs) values proposed by IOM [26] were used, which are quantitative estimates of nutrient intakes to assess and plan diets for healthy people, including the Acceptable Macronutrient Distribution Range (AMDR) values. The prevalence of inadequate macronutrient intake according to the 2020 Nutritional Objectives for Spanish Population proposed by SENC [27] was used.

2.5. Socioeconomic and Lifestyle Determinants

Sociodemographic and lifestyle characteristics were collected from each participant. Educational level was ranked into primary school, secondary school, and university. Physical activity was measured using the validated Spanish version of the Minnesota Leisure Time Physical Activity Questionnaire [28,29]; it was taken by interview with trained research assistants and measured leisure time physical activities (LTPA), including household activities, over the previous 12 months. The Minnesota questionnaire was used to estimate physical activity levels by using metabolic equivalents of tasks (METs) [30]. METs are calculated by multiplying the intensity (showed by the MET-score) and the duration spent on that activity (measured in minutes). The MET-score can be derived from tables (the Compendium of Physical Activities) [31] that show the intensity of the activity relative to resting (METhours/week) spent on physical activity refer to the energy that is spent on activities, over and above existing levels of resting energy expenditure. Finally, information related to individual medical history, current medication use, and smoking status were also obtained.

2.6. Statistical Analyses

Analyses were performed with the SPSS statistical software package version 25.0 (SPSS Inc., Chicago, IL, USA). All analyses were stratified by sex and MetS status. Data are shown as mean, standard deviation (SD), or median and interquartile range (IQR). Normality of data was assessed using Kolmogorov–Smirnov test. Difference in medians between two comparison groups were tested by the Mann-Whitney U-test when variables were not normally distributed, and difference in means between the two comparison groups were tested by unpaired Students' *t*-test when variables were normally distributed. Differences in prevalence of MetS or not among participants were examined using χ^2 (all *p* values are two-tailed). Logistic regression analyses with the calculation of corresponding odds ratio (OR) and the 95% confidence interval (95% Confidence Interval, CI) were also used to assess the association between pathological features of MetS and macronutrients, specific types of fat, and dietary intake. Results were adjusted for sex, age (continuous variable), BMI (continuous variable), energy intake (continuous variable), and total physical activity (continuous variable, expressed as METmin/hour) to control for potential confounders. Results were considered statistically significant if *p*-value (2 tailed) <0.05.

3. Results

Comparison of socioeconomic and lifestyle characteristics between the two study groups stratified by sex are shown in Table 1. Participants with MetS showed higher BMI and lower total physical activity than participants without MetS. As expected, the groups differed in all MetS components, except for blood pressure in women. A higher percentage of patients with MetS showed pathological cut-off values than patients without MetS in all MetS components.

Male MetS patients with high blood pressure plus hyperglycemia plus high abdominal fat comprised 64.5% of the total MetS population; those with high blood pressure plus hypertriglyceridemia plus low HDL-c comprised 42.6% of the MetS population. Female MetS patients with high blood pressure plus hyperglycemia plus high abdominal fat comprised 59.3% of the total MetS population; those with high blood pressure plus hypertriglyceridemia plus low HDL-c comprised 38.7% of the MetS population.

Comparisons of nutrient intakes and food consumption between the two study groups stratified by sex are shown in Tables 2 and 3, respectively. Participants with MetS showed higher total fat and MUFA intake but lower intake of energy, carbohydrates, and fiber than those without MetS ($p < 0.05$). Participants with MetS also showed higher FQI than non-MetS participants. Women with MetS reported higher intake of proteins but lower intake of TFA, ω-3 FA, LA, ALA, and marine and non-marine ω-3 FA than women without MetS. Participants with MetS reported lower consumption of fruits, potatoes, total cereals, whole grain bread, and rice and pasta than participants without MetS. Men with MetS reported lower consumption of ready to-eat-meals than those without MetS. On the other hand, women reported lower consumption of bakery goods and alcohol than those without MetS.

Table 4 shows that participants with MetS, for both men and women, were more likely to be below the AMDR proposed by IOM for carbohydrates and ALA (except for men) and more likely to be above the AMDR for total fat and MUFAs than participants without MetS. Similar results were obtained when the 2020 Nutritional Objectives for the Spanish population were assessed (Table 5). Participants with MetS were also more likely to be below the acceptable nutritional range for carbohydrates and more likely to be above the acceptable nutritional range for total fat and MUFAs than participants without MetS. Finally, participants with MetS were more likely to be below the 2020 Nutritional Objectives for the Spanish population for TFA but also for total fiber, such as in fruits and vegetables.

Multivariate adjusted odds ratio (OR) for the association between pathological features of the MetS components and dietary macronutrient intake in participants with and without MetS showed, after adjustment for potential confounders (i.e., age, sex, BMI, energy and physical activity), that hypertension (equal or higher pathological cut-off value was OR reference: 1.00) is related with lower intake of PUFA (OR: 0.95; 95% CI: 0.91–0.98), SFA (OR: 0.95; 95% CI: 0.92–0.99), TFA (OR: 0.95; 95% CI: 0.91–0.99), LA (OR: 0.94; 95% CI: 0.90–0.98), and ALA (OR: 0.95; 95% CI: 0.91–0.99). However, abdominal obesity (equal or higher pathological cut-off value was OR reference: 1.00) was associated with high PUFA intake (OR: 1.10; 95% CI: 1.01–1.19), LA (OR: 0.12; 95% CI: 1.02–1.23) and vegetable fat (OR: 1.05; 95% CI: 1.01–1.08). No other relationships were found between other pathological components of MetS and dietary macronutrient intake.

Table 1. Socioeconomic and lifestyle characteristics of participants "with Metabolic Syndrome" (n = 333) and "without Metabolic Syndrome" (n = 144) stratified by sex.

	Men					Women				
	Without MetS (n = 63)		With MetS (n = 183)		p-Value *	Without MetS (n = 81)		With MetS (n = 150)		p-Value *
	Mean ± SD	Median (IQR)	Mean ± SD	Median (IQR)		Mean ± SD	Median (IQR)	Mean ± SD	Median (IQR)	
Age (y)	63.8 ± 5.9	64.0 (59.0, 67.0)	64.1 ± 5.9	64.0 (59.0, 69.0)	0.544	66.8 ± 5.0	66.0 (63.0, 70.0)	65.9 ± 4.5	66.0 (62.0, 69.0)	0.340
BMI (kg/m^2)	27.0 ± 3.2	27.5 (24.9, 28.7)	32.0 ± 3.6	31.9 (29.0, 34.5)	<0.001	25.3 ± 3.3	25.6 (22.9, 27.4)	32.8 ± 4.2	32.7 (30.1, 36.1)	<0.001
Current smoking habit (%)					0.081					0.119
Yes		6.3		14.8			6.2		12.8	
No		93.7		85.2			93.8		87.2	
Education (%)					0.660					0.595
Primary		39.7		37.1			53.1		60.0	
Secondary		39.7		36.5			30.9		26.9	
University or graduate		20.6		26.4			16.0		13.1	
Total physical activity (n) [†]		63		158			81		131	
Total physical activity (MET·hour/week) [†]	123 ± 208	84 (60, 117)	61 ± 50	46 (24, 85)	<0.001	88 ± 34	84 (63, 107)	60 ± 46	46 (26, 89)	<0.001
MetS components										
High blood pressure										
Systolic blood pressure (mmHg)	137.0 ± 19.0	134.5 (124, 143)	141.0 ± 16.9	141 (129.7, 148.5)	0.038	135.9 ± 15.8	136 (125.8, 146.3)	138.4 ± 17.3	137.6 (126.7, 148.6)	0.280
Diastolic blood pressure (mmHg)	81.5 ± 9.4	81.5 (74.5, 88.5)	82.8 ± 9.5	83 (75.7, 89.5)	0.362	79.9 ± 9.0	80.5 (74.3, 86.3)	79.6 ± 9.8	79.7 (74.6, 85.3)	0.828
(%) [‡]		76.2		95.6	<0.001 [§]		69.1		88.0	<0.001 [§]
Hyperglycaemia (mg/dL)	98.3 ± 32.2	97 (71, 119)	119.9 ± 39.0	110 (100, 127)	<0.001	89.0 ± 8.0	89 (83, 94)	110.5 ± 23.4	104 (95, 120)	<0.001
(%) [‡]		27.0		81.4	<0.001 [§]		3.7		48.0	<0.001 [§]
Hypertriglyceridemia (mg/dL)	96.2 ± 9.2	95 (93, 100)	155.6 ± 77.1	133 (96, 198)	<0.001	84.5 ± 27.2	80 (64, 100)	135.3 ± 55.5	125 (91, 169.8)	<0.001
(%) [‡]		9.5		53.6	<0.001 [§]		11.0		51.6	<0.001 [§]
Low HDL-cholesterol (mg/dL)	51.5 ± 9.9	50 (45, 55)	41.2 ± 10.0	40 (35, 46)	<0.001	63.3 ± 11.9	63 (55.5, 71)	49.1 ± 10.7	48 (42, 54.5)	<0.001
(%) [‡]		11.1		53.0	<0.001 [§]		22.2		58.0	<0.001 [§]
Abdominal obesity (cm)	92.9 ± 10.1	94 (87.7, 99.2)	112.1 ± 10.3	111.1 (103.9, 120.5)	<0.001	79.9 ± 7.7	80 (75.4, 85.4)	104.6 ± 11.1	105.5 (97.0, 112.3)	<0.001
(%) [‡]		12.7		86.3	<0.001 [§]		11.1		96 0	<0.001 [§]

Abbreviations: BMI, body mass index; FA, fatty acids; FQI, fat quality index; IQR, interquartile range; MetS, Metabolic Syndrome; MET, metabolic equivalent of task; MUFAs, monounsaturated fatty acids; PUFAs, polyunsaturated fatty acids; SD, standard deviation; SFAs, saturated fatty acids. * Differences in means between participants without and with MetS were tested by unpaired Students' t-test. [†] Participants who did not respond to the physical activity questionnaires were excluded from the analysis (i.e., 25 men and 19 women). [‡] Percentage (%) of patients without and with MetS. [§] Differences between participants without and with MetS were tested by χ^2.

Table 2. Nutrient intake in participants "with Metabolic Syndrome" (n = 333) and "without Metabolic Syndrome" (n = 144) stratified by sex.

	Men					Women				
	Without MetS (n = 63)		With MetS (n = 183)		p-Value *	Without MetS (n = 81)		With MetS (n = 150)		p-Value *
	Mean ±SD	Median (IQR)	Mean ±SD	Median (IQR)		Mean ±SD	Median (IQR)	Mean ±SD	Median (IQR)	
Energy intake (kcal/day)	2872 ± 738	2858 (2315, 3282)	2641 ± 689	2561 (2153, 3071)	0.019	2366 ± 698	2323 (1881, 2697)	2071 ± 543	1952 (1713, 2448)	<0.001
Carbohydrate intake (% total E)	44.7 ± 6.2	44.7 (41.3, 48.3)	40.0 ± 6.8	40.7 (34.9, 45.2)	<0.001	44.6 ± 5.2	44.3 (40.7, 47.1)	41.0 ± 6.9	40.9 (36.4, 45.5)	<0.001
Protein intake (% total E)	15.9 ± 2.4	15.6 (14.3, 17.6)	16.3 ± 3.1	15.9 (14.3, 17.7)	0.599	16.9 ± 3.0	16.4 (14.9, 18.5)	18.0 ± 3.2	18.0 (15.7, 20.4)	0.010
Fat intake (% total E)	36.2 ± 6.1	35.6 (31.6, 40.2)	38.9 ± 7.0	38.6 (34.0, 44.0)	0.008	37.6 ± 5.7	37.8 (32.8, 41.3)	40.9 ± 7.6	40.7 (35.5, 46.1)	<0.001
PUFA (% total E)	7.6 ± 3.4	6.3 (5.3, 9.1)	7.5 ± 3.0	6.7 (5.5, 8.8)	0.673	8.0 ± 3.6	6.6 (5.8, 8.9)	8.1 ± 4.1	6.7 (5.6, 9.2)	0.941
MUFA (% total E)	17.5 ± 4.3	16.8 (14.5, 19.7)	19.3 ± 5.0	18.8 (15.9, 22.2)	0.007	18.9 ± 4.4	18.3 (15.5, 21.1)	21.1 ± 5.9	20.3 (17.1, 24.6)	0.003
SFA (% total E)	11.7 ± 3.5	10.9 (9.6, 12.9)	12.0 ± 3.3	11.4 (9.6, 13.3)	0.517	12.5 ± 3.6	11.6 (9.9, 14.4)	12.5 ± 4.0	11.6 (10.1, 13.8)	0.975
Trans FA (g/d)	8.1 ± 8.9	4.7 (2.9, 7.2)	6.8 ± 7.5	3.8 (2.3, 6.5)	0.123	7.8 ± 8.5	4.9 (2.8, 10.3)	6.4 ± 8.5	3.0 (1.5, 5.4)	0.005
Linoleic acid (g/d)	16.2 ± 10.5	12.5 (8.8, 21.2)	14.5 ± 8.9	11.2 (8.5, 18.8)	0.298	14.7 ± 9.8	11.7 (8.7, 16.8)	12.9 ± 9.6	10.0 (6.5, 16.3)	0.034
ω-3 FA (g/d)	26.0 ± 36.0	9.2 (8.9, 18.9)	21.2 ± 29.8	9.2 (1.2, 18.2)	0.135	26.5 ± 34.5	9.4 (8.7, 35.2)	21.8 ± 34.0	8.9 (1.0, 17.9)	0.003
Linolenic acid (g/d)	7.0 ± 9.0	2.8 (2.5, 5.5)	5.8 ± 7.5	2.8 (0.8, 5.1)	0.168	7.1 ± 8.6	3.1 (2.4, 9.2)	5.8 ± 8.5	2.6 (0.6, 4.9)	0.003
Marine ω-3 FA (g/d)	12.7 ± 18.0	4.4 (4.2, 9.1)	10.3 ± 14.9	4.3 (0.3, 8.9)	0.111	13.0 ± 17.3	4.5 (4.1, 17.4)	10.7 ± 17.0	4.2 (0.3, 8.8)	0.009
Non-marine ω-3 FA (g/d)	13.2 ± 18.0	4.9 (4.5, 10)	10.9 ± 14.9	4.9 (0.9, 9.4)	0.161	13.5 ± 17.3	5.1 (4.5, 17.9)	11.1 ± 17.0	4.6 (0.7, 9.2)	0.002
Animal fat (g/d)	49.8 ± 18.2	46.1 (38.5, 59.7)	48.3 ± 19.6	43.7 (34.8, 59.2)	0.307	41.5 ± 23.1	38.6 (27.3, 50.0)	36.0 ± 13.2	35.0 (26.2, 44.1)	0.091
Vegetable fat (g/d)	65.7 ± 23.4	62.3 (45.2, 85.4)	64.9 ± 22.8	62.8 (48.1, 79.9)	0.799	57.7 ± 19.9	56.1 (41.8, 69.2)	58.3 ± 23.9	56.6 (41.9, 70.4)	0.987
FQI score	1.9 ± 0.5	1.7 (1.6, 2.1)	2.0 ± 0.4	1.9 (1.7, 2.3)	0.048	1.8 ± 0.4	1.8 (1.6, 2.0)	2.1 ± 0.5	2.0 (1.7, 2.4)	<0.001
Cholesterol (mg/d)	362 ± 105	358 (289, 423)	348 ± 115	334 (274, 399)	0.146	303 ± 122	286 (243, 349)	288 ± 79	283 (250, 355)	0.819
Fiber intake (g/d)	42.2 ± 17.0	38.2 (28.2, 52.0)	32.9 ± 13.1	31.2 (22.6, 39.5)	<0.001	38.6 ± 16.7	34.0 (28.9, 45.3)	31.2 ± 14.9	27.3 (20.9, 36.2)	<0.001

Abbreviations: E, energy; FA, fatty acids; FQI, fat quality index; IQR, interquartile range; MetS, Metabolic Syndrome; MUFAs, monounsaturated fatty acids; PUFAs, polyunsaturated fatty acids; SD, standard deviation; SFAs, saturated fatty acids. * Difference in means between participants without and with MetS were tested by unpaired Students' t-test.

Table 3. Food consumption in participants "with Metabolic Syndrome" ($n = 333$) and "without Metabolic Syndrome" ($n = 144$) stratified by sex.

	Men						Women					
	Without MetS ($n = 63$)		With MetS ($n = 183$)		p-Value		Without MetS ($n = 81$)		With MetS ($n = 150$)		p-Value *	
	Mean ±SD	Median (IQR)	Mean ±SD	Median (IQR)			Mean ±SD	Median (IQR)	Mean ±SD	Median (IQR)		
Fruits (g/day)	487 ± 205	495 (344, 627)	402 ± 229	364 (220, 546)	0.002		576 ± 218	553 (419, 697)	394 ± 214	352 (242, 499)	<0.001	
Vegetables (g/day)	346 ± 147	341 (232, 426)	311 ± 157	284 (192, 415)	0.075		357 ± 151	334 (258, 431)	343 ± 159	327 (242, 420)	0.407	
Potatoes (g/day)	96.7 ± 45.8	95.7 (57.1, 149.8)	70.2 ± 45.2	56.0 (31.4, 97.4)	<0.001		77.6 ± 45.0	85.7 (38.6, 107.1)	67.3 ± 57.9	49.5 (28.0, 94.1)	0.013	
Legumes (g/day)	20.5 ± 14.7	16.6 (12.0, 25.1)	18.9 ± 12.9	16.1 (12.1, 24.8)	0.901		18.0 ± 12.2	16.0 (12.0, 21.1)	17.8 ± 12.3	16.1 (12.0, 21.6)	0.582	
Olives and EVOO (g/day)	34.7 ± 34.0	28.3 (10.0, 46.4)	39.3 ± 28.2	32.0 (21.0, 50.0)	0.070		24.7 ± 16.5	25.0 (12.4, 32.1)	29.8 ± 24.0	28.3 (10.9, 46.0)	0.289	
Other olives oils	14.3 ± 16.7	10.0 (0.0, 25.0)	13.0 ± 16.4	4.2 (0.0, 25.0)	0.563		15.9 ± 15.4	10.0 (0.0, 25.0)	15.1 ± 14.8	10.0 (0.0, 25.0)	0.724	
Other oils and fats	4.4 ± 9.2	1.3 (0.0, 4.3)	4.9 ± 8.9	0.8 (0.0, 5.0)	0.856		4.7 ± 6.8	2.1 (0.7, 5.8)	3.9 ± 6.6	0.8 (0.0, 5.0)	0.112	
Nuts (g/day)	15.8 ± 17.3	8.6 (4.0, 25.7)	13.3 ± 13.3	8.4 (4.0, 21.0)	0.594		14.7 ± 13.6	8.6 (4.3, 25.7)	11.7 ± 13.5	7.2 (2.0, 16.7)	0.023	
Totalfish (g/day)	96.3 ± 36.2	88.1 (68.1, 120.5)	87.7 ± 45.2	80.3 (56.6, 111.3)	0.049		87.4 ± 37.5	80.7 (60.3, 107.4)	88.1 ± 42.2	80.7 (56.6, 115.1)	0.925	
White fish	25.4 ± 19.7	21 (10, 21)	26.3 ± 22.4	21.0 (10.1, 21.4)	0.620		28.0 ± 21.6	21.4 (10.0, 42.9)	28.3 ± 22.9	21.0 (10.1, 63.0)	0.362	
Bluefish	21.9 ± 19.9	18.6 (8.7, 18.6)	17.2 ± 16.8	8.7 (8.7, 18.2)	0.121		18.1 ± 17.0	18.6 (8.7, 18.6)	20.2 ± 18.7	18.2 (8.7, 18.6)	0.769	
Seafood	35.6 ± 14.6	30.7 (26.7, 45.9)	31.1 ± 23.7	30.8 (17.4, 35.2)	0.096		31.6 ± 17.8	30.7 (26.7, 33.0)	28.9 ± 22.3	30.7 (13.4, 31.9)	0.985	
Canned fish/seafood	11.7 ± 10.5	7.1 (3.3, 21.4)	11.0 ± 9.6	7.0 (3.4, 21.0)	0.215		8.3 ± 7.4	6.7 (3.3, 12.4)	9.4 ± 8.5	7.0 (3.4, 13.0)	0.115	
Total cereal (g/day)	229.3 ± 131.7	222.8 (131.4, 251.6)	159 ± 89	135.9 (91.8, 217.7)	<0.001		149 ± 82	126 (95, 222)	122.8 ± 69.8	102.4 (79.7, 164.3)	0.004	
Whole grain bread	105.2 ± 122.3	75.0 (5.0, 187.5)	61.4 ± 73.8	31.5 (5.0, 75.0)	0.012		66.7 ± 60.0	75.0 (32.1, 75.0)	57.1 ± 63.5	31.5 (5.0, 75.0)	0.019	
Refined grain bread	85.3 ± 108.0	32.1 (5.0, 187.5)	66.6 ± 83.1	31.5 (5.0, 75.0)	0.329		47.2 ± 71.1	10.7 (0.0, 75.0)	39.3 ± 53.6	21.0 (0.0, 75.0)	0.895	
Rice and pasta	34.5 ± 14.7	34.3 (17.1, 51.4)	27.6 ± 18.2	25.2 (12.4, 34.3)	<0.001		28.7 ± 17.5	17.1 (17.1, 34.3)	23.1 ± 15.1	17.0 (12.4, 33.6)	0.001	
Total dairy products (g/day)	295 ± 168	289 (215, 342)	303 ± 216	269 (181, 363)	0.612		312 ± 214	282 (150, 394)	264 ± 164	246 (148, 342)	0.131	
Dairy esserts	31.9 ± 34.6	15.3 (6.7, 51.2)	33.6 ± 47.2	15.3 (6.7, 43.0)	0.930		19.9 ± 27.9	8.7 (6.7, 24.1)	18.4 ± 27.9	6.7 (0.0, 23.4)	0.814	
Cheese	32.9 ± 26.9	24.8 (21.4, 44.5)	32.1 ± 31.2	24.4 (14.0, 42.9)	0.395		33.1 ± 23.2	28.1 (19.6, 48.0)	29.3 ± 22.3	24.4 (10.4, 42.0)	0.179	
Skimmed dairy	84.8 ± 137.6	8.3 (0.0, 125.0)	115 ± 202	52.5 (0.0, 156.0)	0.215		141.6 ± 194.8	53.6 (0.0, 209.5)	114.4 ± 136.5	52.5 (0.0, 200.0)	0.529	
Whole-fat dairy	144.1 ± 141.3	125.0 (8.3, 208.3)	120 ± 141	84.0 (0.0, 200.0)	0.090		112.5 ± 158.6	17.9 (0.0, 200.0)	100 ± 140	17.5 (0.0, 200.0)	0.765	
Total meat (g/day)	152.0 ± 61.1	137 (112, 202)	166.2 ± 71.7	154 (117, 204)	0.247		130 ± 61.7	118 (93, 165)	140 ± 56.6	139 (104, 172)	0.076	
Processed meat	40.7 ± 27.0	34.0 (27.0, 52.0)	46.9 ± 34.7	39.1 (21.0, 62.0)	0.433		31.4 ± 21.4	30.0 (18.2, 39.5)	34.0 ± 28.3	28.7 (16.7, 42.7)	0.869	
Other meats,	108.4 ± 48.8	104.3 (71.4, 135.7)	116 ± 57	107 (76, 149)	0.500		97.2 ± 51.6	87.6 (64.8, 122.9)	103.8± 46.3	103.7 (74.9, 135.8)	0.172	
Bakery godos (g/day)	60.4 ± 44.5	51.2 (26.7, 72.4)	52.1 ± 45.0	44.5 (20.6, 66.7)	0.101		51.0 ± 30.2	46.5 (26.5, 74.2)	37.2 ± 30.6	31.0 (10.4, 53.7)	<0.001	
Ready-to-eat-meals	35.0 ±34.2	26.2 (13.6, 37.6)	27.8 ± 40.3	15.4 (9.4, 30.0)	0.003		19.9 ± 18.7	15.3 (4.3, 26.2)	20.5 ± 23.3	15.4 (2.0, 26.4)	0.357	
Alcohol (g/day)	230 ± 183	198 (82, 337)	291 ± 322	200 (76, 367)	0.753		109 ± 128	47.1 (0.0, 170)	70 ± 101	28.8 (0.0, 100.0)	0.032	

Abbreviations: EVOO, extra virgin olive oil; IQR, interquartile range; MetS, Metabolic Syndrome; SD, standard deviation. * Difference in means between participants without and with MetS were tested by unpaired Students' *t*-test.

Table 4. Percentage of participants "with Metabolic Syndrome" and "without Metabolic Syndrome" below, inside, and above Acceptable Macronutrient Distribution Range (AMDR) proposed by the Institute of Medicine.

Variable	AMDR	Group	% below	% inside	% above	p *
All						
Carbohydrate	45–65%	Without MetS	55.6	44.4	0.0	<0.001
		With MetS	72.7	27.3	0.0	
Protein	10–35%	Without MetS	0.0	100.0	0.0	0.510
		With MetS	0.3	99.7	0.0	
Total fat	20–35%	Without MetS	0.0	39.6	60.4	0.001
		With MetS	0.0	24.9	75.1	
MUFAs	>20%	Without MetS	72.2	-	27.8	0.001
		With MetS	55.6	-	44.4	
LA	5–10%	Without MetS	66.7	20.1	13.2	0.159
		With MetS	64.9	26.4	8.7	
ALA	0.6–1.2%	Without MetS	21.5	29.2	49.3	0.005
		With MetS	36.3	21.0	42.6	
Men						
Carbohydrate	45–65%	Without MetS	52.4	47.6	0.0	0.003
		With MetS	72.7	27.3	0.0	
Protein	10–35%	Without MetS	0.0	100.0	0.0	0.557
		With MetS	0.5	99.5	0.0	
Total fat	20–35%	Without MetS	0.0	46.0	54.0	0.008
		With MetS	0.0	27.9	72.1	
MUFAs	>20%	Without MetS	77.8	-	22.2	0.025
		With MetS	62.3	-	37.7	
LA	5–10%	Without MetS	65.1	22.2	12.7	0.276
		With MetS	66.7	26.8	6.6	
ALA	0.6–1.2%	Without MetS	22.2	38.1	39.7	0.119
		With MetS	35.0	27.3	37.7	
Women						
Carbohydrate	45–65%	Without MetS	58.0	42.0	0.0	0.023
		With MetS	72.7	27.3	0.0	
Protein	10–35%	Without MetS	0.0	100.0	0.0	1.000
		With MetS	0.0	100.0	0.0	
Total fat	20–35%	Without MetS	0.0	34.6	65.4	0.029
		With MetS	0.0	21.3	78.7	
MUFAs	>20%	Without MetS	67.9	-	32.1	0.003
		With MetS	47.3	-	52.7	
LA	5–10%	Without MetS	67.9	18.5	13.6	0.427
		With MetS	62.7	26.0	11.3	
ALA	0.6–1.2%	Without MetS	21.0	22.2	56.8	0.019
		With Met	38.0	13.3	48.7	

Abbreviations: ALA, α-linolenic acid; LA, linoleic acid; MetS, metabolic syndrome; MUFAs, monounsaturated fatty acids. * The differences in prevalence across the two comparison groups was examined using χ^2.

Table 5. Percentage of participants "with Metabolic Syndrome" and "without Metabolic Syndrome" below, inside, and above the 2020 Nutritional Objectives for the Spanish Population proposed by the Spanish Society of Community Nutrition.

Variable	Nutritional Objectives	Group	% Below	% Inside	% Above	p *
Carbohydrate	50–55%	Without MetS	83.3	12.5	4.2	0.004
		With MetS	93.1	5.7	1.2	
Protein	10–20%	Without MetS	0.0	100.0	0.0	1.000
		With MetS	0.0	100.0	0.0	
Total fat	30–35%	Without MetS	9.7	29.9	60.4	0.001
		With MetS	9.3	15.6	75.1	
MUFAs	20%	Without MetS	72.2	-	27.8	0.001
		With MetS	55.6	-	44.4	
PUFAs	5%	Without MetS	14.6	-	85.4	0.774
		With MetS	15.6	-	84.4	
LA	3%	Without MetS	18.1	-	81.9	0.217
		With MetS	23.1	-	76.9	
ALA	1–2%	Without MetS	42.4	30.6	27.1	0.417
		With MetS	48.6	28.5	22.8	
SFA	7–8%	Without MetS	2.8	3.5	93.8	0.952
		With MetS	3.3	3.6	93.1	
Trans FA	<1%	Without MetS	21.5	-	78.5	0.001
		With MetS	36.6	-	63.4	
DHA	300 mg	Without MetS	100.0	-	0.0	1.000
		With MetS	100.0	-	0.0	
Total fiber	M: 35 g/d F: 25 g/d	Without MetS	27.8	-	72.2	<0.001
		With MetS	52.0	-	48.0	
Cholesterol	<300 mg/d	Without MetS	41.0	-	59.0	0.123
		With MetS	48.6	-	51.4	
Fruits	>300 g/d	Without MetS	11.1	-	88.9	<0.001
		With MetS	35.4	-	64.6	
Vegetables	>250g/d	Without MetS	24.3	-	75.7	0.032
		With MetS	34.2	-	65.8	
Sugar foods	<6%	Without MetS	0.7	-	99.3	0.905
		With MetS	0.6	-	99.4	

Abbreviations: ALA, α-linolenic acid; DHA, docosahexaenoic acid; FA, fatty acid; LA, linoleic acid; MetS, metabolic syndrome; MUFA, monounsaturated fatty acids; PUFAs, polyunsaturated fatty acids; SFAs, saturated fatty acids. * Differences in prevalence between groups were assessed by χ^2.

4. Discussion

Subjects with MetS and without MetS showed differences for energy and macronutrient intake, as well as for intake of specific fat subtypes.

Energy and nutrient intake in MetS subjects revealed a diet lower in calories and carbohydrates, but higher in total fat and MUFA than those without MetS. Carbohydrate intake of MetS subjects was below the recommended limits (45–65% of total energy intake) and total fat intake of the same subjects was above the recommended limits (20–35% of total energy intake). Women with MetS showed more energy intake from protein than those without MetS (18% vs. 16.9%, respectively) ($p < 0.01$), but both were within recommended ranges [26,27]. A similar nutrient distribution among Spanish population with MetS [32] and healthy adults has been previously shown [8]. Differences were also previously observed between subjects with and without MetS for total energy intake, sugar intake, dietary glycemic load, percentage of dietary protein, PUFA, and fiber intake [33].

Despite women with MetS reporting lower consumption of bakery goods than those without MetS, differences in sugary food intake (bakery goods, dairy desserts, beverages, fruit juices, breakfast cereals, marmalade, ice creams, chocolate, and ready-to-eat meals) between subjects with and without MetS were not found in our study when the 2020 Nutritional Objectives for the Spanish population were assessed. Total sugar intake was also quantified in the ANIBES study: results were higher in children (17.18%) and adolescents (16.33%) and markedly lower in adults (15.34%) and older adults (12.97%) [8]. The inhabitants of Northern Spain, especially men, consumed more sugar and sweets than adult from other Spanish areas [32]. Conversely, the World Health Organization (WHO) recommended <10% of energy intake be provided by sugars [34], whereas <5% has been recommended in the United Kingdom [35]. It is well known that simple sugar intake is associated with significantly higher risk of developing MetS, including increased blood pressure, central obesity, and serum TG and glucose levels [36–38]. Frequent consumption of sugar-containing foods can also increase the risk of dental caries [39].

This study also demonstrated an association of gender and fat intake for MetS risk. Women showed an inverse association between fat intake and MetS, irrespective of fatty acid type. Women consumed less ω-3 and ω-6 FA, which could be related to the lower consumption of nuts observed in this group. Previously, Bibiloni et al. [40] showed that nut consumers were less likely to be below the estimated average requirement (EAR) for some nutrients and above the adequate intake (AI) for others than non-nut consumers. Other studies showed that European Food Safety Authority (EFSA) recommendations for intake of different types of ω-3 and ω-6 FA, such as LA, ALA, and eicosapentaenoic acid (EPA) + DHA, were not met in around half, one-quarter, and three-quarters of the European countries, respectively [41]. The most recent reviews also concluded that in half of the countries worldwide, the reported average PUFA intake was lower than the recommended range of 6–11% of energy [42–44]. In addition, the ω-3 and ω-6 FA intake was inversely associated with MetS prevalence in females [45]. In our study, total PUFA and specific types of PUFA (LA or ALA) intake were inversely associated with high blood pressure and positively associated with abdominal obesity. Evidence from observational and intervention studies supports the benefits of both ω-3 and ω-6 PUFA in reducing MetS [37,46–49], although other studies showed conflicting results [49–51]. Particularly, the adequate intake of MUFA and PUFAs in the PREvención con DIeta MEDiterránea (PREDIMED) study, mainly due to a high consumption of nuts and olive oil, has been previously associated with better adherence to the Mediterranean diet (MedDiet) [40] and to lower risk of CVD [52]. Moreover, other dietary patterns (Dietary Approaches to Stop Hypertension (DASH), new Nordic and vegetarian diets) have also been proposed as alternatives to the MedDiet for preventing MetS [5].

It is also worth noting that no differences were observed between subjects with and without MetS for SFA and animal fat, although participants without MetS showed higher consumption of bakery goods than those with MetS. Moreover, an association between pathological features of MetS and dietary macronutrient intake showed that hypertensionwas inversely associated with SFA. Contrarily to our results, a positive association between SFA intake and MetS components has been observed in most studies [46,50,53–56], although other studies pointed to a lack of association [49,57]. On the other hand, increased vegetable fat intake was positively associated with abdominal obesity; certain vegetable products may also have high saturated fat contents, such as coconut oil and palm kernel oil, along with many prepared foods [10,58]. Moreover, most of the countries reported an average higher SFA intake than the recommended maximum of 10% of energy [42–44]. A prospective study with an older adult population at high risk of cardiovascular disease also observed an average higher SFA intake (10.3%) [59]. However, there is evidence that the intake of these fats is lower in the adults and older adults in the Mediterranean population, who consume low amounts of processed food; olive oil and meat ranked as the primary individual contributors [8].

Moreover, our findings show that women with MetS consumed more energy from TFA than those without MetS (6.4% versus 7.8%, respectively) ($p < 0.005$). Accordingly, TFA intake was inversely associated with hypertension. In a previous study, plasma TFA concentrations were significantly associated with MetS prevalence and its individual components, except for blood pressure [60]. In another study, the reduction in TFA intake over 1 year was significantly associated with a reduction in low-density lipoprotein particle number (LDL-P), a novel marker of CVD risk [61]. Actually, the 2015–2020 U.S. Dietary Guidelines for Americans and the IOM both recommend that individuals should limit TFA intake as much as possible to avoid their adverse effects on health [62].

Otherwise, the current findings showed that participants with MetS consumed less dietary fiber than the recommended dietary allowances (35 g for males and 25 g for females of this age group), which may be linked to low consumption of fruits and vegetables in our population study. This outcome is according to the outcomes of a previous meta-analysis that provided a potential link between dietary fiber consumption and MetS risk factors [63]. Previous studies also showed a protective effect of fruit intake on MetS development [17,64–66], as well as a protective role on CVD development [67].

Finally, our results also show higher BMI and lower total physical activity in participants with MetS ($p < 0.001$), which is in agreement with a previous study that also showed higher level of physical activity in the control group compared to the MetS group, although this difference disappeared when the subjects were separated by sex and adjusted for total energy intake [16]. Another previous study showed that participants with lower levels of physical activity, being overweight and obese, were associated with higher risk of CVD. Accordingly, the impact of physical activity on CVD might outweigh that of BMI among middle-aged and elderly participants [68]. There is evidence that interventions including regular physical activity practice in patients with MetS improves MetS risk factors [69–75], indicating that maintaining a good physical condition would be essential for a healthy status.

Strengths and Limitations of the Study

This study has several strengths. First, to our knowledge our study provides data on the intake of macronutrients and different types of fat in older adults with MetS or without it, which has been scarcely reported previously. Our research also provides information about dietary fat intake in comparison to national and international recommendations, which may provide references for future public policies.

Some methodological limitations should be acknowledged. First, the cross-sectional study nature; thus, causal inferences cannot be drawn. Second, the relatively small sample size, specifically in the non-MetS group; for this reason, these findings cannot be generalized to the broader community based on this study alone. Third, the FFQ, the source of information to assess dietary fat intake, could overestimate the intake of certain food groups, even those that have been validated. In our study, a trained dietician conducted the interviews to collect the food frequency data; it is hoped that this approach (as compared with self-administration) reduced any potential misclassification bias. Another limitation of this study was that the used food composition databases showed missing or uncalculated data for several fats and fatty acid contents; these missing data are lower than 5% of all analyzed foods (for total fat, SFA, MUFA, PUFA, and cholesterol contents) and lower than 10% of foods (LA, ALA, trans-fat, EPA, DHA, and DPA are mainly from marine species and may change according to season, source, such as wild or from a fish farm, and cooking method) [76].

5. Conclusions

Subjects with MetS were less likely to meet IOM and SENC recommendations for fat and macronutrient intake as compared to non-MetS subjects. A healthy lifestyle is critical to prevent or delay the onset of MetS in older adults and to prevent CVD in those with existing MetS. Thus, healthy diet and lifestyle patternscan be recommended for all people with MetS and should emphasize the consumption of a variety of legumes, cereals (whole grains), fruits, vegetables, fish, and nuts, which have a high nutrient content and are more likely to meet dietary recommendations. This study also raises the possibility that future recommendations and educational campaigns should be most effective in preventing MetS via lifestyle changes.

Author Contributions: M.d.M.B. and J.A.T. designed the study and wrote the protocol. A.J., D.M., and E.A. collected data, conducted literature searches, and provided summaries of previous research studies. M.D.M.B. conducted the statistical analysis. M.D.M.B., A.J., and J.A.T. wrote the first draft of the manuscript. All read and approved the final manuscript.

Acknowledgments: This study was supported by the official funding agency for biomedical research of the Spanish Government, Institute of Health Carlos III (ISCIII) through the Fondo de Investigación para la Salud (FIS), which is co-funded by the European Regional Development Fund (Projects 11/01791, 14/00636, and 17/01827, Red Predimed-RETIC RD06/0045/1004, and CIBEROBN CB12/03/30038), Fundació La Marató TV3 (Spain) project ref. 201630.10, Grant of support to research groups no. 35/2011 and Grant no. AAEE097/2017 (Balearic Islands Gov.), and E.U. Cost ACTION CA16112. The funders had no role in study design, data collection and analysis, decision to publish, or preparation of the manuscript.

Conflicts of Interest: The authors declare that they have no conflict of interest.

References

1. Grundy, S.M.; Hansen, B.; Smith, S.C., Jr.; Cleeman, J.I.; Kahn, R.A.; American Heart Association; National Heart, Lung, and Blood Institute; American Diabetes Association. Clinical management of metabolic syndrome: Report of the American Heart Association/National Heart, Lung, and Blood Institute/American Diabetes Association conference on scientific issues related to management. *Circulation* **2004**, *109*, 551–556. [CrossRef] [PubMed]
2. Alberti, K.G.; Eckel, R.H.; Grundy, S.M.; Zimmet, P.Z.; Cleeman, J.I.; Donato, K.A.; Fruchart, J.C.; James, W.P.; Loria, C.M.; Smith, S.C., Jr.; et al. Harmonizing the metabolic syndrome: A joint interim statement of the International Diabetes Federation Task Force on Epidemiology and Prevention. *Circulation* **2009**, *120*, 1640–1645. [CrossRef] [PubMed]
3. O'Neill, S.; O'Driscoll, L. Metabolic syndrome: A closer look at the growing epidemic and its associated pathologies. *Obes Rev.* **2015**, *16*, 1–12. [CrossRef] [PubMed]
4. Beltran-Sanchez, H.; Harhay, M.O.; Harhay, M.M.; McElligott, S. Prevalence and trends of metabolic syndrome in the adult U.S. population, 1999–2010. *J. Am. Coll. E703Cardiol.* **2013**, *62*, 697–703. [CrossRef] [PubMed]
5. Pérez-Martínez, P.; Mikhailidis, D.P.; Athyros, V.G.; Bullo, M.; Couture, P.; Covas, M.I.; de Koning, L.; Delgado-Lista, J.; Díaz-López, A.; Drevon, C.A.; et al. Lifestyle recommendations for the prevention and management of metabolic syndrome: An international panel recommendation. *Nutr. Rev.* **2017**, *75*, 307–326. [CrossRef] [PubMed]
6. De Carvalho-Vidigal, F.; Bressan, J.; Babio, N.; Salas-Salvadó, J. Prevalence of metabolic syndrome in Brazilian adults: A systematic review. *BMC Public Health* **2013**, *13*, 1198. [CrossRef] [PubMed]
7. Godos, J.; Zappalà, G.; Bernardini, S.; Giambini, I.; Bes-Rastrollo, M.; Martinez-Gonzalez, M. Adherence to the Mediterranean diet is inversely associated with metabolic syndrome occurrence: A meta-analysis of observational studies. *Int. J. Food Sci. Nutr.* **2017**, *68*, 138–148. [CrossRef]
8. Ruiz, E.; Ávila, J.M.; Valero, T.; Del Pozo, S.; Rodriguez, P.; Aranceta-Bartrina, J.; Gil, Á.; González-Gross, M.; Ortega, R.M.; Serra-Majem, L.; et al. Macronutrient Distribution and Dietary Sources in the Spanish Population: Findings from the ANIBES Study. *Nutrients* **2016**, *8*, 177. [CrossRef]

9. Cano-Ibáñez, N.; Gea, A.; Martínez-González, M.A.; Salas-Salvadó, J.; Corella, D.; Zomeño, M.D.; Romaguera, D.; Vioque, J.; Aros, F.; Wärnberg, J.; et al. Dietary Diversity and Nutritional Adequacy among an Older Spanish Population with Metabolic Syndrome in the PREDIMED-PlusStudy: A Cross-Sectional Analysis. *Nutrients* **2019**, *11*, 958. [CrossRef]
10. U.S. Department of Health and Human Services; U.S. Department of Agriculture. *2015–2020 Dietary Guidelines for Americans*, 8th ed.; Government Printing Office: Washington, DC, USA, 2015.
11. McKeown, N.M.; Meigs, J.B.; Liu, S.; Saltzman, E.; Wilson, P.W.; Jacques, P.F. Carbohydrate Nutrition, Insulin Resistance, and the Prevalence of the Metabolic Syndrome in the Framingham Offspring Cohort. *Diabetes Care* **2004**, *27*, 538–546. [CrossRef]
12. Freire, R.D.; Cardoso, M.A.; Gimeno, S.G.; Ferreira, S.R. for the Japanese-Brazilian Diabetes Study Group Dietary Fat Is Associated With Metabolic Syndrome in Japanese Brazilians. *Diabetes Care* **2005**, *28*, 1779–1785. [CrossRef] [PubMed]
13. Bruscato, N.M.; Vieira, J.L.D.C.; Nascimento, N.M.R.D.; Canto, M.E.P.; Stobbe, J.C.; Gottlieb, M.G.; Wagner, M.B.; Dalacorte, R.R. Dietary intake is not associated to the metabolic syndrome in elderly women. *North. Am. J. Med. Sci.* **2010**, *2*, 182–188.
14. Guo, X.F.; Li, X.; Shi, M.; Li, D. n-3 Polyunsaturated Fatty Acids and Metabolic Syndrome Risk: A Meta-Analysis. *Nutr.* **2017**, *9*, 703. [CrossRef] [PubMed]
15. da Cunha, A.T.; Pereira, H.T.; de Aquino, S.L.; Sales, C.H.; Sena-Evangelista, K.C.; Lima, J.G.; Lima, S.C.; Pedrosa, L.F. Inadequacies in the habitual nutrient intakes of patients with metabolic syndrome: A cross-sectional study. *Diabetol. Metab. Syndr.* **2016**, *8*, 32. [CrossRef] [PubMed]
16. Al-Daghri, N.M.; Khan, N.; Alkharfy, K.M.; Al-Attas, O.S.; Alokail, M.S.; Alfawaz, H.A.; Alothman, A.; Vanhoutte, P.M. Selected Dietary Nutrients and the Prevalence of Metabolic Syndrome in Adult Males and Females in Saudi Arabia: A Pilot Study. *Nutrients* **2013**, *5*, 4587–4604. [CrossRef] [PubMed]
17. de Oliveira, E.P.; McLellan, K.C.; Vaz de Arruda Silveira, L.; Burini, R.C. Dietary factors associated with metabolic syndrome in Brazilian adults. *Nutr. J.* **2012**, *11*, 3. [CrossRef] [PubMed]
18. Zhao, M.; Chiriboga, D.; Olendzki, B.; Xie, B.; Li, Y.; McGonigal, L.J.; Maldonado-Contreras, A.; Ma, Y. Substantial Increase in Compliance with Saturated Fatty Acid Intake Recommendations after One Year Following the American Heart Association Diet. *Nutrients* **2018**, *10*, 1486. [CrossRef] [PubMed]
19. Zhang, L.; Pagoto, S.; May, C.; Olendzki, B.; Tucker, L.K.; Ruiz, C.; Cao, Y.; Ma, Y. Effect of AHA dietary counselling on added sugar intake among participants with metabolic syndrome. *Eur. J. Nutr.* **2018**, *57*, 1073–1082. [CrossRef] [PubMed]
20. Rodríguez-Monforte, M.; Sánchez, E.; Barrio, F.; Costa, B.; Flores-Mateo, G. Metabolic syndrome and dietary patterns: A systematic review and meta-analysis of observational studies. *Eur. J. Nutr.* **2017**, *56*, 925–947. [CrossRef]
21. Amor, A.J.; Masana, L.; Soriguer, F.; Goday, A.; Calle-Pascual, A.; Gaztambide, S.; Rojo-Martínez, G.; Valdés, S.; Gomis, R.; Ortega, E.; et al. Estimating Cardiovascular Risk in Spain by the European Guidelines on Cardiovascular Disease Prevention in Clinical Practice. *Rev. Esp. Cardiol. (Engl. Ed)*. **2015**, *68*, 417–425. [CrossRef]
22. Fernandez-Ballart, J.D.; Piñol, J.L.; Zazpe, I.; Corella, D.; Carrasco, P.; Toledo, E.; Perez-Bauer, M.; Martínez-González, M.Á.; Salas-Salvadó, J.; Martín-Moreno, J.M. Relative validity of a semi-quantitative food-frequency questionnaire in an elderly Mediterranean population of Spain. *Br. J. Nutr.* **2010**, *103*, 1808–1816. [CrossRef]
23. Moreiras, O.; Carbajal, A.; Cabrera, L.; Cuadrado, C. *Tablas de Composición de Alimentos*, 17th ed.; Food Composition Tables; Piramide: Madrid, Spain, 2015.
24. BEDCA: Base de Datos Española de Composición de Alimentos. Available online: http://www.bedca.net/ (accessed on 10 February 2019).
25. Sánchez-Tainta, A.; Zazpe, I.; Bes-Rastrollo, M.; Salas-Salvadó, J.; Bullo, M.; Sorlí, J.V.; Corella, D.; Covas, M.I.; Arós, F.; Gutierrez-Bedmar, M. Nutritional adequacy according to carbohydrates and fat quality. *Eur. J. Nutr.* **2016**, *55*, 93–106. [CrossRef] [PubMed]
26. The National Academies of Sciences Engineering Medicine; Institute of Medicine; Food and Nutrition Board. Dietary Reference Intakes (DRIs): Acceptable Macronutrient Distribution Ranges. Available online: http://nationalacademies.org/HMD/Activities/Nutrition/SummaryDRIs/DRI-Tables.aspx (accessed on 11 April 2019).

27. SENC. Objetivosnutricionales para la población española. Consenso de la Sociedad Española de NutriciónComunitaria 2011. *Rev. Esp. Nutr. Com.* **2011**, *17*, 178–199.
28. Elosua, R.; García, M.; Aguilar, A.; Molina, L.; Covas, M.I.; Marrugat, J. Validation of the Minnesota Leisure Time Physical Activity Questionnaire in Spanish Women. *Med. Sci. Sports Exerc.* **2000**, *32*, 1431–1437. [CrossRef]
29. Elosua, R.; Marrugat, J.; Molina, L.; Pons, S.; Pujol, E. Validation of the Minnesota Leisure Time Physical Activity Questionnaire in Spanish Men. *Am. J. Epidemiol.* **1994**, *139*, 1197–1209. [CrossRef] [PubMed]
30. Conway, J.M.; Seale, J.L.; Jacobs, D.R.; Irwin, M.L.; Ainsworth, B.E. Comparison of energy expenditure estimates from doubly labeled water, a physical activity questionnaire, and physical activity records1–3. *Am. J. Clin. Nutr.* **2002**, *75*, 519–525. [CrossRef]
31. Ainsworth, B.E.; Haskell, W.L.; Whitt, M.C.; Irwin, M.L.; Swartz, A.M.; Strath, S.J.; O'brien, W.L.; Bassett, D.R.; Schmitz, K.H.; Emplaincourt, P.O.; et al. Compendium of Physical Activities: An update of activity codes and MET intensities. *Med. Sci. Sports Exerc.* **2000**, *32*, S498–S516. [CrossRef] [PubMed]
32. Cano-Ibáñez, N.; Bueno-Cavanillas, A.; Martínez-González, M.A.; Corella, D.; Salas-Salvadó, J.; Zomeño, M.D.; García-de-la-Hera, M.; Romaguera, D.; Martínez, J.A.; Barón-López, F.J.; et al. Dietary Intake in Population with Metabolic Syndrome: Is the Prevalence of Inadequate Intake Influenced by Geographical Area? Cross-Sectional Analysis from PREDIMED-Plus Study. *Nutrients* **2018**, *10*, 1661. [CrossRef]
33. Cabello-Saavedra, E.; Bes-Rastrollo, M.; Martínez, J.A.; Díez-Espino, J.; Buil-Cosiales, P.; Serrano-Martínez, M.; Martinez-Gonzalez, M.A. Macronutrient Intake and Metabolic Syndrome in Subjects at High Cardiovascular Risk. *Ann. Nutr. Metab.* **2010**, *56*, 152–159. [CrossRef]
34. WHO. Sugars Intake for Adults and Children-Guideline. 2015. Available online: http://www.who.int/nutrition/publications/guidelines/sugars_intake/en/ (accessed on 31 May 2019).
35. Tedstone, A.; Targett, V.; Allen, R. Public Health England-Sugar Reduction. The Evidence for Action. Available online: https://www.gov.uk/government/publications/sugar-reduction-from-evidence-into-action (accessed on 31 May 2019).
36. Barrio-Lopez, M.T.; Martinez-Gonzalez, M.A.; Fernández-Montero, A.; Beunza, J.J.; Zazpe, I.; Bes-Rastrollo, M. Prospective study of changes in sugar-sweetened beverage consumption and the incidence of the metabolic syndrome and its components: The SUN cohort. *Br. J. Nutr.* **2013**, *110*, 1722–1731. [CrossRef]
37. Chan, T.F.; Lin, W.T.; Huang, H.L.; Lee, C.Y.; Wu, P.W.; Chiu, Y.W.; Huang, C.C.; Tsai, S.; Lin, C.L.; Lee, C.H. Consumption of sugar-sweetened beverages is associated with components of the metabolic syndrome in adolescents. *Nutrients* **2014**, *6*, 2088–2103. [CrossRef] [PubMed]
38. Abdelmagid, S.A.; Clarke, S.E.; Roke, K.; Nielsen, D.E.; Badawi, A.; El-Sohemy, A.; Mutch, D.M.; Ma, D.W. Ethnicity, sex, FADS genetic variation, and hormonal contraceptive use influencedelta-5- and delta-6-desaturaseindices and plasma docosahexaenoic acid concentration in young Canadian adults: A cross-sectional study. *Nutr. Metab. (Lond).* **2015**, *12*, 14. [CrossRef] [PubMed]
39. Burt, A.B.; Pai, S. Sugar consumption and caries risk: A systematic review. *J. Dent. Educ.* **2001**, *65*, 1017–1023. [PubMed]
40. Bibiloni, M.D.M.; Julibert, A.; Bouzas, C.; Martínez-González, M.A.; Corella, D.; Salas-Salvadó, J.; Zomeño, M.D.; Vioque, J.; Romaguera, D.; Martínez, J.A.; et al. Nut Consumptions as a Marker of Higher Diet Quality in a Mediterranean Population at High Cardiovascular Risk. *Nutrients* **2019**, *11*, 754. [CrossRef] [PubMed]
41. Sioen, I.; van Lieshout, L.; Eilander, A.; Fleith, M.; Lohner, S.; Szommer, A.; Petisca, C.; Eussen, S.; Forsyth, S.; Calder, P.C.; et al. Systematic Review on N-3 and N-6 Polyunsaturated Fatty Acid Intake in European Countries in Light of the Current Recommendations - Focus on Specific Population Groups. *Ann. Nutr. Metab.* **2017**, *70*, 39–50. [CrossRef] [PubMed]
42. Harika, R.K.; Eilander, A.; Alssema, M.; Osendarp, S.J.; Zock, P.L. Intake of Fatty Acids in General Populations Worldwide Does Not Meet Dietary Recommendations to Prevent Coronary Heart Disease: A Systematic Review of Data from 40 Countries. *Ann. Nutr. Metab.* **2013**, *63*, 229–238. [CrossRef] [PubMed]
43. Micha, R.; Khatibzadeh, S.; Shi, P.; Fahimi, S.; Lim, S.; Andrews, K.G.; Engell, R.E.; Powles, J.; Ezzati, M.; Mozaffarian, D.; et al. Global, regional, and national consumption levels of dietary fats and oils in 1990 and 2010: A systematic analysis including 266 country-specific nutrition surveys. *BMJ.* **2014**, *348*, g2272. [CrossRef] [PubMed]

44. Eilander, A.; Harika, R.K.; Zock, P.L. Intake and sources of dietary fatty acids in Europe: Are current population intakes of fats aligned with dietary recommendations? *Eur. J. Lipid Sci. Technol.* **2015**, *117*, 1370–1377. [CrossRef]
45. Park, S.; Ahn, J.; Kim, N.S.; Lee, B.K. High carbohydrate diets are positively associated with the risk of metabolic syndrome irrespective to fatty acid composition in women: The NHANES 2007–2014. *Int. J. Food Sci. Nutr.* **2017**, *68*, 479–487. [CrossRef] [PubMed]
46. Shab-Bidar, S.; Hosseini-Esfahani, F.; Mirmiran, P.; Hosseinpour-Niazi, S.; Azizi, F. Metabolic syndrome profiles, obesity measures and intake of dietary fatty acids in adults: Tehran Lipid and Glucose Study. *J. Hum. Nutr. Diet* **2014**, *27*, 98–108. [CrossRef]
47. Baik, I.; Abbott, R.D.; Curb, J.D.; Shin, C. Intake of Fish and n-3 Fatty Acids and Future Risk of Metabolic Syndrome. *J. Am. Diet. Assoc.* **2010**, *110*, 1018–1026. [CrossRef]
48. Babio, N.; Toledo, E.; Estruch, R.; Ros, E.; Martínez-González, M.A.; Castañer, O.; Bulló, M.; Corella, D.; Arós, F.; Gómez-Gracia, E.; et al. Mediterranean diets and metabolic syndrome status in the PREDIMED randomized trial. *CMAJ* **2014**, *186*, E649–E657. [CrossRef] [PubMed]
49. Ahola, A.J.; Harjutsalo, V.; Thorn, L.M.; Freese, R.; Forsblom, C.; Mäkimattila, S.; Groop, P.-H. The association between macronutrient intake and the metabolic syndrome and its components in type 1 diabetes. *Br. J. Nutr.* **2017**, *117*, 450–456. [CrossRef]
50. Ebbesson, S.O.E.; Tejero, M.E.; Nobmann, E.D.; Lopez-Alvarenga, J.C.; Ebbesson, L.; Romenesko, T.; Carter, E.A.; Resnick, H.E.; Devereux, R.B.; Maccluer, J.W.; et al. Fatty acid consumption and metabolic syndrome components: The GOCADAN study. *J. Cardio. Metab. Syndr.* **2007**, *2*, 244–249. [CrossRef]
51. Lana, L.Y.; Petrone, A.B.; Pankow, J.S.; Arnett, D.K.; North, K.E.; Ellison, R.C.; Hunt, S.C.; Djoussé, L. Association of dietary omega-3 fatty acids with prevalence of metabolic syndrome: The National Heart, Lung, and Blood Institute Family Heart Study. *Clin. Nutr.* **2013**, *32*, 966–969.
52. PREDIMED Study Investigators; Guasch-Ferré, M.; Babio, N.; Martínez-González, A.M.; Corella, D.; Ros, E.; Martín-Peláez, S.; Estruch, R.; Arós, F.; Gómez-Gracia, E.; et al. Dietary fat intake and risk of cardiovascular disease and all-cause mortality in a population at high risk of cardiovascular disease. *Am. J. Clin. Nutr.* **2015**, *102*, 1563–1573.
53. Hekmatdoost, A.; Mirmiran, P.; Hosseini-Esfahani, F.; Azizi, F. Dietary fatty acid composition and metabolic syndrome in Tehranian adults. *Nutrition* **2011**, *27*, 1002–1007. [CrossRef] [PubMed]
54. Hosseinpour-Niazi, S.; Mirmiran, P.; Fallah-Ghohroudi, A.; Azizi, F. Combined effect of unsaturated fatty acids and saturated fatty acids on the metabolic syndrome: Tehran lipid and glucose study. *J. Health Popul. Nutr.* **2015**, *33*. [CrossRef]
55. Noel, S.E.; Newby, P.K.; Ordovas, J.M.; Tucker, K.L. Adherence to an (n-3) fatty acid/fish intake pattern is inversely associated with metabolic syndrome among Puerto Rican adults in the Greater Boston area. *J. Nutr.* **2010**, *14*, 1846–1854. [CrossRef]
56. Yubero-Serrano, E.M.; Delgado-Lista, J.; Tierney, A.C.; Perez-Martinez, P.; Garcia-Rios, A.; Alcala-Diaz, J.F.; Castaño, J.P.; Tinahones, F.J.; Drevon, C.A.; Defoort, C.; et al. Insulin resistance determines a differential response to changes in dietary fat modification on metabolic syndrome risk factors: The LIPGENE study. *Am. J. Clin. Nutr.* **2015**, *102*, 1509–1517. [CrossRef]
57. Siri-Tarino, P.W.; Sun, Q.; Hu, F.B.; Krauss, R.M. Meta-analysis of prospective cohort studies evaluating the association of saturated fat with cardiovascular disease12345. *Am. J. Clin. Nutr.* **2010**, *91*, 535–546. [CrossRef] [PubMed]
58. Eckel, R.H.; Jakicic, J.M.; Ard, J.D.; de Jesus, J.M.; Houston, M.N.; Hubbard, V.S.; Lee, I.M.; Lichtenstein, A.H.; Loria, C.M.; Millen, B.E.; et al. American College of Cardiology/American Heart Association Task Force on Practice Guidelines.2013 AHA/ACC guideline on lifestyle management to reduce cardiovascular risk: A report of the American College of Cardiology/American Heart Association Task Force on Practice Guidelines. *J. Am. Coll. Cardiol.* **2014**, *63*, 2960–2984.
59. Beulen, Y.; Martínez-González, M.A.; van de Rest, O.; Salas-Salvadó, J.; Sorlí, J.V.; Gómez-Gracia, E.; Fiol, M.; Estruch, R.; Santos-Lozano, J.M.; Schröder, H.; et al. Quality of Dietary Fat Intake and Body Weight and Obesity in a Mediterranean Population: Secondary Analyses within the PREDIMED Trial. *Nutrients* **2018**, *10*, 2011. [CrossRef] [PubMed]

60. Zhang, Z.; Gillespie, C.; Yang, Q. Plasma trans-fatty acid concentrations continue to be associated with metabolic syndrome among US adults after reductions in trans-fatty acid intake. *Nutr. Res.* **2017**, *43*, 51–59. [CrossRef]
61. Garshick, M.; Mochari-Greenberger, H.; Mosca, L. Reduction in dietary trans fat intake is associated with decreased LDL particle number in a primary prevention population. *Nutr. Metab. Cardiovasc. Dis.* **2014**, *24*, 100–106. [CrossRef] [PubMed]
62. Institute of Medicine (U.S.). *Panel on Macronutrients. Dietary Reference Intakes for Energy, Carbohydrate, Fiber, Fat, Fatty Acids, Cholesterol, Protein, and Amino Acids*; National Academies Press: Washington, DC, USA, 2005.
63. Chen, J.P.; Chen, G.C.; Wang, X.P.; Qin, L.; Bai, Y. Dietary Fiber and Metabolic Syndrome: A Meta-Analysis and Review of Related Mechanisms. *Nutrients* **2017**, *10*, 24. [CrossRef]
64. Steemburgo, T.; Dall'Alba, V.; Almeida, J.C.; Zelmanovitz, T.; Gross, J.L.; de Azevedo, M.J. Intake of soluble fibers has a protective role for the presence of metabolic syndrome in patients with type 2 diabetes. *Eur. J. Clin. Nutr.* **2009**, *63*, 127–133. [CrossRef] [PubMed]
65. Esmaillzadeh, A.; Kimiagar, M.; Mehrabi, Y.; Azadbakht, L.; Hu, F.B.; Willett, W.C. Fruit and vegetable intakes, C-reactive protein, and the metabolic syndrome. *Am. J. Clin. Nutr.* **2006**, *84*, 1489–1497. [CrossRef]
66. Shin, A.; Lim, S.Y.; Sung, J.; Shin, H.R.; Kim, J. Dietary Intake, Eating Habits, and Metabolic Syndrome in Korean Men. *J. Am. Diet. Assoc.* **2009**, *109*, 633–640. [CrossRef]
67. Zhu, Y.; Bo, Y.; Liu, Y. Dietary total fat, fatty acids intake, and risk of cardiovascular disease: A dose-response meta-analysis of cohort studies. *Lipids Health Dis.* **2019**, *18*, 91. [CrossRef]
68. Koolhaas, C.M.; Dhana, K.; Schoufour, J.D.; Ikram, M.A.; Kavousi, M.; Franco, O.H. Impact of physical activity on the association of overweight and obesity with cardiovascular disease: The Rotterdam Study. *Eur. J. Prev. Cardiol.* **2017**, *24*, 934–941. [CrossRef] [PubMed]
69. Esposito, K.; Marfella, R.; Ciotola, M. Effect of a Mediterranean-style diet on endothelial dysfunction and markers of vascular inflammation in the metabolic syndrome. A randomized trial. *ACC Curr. J. Rev.* **2004**, *13*, 16–17. [CrossRef]
70. Warburton, D.E.; Nicol, C.W.; Bredin, S.S. Health benefits of physical activity: The evidence. *Can. Med. Assoc. J.* **2006**, *174*, 801–809. [CrossRef]
71. Aizawa, K.; Shoemaker, J.K.; Overend, T.J.; Petrella, R.J. Effects of lifestyle modification on central artery stiffness in metabolic syndrome subjects with pre-hypertension and/or pre-diabetes. *Diabetes Res. Clin. Pr.* **2009**, *83*, 249–256. [CrossRef]
72. Fernández, J.M.; Rosado-Álvarez, D.; Da Silva Grigoletto, M.E.; Rangel-Zúñiga, O.A.; Landaeta-Díaz, L.L.; Caballero-Villarraso, J.; López-Miranda, J.; Pérez-Jiménez, F.; Fuentes-Jiménez, F. Moderate-to-high-intensity training and a hypocaloric Mediterranean diet enhance endothelial progenitor cells and fitness in subjects with the metabolic syndrome. *Clin. Sci. (Lond).* **2012**, *123*, 361–373. [CrossRef]
73. Gremeaux, V.; Drigny, J.; Nigam, A.; Juneau, M.; Guilbeault, V.; Latour, E.; Gayda, M. Long-term Lifestyle Intervention with Optimized High-Intensity Interval Training Improves Body Composition, Cardiometabolic Risk, and Exercise Parameters in Patients with Abdominal Obesity. *Am. J. Phys. Med. Rehabil.* **2012**, *91*, 941–950. [CrossRef] [PubMed]
74. Gomez-Huelgas, R.; Jansen-Chaparro, S.; Baca-Osorio, A.; Mancera-Romero, J.; Tinahones, F.; Bernal-Lopez, M. Effects of a long-term lifestyle intervention program with Mediterranean diet and exercise for the management of patients with metabolic syndrome in a primary care setting. *Eur. J. Intern. Med.* **2015**, *26*, 317–323. [CrossRef]
75. Lee, G.; Choi, H.Y.; Yang, S.J. Effects of Dietary and Physical Activity Interventions on Metabolic Syndrome: A Meta-analysis. *J. Korean Acad. Nurs.* **2015**, *45*, 483. [CrossRef] [PubMed]
76. FESNAD. Dietary Reference Intakes (DRI) for the Spanish Population—2010. *Act. Diet.* **2010**, *14*, 196–197.

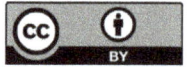

© 2019 by the authors. Licensee MDPI, Basel, Switzerland. This article is an open access article distributed under the terms and conditions of the Creative Commons Attribution (CC BY) license (http://creativecommons.org/licenses/by/4.0/).

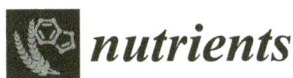

Review

Diet Quality, Saturated Fat and Metabolic Syndrome

Stéphanie Harrison [1,2], Patrick Couture [1,3] and Benoît Lamarche [1,2,*]

1. Centre Nutrition, santé et société (NUTRISS), Institut sur la nutrition et les aliments fonctionnels (INAF), Université Laval, Québec, QC G1V 0A6, Canada; stephanie.harrison.1@ulaval.ca (S.H.); patrick.couture@fmed.ulaval.ca (P.C.)
2. School of Nutrition, Université Laval, Québec, QC G1V 0A6, Canada
3. CHU Research Center, Québec, QC G1V 0A6, Canada
* Correspondence: benoit.lamarche@fsaa.ulaval.ca; Tel.: +1-418-656-2131 (ext. 404355)

Received: 11 September 2020; Accepted: 20 October 2020; Published: 22 October 2020

Abstract: Indices reflecting overall diet quality are used globally in research to predict the risk of various diseases and metabolic disorders such as metabolic syndrome (MetS). Such indices are built to measure adherence to current dietary guidelines or to best assess the diet–disease relationship. Although mostly food-based, dietary guidelines often include recommendations to limit saturated fatty acid (SFA) intake in order to prevent cardiovascular diseases. However, not all diet quality indices consider SFA in their definition of diet quality. Additionally, the relationship between SFA consumption and the development of MetS remains unclear. The purpose of this short review was to explore the association between MetS and various diet quality indices and dietary patterns, with a focus on how SFA contributes to these associations.

Keywords: saturated fatty acids; metabolic syndrome; diet quality; dietary guidelines; cardiovascular disease

---

1. Introduction

Various scores and indices are available to assess overall diet quality in population-based or interventional studies. These scores measure either adherence to certain dietary patterns, such as the Mediterranean diet (MedDiet) or the Dietary Approach to Stop Hypertension (DASH), or to country-specific dietary guidelines, such as Healthy Eating Indices (HEI). As discussed below, dietary patterns and diet quality indices have been associated with the risk of various diseases, including the metabolic syndrome (MetS), a collection of metabolic disorders that increase the risk of cardiovascular diseases (CVD), stroke or type 2 diabetes [1]. The typical features of MetS are central obesity, insulin resistance, dyslipidemia, hypertension, dysglycemia, and a pro-inflammatory/pro-thrombotic state [1]. The dyslipidemic features of the MetS are hypertriglyceridemia (fasting and postprandial) and low high-density lipoprotein cholesterol (HDL-C). While an elevated low-density lipoprotein cholesterol concentration (LDL-C) is not considered a typical feature of MetS, other features of LDL are. Specifically, patients with MetS generally have smaller and denser LDL particles, which are more prone to oxidative stress and are cleared less rapidly from the circulation than larger LDL particles [2].

Dietary patterns are a multidimensional representation of eating and, by definition, do not focus on singled out nutrients or foods. This is also the case for dietary guidelines, which have shifted from mostly nutrient-based to mostly food-based recommendations in recent years [3]. Nevertheless, most dietary guidelines around the globe still include a recommendation to limit intakes of specific nutrients of public health concern, including saturated fatty acids (SFAs). The recommendation to limit the consumption of SFAs is based largely on their well-established cholesterol-raising effects [4,5]. Data from a number of randomized controlled trials (RCTs) have shown that replacing dietary SFA with unsaturated fats reduces the risk of combined CVD events and are also at the basis of the recommendation to limit SFA intakes [5,6]. Replacing dietary SFA with carbohydrates from whole grains foods may also yield cardiovascular benefits, unlike carbohydrates from refined grains [7–9].

Although SFAs have been considered a major nutritional risk factor of CVD for more than 50 years, recent data have provided new challenging evidence suggesting that the SFA–CVD relationship may not be as straightforward as originally thought [10]. For example, the meta-analysis that showed a significant impact of SFA reduction on combined CVD events and showed no significant effect of SFAs on the risk of fatal myocardial infarction (MI) or coronary heart disease (CHD) mortality [5]. The authors of this meta-analysis emphasized the lack of robust, high-quality data to reach definitive conclusions on many of these associations. Others suggest that the recommendations on healthy dietary patterns capture the inherent risk attributed to variations in SFA intake, implying that specific recommendations on SFA intake are, in that context, redundant [11]. The fact that the increase in LDL-C concentrations seen with higher intakes of SFA intake is generally paralleled by an increase in the size of the LDL is another factor complexifying the association between dietary SFA and CVD risk [11]. Finally, the heterogeneity in the health effects of individual types of SFAs (e.g., myristic, lauric, etc.) [7,12] and the important interindividual variation in response to SFA reduction [13] are additional considerations put forward by those against the specific recommendations on SFA [11].

Beyond its well-known LDL-raising effects, the impact of SFA consumption on cardiometabolic health remains controversial. While data from a recent systematic review suggest that increased intake of SFA is associated with an increased risk of MetS, this association appeared to be dependent on the concurrent variations of other nutrients [9]. The purpose of this short review was therefore to explore the association between MetS and various diet quality indices and dietary patterns, with a focus on how SFA may contribute to these associations.

2. Diet Quality and Metabolic Syndrome

2.1. The HEI and MetS

The first HEI was developed in 1995 by the United States Department of Agriculture (USDA) in order to measure adherence to the Dietary Guidelines for Americans (DGA) as well as the Food Guide Pyramid. The HEI's main goal was to serve as a "report card" of Americans' diet, i.e., a measure of overall diet quality. This first HEI had 10 components related to recommendations found in the Food Guide Pyramid (Grains, Vegetables, Fruits, Milk, Meat, and "Other Foods") and in the DGA (Total fat, SFA, Cholesterol, Sodium, and Variety). The HEI-2015 is the most recent healthy eating index in the USA and reflects adherence to the 2015–2020 DGA. It has 13 components, including both adequacy and moderation components (Table 1). The moderation components of the HEI-2015 include a fatty acids sub-score calculated as the ratio of unsaturated fat to SFAs, as well as an SFA sub-score. According to the 2015–2020 DGA, SFA intake should not exceed 10%E per day (the SFA sub-score of the HEI-2015) and should be replaced by unsaturated fats (the fatty acids sub-score of the HEI-2015). As indicated above, those recommendations are based on many studies having shown that replacing SFA with unsaturated fat (notably PUFA) reduces serum levels of total and LDL-cholesterol [4], as well as the risk of CVD events [5]. The rationale for the SFA recommendation (<10% E) in the 2015–2020 DGA is not based on the upper limit instated by the Institute of Medicine. It is based on the notion that in most instances, people with an SFA intake > 10% E cannot meet the recommended intake of all food groups while maintaining an energy balance [3]. SFA intake in the calculation of the HEI-2015 is also partially accounted for in the total protein foods adequacy component, higher fat protein foods receiving fewer points than lower fat protein foods [14]. Finally, the adequacy dairy component of the HEI-2015, which rewards a higher consumption of dairy products irrespective of fat content, as well as the SFA moderation component, which sanctions higher SFA intakes, reflects the 2015–2020 DGA recommendations to favor lower-fat or fat-free dairy products [3].

Surprisingly, very few studies have documented the association between HEIs (2010 or 2015 versions) and the risk of MetS. In a cross-sectional analysis of 1036 Iranian women, participants in the highest quartile of HEI-2010 had a 28% lower risk of MetS compared with those in the first quartile (95% CI 0.50–0.96). Abdominal obesity, high blood pressure, high serum triacylglycerol and low serum HDL-C also decreased across HEI-2010 quartiles [15]. Structural equation modeling analyses of data from a sample of 188 healthy obese adults revealed that the HEI-2015 mediated the association between age and several cardio-metabolic risk factors associated with MetS, including fat mass, fat free mass, systolic blood pressure (SBP) and HDL-C. HEI-2015 scores also mediated the association between gender and waist circumference, SBP, triglyceride and HDL-C [16].

Table 1. Components of different healthy eating indices.

HEI-2015	aHEI	PNNS-GS2
Adequacy		*Adequacy*
1. Total fruits 2. Whole fruits 3. Total vegetables 4. Greens and Beans	1. Fruits 2. Vegetables 3. Nuts/Legumes	1. Vegetables/Fruits 2. Nuts 3. Legumes
5. Whole grains 6. Dairy products 7. Total protein foods 8. Seafood and Plant protein 9. Fatty acids (UFA/SFA ratio)	4. Whole grains 5. Trans fat 6. Long chain n3 fatty acids 7. PUFA	4. Whole grain foods 5. Milk and dairy products 6. Fish and sea foods 7. Added fat (prefer vegetable sources)
Moderation		*Moderation*
	8. Red/Processed meat	8. Red meat 9. Processed meat
10. Refined grains 11. Sodium 12. Added sugars 13. SFA	9. Sodium 10. SSBs 11. Alcohol	10. Sodium 11. Sweet tasting beverages 12. Sugary foods 13. Alcohol

HEI: Healthy Eating Index, PNNS-GS2: Programme National Nutrition Santé-Guideline Score updated to reflect the 2017 French dietary guidelines, UFA: Unsaturated fatty acids, SFA: Saturated fatty acids, PUFA: Polyunsaturated fatty acids, SSBs: Sugar-sweetened beverages. Note: The aHEI does not use the adequacy/moderation classification of its components.

The extent to which each of the HEI-2015 sub-scores, including those related to SFA intake, contribute to modifying individual features of the MetS is a complex question. To the extent that high LDL-C concentrations are not a typical feature of the MetS, adequacy or moderation components of the HEI-2015 having an impact on LDL-C concentrations would not predict changes in the incidence of MetS. However, replacing SFA with PUFA or MUFA slightly reduces HDL-C, total cholesterol, and TG concentrations in healthy adults [4]. Furthermore, replacing SFA by PUFA from different oils or foods reduced HDL-C concentrations in a recently published cross-over randomized controlled trial (RCT) of 36 men and women at risk of CVD, while having no effect on serum TG and glucose levels [17]. The substitution of SFA by PUFA, particularly PUFAs from walnuts, had a small but significant lowering effect on blood pressure but no effect on arterial stiffness in the same RCT [17]. These results suggest that dietary SFA, because of opposing effects on many of the typical features of MetS, cannot explain in and of themselves the favorable association between diet quality, as measured by the HEI-2015, and MetS. On the other hand, consumption of other foods and nutrients accounted for in the HEI-2015 has been more consistently associated with specific features of the MetS. For example, high vs. low dairy consumption has been associated with a lower risk of abdominal obesity and of being overweight [18]. The blood pressure lowering effect of a low sodium diet is well established [19].

Data from observational studies indicate that consumption of fruits and vegetables is associated with a lower risk of MetS [20]. Fruit consumption, independent of vegetable consumption, has also been inversely associated with the incidence of hypertriglyceridemia [21]. Higher consumption of sugar-sweetened beverages (SSBs), one of the main sources of added sugar in the North American diet, has been associated with an increased risk of MetS [22]. Taken together, these results suggest that the SFA component of the HEI-2015 per se cannot explain the favorable association between the HEI-2015 and the risk of MetS.

2.2. The aHEI and MetS

Unlike the HEI-2015, which is meant to measure adherence to dietary guidelines, the Alternate HEI (aHEI) was developed not only as a measure of diet quality but also to entail the diet–disease association. It was first developed in 2002 and included 9 components, including vegetables, fruits, and cereal fiber [23]. While the first version of the aHEI included an SFA component, the updated 2010 version of the aHEI does not (Table 1) [24], reflecting to some extent the inconsistent association between SFA consumption and CVD [11]. This is not to say that SFA is not indirectly accounted for in the aHEI. Indeed, a high score resulting from a high consumption of vegetables and fruits, whole grains, nuts and legumes, and PUFA, combined with a low consumption of SSBs, sodium, and red/processed meat, reflects a healthy food pattern that is very likely to be low in SFA.

In a cross-sectional analysis of 12,406 US Hispanics and Latinos from the multicenter, population-based Hispanic Community Health Study/Study of Latinos cohort, a higher aHEI was associated with lower odds of MetS [25]. Interestingly, the association of the aHEI and cardiometabolic factors varied by ethnic background. Specifically, the aHEI was inversely associated with waist circumference, blood pressure, and glucose among Mexicans and Puerto Ricans and with TG among Mexicans only, and was positively associated with HDL-C among Puerto Ricans and Central Americans [25]. We have also shown a similar inverse association between the aHEI and the prevalence of MetS in a cross-sectional analysis of 998 men and women from the province of Québec, in Canada [26]. In a cross-sectional analysis of 775 healthy women from the Nurses' Health Study, the aHEI was inversely associated with leptin and insulin concentrations but showed no association with other cardiometabolic risk factors traditionally associated with MetS [27]. These associations were, however, no longer present after adjusting for body mass index (BMI). Similar to the HEI-2015, this inverse association between the aHEI and the MetS is unlikely to be explained by variations in dietary SFA intake per se.

2.3. The Programme National Nutrition Santé Guideline Score (PNNSG-GS2) and MetS

The PNNS-GS2 is a score that reflects adherence to the 2017 French nutritional guidelines (Table 1) [28]. Briefly, it includes 13 components, of which seven are considered as adequacy recommendations and six refer to moderation recommendations. Similar to the aHEI, the PNNS-GS2 has no specific sub-score for SFA, but SFA intake is captured by the recommendation on added fat (to favor vegetable sources of fat vs. animal sources of fat) and indirectly by the recommendation on processed meats. Hence, individuals with a higher PNNS-GS2 consumed less SFA than individuals with a lower score [28]. Cross-sectional data from the Nutrinet-Santé Study have shown that a higher PNNS-GS2 was associated with a lower BMI, lower TG and glucose concentrations, lower systolic and diastolic blood pressures, and with higher concentrations of HDL-C in both men and women [28]. Recent data also suggest that higher adherence to the French dietary guidelines is prospectively associated with a lower risk of being overweight or obese [29]. These observations suggest that the PNNS-GS2 is likely to be inversely associated with the risk of incident MetS, but this needs to be formally confirmed with prospective data. The extent to which each of the components of the PNNS-GS2 are associated with individual features of the MetS is also unknown.

2.4. The Dietary Approaches to Stop Hypertension (DASH) Score and MetS

The Dietary Approaches to Stop Hypertension (DASH) score was created to measure adherence to the DASH diet, a healthy eating pattern that has been repeatedly associated with lower blood pressure and reduced CVD risk [30–35]. It was developed in the 1990s for the DASH trial, a randomized controlled trial in which more than 400 participants were randomized to either the control "American" diet, an "American" diet rich in fruits and vegetables or a DASH diet [36]. Most studies available at the time of the trial had shown no clear association between dietary fat (including SFA) and blood pressure [37]. However, it was argued that strict vegetarian diets (i.e., excluding dairy products) that were low in fat and SFA were associated with lower blood pressure. The DASH eating plan as we know it today promotes the consumption of fruits and vegetables, low-fat dairy products, whole grains, legumes, fish, poultry, and nuts and recommends limited intakes of sweets, SSBs, and red meats. Furthermore, individuals wanting to follow a DASH eating plan should choose foods that are low in sodium, SFA and trans-fat and rich in potassium, calcium, magnesium, fiber, and protein [34]. To that extent, the typical DASH diet is also a healthy eating pattern that is low in SFA [34].

Multiple versions of the DASH diet score are available in the literature [35,38–40]. Most scores include some of or all 8 food groups of the DASH eating plan, namely grains, meat/poultry/fish, vegetables, fruits, low-fat dairy products, fats and oils, nuts/legumes, and sweets. Additionally, most versions of the score include a component related to sodium intake. However, even if the recommendation to choose foods low in SFA and to limit consumption of SFA is included in the typical DASH eating plan, not all versions of the DASH score include a component directly related to SFA intake. For example, the DASH score created by Fung et al. does not include a component pertaining to SFA consumption based on the argument that it is already captured, at least partly, by the inclusion of red and processed meat components of the score [35].

In general, a greater adherence to a DASH score is associated with a lower prevalence of MetS [41,42]. Similar to the aHEI, the DASH score showed variable associations with the MetS and its key features among diverse Hispanic/Latino populations [43]. In a cross-sectional analysis among US women, higher adherence to the DASH eating plan was associated with lower TG concentrations, independent of BMI [27]. In a meta-analysis of available RCTs, consumption of the DASH diet over periods ranging from 2 to 24 weeks reduced systolic and diastolic blood pressure as well as LDL-C concentrations, but had no significant effect on TG, HDL-C, and glucose concentrations [44]. Interestingly, the reduction in blood pressure with the DASH diet has been shown to be similar among individuals with and without MetS [45]. Thus, when applied rigorously, the DASH diet is likely to have an impact on MetS, primarily through its important blood pressure lowering effect. Considering that the DASH diet is low in SFA by definition, it is unsurprising to find that adherence to this healthy dietary pattern also reduces serum LDL-C concentration, but this cannot explain the association between the DASH score and MetS.

2.5. The Mediterranean Diet and MetS

The concept of the MedDiet emerged from the Seven Countries Study in the 1950s, which unraveled particularly low CVD mortality rates in countries around the Mediterranean Sea [46]. Such low CVD rates were attributed, at least partly, to the intrinsically low SFA content of the diet of inhabitants around the Mediterranean (<7% E) compared with inhabitants from northern countries such as Finland [47]. It is now recognized that a MedDiet such as the one recommended in dietary guidelines is not just about SFA, although constitutively, a MedDiet is low in SFA. Typically, a MedDiet is characterized by very high intakes of plant-based foods, such as fruits, vegetables, cereals, beans, nuts and seeds, low to moderate intakes of fish and poultry and occasional consumption of eggs and red meat [48]. Olive oil is often considered the main source of fat in the MedDiet. A low to moderate wine consumption is also included in the MedDiet pattern, mostly consumed with meals [48]. The MedDiet is the most documented and researched healthy eating pattern. It has been repeatedly and consistently associated with lower risks of CVD, type 2 diabetes, and some types of cancer as well as cognitive-related diseases [49–52].

Several MedDiet scores have been created to measure adherence to a MedDiet. According to D'Alessandro and De Pergola, there is a certain degree of variability in the different MedDiet scores currently existing [53]. However, Galbete et al. found little differences in disease risk associations when comparing different MedDiet scores [54]. This is not entirely surprising considering that several core foods (fruit, vegetables, legumes, cereals, meat, dairy, fish, alcohol, and healthy fats) are found in most MedDiet scores [53,54]. It must also be stressed that the MedDiet emphasizes consumption of whole foods, with little if no focus on nutrients. Even if SFA is not part of most of the MedDiet scores per se, this healthy eating pattern is intrinsically low in SFA, in part due to the fact that this pattern focuses on fresh foods and because the recommendation to consume almost exclusively olive oil as a source of fat restricts in and of itself SFA consumption.

The PREDIMED study has shown in subjects without MetS at baseline that consumption of a MedDiet supplemented with either nuts or olive oil for five years had no impact on MetS incidence compared with a control diet. However, reversion occurred in almost 3 out of 10 of participants who had MetS at baseline in both groups consuming the MedDiet [55]. MedDiet participants supplemented with olive oil showed significant reductions in abdominal obesity and in fasting glucose while MedDiet participants supplemented with nuts showed a significant reduction in abdominal obesity only. Interestingly, increases in the biomarkers of foods supplied to the Mediterranean diet groups, namely oleic and α-linolenic acids, have been associated with the incidence, reversion, and prevalence of MetS [56]. Similar to the DASH eating plan, higher adherence to the MedDiet has been associated with lower TG concentrations among US women, independent of BMI [27]. Consumption of the MedDiet has also been associated with improvements in several features of the MetS, including blood lipids, blood pressure, glucose-insulin homeostasis, endothelial function, and inflammation markers [57]. Being nutrient-dense and having a low energy density, the MedDiet has often led to weight loss in intervention studies [58], thus potentially amplifying the cardiometabolic changes seen with the MedDiet [59]. Of note, the weight loss achieved with the MedDiet may be more important than with low-fat diets, but similar to low-carbohydrate diets [60]. Others have suggested that consumption of a MedDiet may also reduce central obesity, which in turn may contribute to reduced obesity-related and MetS-related disease risk [61]. To that extent, the contribution of the low SFA content of the MedDiet to its cardiometabolic benefits may be limited to LDL-C and not to features of the MetS.

3. Conclusions

Deciphering the impact of individual foods and nutrients on cardiometabolic risk factors such as those associated with MetS is very challenging because of the numerous food–nutrient interactions found within complex food patterns. This is certainly the case with SFA. In this short narrative review, we have shown that diet quality indices reflecting adherence to dietary guidelines (HEIs) or healthy dietary patterns (DASH, MedDiet) are quite consistently associated with a reduced risk of MetS. Data reviewed here provide indirect evidence that SFA in and of itself may play a rather limited role in the development of MetS. Indeed, while increased SFA intake in place of PUFA is unarguably associated with raised LDL-C concentrations, high LDL-C is not a typical feature of MetS. Moreover, the extent to which variations in SFA intake contribute to the cardiometabolic benefits associated with healthy eating patterns is likely to be diluted within the effects of numerous other nutrients and foods that constitute these patterns and which have been quite consistently associated with features of MetS. However, this may be of little concern since healthy eating scores that do not account for SFA intake per se inevitably capture this component through other components of the scores.

Author Contributions: S.H. and B.L. wrote the paper together. P.C. revised the paper. All authors agreed to the published version of the manuscript.

Funding: This research received no external funding.

Conflicts of Interest: S.H. received the Emerging Scholars Grant from the Canadian Research Data Centre Network (CRDCN) and a Studentship from the Chair of Nutrition, Université Laval. P.C. and B.L. have received funding during the past 5 years from the Canadian Institutes for Health Research, Agriculture and Agri-Food Canada (Growing Forward program supported by the Dairy Farmers of Canada (completion in 2017), Growing Forward program supported by Canola Council of Canada, Flax Council of Canada and Dow Agrosciences (completion in 2017)), National Dairy Council (completion in 2017), and Atrium Innovations. PC has also received funding from Merck Frosst, Pfizer, Amgen, Sanofi, and Kaneka Corporation.

References

1. Desroches, S.; Lamarche, B. The evolving definitions and increasing prevalence of the metabolic syndrome. *Appl. Physiol. Nutr. Metab.* **2007**, *32*, 23–32. [CrossRef] [PubMed]
2. Lamarche, B.; Lemieux, I.; Després, J.P. The small, dense LDL phenotype and the risk of coronary heart disease: Epidemiology, patho-physiology and therapeutic aspects. *Diabetes Metab.* **1999**, *25*, 199–211. [PubMed]
3. Department of Health and Human Services. *Dietary Guidelines for Americans 2015–2020*; Department of Health and Human Services: Washington, DC, USA, 2015; p. 122.
4. Mensink, R. *Effects of Saturated Fatty Acids on Serum Lipids and lipo90proteins: A Systematic Review and Regression Analysis*; WHO: Geneva, Switzerland, 2016.
5. Hooper, L.; Martin, N.; Jimoh, O.F.; Kirk, C.; Foster, E.; Abdelhamid, A.S. Reduction in saturated fat intake for cardiovascular disease. *Cochrane Database Syst. Rev.* **2020**. [CrossRef] [PubMed]
6. Mozaffarian, D.; Micha, R.; Wallace, S. Effects on coronary heart disease of increasing polyunsaturated fat in place of saturated fat: A systematic review and meta-analysis of randomized controlled trials. *PLoS Med.* **2010**, *7*, e1000252. [CrossRef]
7. Briggs, M.A.; Petersen, K.S.; Kris-Etherton, P.M. Saturated Fatty Acids and Cardiovascular Disease: Replacements for Saturated Fat to Reduce Cardiovascular Risk. *Healthcare* **2017**, *5*, 29. [CrossRef]
8. Li, Y.; Hruby, A.; Bernstein, A.M.; Ley, S.H.; Wang, D.D.; Chiuve, S.E.; Sampson, L.; Rexrode, K.M.; Rimm, E.B.; Willett, W.C.; et al. Saturated Fats Compared With Unsaturated Fats and Sources of Carbohydrates in Relation to Risk of Coronary Heart Disease: A Prospective Cohort Study. *J. Am. Coll. Cardiol.* **2015**, *66*, 1538–1548. [CrossRef]
9. Julibert, A.; Bibiloni, M.d.M.; Tur, J.A. Dietary fat intake and metabolic syndrome in adults: A systematic review. *Nutr. Metab. Cardiovasc. Dis.* **2019**, *29*, 887–905. [CrossRef]
10. Lamarche, B.; Couture, P. It is time to revisit current dietary recommendations for saturated fat. *Appl. Physiol. Nutr. Metab.* **2014**, *39*, 1409–1411. [CrossRef]
11. Krauss, R.M.; Kris-Etherton, P.M. Public health guidelines should recommend reducing saturated fat consumption as much as possible: NO. *Am. J. Clin. Nutr.* **2020**, *112*, 19–24. [CrossRef]
12. German, J.B.; Dillard, C.J. Saturated fats: What dietary intake? *Am. J. Clin. Nutr.* **2004**, *80*, 550–559. [CrossRef]
13. Lopez-Miranda, J.; Ordovas, J.M.; Mata, P.; Lichtenstein, A.H.; Clevidence, B.; Judd, J.T.; Schaefer, E.J. Effect of apolipoprotein E phenotype on diet-induced lowering of plasma low density lipoprotein cholesterol. *J. Lipid Res.* **1994**, *35*, 1965–1975. [PubMed]
14. Krebs-Smith, S.M.; Pannucci, T.E.; Subar, A.F.; Kirkpatrick, S.I.; Lerman, J.L.; Tooze, J.A.; Wilson, M.M.; Reedy, J. Update of the Healthy Eating Index: HEI-2015. *J. Acad. Nutr. Diet* **2018**, *118*, 1591–1602. [CrossRef] [PubMed]
15. Saraf-Bank, S.; Haghighatdoost, F.; Esmaillzadeh, A.; Larijani, B.; Azadbakht, L. Adherence to Healthy Eating Index-2010 is inversely associated with metabolic syndrome and its features among Iranian adult women. *Eur. J. Clin. Nutr.* **2017**, *71*, 425–430. [CrossRef] [PubMed]
16. Khodarahmi, M.; Asghari-Jafarabadi, M.; Abbasalizad, M.F. A structural equation modeling approach for the association of a healthy eating index with metabolic syndrome and cardio-metabolic risk factors among obese individuals. *PLoS ONE* **2019**, *14*, e0219193. [CrossRef] [PubMed]
17. Tindall, A.M.; Petersen, K.S.; Skulas-Ray, A.C.; Richter, C.K.; Proctor, D.N.; Kris-Etherton, P.M. Replacing Saturated Fat With Walnuts or Vegetable Oils Improves Central Blood Pressure and Serum Lipids in Adults at Risk for Cardiovascular Disease: A Randomized Controlled-Feeding Trial. *J. Am. Heart Assoc.* **2019**, *8*, e011512. [CrossRef] [PubMed]

18. Schwingshackl, L.; Hoffmann, G.; Schwedhelm, C.; Kalle-Uhlmann, T.; Missbach, B.; Knüppel, S.; Boeing, H. Consumption of Dairy Products in Relation to Changes in Anthropometric Variables in Adult Populations: A Systematic Review and Meta-Analysis of Cohort Studies. *PLoS ONE* **2016**, *11*, e0157461. [CrossRef] [PubMed]
19. Huang, L.; Trieu, K.; Yoshimura, S.; Neal, B.; Woodward, M.; Campbell, N.R.C.; Li, Q.; Lackland, D.T.; Leung, A.A.; Anderson, C.A.M.; et al. Effect of dose and duration of reduction in dietary sodium on blood pressure levels: Systematic review and meta-analysis of randomised trials. *BMJ* **2020**, *368*, m315. [CrossRef]
20. Zhang, Y.; Zhang, D.Z. Associations of vegetable and fruit consumption with metabolic syndrome. A meta-analysis of observational studies. *Public Health Nutr.* **2018**, *21*, 1693–1703. [CrossRef]
21. Kodama, S.; Horikawa, C.; Fujihara, K.; Ishii, D.; Hatta, M.; Takeda, Y.; Kitazawa, M.; Matsubayashi, Y.; Shimano, H.; Kato, K.; et al. Relationship between intake of fruit separately from vegetables and triglycerides—A meta-analysis. *Clin. Nutr. ESPEN* **2018**, *27*, 53–58. [CrossRef]
22. Malik, V.S.; Popkin, B.M.; Bray, G.A.; Després, J.P.; Willett, W.C.; Hu, F.B. Sugar-sweetened beverages and risk of metabolic syndrome and type 2 diabetes: A meta-analysis. *Diabetes Care* **2010**, *33*, 2477–2483. [CrossRef]
23. McCullough, M.L.; Feskanich, D.; Stampfer, M.J.; Giovannucci, E.L.; Rimm, E.B.; Hu, F.B.; Spiegelman, D.; Hunter, D.J.; Colditz, G.A.; Willett, W.C. Diet quality and major chronic disease risk in men and women: Moving toward improved dietary guidance. *Am. J. Clin. Nutr.* **2002**, *76*, 1261–1271. [CrossRef]
24. Chiuve, S.E.; Fung, T.T.; Rimm, E.B.; Hu, F.B.; McCullough, M.L.; Wang, M.; Stampfer, M.J.; Willett, W.C. Alternative dietary indices both strongly predict risk of chronic disease. *J Nutr.* **2012**, *142*, 1009–1018. [CrossRef]
25. Mattei, J.; Sotres-Alvarez, D.; Daviglus, M.L.; Gallo, L.C.; Gellman, M.; Hu, F.B.; Tucker, K.L.; Willett, W.C.; Siega-Riz, A.M.; Van Horn, L.; et al. Diet Quality and Its Association with Cardiometabolic Risk Factors Vary by Hispanic and Latino Ethnic Background in the Hispanic Community Health Study/Study of Latinos. *J. Nutr.* **2016**, *146*, 2035–2044. [CrossRef] [PubMed]
26. Lafrenière, J.; Carbonneau, É.; Laramée, C.; Corneau, L.; Robitaille, J.; Labonté, M.; Lamarche, B.; Lemieux, S. Is the Canadian Healthy Eating Index 2007 an Appropriate Diet Indicator of Metabolic Health? Insights from Dietary Pattern Analysis in the PREDISE Study. *Nutrients* **2019**, *11*, 1597. [CrossRef] [PubMed]
27. AlEssa, H.B.; Malik, V.S.; Yuan, C.; Willett, W.C.; Huang, T.; Hu, F.B.; Tobias, D.K. Dietary patterns and cardiometabolic and endocrine plasma biomarkers in US women. *Am. J. Clin. Nutr.* **2016**, *105*, 432–441. [CrossRef] [PubMed]
28. Chaltiel, D.; Adjibade, M.; Deschamps, V.; Touvier, M.; Hercberg, S.; Julia, C.; Kesse-Guyot, E. Programme National Nutrition Santé—Guidelines score 2 (PNNS-GS2): Development and validation of a diet quality score reflecting the 2017 French dietary guidelines. *Br. J. Nutr.* **2019**, *122*, 331–342. [CrossRef] [PubMed]
29. Chaltiel, D.; Julia, C.; Adjibade, M.; Touvier, M.; Hercberg, S.; Kesse-Guyot, E. Adherence to the 2017 French dietary guidelines and adult weight gain: A cohort study. *PLoS Med.* **2019**, *16*, e1003007. [CrossRef] [PubMed]
30. Sacks, F.M.; Svetkey, L.P.; Vollmer, W.M.; Appel, L.J.; Bray, G.A.; Harsha, D.; Obarzanek, E.; Conlin, P.R.; Miller, E.R.; Simons-Morton, D.G., 3rd; et al. Effects on blood pressure of reduced dietary sodium and the Dietary Approaches to Stop Hypertension (DASH) diet. DASH-Sodium Collaborative Research Group. *N. Engl. J. Med.* **2001**, *344*, 3–10. [CrossRef]
31. Hu, E.A.; Steffen, L.M.; Coresh, J.; Appel, L.J.; Rebholz, C.M. Adherence to the Healthy Eating Index-2015 and Other Dietary Patterns May Reduce Risk of Cardiovascular Disease, Cardiovascular Mortality, and All-Cause Mortality. *J. Nutr.* **2020**, *150*, 312–321. [CrossRef]
32. Saneei, P.; Salehi-Abargouei, A.; Esmaillzadeh, A.; Azadbakht, L. Influence of Dietary Approaches to Stop Hypertension (DASH) diet on blood pressure: A systematic review and meta-analysis on randomized controlled trials. *Nutr. Metab. Cardiovasc. Dis.* **2014**, *24*, 1253–1261. [CrossRef]
33. Appel, L.J.; Champagne, C.M.; Harsha, D.W.; Cooper, L.S.; Obarzanek, E.; Elmer, P.J.; Stevens, V.J.; Vollmer, W.M.; Lin, P.H.; Svetkey, L.P.; et al. Effects of comprehensive lifestyle modification on blood pressure control: Main results of the PREMIER clinical trial. *JAMA* **2003**, *289*, 2083–2093. [CrossRef] [PubMed]
34. National Heart Lung and Blood Institute. *DASH Eating Plan*; National Heart Lung and Blood Institute: Bethesda, MD, USA, 2020.

35. Fung, T.T.; Chiuve, S.E.; McCullough, M.L.; Rexrode, K.M.; Logroscino, G.; Hu, F.B. Adherence to a DASH-Style Diet and Risk of Coronary Heart Disease and Stroke in Women. *Arch. Intern. Med.* **2008**, *168*, 713–720. [CrossRef] [PubMed]
36. Appel, L.J.; Moore, T.J.; Obarzanek, E.; Vollmer, W.M.; Svetkey, L.P.; Sacks, F.M.; Bray, G.A.; Vogt, T.M.; Cutler, J.A.; Windhauser, M.M.; et al. A Clinical Trial of the Effects of Dietary Patterns on Blood Pressure. *N. Engl. J. Med.* **1997**, *336*, 1117–1124. [CrossRef] [PubMed]
37. Sacks, F.M.; Obarzanek, E.; Windhauser, M.M.; Svetkey, L.P.; Vollmer, W.M.; McCullough, M.; Karanja, N.; Lin, P.-H.; Steele, P.; Proschan, M.A.; et al. Rationale and design of the Dietary Approaches to Stop Hypertension trial (DASH): A multicenter controlled-feeding study of dietary patterns to lower blood pressure. *Ann. Epidemiol.* **1995**, *5*, 108–118. [CrossRef]
38. Dixon, L.B.; Subar, A.F.; Peters, U.; Weissfeld, J.L.; Bresalier, R.S.; Risch, A.; Schatzkin, A.; Hayes, R.B. Adherence to the USDA Food Guide, DASH Eating Plan, and Mediterranean dietary pattern reduces risk of colorectal adenoma. *J. Nutr.* **2007**, *137*, 2443–2450. [CrossRef]
39. Günther, A.L.; Liese, A.D.; Bell, R.A.; Dabelea, D.; Lawrence, J.M.; Rodriguez, B.L.; Standiford, D.A.; Mayer-Davis, E.J. Association between the dietary approaches to hypertension diet and hypertension in youth with diabetes mellitus. *Hypertension* **2009**, *53*, 6–12. [CrossRef]
40. Mellen, P.B.; Gao, S.K.; Vitolins, M.Z.; Goff, D.C., Jr. Deteriorating dietary habits among adults with hypertension: DASH dietary accordance, NHANES 1988-1994 and 1999-2004. *Arch. Intern. Med.* **2008**, *168*, 308–314. [CrossRef] [PubMed]
41. Kang, S.H.; Cho, K.H.; Do, J.Y. Association Between the Modified Dietary Approaches to Stop Hypertension and Metabolic Syndrome in Postmenopausal Women Without Diabetes. *Metab. Syndr. Relat. Disord.* **2018**, *16*, 282–289. [CrossRef]
42. Saneei, P.; Fallahi, E.; Barak, F.; Ghasemifard, N.; Keshteli, A.H.; Yazdannik, A.R.; Esmaillzadeh, A. Adherence to the DASH diet and prevalence of the metabolic syndrome among Iranian women. *Eur. J. Nutr.* **2015**, *54*, 421–428. [CrossRef]
43. Joyce, B.T.; Wu, D.; Hou, L.; Dai, Q.; Castaneda, S.F.; Gallo, L.C.; Talavera, G.A.; Sotres-Alvarez, D.; Van Horn, L.; Beasley, J.M.; et al. DASH diet and prevalent metabolic syndrome in the Hispanic Community Health Study/Study of Latinos. *Prev. Med. Rep.* **2019**, *15*, 100950. [CrossRef]
44. Siervo, M.; Lara, J.; Chowdhury, S.; Ashor, A.; Oggioni, C.; Mathers, J.C. Effects of the Dietary Approach to Stop Hypertension (DASH) diet on cardiovascular risk factors: A systematic review and meta-analysis. *Br. J. Nutr.* **2015**, *113*, 1–15. [CrossRef] [PubMed]
45. Hikmat, F.; Appel, L.J. Effects of the DASH diet on blood pressure in patients with and without metabolic syndrome: Results from the DASH trial. *J. Hum. Hypertens.* **2014**, *28*, 170–175. [CrossRef] [PubMed]
46. Toshima, H.; Keys, A.; Koga, Y.; Blackburn, H. *Lessons for Science from the Seven Countries Study: A 35-Year Collaborative Experience in Cardiovascular Disease Epidemiology*; Springer: Tokyo, Japan, 2012.
47. Keys, A.; Menotti, A.; Karvonen, M.J.; Aravanis, C.; Blackburn, H.; Buzina, R.; Djordjevic, B.S.; Dontas, A.S.; Fidanza, F.; Keys, M.H.; et al. The Diet and 15-Year Death Rate in the Seven Countries Study. *Am. J. Epidemiol.* **2017**, *185*, 1130–1142. [CrossRef] [PubMed]
48. Willett, W.C.; Sacks, F.; Trichopoulou, A.; Drescher, G.; Ferro-Luzzi, A.; Helsing, E.; Trichopoulos, D. Mediterranean diet pyramid: A cultural model for healthy eating. *Am. J. Clin. Nutr.* **1995**, *61* (Suppl. 6), 1402s–1406s. [CrossRef] [PubMed]
49. Singh, B.; Parsaik, A.; Mielke, M.M.; Erwin, P.; Knopman, D.; Petersen, R.C.; Roberts, R. Association of Mediterranean Diet with Mild Cognitive Impairment and Alzheimer's Disease: A Systematic Review and Meta-Analysis. *J. Alzheimers Dis.* **2014**, *39*, 271–282. [CrossRef] [PubMed]
50. Schwingshackl, L.; Schwedhelm, C.; Galbete, C.; Hoffmann, G. Adherence to Mediterranean Diet and Risk of Cancer: An Updated Systematic Review and Meta-Analysis. *Nutrients* **2017**, *9*, 63. [CrossRef]
51. Schwingshackl, L.; Missbach, B.; König, J.; Hoffmann, G. Adherence to a Mediterranean diet and risk of diabetes: A systematic review and meta-analysis. *Public Health Nutr.* **2015**, *18*, 1292–1299. [CrossRef]
52. Rosato, V.; Temple, N.J.; La Vecchia, C.; Castellan, G.; Tavani, A.; Guercio, V. Mediterranean diet and cardiovascular disease: A systematic review and meta-analysis of observational studies. *Eur. J. Nutr.* **2019**, *58*, 173–191. [CrossRef]
53. D'Alessandro, A.; De Pergola, G. The Mediterranean Diet: Its definition and evaluation of a priori dietary indexes in primary cardiovascular prevention. *Int. J. Food Sci. Nutr.* **2018**, *69*, 647–659. [CrossRef]

54. Galbete, C.; Schwingshackl, L.; Schwedhelm, C.; Boeing, H.; Schulze, M.B. Evaluating Mediterranean diet and risk of chronic disease in cohort studies: An umbrella review of meta-analyses. *Eur. J. Epidemiol.* **2018**, *33*, 909–931. [CrossRef]
55. Babio, N.; Toledo, E.; Estruch, R.; Ros, E.; Martínez-González, M.A.; Castañer, O.; Bulló, M.; Corella, D.; Arós, F.; Gómez-Gracia, E.; et al. Mediterranean diets and metabolic syndrome status in the PREDIMED randomized trial. *CMAJ* **2014**, *186*, E649–E657. [CrossRef]
56. Mayneris-Perxachs, J.; Sala-Vila, A.; Chisaguano, M.; Castellote, A.I.; Estruch, R.; Covas, M.I.; Fitó, M.; Salas-Salvadó, J.; Martínez-González, M.A.; Lamuela-Raventós, R.; et al. Effects of 1-year intervention with a Mediterranean diet on plasma fatty acid composition and metabolic syndrome in a population at high cardiovascular risk. *PLoS ONE* **2014**, *9*, e85202. [CrossRef]
57. Kastorini, C.-M.; Milionis, H.J.; Esposito, K.; Giugliano, D.; Goudevenos, J.A.; Panagiotakos, D.B. The Effect of Mediterranean Diet on Metabolic Syndrome and its Components: A Meta-Analysis of 50 Studies and 534,906 Individuals. *J. Am. Coll. Cardiol.* **2011**, *57*, 1299–1313. [CrossRef]
58. Esposito, K.; Kastorini, C.M.; Panagiotakos, D.B.; Giugliano, D. Mediterranean diet and weight loss: Meta-analysis of randomized controlled trials. *Metab. Syndr. Relat. Disord.* **2011**, *9*, 1–12. [CrossRef]
59. Richard, C.; Couture, P.; Desroches, S.; Charest, A.; Lamarche, B. Effect of the Mediterranean diet with and without weight loss on cardiovascular risk factors in men with the metabolic syndrome. *Nutr. Metab. Cardiovasc. Dis.* **2011**, *21*, 628–635. [CrossRef]
60. Mancini, J.G.; Filion, K.B.; Atallah, R.; Eisenberg, M.J. Systematic Review of the Mediterranean Diet for Long-Term Weight Loss. *Am. J. Med.* **2016**, *129*, 407–415.e4. [CrossRef]
61. Bendall, C.L.; Mayr, H.L.; Opie, R.S.; Bes-Rastrollo, M.; Itsiopoulos, C.; Thomas, C.J. Central obesity and the Mediterranean diet: A systematic review of intervention trials. *Crit. Rev. Food Sci. Nutr.* **2018**, *58*, 3070–3084. [CrossRef]

Publisher's Note: MDPI stays neutral with regard to jurisdictional claims in published maps and institutional affiliations.

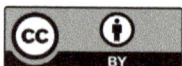

© 2020 by the authors. Licensee MDPI, Basel, Switzerland. This article is an open access article distributed under the terms and conditions of the Creative Commons Attribution (CC BY) license (http://creativecommons.org/licenses/by/4.0/).

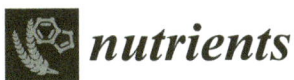

Review

Sleep Apnea and Sleep Habits: Relationships with Metabolic Syndrome

Anne-Laure Borel [1,2]

[1] Department of Endocrinology, Diabetes and Nutrition, Grenoble Alpes University Hospital, 38043 Grenoble, France; alborel@chu-grenoble.fr; Tel.: +33-4-7676-55-09

[2] "Hypoxia, Pathophysiology" (HP2) Laboratory INSERM U1042, Grenoble Alpes University, 38043 Grenoble, France

Received: 2 September 2019; Accepted: 16 October 2019; Published: 2 November 2019

Abstract: Excess visceral adiposity is a primary cause of metabolic syndrome and often results from excess caloric intake and a lack of physical activity. Beyond these well-known etiologic factors, however, sleep habits and sleep apnea also seem to contribute to abdominal obesity and metabolic syndrome: Evidence suggests that sleep deprivation and behaviors linked to evening chronotype and social jetlag affect eating behaviors like meal preferences and eating times. When circadian rest and activity rhythms are disrupted, hormonal and metabolic regulations also become desynchronized, and this is known to contribute to the development of metabolic syndrome. The metabolic consequences of obstructive sleep apnea syndrome (OSAS) also contribute to incident metabolic syndrome. These observations, along with the first sleep intervention studies, have demonstrated that sleep is a relevant lifestyle factor that needs to be addressed along with diet and physical activity. Personalized lifestyle interventions should be tested in subjects with metabolic syndrome, based on their specific diet and physical activity habits, but also according to their circadian preference. The present review therefore focuses (i) on the role of sleep habits in the development of metabolic syndrome, (ii) on the reciprocal relationship between sleep apnea and metabolic syndrome, and (iii) on the results of sleep intervention studies.

Keywords: metabolic syndrome; sleep; sleep apnea; sleep habit; sleep duration; chronotype; social jetlag

1. Introduction

Metabolic syndrome defines a group of risk factors underlying cardiovascular and metabolic diseases: abdominal obesity, atherogenic dyslipidemia, elevated blood pressure, and fasting plasma glucose [1]. The combined criteria used to define this syndrome identify a phenotype which is related to a greatest risk of developing cardiovascular and metabolic diseases than the simple addition of risks associated with each criterion [2].

Excess visceral adipose tissue is believed to be a primary driver of the cardiometabolic complications of metabolic syndrome [3]. An increase in visceral adiposity is thought to reflect the relative inability of the subcutaneous adipose tissue depot to sufficiently metabolize and store excess calories [2]. The specific characteristics of visceral adiposity, as opposed to subcutaneous adiposity elsewhere in the body, drive altered glucose homeostasis, proinflammatory adipocytokine release, and endothelial dysfunction that are the primary causes of metabolic syndrome [3].

Excess visceral fat is a modifiable risk factor that is usually associated with both excess caloric intake and a lack of physical activity [4]. Beyond these well-known, lifestyle-related etiologies, it also seems reasonable to assume that sleep habits could also contribute to abdominal obesity and, thus, metabolic syndrome. In addition, sleep apnea has been shown to increase the risk of cardiometabolic disease, and patients with metabolic syndrome are prone to develop sleep apnea [5].

The present narrative review focuses (i) on the role of sleep habits in the development of metabolic syndrome and (ii) on the reciprocal relationship between sleep apnea and metabolic syndrome. Finally, emerging evidence is reviewed regarding sleep intervention studies and how targeting of one specific lifestyle habits may impact other behaviors.

2. Sleep Habits and Metabolic Syndrome

2.1. Definitions

Metabolic syndrome: In 1998, the World Health Organization (WHO) became the first organization to introduce the term metabolic syndrome, with a primary focus on insulin resistance and hyperglycemia [3]. In 2001, the National Cholesterol Education Program's Adult Treatment Panel III (NCEP-ATP III) released its own definition, adding abdominal adiposity, specifically an increased waist circumference, as a major component of the syndrome [4]. Several definitions followed, issued from different societies, which mainly diverged on the clinical evaluation of abdominal adiposity. In 2009, the International Diabetes Federation Task Force on Epidemiology and Prevention; the National Heart, Lung, and Blood Institute; the American Heart Association; the World Heart Federation; and the International Atherosclerosis Society joined to release a statement harmonizing the criteria for defining the metabolic syndrome. This is the definition that is in use today, and it takes into account population-specific cutoffs for waist circumference [5]. Metabolic syndrome is defined by three of five criteria, with dyslipidemia being two criteria among: Fasting glucose ≥ 100 mg/dL or antidiabetic therapy, increased waist circumference, TG ≥ 150 mg/dl, and/or HDL-C < 40/50 in men/women or antilipidic therapy, ≥130/85 mmHg or therapy.

Sleep characteristics: Recent research has indicated that people's sleep habits are changing. In this paper, we use the following definitions for terms commonly used in this field [6,7]:

'Sleep duration' is the time between falling asleep and waking up.

'Sleep debt' is a value calculated as the weekend sleep duration (i.e., Friday and Saturday nights) minus the sleep duration during the rest of the week.

'Chronotype' defines an individual's circadian preference: 'early' or 'morning' people tend to go to bed and wake up early, whereas 'late' or 'evening' people go to bed and wake up late [8,9]. The chronotype is calculated as follows [10]:

$$\text{Chronotype} = \text{Mid-sleep time on free days (MSF)} - 0.5 \times \text{sleep debt}$$

MSF represents the 'mid sleep time' that is calculated as the mid-point between sleep onset and wake time on free days, i.e., days when people do not have to get up for work.

Whether people are a 'night owl' or an 'early bird' can also be assessed using the Morningness–Eveningness Questionnaire, a 19-item scale validated by Horne and Östberg that addresses the timing preference for different daily activities [11].

'Social jetlag' refers to a misalignment of sleep timing between work and free days. Work, school, and other schedules often interfere with an individual's sleep preferences. Evening people, for example, are more likely to accumulate a sleep debt during the workdays which will be recovered during work-free days. This is calculated as the absolute difference between mid-sleep time on free days (MSF) and week days (MSW) i.e., social jetlag = |MSF − MSW| [12].

2.2. Epidemiological Evidence Related to Metabolic Syndrome

A normal amount of sleep is considered to be 7 to 8 h per night. Fewer than 6 h per night is classed as sleep deprivation and more than 9 h per night is considered as oversleeping. Sleep duration has decreased over the last 50 years in industrialized countries: In the USA, the percentage of those who self-reported that they did not sleep enough increased during this period from about 15% to 30% [13]. In France, it is estimated that average sleep duration has shown a 1 h 30 min reduction in the last 50 years (https://www.inserm.fr/en/health-information/health-and-research-from-z/sleep). In a 2017 telephone survey to investigate public health in France called the "Baromètre de Santé publique France 2017" (Public health barometer France 2017), 12,637 men and women aged between 18 and 75 years answered questions about their sleeping habits; 36% reported sleeping fewer than 6 h per night.

Several epidemiological studies and their meta-analysis have revealed sleep restriction to be associated with an increased prevalence of obesity [14]. Children seem particularly vulnerable: Reviews of child and adolescent data demonstrated an increased incidence of obesity in groups sleeping less than the time recommended for their age group [15]; this association was not so clearly marked in adults [16].

Regarding the specific association between sleep deprivation and metabolic syndrome, numerous studies have reported an association between a short sleep duration and an increased prevalence of metabolic syndrome. Some, but not all, research has also reported a similar association with long sleep duration. Eighteen such cross-sectional studies were included in a recent meta-analysis into (sleep) dose–(metabolic) response association [16]. A total of 75,657 adults were included, 51% of whom were men, and the age range was 18–96 years. Most studies reported odds ratios (OR) adjusted for age, sex, smoking, and alcohol intake. Short sleep was associated with metabolic syndrome, with a pooled estimate of the OR of 1.23 (95% CI, 1.11–1.37; $p < 0.001$; I^2, 71%). Thus, there was a significantly higher proportion of metabolic syndrome in those who had short sleep durations, with low heterogeneity between studies. In addition, a dose–response relationship was found for durations of sleep <5 h, 5–6 h, and 6–7 h: Pooled ORs for having metabolic syndrome for these sleep groups were 1.51 (95% CI, 1.10–2.08; $p = 0.01$; I^2, 88%), 1.28 (95% CI, 1.11–1.48; $p < 0.001$; I^2, 67%), and 1.16 (95% CI, 1.02–1.31; $p = 0.02$; I^2, 81%), respectively. There was no significant association with long sleep durations (pooled OR of 15 studies = 1.13, 95% CI, 0.97–1.32; $p = 0.10$; I^2, 89%). These results were consistent with a previous meta-analysis [17].

In children, sleep deprivation has also been associated with an increase in cardiometabolic risk. This pattern has been seen in cross-sectional analyses based on both self-reported sleeping habits [18] and objective, actimetry-measured sleep patterns [19].

Although these relationships found in cross-sectional studies appear to be robust, there is less evidence for longitudinal associations. A large-scale prospective study into the risk of developing metabolic syndrome used data collected from 162,121 adults aged 20–80 years (men 47.4%) who had participated in a medical screening program in Taiwan [20]. At the start of the screening, no participant was either obese or had any characteristic of metabolic syndrome. Follow-up data were available annually from 98% of participants, and the number of visits made by each participant ranged from 2 to 19. Of these, 18.6% of people were short sleepers (<6 h/day), 72.8% were regular sleepers (6–8 h/day, control values) and 8.6% were long sleepers (>8 h/day). More than half of the participants (57.6%) reported that they had insomnia symptoms. Compared to regular sleep data, short sleep duration was associated with a 12% (adjusted HR 1.12 [1.07–1.17]) increase in risk of becoming centrally obese during the follow-up period. Short sleepers were also more likely to develop metabolic syndrome (adjusted HR 1.09 [1.05–1.13]) compared to regular sleepers ($p < 001$). By contrast, long sleep was associated with a decreased risk of metabolic syndrome (adjusted HR 0.93 [0.88–0.99]). Similar results were found in two other longitudinal studies [21,22].

It is also interesting to note that in 1344 participants of the Penn State Adult Cohort, the cardiovascular mortality associated with metabolic syndrome showed an interaction with sleep duration as measured in a single polysomnography. In this sample, the mean age was 48.8 (14.2) years, and 57.8% were women and 9.5% black. The initial prevalence of metabolic syndrome was 39.2%. Overall, those with metabolic syndrome had a higher crude mortality rate than those without (32.7% versus 15.1%); $p < 0.01$ after 16.6 (4.2) years of follow-up. The mean sleep duration for the entire sample was 5.9 (1.3) h. There was a significant interaction between metabolic syndrome and objective sleep duration for mortality risk. The risk of cardiovascular mortality associated with metabolic syndrome as a function of objective short sleep duration was 1.49 (95% CI = 0.75–2.97) for subjects who slept ≥6 h/night and 2.10 (95% CI = 1.39–3.16) for those who slept <6 h per night [23].

The impact of work on sleep quality has been shown as a major contributor on occupational health disparities. For instance, the 2011–2012 US National Health and Nutrition Examination Survey (NHANES) compared the metabolic health of 260 long-haul truck drivers from North Carolina with the general population. The results showed that more years of driving and poorer quality sleep were statistically significant predictors for the higher cardiometabolic risk that was observed in the drivers [24]. In 39,182 male employees in Japan that were followed up for up to seven years, it was also found that short sleep duration and shift work were independently associated with the development of metabolic syndrome [25].

Numerous studies have also found that subjects with late chronotypes tend to have poorer metabolic health as compared with those with early chronotypes: They present more often with obesity [26–28], central repartition of adiposity [29,30], and with metabolic syndrome [19,30,31]. Indeed, in the Obesity, Nutrigenetics, Timing, and Mediterranean (ONTIME) study of 404 men and 1722 women, all of whom were overweight or obese, those with late chronotypes had higher BMI scores, higher triglycerides, lower HDL-cholesterol, higher levels of homeostasis model assessment for insulin resistance (HOMA-IR), and higher total metabolic syndrome scores [31].

In 1620 subjects derived from the Ansan cohort of the Korean Genome Epidemiology Study(KoGES), metabolic characteristics, body composition assessed by Dual-energy X-ray absorptiometry (DEXA), and visceral adiposity measured by computed tomography were collected and compared according to "morningness/eveningness" preference (Horne-Ostberg Morningness-Eveningness Questionnaire). In men, eveningness was associated with higher triglycerides levels but surprisingly lower systolic blood pressure. Anthropometrics measurements found less muscle mass in men with evening preference. In women, eveningness was associated with lower HDL-cholesterol and higher triglycerides and C-reactive protein (CRP) levels. Anthropometrics showed more visceral fat in women with evening preference [30].

Social jetlag, which is of greater amplitude in subjects with late chronotype, has also been independently linked with obesity [12,29] and metabolic disturbances [7]. However, few studies did not find such an association [32,33]. For instance, chronotype and social jetlag, objectively measured by wrist actimetry in 390 healthy young adults (21–35 years old), did not show any association with excess body weight, nor with elevated blood pressure [32].

2.3. Mechanisms of Action

Environmental cues, or "natural zeitgebers", like the alternation between day and night or cycles in external temperatures, usually synchronize circadian rhythms including patterns of rest and activity, food intake, and daily variations in metabolic fluxes and levels of hormones [34]. The timing of such patterns also varies with a normal distribution according to individuals' circadian preferences or chronotype. This normal distribution is in part dependent on genetic variations. In a twin study that measured circadian variations by wrist temperature, the results showed that between 46% and 70% of the observed circadian variance in temperatures could be attributed to genetic factors [35]. Three genome wide association studies (GWAS) performed in participants of European descent using data from the UK Biobank and the US genetics company 23andMe have also reported several single-nucleotide polymorphisms (SNPs) that are associated with chronotype [36–38]. Variations in other sleep characteristics, including sleep duration, have also been linked with polymorphisms at other loci [39].

However, sleep timing is also dependent upon extrinsic or "social zeitgebers" which may be related to work or leisure activities whose schedules conflict with intrinsic factors. A typical example of this conflict is found in shift workers: The work activities, food intake, and exposure to artificial lights at night cause a loss of internal synchrony and, in consequence, adverse effects on body weight and metabolism [40].

It has been shown that subjects with late chronotype have a tendency to eat less in the morning, while in the evening, they have higher global energy intakes and also higher intakes in sucrose, fat, and saturated fatty acids than subjects with morning chronotypes [41]. A daily caloric distribution with larger evening meals has been associated with a higher risk of obesity, particularly in those with evening chronotypes [42]. In patients with type 2 diabetes, late chronotypes have been associated with higher levels of glycated hemoglobin compared to early chronotypes and also with behaviors such as more frequently skipping breakfast [43]. Furthermore, food addiction, defined as an addictive behavior towards palatable foods, seems to be more frequent in subjects with late chronotype and is reported to be mediated by a higher frequency of insomnia and impulsivity [44]. Multiple studies have shown that an evening chronotype is associated with unhealthier diets and behaviors, such as smoking or drinking more alcohol [45–47]. People who are evening chronotypes are also more likely to be less physically active and to have more sedentary activities [45,47–49].

The role of gene variants that are associated with a latter chronotype to explain higher BMI and unfavorable metabolic traits has been evaluated in the GWAS based on UK-biobank data [37]. A reciprocal Mendelian randomization analysis, using a genetic risk score based on the 13 known variants of chronotype-linked genes, found no consistent evidence that early or late chronotypes led to higher BMI. This contrasts with another study that showed that a genetic risk score (GRS) for longer sleep duration was negatively associated with obesity [50].

The ONTIME study, reported by Vera et al. [31], addressed the question of the respective role gene versus behaviors to explain the deleterious metabolic profile of subjects with late chonotype. Firstly, the study showed that the GRS related to late chronotype, derived from GWAS studies, provided a reliable indication of subjects' circadian preferences. Second, the study identified that people with late chronotype had a higher metabolic risk score than people with an early chronotype. The analyses then showed that lifestyle factors, not chronotype GRS, underlay the relationship between evening chronotypes and metabolic alterations. Late chronotypes ate all three main meals later in the day, were more likely to have larger portion sizes, second helpings, to choose energy-dense foods, and to have a higher emotional eating score. However, evening types did not have a higher caloric intake, but they were less physically active and spent longer sitting down each day. These data therefore suggest that while the GRS can capture late chronotype, it does not associate with their metabolic risks. Metabolic alterations in people with late chronotype seem linked to unhealthy behaviors rather than to genetic predisposition.

Therefore, based on current knowledge, it seems that extrinsic factors linked to circadian preference, rather than intrinsic factors, are implicated in the cardiometabolic risk profile of an individual (Figure 1).

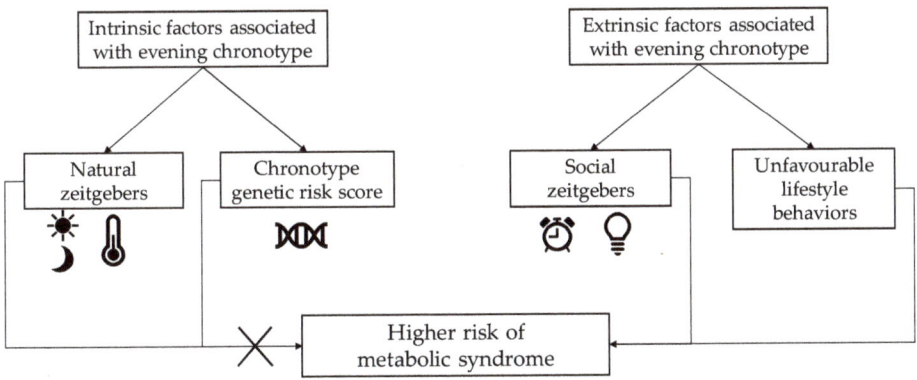

Figure 1. Schema showing the roles of intrinsic and extrinsic factors associated with evening chronotype in the risk of developing metabolic syndrome.

However, there are several data that suggest a gene–environment interaction between genetic traits that underlie our sleep characteristics and the risk of developing metabolic diseases under exposition to unhealthy food or physical inactivity. For instance, in the PREVIMED study, a significant association between the CLOCK-rs4580704 SNP and the risk of developing type 2 diabetes was observed after 4.8 years of follow-up. A gene–diet effect was found since only patients in the intervention group had a protective effect of the G variant for type 2 diabetes incidence and not the control group [51].

Dashti et al. [52] performed cross-sectional meta-analyses of population-based cohorts using data from the CHARGE (Cohorts for Heart and Aging Research in Genomic Epidemiology) Consortium. They studied whether dietary intake and sleep duration modified associations between five common circadian-related gene variants (CLOCK-rs1801260, CRY2-rs11605924, MTNR1B-rs1387153, MTNR1Brs10830963, and NR1D1-rs2314339) and glycemic traits, anthropometrics, and HDL-c levels. They found that higher intakes of carbohydrates and lower intakes of fat were linked to lower fasting glucose and HOMA-IR levels. Both short and long sleep durations were associated with higher fasting glucose levels, increased BMI, and greater waist circumference. Accordingly, known associations of selected SNPs on cardiometabolic traits were essentially replicated, but no diet–gene or sleep–gene interactions were found at the prespecified Bonferroni-corrected significance level of $p < 0.003$.

Thus, some evidence argues for a gene–environment interaction with circadian-related genes. It suggests a different metabolic answer to unhealthy behaviors as well as a different benefit from lifestyle interventions according to circadian genetic traits. If confirmed in further studies, such interactions will allow personalized risk prediction and personalized lifestyle intervention.

3. Obstructive Sleep Apnea and Metabolic Syndrome

3.1. Definition

Obstructive sleep apnea syndrome (OSAS) is caused by the complete or partial collapse of the pharynx repeatedly during sleep. These repeated collapses have four main consequences: desaturation–reoxygenation sequences, transitory episodes of hypercapnia, increased respiratory effort, and repeated micro-awakenings that end the respiratory event. Central obesity predisposes individuals to OSAS due to an infiltration of fat in the neck that causes upper airway collapse and increases abdominal pressure, leading to a reduction in lung volume. It has also been suggested that adipose tissue accumulation alters the neuromechanical control of the upper airway via the effects of leptin on central respiratory drive [5,53].

OSAS is defined as the presence of apnea (a 10-second interruption in airflow) and/or hypopnea (a ≤30% decrease in respiratory airflow with an associated oxygen desaturation >3% and/or micro-arousals). It is considered as mild if the Apnea–Hypopnea Index (AHI: the sum of the number of apnea and hypopnea events per hour) is between 5 and 14.9, as moderate if the score is between 15 and 29.9, and severe if the score is >30 events per hour. Clinical signs of OSAS include daytime fatigue and sleepiness, severe and daily snoring, reported sensations of choking or suffocation during sleep, nycturia, and morning headaches. The associated daytime loss of vigilance can be dangerous due to the risk of falling asleep while driving or at work [54,55]. It also causes cognitive disorders as a result of loss of attention, memory, and concentration [56].

3.2. Epidemiological Evidence Relating OSAS to Metabolic Syndrome

Metabolic syndrome and OSAS share a common risk factor, abdominal obesity, and 50%–60% of people with metabolic syndrome also have OSAS [57,58]. However, studies have also shown an association, independent of obesity, between OSAS and cardiometabolic risk factors, including hypertension [59], insulin resistance [60], and type 2 diabetes [61]. OSAS has been found to be associated with metabolic syndrome in several case-control and cross-sectional studies: A meta-analysis of 13 studies ($n = 7934$ subjects) reported an increased risk of metabolic syndrome in patients with OSAS with a pooled odds ratio (OR) of 1.72 (95% CI: 1.31–2.26, $p < 0.001$) and with a BMI-adjusted pooled OR of 1.97 (95% CI: 1.34–2.88, $p < 0.001$) [62].

A recent cohort study evaluated the influence of OSAS on the incidence of metabolic syndrome in a multiethnic sample of 1853 people from two population-based samples (Episono in Brazil and

HypnoLaus in Switzerland) [63]. Participants included in the analysis were mainly female (56%) and Caucasian (88%), with an average age of 51.9 (±13.1) years and a BMI of 24.9 (±3.7) kg/m^2. The mean follow-up duration was 5.9 (±1.3) years, and 17.2% developed a metabolic syndrome during this time. The OR for developing metabolic syndrome when having moderate-to-severe OSAS was 2.245 (95%CI: 1.214 - 4.149), $p = 0.010$) after adjustments for cohort, age, BMI, and the number of metabolic syndrome components present at baseline. Of note, to assess whether the relationship between OSAS and metabolic syndrome could be bidirectional, a subset analysis was performed on 547 participants free of OSAS at baseline from the Episono cohort. After adjustment for sex, age, and baseline AHI and BMI, metabolic syndrome was not found a significant predictor of incident OSAS.

3.3. Mechanism of Action

The immediate consequences of OSAS-related respiratory events are intermittent hypoxia and fragmented sleep. These intermittent hypoxic respiratory events lead to the development of chronic adaptative mechanisms.

Studies in animals and humans have shown that intermittent exposure to hypoxia leads to sympathetic hyperactivity [64,65], to systemic and vascular inflammation via NFkB [66–69], to oxidative stress [70], and to pro-inflammatory stimulation of the adipose tissue via hypoxia and hypoxia inducible factor 1 (HIF-1) [71,72]. Sleep fragmentation also disrupts the nychthemeral cycle of cortisol secretion and the somatotropic axis, leading to an increase in nocturnal cortisol and a decrease in IGF-1 [73–76].

These mechanisms are involved in the development of insulin resistance, endothelial dysfunction, and vascular remodeling that is characterized by increased arterial rigidity. OSAS also alters the nictemeral cycle of arterial pressure: Patients lose the normal nocturnal reduction in arterial pressure of 10%–20% in comparison to daytime pressure, and this is responsible for the so-called 'non-dipper' or 'reverse dipper' blood pressure profile [49–51] which can evolve toward permanent, 24 h hypertension [54–56].

The above mechanisms may, at least in part, explain the development of cardiometabolic abnormalities in patients with OSAS. Nevertheless, the relationship between the two disorders is bidirectional (Figure 2): Visceral adiposity is strongly associated with development of OSAS. Central obesity, as described above, is associated with an increase in neck fat infiltration that reduces upper airway volume. Excess intraabdominal fat accumulation increases abdominal pressure, leading to lung volume reduction [5]. In addition to these mechanical effects, visceral adiposity generates low-grade inflammation [77]. Visceral fat adipocytes secrete low levels of TNF-alpha, which then stimulates preadipocytes and surrounding endothelial cells to produce monocyte chemoattract protein-1 (MCP-1). MCP-1, in turn, promotes macrophage recruitment and adhesion to endothelial cells [78] where they secrete proinflammatory cytokines like TNF-alpha, IL-6, and IL-1b, which results in increased plasma C-reactive protein (CRP).

It has been shown that anti-inflammatory therapy can modestly reduce OSAS severity in the absence of other treatments: A placebo-controlled, double-blind study of eight men with obesity and severe OSAS found that a three-week trial of the TNF-alpha antagonist etanercept significantly reduced AHI, IL-6 levels, and objectively measured daytime sleepiness [79]. These data therefore suggest systemic inflammation plays a role in the pathogenesis of OSAS.

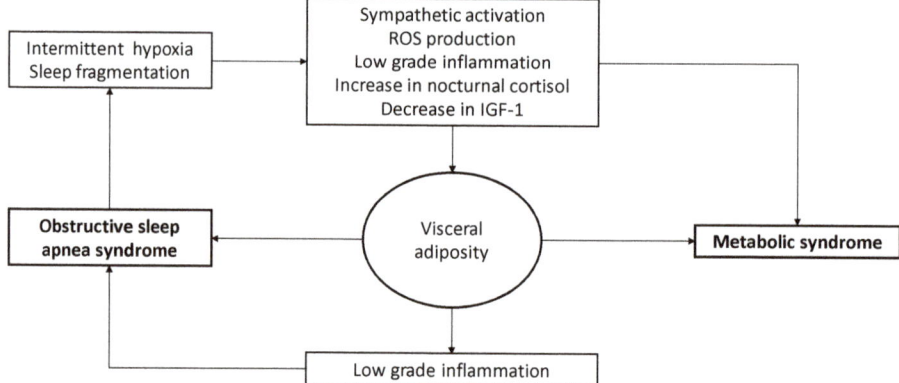

Figure 2. Bidirectional relationship between obstructive sleep apnea syndrome and metabolic syndrome. ROS, reactive oxygen species; IGF-1, insulin-like growth factor 1.

4. Sleep as a Component of a Comprehensive Lifestyle Intervention

4.1. First Steps of Chronotherapy as a Lifestyle Intervention

With regard to the timing of food intake, people with an evening chronotype have a later intake of all three main meals. The timing and daily distribution of this energy intake has been linked to a deleterious cardiometabolic risk profile, as described above. Thus, emerging evidence suggests that meal timing (when) is a dimension of dietary intake that matters, in addition to meal composition (what) and eating behaviors (how) [31,80].

Few works have studied the role of food intake timing. One study that included 32 young, normal weight women in a randomized, crossover protocol compared two different lunch-eating conditions: early lunch eating at 13:00 and late lunch eating at 16:30 [81]. Breakfast, lunch, and dinner composition were standardized. Those who ate lunch later had a lower pre-meal resting energy expenditure and glucose tolerance. Early eating, by contrast, was associated with improved circadian cortisol and temperature profiles.

A second study recruited eight overweight individuals who had an average eating duration (time range between the first and last daily food intake) >14 h [82]. The study consisted in a 16-week pilot intervention where participants were asked to restrict their eating duration to a self-selected window of 10–12 h and then to maintain this pattern during both weekdays and weekends to minimize metabolic jetlag. After 16 weeks, the participants had successfully reduced their eating time range and had lost a mean of 3.3 kg (95% CI: 0.9–5.6). Unexpectedly, they also reported greater sleep satisfaction. These results were maintained one year after the intervention. Thus, it appeared that changing the timing of meals not only may affect body weight, resting energy expenditure, and metabolic health but that it may also improve sleep quality.

Fewer studies have investigated the cardiometabolic effect of interventions aiming at improving sleep. A recent review [83] found only seven studies using a variety of interventions to extend sleep that also described the effects of this sleep extension on at least one cardiometabolic risk factor. The research was conducted in both subjects who were healthy and those who were hypertensive. Most had short sleep, although in one study, the subjects had normal sleep ($n = 14$). The interventions were short-term, lasting from 3 days to 6 weeks. These interventions were successful to increase sleep duration from 21 to 177 min. In intervention arms, subjects reported a reduction in their overall appetite, a decreased desire for sweet and salty foods, a lowered daily intake of free sugar, and less caloric intake from protein. Metabolically, insulin sensitivity improved in two studies [84,85].

An additional cross-over study, published since that review, included 21 nondiabetic subjects that usually slept <6 h per night. In the intention-to-treat analysis, the sleep extension group had their sleep extended by 36.0 (45.2) min. There was no improvement in plasma glucose/insulin homeostasis (as measured by oral glucose tolerance tests), but per-protocol analysis of the eight subjects who achieved a sleep duration >6 h during the sleep extension phase showed that sleep extension was associated with improved insulin sensitivity and insulin secretion [86].

Finally, physical activity has also been proven to have a positive impact on both sleep quality and sleep latency, the time in bed before falling asleep, without changing sleep duration [87]. It appears that the timing of physical activity is also important with regard to the cardiometabolic benefit: For instance, postprandial glucose increases were lower if patients with type 2 diabetes carried out physical activity after meals rather than before [88,89]. Thus, the introduction of chronotherapy in either diet or physical activity interventions could improve the cardiometabolic benefits. These interventions do not only change the targeted behavior but also have a positive impact on other behaviors: Changing food timing and increasing physical activity improve sleep quality and promoting sleep extension positively impacts food choices.

4.2. Effect of OSAS Treatment

Continuous positive airway pressure (CPAP) is currently the main treatment for moderate-to-severe OSAS. CPAP provides a pneumatic splint to prevent pharyngeal collapse, and it must be applied to the upper airways via a nasal or oronasal mask for ≥4 h per night in order to achieve its therapeutic goals [90]. The beneficial effects of CPAP on daily sleepiness and quality of life have been clearly demonstrated in patients with moderate-to-severe forms of OSAS [91].

Whereas the severity of OSAS is clearly parallel to the severity of excess weight [92], CPAP treatment in itself does not allow body weight reduction and was even associated with a small increase in body weight in a meta-analysis of randomized controlled trials (RCTs) [93]. Accordingly, CPAP did not impact visceral adiposity accumulation or body composition in a three-month RCT [94].

Regarding the cardiometabolic impact of CPAP treatment, the most robust evidence is related to blood pressure. Regular CPAP therapy results in modest reductions in blood pressure [95]. This is supported by a recent meta-analysis that pooled the results of 24 h recordings from five randomized trials and found a reduction in systolic and diastolic blood pressure of 4.78 mmHg (IC95%: −7.95 to −1.61) and 2.95 mmHg (IC 95%: −5.37 to −0.53), respectively, in patients with resistant hypertension who had been treated with CPAP [96]. CPAP also modestly improves insulin sensitivity. This was shown in a meta-analysis that included 12 observational studies: CPAP significantly improved the HOMA-IR index [97]. A modest, but significant, effect on insulin sensitivity was also found in a meta-analysis that included 244 patients without diabetes in five RCTs that compared the effects of CPAP and a placebo treatment applied between 6 weeks and 6 months [94,98–100]. In patients with type 2 diabetes, CPAP did not improve HbA1c in RCTs, although there was some evidence to suggest that CPAP decreased nocturnal glucose levels and insulin sensitivity [61].

The hypothesis that CPAP might reduce the rate of cardiovascular events was tested in four RCTs. The results all showed that CPAP did not impact the rate of cardiovascular events. This finding was further confirmed by a meta-analysis of 10 RCTs which involved comparison of CPAP to placebo treatments in studies with various main objectives, not only those related to cardiovascular events [101].

Despite the neutral or slightly negative effect of CPAP on body weight per se, it has been suggested that CPAP treatment could be a useful adjunct to improve the overall success of a lifestyle intervention. For example, a diet and physical activity intervention aimed at viscerally obese men (an ancillary study of the SYNERGY trial) found that those who did not have sleep apnea had all-round better results following the intervention than men who had presented with untreated apnea. Despite a similar level of adherence to the diet and physical activity recommendations, the men with apnea showed smaller reductions in BMI, waist circumference, and plasma triglycerides as well as smaller increases in HDL cholesterol and adiponectin [102].

Chirinos et al. [103] have treated people having OSAS by CPAP, weight loss intervention or both combined. When both interventions were cumulated, an incremental reduction in insulin resistance and serum triglyceride levels was obtained compared to weight loss intervention alone. In addition, providing a good adherence to a regimen of weight loss and CPAP resulted in incremental reductions in blood pressure as compared to either intervention alone.

5. Conclusions

This review provides evidence that sleep matters in terms of cardiometabolic health, and more specifically, metabolic syndrome. Sleep deprivation, behaviors linked to an evening chronotype, and social jetlag impact food timing, food preference, and food behavior. In addition, when an individual does not respect their own intrinsic circadian rhythm of rest and activity, dysregulation of hormonal and metabolic regulations occurs, and this strongly contributes to the development of metabolic syndrome.

In addition to sleep habits, the metabolic consequences of OSAS also contribute to metabolic syndrome: Both conditions are linked by a bidirectional autoaggravating relationship through the excess of visceral fat. Central obesity promotes sleep apnea through mechanical action and low-grade inflammation, while OSAS promotes metabolic syndrome through sympathetic nervous overactivity, reactive oxygen production, low-grade inflammation, and alterations in cortisol and IGF-1 circadian fluctuations.

From these observations, sleep has emerged as a relevant lifestyle factor that needs to be addressed along with diet and physical activity as part of a holistic treatment plan for those with metabolic syndrome. Recent intervention studies have demonstrated that improving one behavior, be it diet, physical activity or sleep, may positively impact the others. Early research on the first interventions targeting sleep extension or food timing seem promising. Further interventional studies should address comprehensive interventions, including chronotherapy through sleep, food, and physical activity timing. Personalized behavioral interventions should be tested in subjects with metabolic syndrome, based on their specific diet and physical activity habits, but also according to their circadian preference.

Funding: This research received no external funding.

Acknowledgments: I thank J.R. and J.D.P. for English revision.

Conflicts of Interest: The author declares no conflict of interest.

References

1. Alberti, K.G.; Eckel, R.H.; Grundy, S.M.; Zimmet, P.Z.; Cleeman, J.I.; Donato, K.A.; Fruchart, J.C.; James, W.P.; Loria, C.M.; Smith, S.C., Jr. Harmonizing the Metabolic Syndrome: A Joint Interim Statement of the International Diabetes Federation Task Force on Epidemiology and Prevention; National Heart, Lung, and Blood Institute; American Heart Association; World Heart Federation; International Atherosclerosis Society; and International Association for the Study of Obesity. *Circulation* **2009**, *120*, 1640–1645.
2. Sperling, L.S.; Mechanick, J.I.; Neeland, I.J.; Herrick, C.J.; Despres, J.P.; Ndumele, C.E.; Vijayaraghavan, K.; Handelsman, Y.; Puckrein, G.A.; Araneta, M.R.; et al. The CardioMetabolic Health Alliance: Working Toward a New Care Model for the Metabolic Syndrome. *J. Am. Coll. Cardiol.* **2015**, *66*, 1050–1067. [CrossRef] [PubMed]
3. Despres, J.P.; Lemieux, I. Abdominal Obesity and Metabolic Syndrome. *Nature* **2006**, *444*, 881–887. [CrossRef] [PubMed]
4. Neeland, I.J.; Poirier, P.; Despres, J.P. Cardiovascular and Metabolic Heterogeneity of Obesity: Clinical Challenges and Implications for Management. *Circulation* **2018**, *137*, 1391–1406. [CrossRef] [PubMed]
5. Levy, P.; Kohler, M.; McNicholas, W.T.; Barb, F.; Mcevoy, R.D.; Somers, V.K.; Lavie, L.; Pepin, J.L. Obstructive Sleep Apnoea Syndrome. *Nat. Rev. Dis. Primers* **2015**, *1*, 15015. [CrossRef] [PubMed]
6. Larcher, S.; Benhamou, P.Y.; Pepin, J.L.; Borel, A.L. Sleep Habits and Diabetes. *Diabetes Metab.* **2015**, *41*, 263–271. [CrossRef]
7. Larcher, S.; Gauchez, A.S.; Lablanche, S.; Pepin, J.L.; Benhamou, P.Y.; Borel, A.L. Impact of Sleep Behavior on Glycemic Control in Type 1 Diabetes: The Role of Social Jetlag. *Eur. J. Endocrinol.* **2016**, *175*, 411–419. [CrossRef]

8. Baehr, E.K.; Revelle, W.; Eastman, C.I. Individual Differences in the Phase and Amplitude of the Human Circadian Temperature Rhythm: With an Emphasis on Morningness-Eveningness. *J. Sleep Res.* **2000**, *9*, 117–127. [CrossRef]
9. Roenneberg, T.; Kuehnle, T.; Juda, M.; Kantermann, T.; Allebrandt, K.; Gordijn, M.; Merrow, M. Epidemiology of the Human Circadian Clock. *Sleep Med. Rev.* **2007**, *11*, 429–438. [CrossRef]
10. Roenneberg, T.; Wirz-Justice, A.; Merrow, M. Life between Clocks: Daily Temporal Patterns of Human Chronotypes. *J. Biol. Rhythm.* **2003**, *18*, 80–90. [CrossRef]
11. Horne, J.A.; Ostberg, O. A Self-Assessment Questionnaire to Determine Morningness-Eveningness in Human Circadian Rhythms. *Int. J. Chronobiol.* **1976**, *4*, 97–110. [PubMed]
12. Roenneberg, T.; Allebrandt, K.V.; Merrow, M.; Vetter, C. Social Jetlag and Obesity. *Curr. Biol.* **2012**, *22*, 939–943. [CrossRef] [PubMed]
13. Knutson, K.L.; Van Cauter, E.; Rathouz, P.J.; DeLeire, T.; Lauderdale, D.S. Trends in the Prevalence of Short Sleepers in the USA: 1975–2006. *Sleep* **2010**, *33*, 37–45. [CrossRef] [PubMed]
14. Cappuccio, F.P.; Taggart, F.M.; Kandala, N.B.; Currie, A.; Peile, E.; Stranges, S.; Miller, M.A. Meta-Analysis of Short Sleep Duration and Obesity in Children and Adults. *Sleep* **2008**, *31*, 619–626. [CrossRef]
15. Miller, M.A.; Kruisbrink, M.; Wallace, J.; Ji, C.; Cappuccio, F.P. Sleep Duration and Incidence of Obesity in Infants, Children, and Adolescents: A Systematic Review and Meta-Analysis of Prospective Studies. *Sleep* **2018**, *41*. [CrossRef]
16. Magee, L.; Hale, L. Longitudinal Associations between Sleep Duration and Subsequent Weight Gain: A Systematic Review. *Sleep Med. Rev.* **2012**, *16*, 231–241. [CrossRef]
17. Xi, B.; He, D.; Zhang, M.; Xue, J.; Zhou, D. Short Sleep Duration Predicts Risk of Metabolic Syndrome: A Systematic Review and Meta-Analysis. *Sleep Med. Rev.* **2014**, *18*, 293–297. [CrossRef]
18. Pulido-Arjona, L.; Correa-Bautista, J.E.; Agostinis-Sobrinho, C.; Mota, J.; Santos, R.; Correa-Rodriguez, M.; Garcia-Hermoso, A.; Ramirez-Velez, R. Role of Sleep Duration and Sleep-Related Problems in the Metabolic Syndrome Among Children and Adolescents. *Ital. J. Pediatr.* **2018**, *44*, 9. [CrossRef]
19. Lucas-De La Cruz, L.; Martin-Espinosa, N.; Cavero-Redondo, I.; Gonzalez-Garcia, A.; Diez-Fernandez, A.; Martinez-Vizcaino, V.; Notario-Pacheco, B. Sleep Patterns and Cardiometabolic Risk in Schoolchildren from Cuenca, Spain. *PLoS ONE* **2018**, *13*, e0191637. [CrossRef]
20. Deng, H.B.; Tam, T.; Zee, B.C.; Chung, R.Y.; Su, X.; Jin, L.; Chan, T.C.; Chang, L.Y.; Yeoh, E.K.; Lao, X.Q. Short Sleep Duration Increases Metabolic Impact in Healthy Adults: A Population-Based Cohort Study. *Sleep* **2017**, *40*. [CrossRef]
21. Kim, J.Y.; Yadav, D.; Ahn, S.V.; Koh, S.B.; Park, J.T.; Yoon, J.; Yoo, B.S.; Lee, S.H. A Prospective Study of Total Sleep Duration and Incident Metabolic Syndrome: The ARIRANG Study. *Sleep Med.* **2015**, *16*, 1511–1515. [CrossRef] [PubMed]
22. Song, Q.; Liu, X.; Zhou, W.; Wang, X.; Wu, S. Changes in sleep Duration and Risk of Metabolic Syndrome: The Kailuan Prospective Study. *Sci. Rep.* **2016**, *6*, 36861. [CrossRef] [PubMed]
23. Fernandez-Mendoza, J.; He, F.; LaGrotte, C.; Vgontzas, A.N.; Liao, D.; Bixler, E.O. Impact of the Metabolic Syndrome on Mortality is Modified by Objective Short Sleep Duration. *J. Am. Heart Assoc.* **2017**, *6*. [CrossRef] [PubMed]
24. Hege, A.; Lemke, M.K.; Apostolopoulos, Y.; Sonmez, S. Occupational Health Disparities among U.S. long-Haul Truck Drivers: The Influence of Work Organization and Sleep on Cardiovascular and Metabolic Disease Risk. *PLoS ONE* **2018**, *13*, e0207322. [CrossRef] [PubMed]
25. Itani, O.; Kaneita, Y.; Tokiya, M.; Jike, M.; Murata, A.; Nakagome, S.; Otsuka, Y.; Ohida, T. Short Sleep Duration, Shift Work, and Actual Days Taken off Work are Predictive Life-Style Risk Factors for New-Onset Metabolic Syndrome: A Seven-Year Cohort Study of 40,000 Male Workers. *Sleep Med.* **2017**, *39*, 87–94. [CrossRef] [PubMed]
26. Maukonen, M.; Kanerva, N.; Partonen, T.; Mannisto, S. Chronotype and Energy Intake Timing in Relation to Changes in Anthropometrics: A 7-Year Follow-Up Study in Adults. *Chronobiol. Int.* **2019**, *36*, 27–41. [CrossRef]
27. Zhang, Y.; Xiong, Y.; Dong, J.; Guo, T.; Tang, X.; Zhao, Y. Caffeinated Drinks Intake, Late Chronotype, and Increased Body Mass Index among Medical Students in Chongqing, China: A Multiple Mediation Model. *Int. J. Environ. Res. Public Health* **2018**, *15*, 1721. [CrossRef]

28. Ruiz-Lozano, T.; Vidal, J.; De Hollanda, A.; Canteras, M.; Garaulet, M.; Izquierdo-Pulido, M. Evening Chronotype Associates with Obesity in Severely Obese Subjects: Interaction with CLOCK 3111T/C. *Int. J. Obes.* **2016**, *40*, 1550–1557. [CrossRef]
29. Malone, S.K.; Zemel, B.; Compher, C.; Souders, M.; Chittams, J.; Thompson, A.L.; Pack, A.; Lipman, T.H. Social Jet Lag, Chronotype and Body Mass Index in 14–17-Year-Old Adolescents. *Chronobiol. Int.* **2016**, *33*, 1255–1266. [CrossRef]
30. Yu, J.H.; Yun, C.H.; Ahn, J.H.; Suh, S.; Cho, H.J.; Lee, S.K.; Yoo, H.J.; Seo, J.A.; Kim, S.G.; Choi, K.M.; et al. Evening Chronotype is Associated with Metabolic Disorders and Body Composition in Middle-Aged Adults. *J. Clin. Endocrinol. Metab.* **2015**, *100*, 1494–1502. [CrossRef]
31. Vera, B.; Dashti, H.S.; Gomez-Abellan, P.; Hernandez-Martinez, A.M.; Esteban, A.; Scheer, F.; Saxena, R.; Garaulet, M. Modifiable Lifestyle Behaviors, but not a Genetic Risk Score, Associate with Metabolic Syndrome in Evening Chronotypes. *Sci. Rep.* **2018**, *8*, 945. [CrossRef] [PubMed]
32. McMahon, D.M.; Burch, J.B.; Youngstedt, S.D.; Wirth, M.D.; Hardin, J.W.; Hurley, T.G.; Blair, S.N.; Hand, G.A.; Shook, R.P.; Drenowatz, C.; et al. Relationships between Chronotype, Social Jetlag, Sleep, Obesity and Blood Pressure in Healthy Young Adults. *Chronobiol. Int.* **2019**, *36*, 493–509. [CrossRef] [PubMed]
33. Marinac, C.R.; Quante, M.; Mariani, S.; Weng, J.; Redline, S.; Cespedes Feliciano, E.M.; Hipp, J.A.; Wang, D.; Kaplan, E.R.; James, P.; et al. Associations between Timing of Meals, Physical Activity, Light Exposure, and Sleep With Body Mass Index in Free-Living Adults. *J. Phys. Act. Health* **2019**, *16*, 214–221. [CrossRef] [PubMed]
34. Yetish, G.; Kaplan, H.; Gurven, M.; Wood, B.; Pontzer, H.; Manger, P.R.; Wilson, C.; McGregor, R.; Siegel, J.M. Natural Sleep and its Seasonal Variations in Three Pre-Industrial Societies. *Curr. Biol.* **2015**, *25*, 2862–2868. [CrossRef]
35. Lopez-Minguez, J.; Ordonana, J.R.; Sanchez-Romera, J.F.; Madrid, J.A.; Garaulet, M. Circadian System Heritability as Assessed by Wrist Temperature: A Twin Study. *Chronobiol. Int.* **2015**, *32*, 71–80. [CrossRef]
36. Lane, J.M.; Vlasac, I.; Anderson, S.G.; Kyle, S.D.; Dixon, W.G.; Bechtold, D.A.; Gill, S.; Little, M.A.; Luik, A.; Loudon, A.; et al. Genome-Wide Association Analysis Identifies Novel Loci for Chronotype in 100,420 Individuals from the UK Biobank. *Nat. Commun.* **2016**, *7*, 10889. [CrossRef]
37. Jones, S.E.; Tyrrell, J.; Wood, A.R.; Beaumont, R.N.; Ruth, K.S.; Tuke, M.A.; Yaghootkar, H.; Hu, Y.; Teder-Laving, M.; Hayward, C.; et al. Genome-Wide Association Analyses in 128,266 Individuals Identifies New Morningness and Sleep Duration Loci. *PLoS Genet.* **2016**, *12*, e1006125. [CrossRef]
38. Hu, Y.; Shmygelska, A.; Tran, D.; Eriksson, N.; Tung, J.Y.; Hinds, D.A. GWAS of 89,283 Individuals Identifies Genetic Variants Associated with Self-Reporting of being a Morning Person. *Nat. Commun.* **2016**, *7*, 10448. [CrossRef]
39. Goel, N. Genetic Markers of Sleep and Sleepiness. *Sleep Med. Clin.* **2017**, *12*, 289–299. [CrossRef]
40. Guerrero-Vargas, N.N.; Espitia-Bautista, E.; Buijs, R.M.; Escobar, C. Shift-Work: Is Time of Eating Determining Metabolic Health? Evidence from Animal Models. *Proc. Nutr. Soc.* **2018**, *77*, 199–215. [CrossRef]
41. Maukonen, M.; Kanerva, N.; Partonen, T.; Kronholm, E.; Tapanainen, H.; Kontto, J.; Mannisto, S. Chronotype Differences in Timing of Energy and Macronutrient Intakes: A Population-Based Study in Adults. *Obesity* **2017**, *25*, 608–615. [CrossRef] [PubMed]
42. Xiao, Q.; Garaulet, M.; Scheer, F. Meal Timing and Obesity: Interactions with Macronutrient Intake and Chronotype. *Int. J. Obes.* **2019**, *43*, 1701–1711. [CrossRef] [PubMed]
43. Reutrakul, S.; Hood, M.M.; Crowley, S.J.; Morgan, M.K.; Teodori, M.; Knutson, K.L. The Relationship between Breakfast Skipping, Chronotype, and Glycemic Control in Type 2 Diabetes. *Chronobiol. Int.* **2014**, *31*, 64–71. [CrossRef] [PubMed]
44. Kandeger, A.; Selvi, Y.; Tanyer, D.K. The Effects of Individual Circadian Rhythm Differences on Insomnia, Impulsivity, and Food Addiction. *Eat. Weight Disord.* **2019**, *24*, 47–55. [CrossRef]
45. Maukonen, M.; Kanerva, N.; Partonen, T.; Kronholm, E.; Konttinen, H.; Wennman, H.; Mannisto, S. The Associations between Chronotype, a Healthy Diet and Obesity. *Chronobiol. Int.* **2016**, *33*, 972–981. [CrossRef] [PubMed]
46. Mota, M.C.; Waterhouse, J.; De-Souza, D.A.; Rossato, L.T.; Silva, C.M.; Araujo, M.B.; Tufik, S.; De Mello, M.T.; Crispim, C.A. Association between Chronotype, Food Intake and Physical Activity in Medical Residents. *Chronobiol. Int.* **2016**, *33*, 730–739. [CrossRef] [PubMed]

47. Patterson, F.; Malone, S.K.; Lozano, A.; Grandner, M.A.; Hanlon, A.L. Smoking, Screen-Based Sedentary Behavior, and Diet Associated with Habitual Sleep Duration and Chronotype: Data from the UK Biobank. *Ann. Behav. Med.* **2016**, *50*, 715–726. [CrossRef]
48. Wennman, H.; Kronholm, E.; Partonen, T.; Peltonen, M.; Vasankari, T.; Borodulin, K. Evening Typology and Morning Tiredness Associates with Low Leisure Time Physical Activity and High Sitting. *Chronobiol. Int.* **2015**, *32*, 1090–1100. [CrossRef]
49. Olds, T.S.; Maher, C.A.; Matricciani, L. Sleep Duration or Bedtime? Exploring the Relationship between Sleep Habits and Weight Status and Activity Patterns. *Sleep* **2011**, *34*, 1299–1307. [CrossRef]
50. Dashti, H.S.; Redline, S.; Saxena, R. Polygenic Risk Score Identifies Associations between Sleep Duration and Diseases Determined from an Electronic Medical Record Biobank. *Sleep* **2019**, *42*. [CrossRef]
51. Corella, D.; Asensio, E.M.; Coltell, O.; Sorli, J.V.; Estruch, R.; Martinez-Gonzalez, M.A.; Salas-Salvado, J.; Castaner, O.; Aros, F.; Lapetra, J.; et al. CLOCK Gene Variation is Associated with Incidence of Type-2 Diabetes and Cardiovascular Diseases in Type-2 Diabetic Subjects: Dietary Modulation in the PREDIMED Randomized Trial. *Cardiovasc. Diabetol.* **2016**, *15*, 4. [CrossRef] [PubMed]
52. Dashti, H.S.; Follis, J.L.; Smith, C.E.; Tanaka, T.; Garaulet, M.; Gottlieb, D.J.; Hruby, A.; Jacques, P.F.; Kiefte-De Jong, J.C.; Lamon-Fava, S.; et al. Gene-Environment Interactions of Circadian-Related Genes for Cardiometabolic Traits. *Diabetes Care* **2015**, *38*, 1456–1466. [CrossRef] [PubMed]
53. Balachandran, J.S.; Patel, S.R. In the Clinic. Obstructive Sleep Apnea. *Ann. Intern. Med.* **2014**, *161*. [CrossRef] [PubMed]
54. Tregear, S.; Reston, J.; Schoelles, K.; Phillips, B. Obstructive Sleep Apnea and Risk of Motor Vehicle Crash: Systematic Review and Meta-Analysis. *J. Clin. Sleep Med.* **2009**, *5*, 573–581. [PubMed]
55. Mulgrew, A.T.; Nasvadi, G.; Butt, A.; Cheema, R.; Fox, N.; Fleetham, J.A.; Ryan, C.F.; Cooper, P.; Ayas, N.T. Risk and Severity of Motor Vehicle Crashes in Patients with Obstructive Sleep Apnoea/Hypopnoea. *Thorax* **2008**, *63*, 536–541. [CrossRef] [PubMed]
56. Mazza, S.; Pepin, J.L.; Naegele, B.; Rauch, E.; Deschaux, C.; Ficheux, P.; Levy, P. Driving Ability in Sleep Apnoea Patients before and after CPAP Treatment: Evaluation on a Road Safety Platform. *Eur. Respir. J.* **2006**, *28*, 1020–1028. [CrossRef]
57. Drager, L.F.; Togeiro, S.M.; Polotsky, V.Y.; Lorenzi-Filho, G. Obstructive Sleep Apnea: A Cardiometabolic Risk in Obesity and the Metabolic Syndrome. *J. Am. Coll. Cardiol.* **2013**, *62*, 569–576. [CrossRef]
58. Resta, O.; Foschino-Barbaro, M.P.; Legari, G.; Talamo, S.; Bonfitto, P.; Palumbo, A.; Minenna, A.; Giorgino, R.; De Pergola, G. Sleep-Related Breathing Disorders, Loud Snoring and Excessive Daytime Sleepiness in Obese Subjects. *Int. J. Obes. Relat. Metab. Disord.* **2001**, *25*, 669–675. [CrossRef]
59. Pepin, J.L.; Borel, A.L.; Tamisier, R.; Baguet, J.P.; Levy, P.; Dauvilliers, Y. Hypertension and Sleep: Overview of a Tight Relationship. *Sleep Med. Rev.* **2014**, *18*, 509–599. [CrossRef]
60. Borel, A.L.; Monneret, D.; Tamisier, R.; Baguet, J.P.; Faure, P.; Levy, P.; Halimi, S.; Pepin, J.L. The Severity of Nocturnal Hypoxia but not Abdominal Adiposity is Associated with Insulin Resistance in non-Obese Men with Sleep Apnea. *PLoS ONE* **2013**, *8*, e71000. [CrossRef]
61. Borel, A.L.; Tamisier, R.; Bohme, P.; Priou, P.; Avignon, A.; Benhamou, P.Y.; Hanaire, H.; Pepin, J.L.; Kessler, L.; Valensi, P.; et al. Obstructive Sleep Apnoea Syndrome in Patients Living with Diabetes: Which Patients should be Screened? *Diabetes Metab.* **2018**. [CrossRef] [PubMed]
62. Qian, Y.; Xu, H.; Wang, Y.; Yi, H.; Guan, J.; Yin, S. Obstructive Sleep Apnea Predicts Risk of Metabolic Syndrome Independently of Obesity: A Meta-Analysis. *Arch. Med. Sci.* **2016**, *12*, 1077–1087. [CrossRef] [PubMed]
63. Hirotsu, C.; Haba-Rubio, J.; Togeiro, S.M.; Marques-Vidal, P.; Drager, L.F.; Vollenweider, P.; Waeber, G.; Bittencourt, L.; Tufik, S.; Heinzer, R. Obstructive Sleep Apnoea as a Risk Factor for Incident Metabolic Syndrome: A Joined Episono and HypnoLaus Prospective Cohorts Study. *Eur. Respir. J.* **2018**, *52*. [CrossRef] [PubMed]
64. Fletcher, E.C. Sympathetic over Activity in the Etiology of Hypertension of Obstructive Sleep Apnea. *Sleep* **2003**, *26*, 15–19. [CrossRef]
65. Somers, V.K.; Dyken, M.E.; Clary, M.P.; Abboud, F.M. Sympathetic Neural Mechanisms in Obstructive Sleep Apnea. *J. Clin. Investig.* **1995**, *96*, 1897–1904. [CrossRef]
66. Ryan, S.; Mc Nicholas, W.T. Intermittent Hypoxia and Activation of Inflammatory Molecular Pathways in OSAS. *Arch. Physiol. Biochem.* **2008**, *114*, 261–266. [CrossRef]

67. Ryan, S.; Taylor, C.T.; Mc Nicholas, W.T. Selective Activation of Inflammatory Pathways by Intermittent Hypoxia in Obstructive Sleep Apnea Syndrome. *Circulation* **2005**, *112*, 2660–2667. [CrossRef]
68. Ryan, S.; Taylor, C.T.; Mc Nicholas, W.T. Systemic Inflammation: A Key Factor in the Pathogenesis of Cardiovascular Complications in Obstructive Sleep Apnoea Syndrome? *Thorax* **2009**, *64*, 631–636. [CrossRef]
69. Arnaud, C.; Beguin, P.C.; Lantuejoul, S.; Pepin, J.L.; Guillermet, C.; Pelli, G.; Burger, F.; Buatois, V.; Ribuot, C.; Baguet, J.P.; et al. The Inflammatory Preatherosclerotic Remodeling Induced by Intermittent Hypoxia is Attenuated by RANTES/CCL5 inhibition. *Am. J. Respir. Crit. Care. Med.* **2011**, *184*, 724–731. [CrossRef]
70. Jelic, S.; Padeletti, M.; Kawut, S.M.; Higgins, C.; Canfield, S.M.; Onat, D.; Colombo, P.C.; Basner, R.C.; Factor, P.; LeJemtel, T.H. Inflammation, Oxidative Stress, and Repair Capacity of the Vascular Endothelium in Obstructive Sleep Apnea. *Circulation* **2008**, *117*, 2270–2278. [CrossRef]
71. Lee, Y.S.; Kim, J.W.; Osborne, O.; Oh, D.Y.; Sasik, R.; Schenk, S.; Chen, A.; Chung, H.; Murphy, A.; Watkins, S.M.; et al. Increased Adipocyte O_2 Consumption Triggers HIF-1alpha, Causing Inflammation and Insulin Resistance in Obesity. *Cell* **2014**, *157*, 1339–1352. [CrossRef] [PubMed]
72. Poulain, L.; Thomas, A.; Rieusset, J.; Casteilla, L.; Levy, P.; Arnaud, C.; Dematteis, M. Visceral white Fat Remodelling Contributes to Intermittent Hypoxia-Induced Atherogenesis. *Eur. Respir. J.* **2014**, *43*, 513–522. [CrossRef] [PubMed]
73. Leproult, R.; Copinschi, G.; Buxton, O.; Van Cauter, E. Sleep Loss Results in an Elevation of Cortisol Levels the next Evening. *Sleep* **1997**, *20*, 865–870.
74. Vgontzas, A.N.; Pejovic, S.; Zoumakis, E.; Lin, H.M.; Bentley, C.M.; Bixler, E.O.; Sarrigiannidis, A.; Basta, M.; Chrousos, G.P. Hypothalamic-Pituitary-Adrenal Axis Activity in Obese Men with and without Sleep Apnea: Effects of Continuous Positive Airway Pressure Therapy. *J. Clin. Endocrinol. Metab.* **2007**, *92*, 4199–4207. [CrossRef] [PubMed]
75. Bratel, T.; Wennlund, A.; Carlstrom, K. Pituitary Reactivity, Androgens and Catecholamines in Obstructive Sleep Apnoea. Effects of Continuous Positive Airway Pressure Treatment (CPAP). *Respir. Med.* **1999**, *93*, 1–7. [CrossRef]
76. Leproult, R.; Van Cauter, E. Role of Sleep and Sleep Loss in Hormonal Release and Metabolism. *Endocr. Dev.* **2010**, *17*, 11–21. [PubMed]
77. Hotamisligil, G.S. Inflammation and Metabolic Disorders. *Nature* **2006**, *444*, 860–867. [CrossRef] [PubMed]
78. Xu, H.; Barnes, G.T.; Yang, Q.; Tan, G.; Yang, D.; Chou, C.J.; Sole, J.; Nichols, A.; Ross, J.S.; Tartaglia, L.A.; et al. Chronic Inflammation in Fat Plays a Crucial Role in the Development of Obesity-Related Insulin Resistance. *J. Clin. Investig.* **2003**, *112*, 1821–1830. [CrossRef]
79. Vgontzas, A.N.; Zoumakis, E.; Lin, H.M.; Bixler, E.O.; Trakada, G.; Chrousos, G.P. Marked Decrease in Sleepiness in Patients with Sleep Apnea by Etanercept, a Tumor Necrosis Factor-Alpha Antagonist. *J. Clin. Endocrinol. Metab.* **2004**, *89*, 4409–4413. [CrossRef]
80. Jiang, P.; Turek, F.W. Timing of Meals: When is as Critical as what and how much. *Am. J. Physiol. Endocrinol. Metab.* **2017**, *312*, E369–E380. [CrossRef]
81. Bandin, C.; Scheer, F.A.; Luque, A.J.; Avila-Gandia, V.; Zamora, S.; Madrid, J.A.; Gomez-Abellan, P.; Garaulet, M. Meal Timing Affects Glucose Tolerance, Substrate Oxidation and Circadian-Related Variables: A Randomized, Crossover Trial. *Int. J. Obes.* **2015**, *39*, 828–833. [CrossRef] [PubMed]
82. Gill, S.; Panda, S. A Smartphone App Reveals Erratic Diurnal Eating Patterns in Humans that Can Be Modulated for Health Benefits. *Cell Metab.* **2015**, *22*, 789–798. [CrossRef] [PubMed]
83. Henst, R.H.P.; Pienaar, P.R.; Roden, L.C.; Rae, D.E. The Effects of Sleep Extension on Cardiometabolic Risk Factors: A Systematic Review. *J. Sleep Res.* **2019**, e12865. [CrossRef] [PubMed]
84. Al Khatib, H.K.; Hall, W.L.; Creedon, A.; Ooi, E.; Masri, T.; McGowan, L.; Harding, S.V.; Darzi, J.; Pot, G.K. Sleep Extension is a Feasible Lifestyle Intervention in Free-Living Adults who are Habitually Short Sleepers: A Potential Strategy for Decreasing Intake of Free Sugars? A Randomized Controlled Pilot Study. *Am. J. Clin. Nutr.* **2018**, *107*, 43–53. [CrossRef] [PubMed]
85. Tasali, E.; Chapotot, F.; Wroblewski, K.; Schoeller, D. The Effects of Extended Bedtimes on Sleep Duration and Food Desire in Overweight Young Adults: A Home-Based Intervention. *Appetite* **2014**, *80*, 220–224. [CrossRef]
86. So-Ngern, A.; Chirakalwasan, N.; Saetung, S.; Chanprasertyothin, S.; Thakkinstian, A.; Reutrakul, S. Effects of Two-Week Sleep Extension on Glucose Metabolism in Chronically Sleep-Deprived Individuals. *J. Clin. Sleep Med.* **2019**, *15*, 711–718. [CrossRef]

87. Yang, P.Y.; Ho, K.H.; Chen, H.C.; Chien, M.Y. Exercise Training Improves Sleep Quality in Middle-Aged and Older Adults with Sleep Problems: A Systematic Review. *J. Physiother.* **2012**, *58*, 157–163. [CrossRef]
88. Reynolds, A.N.; Mann, J.I.; Williams, S.; Venn, B.J. Advice to Walk after Meals is more Effective for Lowering Postprandial Glycaemia in Type 2 Diabetes Mellitus than Advice that does not Specify Timing: A Randomised Crossover Study. *Diabetologia* **2016**, *59*, 2572–2578. [CrossRef]
89. Borror, A.; Zieff, G.; Battaglini, C.; Stoner, L. The Effects of Postprandial Exercise on Glucose Control in Individuals with Type 2 Diabetes: A Systematic Review. *Sports Med.* **2018**, *48*, 1479–1491. [CrossRef]
90. Sullivan, C.E.; Issa, F.G.; Berthon-Jones, M.; Eves, L. Reversal of Obstructive Sleep Apnoea by Continuous Positive Airway Pressure Applied Through the Nares. *Lancet* **1981**, *1*, 862–865. [CrossRef]
91. McDaid, C.; Griffin, S.; Weatherly, H.; Duree, K.; Van Der Burgt, M.; Van Hout, S.; Akers, J.; Davies, R.J.; Sculpher, M.; Westwood, M. Continuous Positive Airway Pressure Devices for the Treatment of Obstructive Sleep Apnoea-Hypopnoea Syndrome: A Systematic Review and Economic Analysis. *Health Technol. Assess.* **2009**, *13*, iii–iv, xi–xiv, 1–119, 143–274. [CrossRef] [PubMed]
92. Peppard, P.E.; Young, T.; Palta, M.; Dempsey, J.; Skatrud, J. Longitudinal Study of Moderate Weight Change and Sleep-Disordered Breathing. *JAMA* **2000**, *284*, 3015–3021. [CrossRef] [PubMed]
93. Drager, L.F.; Brunoni, A.R.; Jenner, R.; Lorenzi-Filho, G.; Bensenor, I.M.; Lotufom, P.A. Effects of CPAP on Body Weight in Patients with Obstructive Sleep Apnoea: A Meta-Analysis of Randomised Trials. *Thorax* **2015**, *70*, 258–264. [CrossRef] [PubMed]
94. Hoyos, C.M.; Killick, R.; Yee, B.J.; Phillips, C.L.; Grunstein, R.R.; Liu, P.Y. Cardiometabolic Changes after Continuous Positive Airway Pressure for Obstructive Sleep Apnoea: A Randomised Sham-Controlled Study. *Thorax* **2012**, *67*, 1081–1089. [CrossRef]
95. Furlan, S.F.; Braz, C.V.; Lorenzi-Filho, G.; Drager, L.F. Management of Hypertension in Obstructive Sleep Apnea. *Curr. Cardiol. Rep.* **2015**, *17*, 108. [CrossRef]
96. Liu, L.; Cao, Q.; Guo, Z.; Dai, Q. Continuous Positive Airway Pressure in Patients With Obstructive Sleep Apnea and Resistant Hypertension: A Meta-Analysis of Randomized Controlled Trials. *J. Clin. Hypertens.* **2016**, *18*, 153–158. [CrossRef]
97. Yang, D.; Liu, Z.; Yang, H.; Luo, Q. Effects of Continuous Positive Airway Pressure on Glycemic Control and Insulin Resistance in Patients with Obstructive Sleep Apnea: A Meta-Analysis. *Sleep Breath.* **2013**, *17*, 33–38. [CrossRef]
98. Weinstock, T.G.; Wang, X.; Rueschman, M.; Ismail-Beigi, F.; Aylor, J.; Babineau, D.C.; Mehra, R.; Redline, S. A Controlled Trial of CPAP Therapy on Metabolic Control in Individuals with Impaired Glucose Tolerance and Sleep Apnea. *Sleep* **2012**, *35*, 617–625B. [CrossRef]
99. Coughlin, S.R.; Mawdsley, L.; Mugarza, J.A.; Wilding, J.P.; Calverley, P.M. Cardiovascular and Metabolic Effects of CPAP in Obese Males with OSA. *Eur. Respir. J.* **2007**, *29*, 720–727. [CrossRef]
100. Craig, S.E.; Kohler, M.; Nicoll, D.; Bratton, D.J.; Nunn, A.; Davies, R.; Stradling, J. Continuous Positive Airway Pressure Improves Sleepiness but not Calculated Vascular Risk in Patients with Minimally Symptomatic Obstructive Sleep Apnoea: The MOSAIC Randomised Controlled Trial. *Thorax* **2012**, *67*, 1090–1096. [CrossRef]
101. Yu, J.; Zhou, Z.; McEvoy, R.D.; Anderson, C.S.; Rodgers, A.; Perkovic, V.; Neal, B. Association of Positive Airway Pressure with Cardiovascular Events and Death in Adults With Sleep Apnea: A Systematic Review and Meta-analysis. *JAMA* **2017**, *318*, 156–166. [CrossRef] [PubMed]
102. Borel, A.L.; Leblanc, X.; Almeras, N.; Tremblay, A.; Bergeron, J.; Poirier, P.; Despres, J.P.; Series, F. Sleep Apnoea Attenuates the Effects of a Lifestyle Intervention Programme in Men with Visceral Obesity. *Thorax* **2012**, *67*, 735–741. [CrossRef] [PubMed]
103. Chirinos, J.A.; Gurubhagavatula, I.; Teff, K.; Rader, D.J.; Wadden, T.A.; Townsend, R.; Foster, G.D.; Maislin, G.; Saif, H.; Broderick, P.; et al. CPAP, Weight Loss, or Both for Obstructive Sleep Apnea. *N. Engl. J. Med.* **2014**, *370*, 2265–2275. [CrossRef] [PubMed]

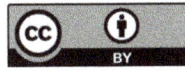

© 2019 by the author. Licensee MDPI, Basel, Switzerland. This article is an open access article distributed under the terms and conditions of the Creative Commons Attribution (CC BY) license (http://creativecommons.org/licenses/by/4.0/).

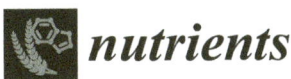

Article

Waist Circumference and Abdominal Volume Index Can Predict Metabolic Syndrome in Adolescents, but only When the Criteria of the International Diabetes Federation are Employed for the Diagnosis

Javier S. Perona [1], Jacqueline Schmidt-RioValle [2,*], Ángel Fernández-Aparicio [2], María Correa-Rodríguez [2], Robinson Ramírez-Vélez [3] and Emilio González-Jiménez [2]

1. Instituto de la Grasa-CSIC, Campus Universidad Pablo de Olavide, Edificio 46, 41013 Seville, Spain; perona@ig.csic.es
2. Department of Nursing, University of Granada, Av. Ilustración, 60, 18016 Granada, Spain; anfeapa@ugr.es (Á.F.-A.); macoro@ugr.es (M.C.-R.); emigoji@ugr.es (E.G.-J.)
3. Department of Health Sciences, Public University of Navarra, Navarrabiomed- IdiSNA, Pamplona, 31006 Navarra, Spain; robin640@hotmail.com
* Correspondence: jschmidt@ugr.es; Tel.: +34-958-243-495; Fax: +34-958-243-495

Received: 27 May 2019; Accepted: 14 June 2019; Published: 18 June 2019

Abstract: We previously reported, using the diagnostic criteria of the International Diabetes Federation (IDF), that waist circumference (WC) and abdominal volume index (AVI) were capable of predicting metabolic syndrome (MetS) in adolescents. This study was aimed at confirming this finding when other diagnostic criteria are used. A cross-sectional study was performed on 981 Spanish adolescents (13.2 ± 1.2 years). MetS was diagnosed by eight different criteria. Ten anthropometric indexes were calculated and receiver-operator curves (ROC) were created to determine their discriminatory capacity for MetS. Of all diagnostic criteria, the ones proposed by the IDF showed the highest mean values for weight, WC and systolic blood pressure in boys and girls with MetS, and the lowest for glucose and triglycerides in boys. ROC analysis showed that only WC, AVI and body roundness index (BRI) achieved area under the curve (AUC) values above 0.8 in boys, and that fat content, body mass index (BMI), WC, AVI, BRI and pediatric body adiposity index (BAIp) showed AUC values above 0.8 in girls. Importantly, this occurred only when diagnosis was carried out using the IDF criteria. We confirm that WC and AVI can predict MetS in adolescents but only when the IDF's diagnostic criteria are employed.

Keywords: anthropometric indexes; diagnosis criteria; metabolic syndrome; adolescents; obesity

1. Introduction

Metabolic syndrome (MetS) is defined as the clustering of risk factors for cardiovascular disease (CVD) and type 2 diabetes mellitus, such as hypertension, central obesity, atherogenic dyslipidemia, and insulin resistance [1]. It is now recognized that MetS is not only a problem of adulthood. Children that suffer changes in their metabolic profile present a higher risk of developing this condition in early stages of their lives, like adolescence [2,3], with the resulting risk of developing type 2 diabetes mellitus and cardiovascular disease [4].

For this reason, it is necessary to identify early changes in the metabolic profile for the diagnosis of this condition in children and adolescents [5]. In addition, scientific evidence shows that the use of anthropometric indexes is a simple and innocuous method that can discriminate regional fat to predict disorders as MetS in adolescents. In a previous study with 981 Spanish adolescents, we concluded that waist circumference (WC) and abdominal volume index (AVI) are the anthropometric indexes that best predict MetS in this population Perona et al. [6]. In that study, however, only the criteria of the International Diabetes Federation (IDF) for the diagnosis of MetS [7] were considered.

There is currently no consensus over the most effective criterion for the diagnosis of MetS in the adolescent population [8,9], in all likelihood because of the different sets of components used in the different diagnostic criteria [10]. In recent years, adaptations of the criteria established for the diagnosis of MetS in adults, such as the National Cholesterol Education Program—Adult Treatment Panel III (NCEP–ATP III) [11], modified by Cook et al. [12], Weiss et al. [13], Duncan et al. [14], and de Ferranti et al. [15], have been used. Unlike others, the criteria established by the IDF [7] consider the presence of abdominal obesity as a pre-requisite for the diagnosis of MetS. In contrast, Cook et al. [12], Cruz and Goran [16], de Ferranti et al. [15], and Rodríguez et al. [17] consider the presence of three or more impaired components for the diagnosis, even if adolescents do not have abdominal obesity. Viner et al. [18], following modified WHO criteria adapted for children (Alberti and Zimmet [19]), considered the presence of at least four impaired components as necessary for the diagnosis of MetS.

This variability in the criteria leads to striking differences in the diagnosis of MetS and might affect the results of our previous study. Therefore, the present study is aimed at verifying whether WC and AVI still maintain their predictive capacity for MetS in adolescents when other criteria, such as those aforementioned, are used together with the ones proposed by the IDF.

2. Materials and Methods

2.1. Study Design and Participants

This cross-sectional study included 981 adolescents (456 boys and 525 girls) with a mean age of 13.2 ± 1.2 years (11–16 years old). All of the participants had been born in Spain and also resided there. They came from families of a similar socio-economic level and attended 18 educational centers in the provinces of Granada and Almeria (southeastern Spain). Ten of these schools were public, and eight were private. The principals were sent a letter inviting their schools to participate in the study. In all cases, the invitation was accepted. In each school, two classes of a total of three per grade were randomly selected for participation. The flow diagram in Figure 1 shows the recruiting process. The Education Boards of Granada and Almeria gave their approval to the research study before it was carried out. The study also received the authorization of the principals of the participating school.

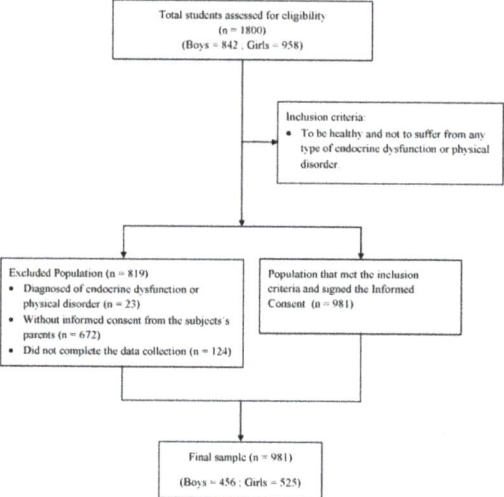

Figure 1. Flow diagram of the recruitment progress.

The Ethics Committee of the University of Granada approved both the study and the model of informed consent used. The parents and legal guardians of the participants gave their written informed consent at the beginning of the study. In addition, the study complied with the International Code of Medical Ethics of the World Medical Association and the Helsinki Declaration. To be included in the study, students had to be healthy and not suffer from any endocrine or physical disorder.

2.2. Anthropometric Measurements

All participants underwent an anthropometric evaluation, which was performed by a member of the research team, trained for that purpose. The evaluation was carried out according to the criteria established by the International Society for the Advancement of Kinanthropometry (ISAK) [20]. All body measurements were taken in the morning after a 12-h fasting period and 24-h without any physical exercise. The body weight of each participant was measured twice on a self-calibrating SECA 861 class (III) digital floor scale (Saint Paul, MI, USA) with a precision of up to 100 g. All participants were asked to wear light clothes and to remove their shoes beforehand.

Height measurements were taken with a SECA anthropometer (Model 214). Participants without shoes were measured in an upright position with their back and heels in permanent contact with the vertical height rod of the anthropometer and their head oriented in the Frankfurt plane. The horizontal headpiece was then placed on top of their heads. In all cases, the participants' height and weight were measured twice. The final value was the average of the two measurements.

In addition, the BMI was calculated as the participant's weight divided by the square of his/her height (kg/m^2). The WC and hip circumference were measured with a SECA flexible, inextensible measuring tape with an accuracy of 1mm. The WC was measured on a horizontal plane at a point that was equidistant from the lowest floating rib and the upper border of the iliac crest. In all cases, this measurement was taken after exhalation.

Hip circumference was also measured on the horizontal plane and at the maximum protuberance of the buttocks, which coincides in the front with the ischiopubic symphysis. The waist-to-hip ratio (WHR) was calculated by dividing the waist perimeter by the hip perimeter. Also measured were the triceps, biceps, subscapular, and suprailiac skinfolds. The instrument used for this purpose was a Holtain skinfold caliper (Holtain Ltd., Crymych, UK), with an accuracy of 0.1–0.2 mm. The percentage of body fat was based on these skinfold measurements.

Previously, the Brook equation was used to calculate body density [21]. Once the body density value had been obtained, the body fat percentage was determined with the Siri equation [22]. In each educational center, all anthropometric measurements were taken in a classroom that had been especially prepared for this purpose. The privacy of the students was thus guaranteed.

The rest of the anthropometric indexes, abdominal volume index (AVI), body roundness index (BRI), body adiposity index (BAI), body adiposity index for pediatrics (BAIp), conicity index (C-Index), and body shape index (ABSI), were calculated using the following Equations [23–28]:

$$AVI = (2\text{Waist Circumference}^2 \text{ (cm)} + 0.7(\text{Waist Circumference} - \text{Hip Circumference})^2 \text{ (cm)})/1000$$

$$BRI = 364.2 - 365.5 \left[1 - \pi^{-2} \text{ Waist Circumference}^2 \text{ (m) Height}^{-2} \text{ (m)}\right]^{1/2}$$

$$BAI = [\text{Hip circumference (m)/Height}^{2/3} \text{ (m)}] - 18$$

$$BAIp = \text{Hip circumference (cm)/Height (m)}^{0.8} - 38$$

$$\text{C-Index} = 0.109^{-1} \text{ Waist Circumference (m) } [\text{Weight (kg)/Height (m)}]^{-1/2}$$

$$ABSI = WC \text{ (m)}/(BMI^{2/3}(kg/m2)\text{Height}^{1/2} \text{ (m)})$$

2.3. Serum Biochemical Examination

Blood collection was performed after a 12-h fast. At 8:00 a.m., a nurse member of the research team extracted 10 mL of blood from the median cubital vein of the right arm. For this purpose, a vacutainer system was used with a vacuum blood collection tube. Once the blood had been collected, the glucose concentration was measured with an enzymatic colorimetric method (glucose oxidase-phenol aminophenazone (GOD-PAP); Human Diagnostics, Germany). Also measured were concentrations of HDL-C, total cholesterol, and triglycerides by means of enzymatic colorimetric methods. This was done with an Olympus analyzer.

Four hours after the blood extraction, the samples were centrifuged at 1300 g for 15 minutes (Z400 K, Hermle, Wehingen, Germany). This process separated the red blood cells from the serum, which was then frozen at −80 °C for subsequent analysis. The estimation of low-density-lipoprotein cholesterol (LDL-C) was obtained with the Friedewald equation:

$$LDL\text{-}C = \text{Total Cholesterol} - HDL\text{-}C - (TG/5)$$

where TG = concentration of triglycerides. Serum insulin was determined by radioimmunoanalysis (Insulin Kit; DPC, Los Angeles, EEUU). Insulin resistance was quantified by Homeostatic Model Assessment (HOMA) [29] with the following equation: fasting glucose (mmol/L) × fasting insulin (mU/L)/22.5.

2.4. Blood Pressure Determination

Blood pressure levels were measured by a calibrated aneroid sphygmomanometer and a Littmann® stethoscope (Saint Paul, MI, USA), according to most widely accepted international recommendations [30]. Systolic blood pressure (SBP) ≥130 and/or diastolic blood pressure (DBP) ≥85 mm Hg were considered to be a risk factor of MetS.

2.5. Diagnostic Criteria of Metabolic Syndrome

Eight different criteria were used to diagnose MetS in the adolescent sample studied: Cook et al. [12], Weiss et al. [13], Duncan et al. [14], de Ferranti et al. [15], Cruz and Goran [16], Rodríguez-Morán et al. [17], and Viner et al. [18], as well as the IDF criteria as published by Zimmet et al. [7]. The details of the criteria employed may be consulted in Table 1.

2.6. Statistical Analysis

The normality of the distribution was assessed using the Kolmogorov-Smirnov test. Results were reported as mean ± SD, except for the number of girls and boys with or without MetS, which was expressed as a number. Student's t-test was used to assess mean differences between boys and girls. The area under receiver operating characteristic (ROC) curves was calculated to evaluate the abilities of the anthropometric indices to predict MetS. Cutoff points were proposed after calculation of the Youden's Index (sensitivity+specificity-1). The areas under the ROC curves were compared using DeLong et al.'s [31] non-parametric approach. Based on the assumption that abdominal obesity is a component of MetS, we conducted a multicollinearity test for the anthropometric indexes that included WC (AVI, BRI and ABSI), and the variance inflation factor (VIF) was calculated. Comparisons of means were assessed by ANOVA, followed by Tukey's test. SPSS v24.0 (IBM, Armonk, NY, USA) was used to perform statistical analyses. Statistical significance was defined as $p < 0.05$.

Table 1. Diagnostic criteria for the MetS in adolescents.

	IDF	Cook	De Ferranti	Weiss	Viner	Duncan	Rodríguez-Morán	Cruz & Goran
Age (years)	10–16	12–19	≥12	4–20	2–18	12–19	10–18	8–13
Number of components	Obesity + 2 components	≥3	≥3	≥3	≥4	≥3	≥3	≥3
Obesity	WC > 90 percentile	WC > 90 percentile	WC > 75 percentile	BMI z-score ≥ 2	BMI ≥ 95 percentile	WC ≥ 90 percentile	WC ≥ 90 percentile	WC ≥ 90 percentile
Glucose (mg/dL)	≥100	≥110	≥110	≥140	≥110	≥110	≥110	<100
TG (mg/dL)	≥150	≥110	≥100	>95 percentile	≥150	≥110	≥90 percentile	≥90 percentile
HDL-cholesterol (mg/dL)	≤40	≤40	<50 girls <45 boys	<5 percentile	≤35	<40	-	<10 percentile
SBP (mmHg)	≥130	>90 percentile	>90 percentile	>95 percentile	>95 percentile	≥90 percentile	≥90 percentile	≥90 percentile
DBP (mmHg)	≥85	-	-	-	-	-	-	-

Notes: IDF, International Diabetes Federation; TG, triglycerides; HDL, high-density lipoprotein; SBP, systolic blood pressure; DBP, diastolic blood pressure; WC, waist circumference; BMI, body mass index.

3. Results

3.1. Baseline Characteristics of the Participants

Table 2 shows the characteristics of the participants, including anthropometric and biochemical measures, including HOMA-IR. On average, variables were within normal limits, and for most of them, no differences were observed between boys and girls. However, girls showed significantly lower body weight, WC and SBP and higher fat content.

Table 2. Baseline characteristics of participants.

Variables	Boys (n = 456)		Girls (n = 525)	
	Mean	SD	Mean	SD
Age (years)	13.2	1.2	13.3	1.2
Weight (kg)	57.1	14.1	53.1	11.0 ***
Fat (%)	27.3	8.3	29.6	7.8 ***
BMI (kg/m^2)	21.5	4.0	21.1	3.6
WC (cm)	73.7	11.8	71.3	9.6 ***
Glucose (mg/dL)	86.2	31.2	85.2	28.7
TG (mg/dL)	129.2	59.3	125.0	46.2
Cholesterol (mg/dL)	81.8	17.3	81.4	15.7
LDL-c (mg/dL)	93.4	23.6	92.9	22.5
HDL-c (mg/dL)	40.1	2.8	40.0	3.1
SBP (mmHg)	119.6	15.7	116.9	15.1 **
DBP (mmHg)	64.5	9.2	63.9	8.8
Insulin (mU/mL)	21.0	10.2	20.2	9.0
HOMA-IR	4.5	2.9	4.3	3.1

Notes: Fat (%), body fat percentage; BMI, body mass index; WC, waist circumference; TG, triglycerides; LDL-c, low-density lipoprotein cholesterol; HDL-c, high-density lipoprotein cholesterol; SBP, systolic blood pressure, DBP, diastolic blood pressure, HOMA-IR, homeostatic model assessment of insulin resistance. Differences between means were assessed by an unpaired Student's t-test. **, $p < 0.05$; ***, $p < 0.001$.

Tables 3 and 4 show the characteristics of boys and girls, respectively, diagnosed of MetS according to the different diagnostic criteria studied. The number of diagnosed participants varied with the criteria from 25 to 68 boys. In these subjects, the criteria proposed by Viner et al. [18] resulted in 25 individuals with MetS, while those proposed by Duncan et al. [14], Rodriguez-Moran et al. [17] and Cruz and Goran [16] resulted in 68 individuals. Since these latter subjects were actually the same, the mean values of all variables studied (weight, fat %, BMI, WC, fasting glucose, triglycerides, cholesterol, LDL-cholesterol, HDL-cholesterol, SBP, DBP, insulin and HOMA-IR) were also the same. The criteria proposed by the IDF consistently showed the highest mean values for weight, WC, HDL-cholesterol, SBP, DBP and insulin and the lowest for glucose, triglycerides, cholesterol and LDL-cholesterol. In contrast, using the criteria proposed by Viner et al. [18], resulted in the highest mean levels of glucose, triglycerides, cholesterol, LDL-cholesterol and HOMA-IR. Among the components of the MetS, the highest mean values for WC, HDL-cholesterol and SBP were 86.0 cm, 35.7 mg/dL and 137.2 mmHg, respectively, (IDF) and for glucose and triglycerides, 193.7 mg/dL and 338.9 mg/dL, respectively [18]. The lowest mean values for WC, HDL-cholesterol and SBP were 74.6 cm (Cook et al. [12]), 32.4 mg/dL (Viner et al. [18]) and 121.6 mmHg (Cook et al. [12]), respectively. No significant differences were observed in age, fat content and BMI among adolescent boys with MetS, regardless of the criteria used.

Table 3. Characteristics of boys diagnosed of MetS according to the different diagnostic criteria.

Variables	IDF		Cook		De Ferranti		Weiss		Viner		Duncan		Rodríguez-Moran		Cruz & Goran	
	Mean	SD	Mean	SD	Mean	SD	Mean	SD	Mean	SD	Mean	SD	Mean	SD	Mean	SD
MetS (number)	41		39		63		32		25		68		68		68	
Age (y)	13.6 [a]	1.0	12.9 [a]	1.2	13.0 [a]	1.0	13.2 [a]	1.2	13.0 [a]	1.2	13.1 [a]	1.1	13.1 [a]	1.1	13.1 [a]	1.1
Weight (kg)	69.3 [a]	13.6	54.9 [b]	14.3	59.8 [b]	15.6	59.3 [ab]	17.4	59.1 [ab]	17.0	60.3 [ab]	15.3	60.3 [ab]	15.3	60.3 [ab]	15.3
Fat (%)	34.1 [a]	6.5	29.3 [a]	7.8	32.1 [a]	7.7	29.4 [a]	8.4	30.3 [a]	8.1	31.3 [a]	7.8	31.3 [a]	7.8	31.3 [a]	7.8
BMI (kg/m^2)	25.2 [a]	4.3	21.8 [a]	4.2	23.6 [a]	4.7	22.4 [a]	5.5	22.4 [a]	5.0	23.4 [a]	4.5	23.4 [a]	4.5	23.4 [a]	4.5
WC (cm)	86.0 [a]	9.9	74.6 [b]	11.7	80.2 [ab]	12.7	76.9 [b]	14.0	77.8 [ab]	13.5	79.5 [ab]	12.4	79.5 [ab]	12.4	79.5 [ab]	12.4
Glucose (mg/dL)	128.4 [a]	53.5	172.9 [b]	47.4	139.5 [a]	56.9	191.4 [b]	27.8	193.7 [b]	24.4	136.0 [a]	56.2	136.0 [a]	56.2	136.0 [a]	56.2
TG (mg/dL)	193.0 [a]	120.1	257.9 [a]	146.4	210.1 [ac]	133.9	295.0 [bc]	143.9	338.9 [b]	132.5	204.0 [a]	130.6	204.0 [a]	130.6	204.0 [a]	130.6
Chol (mg/dL)	129.6 [a]	35.6	151.6 [ab]	27.1	134.6 [a]	35.7	163.0 [b]	7.3	163.2 [b]	8.1	133.4 [a]	35.4	133.4 [a]	35.4	133.4 [a]	35.4
LDL-c (mg/dL)	101.9 [a]	23.8	119.7 [b]	24.9	107.2 [ab]	26.7	126.3 [c]	19.8	126.0 [c]	21.3	107.2 [ab]	25.3	107.2 [ab]	25.3	107.2 [ab]	25.3
HDL-c (mg/dL)	35.7 [a]	3.4	33.1 [bc]	2.2	35.0 [a]	3.4	32.3 [c]	1.6	32.4 [c]	1.8	34.9 [ab]	3.2	34.9 [ab]	3.2	34.9 [ab]	3.2
SBP (mmHg)	137.2 [a]	14.7	121.6 [b]	17.0	123.5 [b]	17.3	122.9 [b]	17.9	123.4 [b]	18.8	124.0 [b]	16.6	124.0 [b]	16.6	124.0 [b]	16.6
DBP mmHg)	74.1 [a]	11.4	64.6 [b]	8.6	65.5 [b]	9.0	65.1 [b]	9.0	63.9 [b]	9.2	66.3 [b]	8.7	66.3 [b]	8.7	66.3 [b]	8.7
Insulin (mU/mL)	28.7 [a]	15.1	20.9 [a]	10.4	25.5 [a]	13.6	23.7 [a]	14.2	24.0 [a]	14.3	24.9 [a]	13.3	24.9 [a]	13.3	24.9 [a]	13.3
HOMA-IR	8.8 [a]	6.0	9.1 [a]	5.7	8.3 [a]	5.1	10.7 [a]	5.6	11.1 [a]	6.2	8.0 [a]	5.0	8.0 [a]	5.0	8.0 [a]	5.0

Notes: Fat (%), body fat percentage; BMI, body mass index; WC, waist circumference; TG, triglycerides; Chol, cholesterol; LDL-c, low-density lipoprotein cholesterol; HDL-c, high-density lipoprotein cholesterol; SBP, systolic blood pressure; DBP, diastolic blood pressure; HOMA-IR, homeostatic model assessment of insulin resistance. Differences between means that share a letter are not statistically significant ($p < 0.05$).

Table 4. Characteristics of girls diagnosed of MetS according to the different diagnostic criteria.

Variables	IDF		Cook		de Ferranti		Weiss		Viner		Duncan		Rodriguez-Moran		Cruz & Goran	
	Mean	SD	Mean	SD	Mean	SD	Mean	SD	Mean	SD	Mean	SD	Mean	SD	Mean	SD
MetS (number)	32		58		97		18		21		134		86		171	
Age (years)	13.3 [a]	1.1	12.9 [a]	1.1	12.9 [a]	1.1	13.1 [a]	1.4	13.2 [a]	1.3	13.0 [a]	1.1	13.1 [a]	1.1	13.1 [a]	1.1
Weight (kg)	67.1 [a]	10.1	51.8 [b]	12.8	55.4 [bc]	11.9	57.0 [ab]	18.0	59.2 [ab]	16.6	54.1 [b]	10.4	60.3 [ac]	15.3	54.8 [b]	11.0
Fat (%)	38.1 [a]	6.6	30.0 [a]	8.4	32.6 [a]	8.0	31.9 [a]	11.3	33.0 [a]	9.9	31.9 [a]	7.5	31.3 [a]	7.8	32.0 [a]	7.6
BMI (kg/m^2)	25.8 [a]	3.5	21.1 [b]	4.3	22.5 [bc]	4.0	22.4 [ab]	5.9	23.1 [ab]	5.2	22.1 [bc]	3.6	23.4 [a]	4.5	22.1 [bc]	3.7
WC (cm)	83.2 [a]	7.5	70.5 [b]	10.4	75.2 [bc]	10.3	73.7 [bc]	14.8	75.5 [ab]	13.3	73.6 [b]	9.1	79.5 [ac]	12.4	73.7 [b]	9.5
Glucose (mg/dL)	132.0 [abc]	52.2	148.3 [b]	51.8	121.1 [a]	52.3	194.4 [d]	7.1	188.2 [d]	22.5	110.0 [c]	48.2	136.0 [ab]	56.2	104.5	43.9 [c]
TG (mg/dL)	196.2 [ab]	120.9	191.6 [ab]	114.9	164.5 [ab]	98.1	329.8 [c]	121.9	312.9 [c]	128.1	151.9 [a]	85.9	204.0 [b]	130.6	145.5 [a]	77.0
Chol (mg/dL)	132.3 [ab]	33.2	139.9 [a]	30.9	122.1 [b]	35.8	161.4 [a]	4.8	160.0 [a]	4.9	114.1 [c]	34.8	133.4 [a]	35.4	109.3 [c]	32.5
LDL-c (mg/dL)	106.3 [ab]	20.0	109.3 [a]	21.2	98.2 [b]	23.3	126.1 [a]	16.1	122.8 [a]	15.9	92.9 [c]	22.3	107.2 [a]	25.3	90.1 [c]	21.2
HDL-c (mg/dL)	35.3 [ab]	2.6	33.7 [a]	4.5	36.1 [b]	4.8	32.8 [a]	1.3	33.1 [a]	1.3	37.2 [c]	4.6	34.9	3.2 [a]	38.0	4.3 [c]
SBP (mmHg)	132.3 [a]	10.2	113.4 [b]	17.1	117.7 [bc]	17.0	116.4 [bc]	20.8	118.8 [ab]	19.5	117.2 [b]	15.5	124.0 [ac]	16.6	117.5 [b]	15.3
DBP mmHg)	70.7 [a]	8.8	62.1 [a]	8.8	62.6 [a]	9.5	64.4 [a]	10.2	64.4 [a]	10.1	63.0 [a]	9.0	66.3 [a]	8.7	63.7 [a]	8.9
Insulin (mU/mL)	11.0 [a]	8.0	8.4 [b]	6.6	7.1 [bc]	5.6	13.8 [a]	8.7	13.6 [a]	8.5	6.1 [b]	5.0	8.0 [ab]	5.0	5.8 [c]	4.6
HOMA-IR	32.5 [a]	15.8	22.0 [b]	12.2	23.6 [b]	12.3	28.8 [ab]	17.9	28.8 [ab]	17.1	21.7 [b]	10.4	24.9 [ab]	13.3	21.8 [c]	10.5

Notes: Fat (%), body fat percentage; BMI, body mass index; WC, waist circumference; TG, triglycerides; Chol, cholesterol; LDL-c, low-density lipoprotein cholesterol; HDL-c, high-density lipoprotein cholesterol; SBP, systolic blood pressure; DBP, diastolic blood pressure, HOMA-IR, homeostatic model assessment of insulin resistance. Differences between means that share a letter are not statistically significant ($p < 0.05$).

In girls, the variability in the number of diagnosed individuals was much higher. The criteria proposed by Weiss et al. [13] resulted in the diagnostic of only 18 individuals with MetS, while those proposed by Cruz and Goran [16] resulted in 171 individuals. The criteria proposed by the IDF consistently showed the highest mean values for weight, BMI, WC and SBP, while the lowest were found when the criteria by Cook et al. [12] were employed. Regarding mean biochemical parameters (glucose, triglycerides, cholesterol and LDL-cholesterol), the highest values were observed in individuals diagnosed using the criteria by Weiss et al. [13], while the lowest corresponded to individuals diagnosed using the criteria by Cruz and Goran [16]. Among the components of the MetS, the highest mean values for WC and SBP were 83.2 cm, and 132.3 mmHg, respectively (IDF), for HDL-cholesterol was 38.0 mg/dL (Cruz and Goran [16]) and for glucose and triglycerides, 194.4 mg/dL and 329.8 mg/dL, respectively (Weiss et al. [13]). The lowest mean values for WC and SBP were 70.5 cm and 113.4 mmHg, respectively (Cook et al. [12]), for HDL-cholesterol was 32.8 (Weiss et al. [13]) and for glucose and triglycerides, 104.5 mg/dL and 145.5 mg/dL, respectively (Cruz and Goran [16]). No significant differences were observed in age, fat content and DBP among girls with MetS regardless the criteria used.

3.2. Area under the Curve Values of the Anthropometric Indexes for the Diagnosis of Metabolic Syndrome

Tables 5 and 6 show the area under the curve (AUC) values obtained from ROC analyses of the different anthropometric indexes for predicting MetS in adolescent boys and girls, respectively, according to the different diagnostic criteria employed. In boys, only WC, AVI and BRI achieved AUC values above 0.8, thus showing a high predictive capacity. These values were obtained when the diagnosis of MetS was performed using the IDF criteria. When using any of the other criteria studied, AUC values were always below 0.8. The lowest AUC values observed, i.e., the lowest predictive capacity of all of the anthropometric indexes, were found when the criteria used for the diagnosis were those proposed by Weiss et al. [13] and Cook et al. [12].

In girls, fat content, BMI, WC, AVI, BRI and BAIp showed AUC values for MetS above 0.8 and in all cases when the diagnostic was carried out using the IDF criteria. WHR, ABSI and BAI were unable to predict the MetS in girls with a high level of certainty, as AUC values were below 0.8 for all diagnostic criteria employed. In particular, the highest AUC value for ABSI was obtained when the criteria proposed by de Ferranti et al. [15] were used, although it was only 0.590. The lowest AUC values observed corresponded to anthropometric indexes when using the criteria recommended by Weiss et al. [13].

The collinearity test for all anthropometric indexes that included WC for their calculation was found to be negative for WC and AVI (VIF < 3) and positive for, BRI and ABSI (VIF > 3).

Table 5. Area under the curve (AUC) in receiver-operator curve (ROC) analysis of different anthropometric indexes for predicting MetS components in boys according to diagnostic criteria.

Variables	IDF	Cook	De Ferranti	Weiss	Viner	Duncan	Rodríguez-Morán	Cruz & Goran	Maximum	Author	Minimum	Author
Fat (%)	0.757	0.582	0.696	0.576	0.612	0.666	0.666	0.666	0.757	IDF	0.576	Weiss
BMI	0.783	0.523	0.663	0.523	0.542	0.657	0.657	0.657	0.783	IDF	0.523	Weiss and Cook
WC	0.831	0.526	0.680	0.564	0.601	0.669	0.669	0.669	0.831	IDF	0.526	Cook
WHR	0.789	0.609	0.715	0.635	0.690	0.655	0.655	0.655	0.789	IDF	0.609	Cook
ABSI	0.663	0.559	0.652	0.564	0.617	0.615	0.615	0.615	0.663	IDF	0.559	Cook
BAI	0.686	0.559	0.689	0.496	0.512	0.664	0.664	0.664	0.689	de Ferranti	0.496	Weiss
AVI	0.831	0.524	0.678	0.562	0.599	0.668	0.668	0.668	0.831	IDF	0.524	Cook
BRI	0.800	0.590	0.728	0.572	0.615	0.700	0.700	0.700	0.800	IDF	0.572	Weiss
CI	0.767	0.577	0.706	0.593	0.644	0.675	0.675	0.675	0.767	IDF	0.577	Cook
BAIp	0.752	0.521	0.671	0.499	0.515	0.668	0.668	0.668	0.752	IDF	0.499	Weiss

Notes: ABSI, a body shape index; AVI, abdominal volume index; BAI, body adiposity index; BAIp, pediatric body adiposity index; BMI, body mass index; BRI, body roundness index; C-Index, conicity index; Fat (%), body fat percentage; WC, waist circumference; WHR, waist-to-hip ratio. Maximum and minimum indicate the highest and lowest AUC values observed, together with the corresponding author of the diagnostic criteria.

Table 6. Area under the curve (AUC) in receiver-operator curve (ROC) analysis of different anthropometric indexes for predicting MetS components in girls according to diagnostic criteria.

Variables	IDF	Cook	De Ferranti	Weiss	Viner	Duncan	Rodríguez-Morán	Cruz & Goran	Maximum	Author	Minimum	Author
Fat (%)	0.812	0.638	0.638	0.559	0.605	0.619	0.557	0.634	0.812	IDF	0.557	Rodriguez-Moran
BMI	0.855	0.635	0.635	0.517	0.607	0.627	0.557	0.636	0.855	IDF	0.517	Weiss
WC	0.866	0.645	0.645	0.535	0.614	0.616	0.554	0.626	0.866	IDF	0.535	Weiss
WHR	0.717	0.662	0.662	0.528	0.557	0.536	0.533	0.537	0.717	IDF	0.528	Weiss
ABSI	0.585	0.590	0.590	0.489	0.496	0.541	0.511	0.539	0.590	de Ferranti	0.489	Weiss
BAI	0.797	0.651	0.651	0.513	0.585	0.714	0.590	0.702	0.797	IDF	0.513	Weiss
AVI	0.867	0.643	0.643	0.535	0.616	0.619	0.554	0.629	0.867	IDF	0.535	Weiss
BRI	0.848	0.677	0.677	0.519	0.594	0.663	0.575	0.661	0.848	IDF	0.519	Weiss
CI	0.730	0.642	0.642	0.520	0.552	0.597	0.542	0.593	0.730	IDF	0.520	Weiss
BAIp	0.840	0.624	0.624	0.525	0.608	0.687	0.575	0.688	0.840	IDF	0.525	Weiss

Notes: ABSI, a body shape index; AVI, abdominal volume index; BAI, body adiposity index; BAIp, pediatric body adiposity index; BMI, body mass index; BRI, body roundness index; C-Index, conicity index; Fat (%), body fat percentage; WC, waist circumference; WHR, waist-to-hip ratio. Maximum and minimum indicate the highest and lowest AUC values observed, together with the corresponding author of the diagnostic criteria.

4. Discussion

In this study, eight different criteria for the diagnosis of MetS in adolescents were used, which resulted in a high variability in prevalence both in boys and girls, but no significant differences in age, fat content or in BMI, which is in agreement with Pergher et al. [8]. In boys, the number of diagnosed individuals ranged from 25 cases when the criteria of Viner et al. [18] were used, up to 68 cases when applying the criteria of Duncan et al. [14], Rodriguez-Moran et al. [17] and Cruz and Goran [16]. This variability could be explained by differences in the cut-off points of the components that make up each of the criteria to define MetS in the adolescent population [32]. There is also a high variability in terms of the components that are considered to be altered for each of the criteria used, which makes it difficult to establish comparisons [33]. Among the criteria used, those proposed by the IDF resulted in the highest average values for the variables weight, WC, HDL cholesterol, SBP, DBP and insulin and the lowest values for glucose, triglycerides, cholesterol and LDL cholesterol. These results differ partially from those obtained in other studies. Sarrafzadegan et al. [34], in their study of an Iranian adolescent population, used the criteria proposed by the IDF and found higher blood pressure levels but lower HDL-c levels compared with our study. On the other hand, Ramírez-Vélez et al. [35], in their study of adolescents from Colombia, also applying the criteria of the IDF, found that the most prevalent altered components were low levels of HDL-c and high levels of triglycerides, whereas the less prevalent components were elevated waist circumference and hyperglycemia. In our study, using the criteria proposed by Viner et al. [18], higher mean levels of glucose, triglycerides, cholesterol, LDL-c and HOMA-IR were obtained.

In girls, the variability of individuals diagnosed with MetS was even higher, ranging from 18 diagnosed subjects with the criteria of Weiss et al. [13] to 171 with the criteria of Cruz and Goran [16]. According to Nasreddine et al. [36], in their study of adolescents in Lebanon, the differences in the prevalence of MetS among boys and girls could be explained, in part, by the variations in the body composition of the human species, in particular due to a higher fat content in girls. This was also observed in our study, as girls presented a significantly higher fat content, expressed as percentage (Table 2). In addition, in line with Nasreddine et al. [36], the criteria proposed by the IDF showed higher mean values for the variables weight, BMI, WC and SBP in girls.

Regarding the discriminatory capacity for MetS of the anthropometric indexes studied and according to the different diagnostic criteria used, the ROC analysis showed that in boys, only WC, AVI and BRI reached AUC values higher than 0.8, indicating a high predictive capacity. Interestingly, this occurred only when the diagnosis of MetS was performed using the IDF criteria. Consequently, these results show the importance of these indices in the assessment of fat tissue distribution in the body and its relationship with the development of metabolic and cardiovascular disorders at an early age [37].

For the rest of the criteria studied, AUC values lower than 0.8 were obtained, indicating a lower predictive capacity of all anthropometric indexes. Values were particularly low when the criteria used for diagnosis were those proposed by Weiss et al. [13] and Cook et al. [12].

In girls, fat content, BMI, WC, AVI, BRI and BAIp showed values of AUC for the MetS above 0.8 and in all cases when the diagnosis was made using the criteria of the IDF, but not when other criteria were used. On the other hand, WHR, ABSI and BAI showed a lower predictive capacity against MetS in girls, with AUC values below 0.8 for all of the diagnostic criteria used. Based on these findings, it is worth noting the importance of using the IDF criteria for the diagnosis of MetS in adolescents compared to the other criteria in adolescents, in particular when trying to estimate the presence of MetS from anthropometric indexes. These results are in contrast with those obtained by Xu et al. [38], in Chinese male adolescents, who, using the criteria of Cook et al. [12], found AUC values of 0.79 for WHR, higher than those observed in our study. Similarly, Zaki et al. [39], in Egyptian adolescents and using the IDF criteria, found AUC values considerably higher than 0.80 for WHR, while in our study, values were slightly below 0.8 in both boys and girls. These results could suggest a possible influence of factors such as ethnicity and culture on the usefulness of the different criteria to define MetS in adolescents.

It is noteworthy that, for the ABSI index, the highest value of AUC was obtained only when the criteria proposed by de Ferranti et al. [15] were applied, and was lower than 0.6, indicating a very low predictive capacity. Consequently, and in line with previous studies in adults [40,41] and our previous report in adolescents [6], ABSI should not be used as a predictive index for MetS in adolescents of both genders. As with boys, the lowest values of AUC observed corresponded to the anthropometric indexes after using the criteria recommended by Weiss et al. [13]. At the same time, assuming that WC is used as a component of the MetS, the collinearity test for all the anthropometric indexes that included the WC for calculation showed negative results for WC and AVI (VIF <3) and positive for BRI and ABSI (VIF >3). These results show, once again, that WC and AVI are appropriate anthropometric indicators and of great clinical utility for the diagnosis of MetS in the adolescent population. Cutoff points obtained from ROC analysis for the diagnosis of MetS showed a high variability among the different criteria. Only the cutoff points for WHR and BRI showed a variation coefficient lower than 2% in boys (Supplementary Materials Table S1). In girls, variability was even higher, and Fat (%), BMI, BAI, BAIp and BRI showed variation coefficients above 10% (Supplementary Materials Table S2).

The present study has some strengths and limitations. To the best of our knowledge, this study is the first to use eight different criteria for the diagnosis of MetS in adolescents. In addition, we would like to emphasize the usefulness of the large sample size, which allowed us to obtain solid results that are comparable to those of other studies. Furthermore, the acquisition of a representative sample for the age groups contemplated in each region gave this study even greater epidemiological value. Moreover, the fact that all of the adolescents came from the same geographic area and shared the same culture, life style, and nutritional habits increased the homogeneity of sample. This study had various limitations, such as its transversal design, which does not permit causal inference. In addition, there is also a lack of information regarding the puberty status of the participants. For these reasons, the results should be interpreted with caution.

5. Conclusions

In conclusion, the results confirm that AVI and WC are the anthropometric indexes that best discriminate between MetS and non-MetS individuals when the criteria proposed by the IDF are used for diagnosis in adolescents. Importantly, the other seven diagnostic criteria were not helpful for this purpose, despite the fact that some of them (Duncan et al. [14] and Cruz and Goran [16], in particular) resulted in a large number of diagnosed individuals, especially in girls. These findings should be considered in future studies and in daily clinical practice, and health professionals should apply the criteria proposed by the IDF. The health authorities should promote the implementation of individual anthropometric indicators in the physical examination that takes place during periodic health checks in the adolescent population. At the same time, new studies with ethnically and culturally different populations are necessary in order to explore in greater depth the usefulness of the different criteria for the diagnosis of MetS and the predictive capacity of all the anthropometric indices studied.

Supplementary Materials: The following are available online at http://www.mdpi.com/2072-6643/11/6/1370/s1, Table S1: Optimal cutoff points in receiver-operator curves (ROC) analysis of different anthropometric indexes for predicting MetS in boys according to diagnostic criteria, Table S2: Optimal cutoff points in receiver-operator curves (ROC) analysis of different anthropometric indexes for predicting MetS in girls according to diagnostic criteria.

Author Contributions: E.G.-J. and J.S.P. conceived and designed the study. M.C.-R. and A.F.-A. collected and analyzed the data. J.S.-R. and R.R.-V. interpreted the data. E.G.-J. and J.S.P. drafted the manuscript. All authors have revised and approved the submitted manuscript.

Funding: This work was supported by funds from Grant CEI2015-MP-BS23 from Campus of International Excellence CEIBioTic Granada and by funds from Ministry of Economy and Competitiveness (AGL2011-23810).

Acknowledgments: The authors are grateful to schools, parents, and guardians as well as to participant students for their collaboration in the development of this study. This work was supported by funds from Grant CEI2015-MP-BS23 from Campus of International Excellence CEIBioTic Granada and by funds from Ministry of Economy and Competitiveness (AGL2011-23810).

Conflicts of Interest: The authors declare no conflict of interest.

References

1. Eisenmann, J.C.; Laurson, K.R.; Dubose, K.D.; Smith, B.K.; Donnelly, J.E. Construct validity of a continuous metabolic syndrome score in children. *Diabetol. Metab. Syndr.* **2010**, *2*, 8. [CrossRef] [PubMed]
2. Costa, R.F.; Santos, N.S.; Goldraich, N.P.; Barski, T.F.; Andrade, K.S.; Kruel, L.F.M. Metabolic syndrome in obese adolescents: A comparison of three different diagnostic criteria. *J. Pediatr.* **2012**, *88*, 303–309. [CrossRef] [PubMed]
3. Kim, J.; Lee, I.; Lim, S. Overweight or obesity in children aged 0 to 6 and the risk of adultmetabolic-syndrome: A systematic review and meta-analysis. *J. Clin. Nurs.* **2017**, *26*, 3869–3880. [CrossRef] [PubMed]
4. Kaur, J. A comprehensive review on metabolic syndrome. *Cardiol. Res. Pract.* **2014**, *2014*, 1–21. [CrossRef] [PubMed]
5. Vanlancker, T.; Schaubroeck, E.; Vyncke, K.; Cadenas-Sanchez, C.; Breidenassel, C.; González-Gross, M.; Gottrand, F.; Moreno, L.A.; Beghin, L.; Molnár, D.; et al. Comparison of definitions for the metabolic syndrome in adolescents. The HELENA study. *Eur. J. Pediatr.* **2017**, *176*, 241–252. [CrossRef]
6. Perona, J.S.; Schmidt Rio-Valle, J.; Ramírez-Vélez, R.; Correa-Rodríguez, M.; Fernández-Aparicio, Á.; González-Jiménez, E. Waist circumference and abdominal volume index are the strongest anthropometric discriminators of metabolic syndrome in Spanish adolescents. *Eur. J. Clin. Investig.* **2019**, *49*, e13060. [CrossRef]
7. Zimmet, P.; Alberti, K.G.; Kaufman, F.; Tajima, N.; Silink, M.; Arslanian, S.; Wong, G.; Bennett, P.; Shaw, J.; Caprio, S. The metabolic syndrome in children and adolescents—An IDF consensus report. *Pediatr. Diabetes* **2007**, *8*, 299–306. [CrossRef]
8. Pergher, R.N.; Melo, M.E.; Halpern, A. Is a diagnosis of metabolic syndrome applicable to children? *J. Pediatr.* **2010**, *86*, 101–108. [CrossRef]
9. Weiss, R.; Bremer, A.; Lustig, R.H. What is metabolic syndrome, and why are children getting it? *Ann. N. Y. Acad. Sci.* **2013**, *1281*, 123–140. [CrossRef]
10. Goodman, E.; Daniels, S.R.; Meigs, J.B.; Dolan, L.M. Instability in the diagnosis of metabolic syndrome in adolescents. *Circulation* **2007**, *115*, 2316–2322. [CrossRef]
11. National Institutes of Health/National Heart, Lung, and Blood Institute. Third Report of the National Cholesterol Education Program (NCEP). In *Expert Panel on Detection, Evaluation, and Treatment of High Blood Cholesterol in Adults (Adult Treatment Panel III)*; Final Report; National Institutes of Health: Bethesda, MD, USA, 2002.
12. Cook, S.; Weitzman, M.; Auinger, P.; Nguyen, M.; Dietz, W.H. Prevalence of a metabolic syndrome phenotype in adolescents: Findings from the third National Health and Nutrition Examination Survey, 1988-1994. *Arch. Pediatr. Adolesc. Med.* **2003**, *157*, 821–827. [CrossRef] [PubMed]
13. Weiss, R.; Dziura, J.; Burgert, T.S.; Tamborlane, W.V.; Taksali, S.E.; Yeckel, C.W.; Allen, K.; Lopes, M.; Savoye, M.; Morrison, J.; et al. Obesity and the metabolic syndrome in children and adolescents. *N. Engl. J. Med.* **2004**, *350*, 2362–2374. [CrossRef] [PubMed]
14. Duncan, G.E.; Li, S.M.; Zhou, X.H. Prevalence and trends of a metabolic syndrome phenotype among U.S. adolescents, 1999–2000. *Diabetes Care* **2004**, *27*, 2438–2443. [CrossRef] [PubMed]
15. De Ferranti, S.D.; Gauvreau, K.; Ludwig, D.S.; Neufeld, E.J.; Newburger, J.W.; Rifai, N. Prevalence of the metabolic syndrome in American adolescents: Findings from the Third National Health and Nutrition Examination Survey. *Circulation* **2004**, *110*, 2494–2497. [CrossRef] [PubMed]
16. Cruz, M.L.; Goran, M.I. The metabolic syndrome in children and adolescents. *Curr. Diabetes Rep.* **2004**, *4*, 53–62. [CrossRef]
17. Rodríguez, M.; Salazar, B.; Violante, R.; Guerrero, F. Metabolic syndrome among children and adolescents aged 10–18 years. *Diabetes Care* **2004**, *27*, 2516–2517. [CrossRef] [PubMed]

18. Viner, R.M.; Segal, T.Y.; Lichtarowicz-Krynska, E.; Hindmarsh, P. Prevalence of the insulin resistance syndrome in obesity. *Arch. Dis. Child.* **2005**, *90*, 10–14. [CrossRef]
19. Alberti, K.G.; Zimmet, P.Z. Definition, diagnosis and classification of diabetes mellitus and its complications. Part 1: Diagnosis and classification of diabetes mellitus provisional report of a WHO consultation. *Diabetes Med.* **1998**, *15*, 539–553. [CrossRef]
20. Marfell-Jones, M.; Olds, T.; Stewart, A. *International Standards for Anthropometric Assessment*; ISAK: Potchefstroom, South Africa, 2006.
21. Brook, C.G.D. Determination of body composition of children from skinfold measurements. *Arch. Dis. Child.* **1971**, *46*, 182–184. [CrossRef]
22. Siri, W.E. Body composition from fluid spaces and density: Analysis of methods. In *Techniques for Measuring Body Composition*; Brozeck, J., Henschel, A., Eds.; National Academies Sciences National Research Council: Washington, DC, USA, 1961.
23. Guerrero-Romero, F.; Rodríguez-Morán, M. Abdominal volume index. An anthropometry-based index for estimation of obesity is strongly related to impaired glucose tolerance and type 2 diabetes mellitus. *Arch. Med. Res.* **2003**, *34*, 428–432. [CrossRef]
24. Thomas, D.M.; Bredlau, C.; Bosy-Westphal, A.; Mueller, M.; Shen, W.; Gallagher, D.; Maeda, Y.; McDougall, A.; Peterson, C.M.; Ravussin, E.; et al. Relationships between body roundness with body fat and visceral adipose tissue emerging from a new geometrical model. *Obesity* **2013**, *21*, 2264–2271. [CrossRef] [PubMed]
25. Bergman, R.N.; Stefanovski, D.; Buchanan, T.A.; Sumner, A.E.; Reynolds, J.C.; Sebring, N.G.; Xiang, A.H.; Watanabe, R.M. A better index of body adiposity. *Obesity* **2011**, *19*, 1083–1089. [CrossRef] [PubMed]
26. El Aarbaoui, T.; Samouda, H.; Zitouni, D.; di Pompeo, C.; de Beaufort, C.; Trincaretto, F.; Mormentyn, A.; Hubert, H.; Lemdani, M.; Guinhouya, B.C. Does the body adiposity index (BAI) apply to paediatric populations? *Ann. Hum. Biol.* **2013**, *40*, 451–458. [CrossRef] [PubMed]
27. Valdez, R. A simple model-based index of abdominal adiposity. *J. Clin. Epidemiol.* **1991**, *44*, 955–956. [CrossRef]
28. Krakauer, N.Y.; Krakauer, J.C. A new body shape index predicts mortality hazard independently of body mass index. *PLoS ONE* **2012**, *7*, e39504. [CrossRef] [PubMed]
29. Matthews, D.; Hosker, J.; Rudenski, A.; Naylor, B.; Treacher, D.; Turner, R. Homeostasis model assessment: Insulin resistance and B-cell function from fasting plasma glucose and insulin concentrations in man. *Diabetologia* **1985**, *28*, 412–419. [CrossRef] [PubMed]
30. Pickering, T.G.; Hall, J.E.; Appel, L.J.; Falkner, B.E.; Graves, J.; Hill, M.N.; Jones, D.W.; Kurtz, T.; Sheps, S.G.; Roccella, E.J. Subcommittee of Professional and Public Education of the American Heart Association Council on High Blood Pressure Research. Recommendations for blood pressure measurement in humans and experimental animals, part 1: Blood pressure measurement in humans: A statement for professionals from the Subcommittee of Professional and Public Education of the American Heart Association Council on High Blood Pressure Research. *Hypertension* **2005**, *45*, 142–161. [PubMed]
31. DeLong, E.R.; DeLong, D.M.; Clarke-Pearson, D.L. Comparing the areas under two or more correlated receiver operating characteristic curves: A nonparametric approach. *Biometrics* **1988**, *44*, 837–845. [CrossRef]
32. Braga-Tavares, H.; Fonseca, H. Prevalence of metabolic syndrome in a Portuguese obese adolescent population according to three different definitions. *Eur. J. Pediatr.* **2010**, *169*, 935–940. [CrossRef]
33. Saffari, F.; Jalilolghadr, S.; Esmailzadehha, N.; Azinfar, P. Metabolic syndrome in a sample of the 6- to 16-year-old overweight or obese pediatric population: A comparison of two definitions. *Ther. Clin. Risk Manag.* **2012**, *8*, 55–63. [CrossRef]
34. Sarrafzadegan, N.; Gharipour, M.; Sadeghi, M.; Nouri, F.; Asgary, S.; Zarfeshani, S. Differences in the prevalence of metabolic syndrome in boys and girls based on various definitions. *ARYA Atheroscler.* **2013**, *9*, 70–76. [PubMed]
35. Ramírez-Vélez, R.; Anzola, A.; Martinez-Torres, J.; Vivas, A.; Tordecilla-Sanders, A.; Prieto-Benavides, D.; Izquierdo, M.; Correa-Bautista, J.E.; Garcia-Hermoso, A. Metabolic Syndrome and Associated Factors in a Population-Based Sample of Schoolchildren in Colombia: The FUPRECOL Study. *Metab. Syndr. Relat. Disord.* **2016**, *14*, 455–462. [CrossRef] [PubMed]
36. Nasreddine, L.; Naja, F.; Tabet, M.; Habbal, M.; El-Aily, A.; Haikal, C.; Sidani, S.; Adra, N.; Hwalla, N. Obesity is associated with insulin resistance and components of the metabolic syndrome in Lebanese adolescents. *Ann. Hum. Biol.* **2012**, *39*, 122–128. [CrossRef] [PubMed]

37. Shashaj, B.; Bedogni, G.; Graziani, M.P.; Tozzi, A.E.; DiCorpo, M.L.; Morano, D.; Tacconi, L.; Veronelli, P.; Contoli, B.; Manco, M. Origin of cardiovascular risk in overweight preschool children: A cohort study of cardiometabolic risk factors at the onset of obesity. *JAMA Pediatr.* **2014**, *168*, 917–924. [CrossRef] [PubMed]
38. Xu, T.; Liu, J.; Liu, J.; Zhu, G.; Han, S. Relation between metabolic syndrome and body compositions among Chinese adolescents and adults from a large-scale population survey. *BMC Public Health* **2017**, *17*, 337. [CrossRef] [PubMed]
39. Zaki, M.E.; El-Bassyouni, H.T.; El-Gammal, M.; Kamal, S. Indicators of the metabolic syndrome in obese adolescents. *Arch. Med. Sci.* **2015**, *11*, 92–98. [CrossRef] [PubMed]
40. Haghighatdoost, F.; Sarrafzadegan, N.; Mohammadifard, N.; Asgary, S.; Boshtam, M.; Azadbakht, L. Assessing body shape index as a risk predictor for cardiovascular diseases and metabolic syndrome among Iranian adults. *Nutrition* **2014**, *30*, 636–644. [CrossRef]
41. Behboudi-Gandevani, S.; Ramezani Tehrani, F.; Cheraghi, L.; Azizi, F. Could, "a body shape index" and "waist to height ratio" predict insulin resistance and metabolic syndrome in polycystic ovary syndrome? *Eur. J. Obstet. Gynecol. Reprod. Biol.* **2016**, *205*, 110–114. [CrossRef]

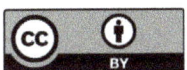 © 2019 by the authors. Licensee MDPI, Basel, Switzerland. This article is an open access article distributed under the terms and conditions of the Creative Commons Attribution (CC BY) license (http://creativecommons.org/licenses/by/4.0/).

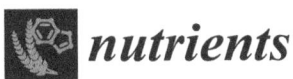

Article

Validation of Surrogate Anthropometric Indices in Older Adults: What Is the Best Indicator of High Cardiometabolic Risk Factor Clustering?

Robinson Ramírez-Vélez [1,*], Miguel Ángel Pérez-Sousa [2], Mikel Izquierdo [1,3], Carlos A. Cano-Gutierrez [4], Emilio González-Jiménez [5], Jacqueline Schmidt-RioValle [5], Katherine González-Ruíz [6] and María Correa-Rodríguez [5]

1. Department of Health Sciences, Public University of Navarra, Navarrabiomed-Biomedical Research Centre, IDISNA-Navarra's Health Research Institute, C/irunlarrea 3, Complejo Hospitalario de Navarra, 31008 Pamplona, Navarra, Spain
2. Faculty of Sport Sciences, University of Huelva, Avenida de las Fuerzas Armadas s/n, 21007 Huelva, Spain
3. Centro de Investigación Biomédica en Red de Fragilidad y Envejecimiento Saludable (CIBERFES), Instituto de Salud Carlos III, 28029 Madrid, Spain
4. Hospital Universitario San Ignacio – Aging Institute, Pontificia Universidad Javeriana, Bogotá 110111, Colombia
5. Department of Nursing, Faculty of Health Sciences, University of Granada, Av. Ilustración, 60, 18016 Granada, Spain
6. Grupo de Ejercicio Físico y Deportes, Vicerrectoría de Investigaciones, Facultad de Salud, Universidad Manuela Beltrán, Bogotá 110231, DC, Colombia
* Correspondence: robin640@hotmail.com; Tel.: +34-699-993-920

Received: 5 July 2019; Accepted: 22 July 2019; Published: 24 July 2019

Abstract: The present study evaluated the ability of five obesity-related parameters, including a body shape index (ABSI), conicity index (CI), body roundness index (BRI), body mass index (BMI), and waist-to-height ratio (WtHR) for predicting increased cardiometabolic risk in a population of elderly Colombians. A cross-sectional study was conducted on 1502 participants (60.3% women, mean age 70 ± 7.6 years) and subjects' weight, height, waist circumference, serum lipid indices, blood pressure, and fasting plasma glucose were measured. A cardiometabolic risk index (CMRI) was calculated using the participants' systolic and diastolic blood pressure, triglycerides, high-density lipoprotein and fasting glucose levels, and waist circumference. Following the International Diabetes Federation definition, metabolic syndrome was defined as having three or more metabolic abnormalities. All surrogate anthropometric indices correlated significantly with CMRI ($p < 0.01$). Receiver operating characteristic curve analysis of how well the anthropometric indices identified high cardiometabolic risk showed that WtHR and BRI were the most accurate indices. The best WtHR and BRI cut-off points in men were 0.56 (area under curve, AUC 0.77) and 4.71 (AUC 0.77), respectively. For women, the WtHR and BRI cut-off points were 0.63 (AUC 0.77) and 6.20 (AUC 0.77), respectively. In conclusion, BRI and WtHR have a moderate discriminating power for detecting high cardiometabolic risk in older Colombian adults, supporting the idea that both anthropometric indices are useful screening tools for use in the elderly.

Keywords: anthropometric indices; diagnosis criteria; metabolic syndrome; cardiometabolic risk; elderly

1. Introduction

Metabolic syndrome (MetS) is a complex cluster of cardiovascular risk factors associated with a sedentary lifestyle, poor nutrition, and consequent overweight. It is also strongly associated with other abnormalities linked to cardiovascular disease (CVD), including glucose intolerance (type 2 diabetes, impaired glucose tolerance, or impaired fasting glycemia), insulin resistance, abdominal obesity, dyslipidemia, and hypertension [1]. Accordingly, MetS increases the risk of developing diseases of cardiovascular origin, such as acute myocardial infarction, ischemic stroke, or coronary heart disease [2]. Indeed, the prevalence of CVD attributable to MetS is estimated at around 12–17% [3]. Several studies have examined the presence of MetS in Latin America, reporting associated factors including advanced age, having Hispanic or indigenous heritage, physical inactivity, high alcohol intake, smoking, history of hypertension or type 2 diabetes (first-degree family members), and having a low socioeconomic status (reviewed in [4]). The general prevalence of MetS in Latin-American countries has been established as 24.9% (range: 18.8–43.3%) and is slightly more frequent in women (25.3%) than in men (23.2%).

The clinical utility of identifying MetS in older adults has been much debated because, among the issues raised, it has been argued that there is no consensus on the clinical criteria for screening the elderly population to identify patients likely to be characterized with MetS. In this line, several clinical criteria and cut-off points have been proposed. For instance, the cardiometabolic risk index (CMRI) in older adults, measured as a continuous summary score, might represent an important intermediate or preclinical outcome that can be measured prior to the onset of disease, and could provide opportunities for prevention. As a marker of cardiometabolic disease risk, the use of adult CMRI severity z-scores has been suggested as an accurate method to detect overall metabolic changes [5]. This continuous score would be more sensitive to small and large changes that do not modify the most recent Joint Interim Statement of the International Diabetes Federation (IDF) Task Force on Epidemiology and Prevention criteria [6]. Thus, an increase in cholesterol from 150 to 250 mg/dl would have no impact on the IDF score, but would be reflected as a non-trivial change in the continuous CMRI [7]. Nevertheless, there is no validated or harmonized consensus for defining CMRI in older adults, and several continuous CMRI scores have been reported in the literature, as described in previous narrative reviews.

Measurements of anthropometric indices are inexpensive and non-invasive, and are easily conducted as part of normal health exams. Interestingly, anthropometric measurements such as body mass index (BMI), waist circumference (WC), and waist-to-height ratio (WtHR) show a close correlation with MetS components and could thus be useful surrogate markers for predicting MetS [8–10]. That being said, there remains controversy over which anthropometric indices [11] are the most appropriate predictors of cardiometabolic disease [12]. In 2012, Krakauer and Krakauer developed "A Body Shape Index" (ABSI), based on WC adjusted for height and weight [13], and demonstrated that a high ABSI is associated with the accumulation of excess abdominal adipose tissue and seems to be a substantial risk factor for premature mortality in the general population [13]. In a similar vein, the conicity index (CI), an index of abdominal obesity, has been considered useful for detecting central obesity, and has been studied as a predictor for alterations in fasting insulin, blood pressure, and triglyceride levels [14]. Lastly, in 2013, Thomas and colleagues [15] developed the body roundness index (BRI), which combines height and WC to predict the percentage of body fat. When compared with other anthropometric indices, BRI was optimal for identifying MetS, insulin resistance, inflammatory factors [16], and arterial stiffness [17] in obese and overweight populations. However, to date, few studies have evaluated the predictive ability of BRI, ABSI, or CI compared with traditional metrics, such as BMI and WtHR, with regard to CMRI in older adults [18–20].

South America has undergone a rapid epidemiologic transition, including a non-communicable disease epidemic [21] and adverse lifestyle changes that could contribute to increase a cluster of cardiometabolic risk factors such as MetS [4]. To the best of our knowledge, the predictive power of anthropometric measurements, which can be measured easily in a routine health exam, has not been assessed in elderly Latin-American individuals with high cardiovascular risk, for whom the early detection of risk factors is essential for prevention of CVD. This is particularly true in Colombia, where anthropometric index measurements and blood collection are not usually standard in the annual health exam, and, to date, there have been few studies conducted in the general older population.

For these reasons, the aim of the present study was to evaluate the prevalence of MetS using a CMRI among older adults from Colombia, and validate the associated anthropometric surrogate markers. We also compared the predictive ability of BRI, ABSI, CI, BMI, and WtHR to determine whether there is a single best CMRI predictor.

2. Materials and Methods

2.1. Study Design and Participants

The data for this secondary cross-sectional study was obtained from the 2015 Colombian Health, Well-Being and Aging Survey (SABE 2015, from the Spanish: SAlud, Bienestar and Envejecimiento, 2015), a multicenter project conducted from 2014 to 2015 by the Pan-American Health Organization and supported by the Epidemiological Office of the Ministry of Health and Social Protection of Colombia (https://www.minsalud.gov.co/). The survey is a cross-sectional tool for exploring and evaluating several aspects that intervene in the phenomenon of aging and old age in the Colombian population [19]. Details of the survey have been previously published [19]. SABE 2015 was a joint venture between the Ministry of Health and Social Protection and the Administrative Department of Science, Technology and Innovation in Colombia.

The sample was regionally representative and involved self-representation in large cities, with urban-rural stratification of the sample and stage selection in accordance with the municipal map available from the Ministry of Health and Social Protection, with the following hierarchy: municipalities, urban/rural segments, homes or sidewalks, homes, and people. The study included the Colombian population ≥60 years old, and the indicators were disaggregated by age range, sex, ethnicity, and socioeconomic level. To calculate the original sample size, the non-institutionalized Colombian population aged ≥60 years was considered, and the following parameters were used: minimum estimable proportion = 0.03, design effect = 1.2, and Relative Standard Error = 0.05 (1.2). The universe of study comprised 99% of the population residing in private homes in both urban and rural areas.

A total of 23,694 surveys were conducted across the country and 6365 total population segments were investigated in 246 municipalities. As Bogotá is the capital it was independently selected, with a total of 545 urban segments and one rural segment. The average number of adults per segment was 4.2. The estimation of means or proportions was conducted to a level of precision of up to 6% of the maximum expected error, at a level of national disaggregation only. The basic procedure for the population survey was a face-to-face interview using a structured questionnaire. The interviewers visited the selected homes, carrying the appropriate identification. At each home visited, the standardized process involved the following: identifying the participants, registering the demographic data, obtaining the signed informed consent, applying the established filters and selection criteria, obtaining a signed assent form when necessary, and completion of the questionnaire by the interviewer. A total of 1502 participants from 86 municipalities were included in this analysis.

The institutional review boards involved in developing the SABE 2015 study (the University of Caldas, ID protocol CBCS-021-14, and the University of Valle, ID protocol 09-014 and O11-015) reviewed and approved the study protocol. Written informed consent was obtained from each individual before inclusion and completion of the first examination. One of the authors (C.A.C.-G.) applied to the Ministry of Health and Social Protection of Colombia and obtained permission to use publicly available data for research and teaching purposes (permission and details available at https://www.minsalud.gov.co/). The study protocol for the secondary analysis was approved by the Human Subjects Committee at the Pontificia Universidad Javeriana (ID protocol 20/2017-2017/180, FM-CIE-0459-17) in accordance with the Declaration of Helsinki (World Medical Association) and Resolution 8430 from 1993, of the then Colombian Ministry of Health, on technical, scientific, and administrative standards for conducting research with humans.

2.2. Anthropometric Measurements

The research teams of the coordinating centers (Caldas and Valle universities, Colombia) trained the data collection staff to carry out the face-to-face interviews and physical measurements. Anthropometric measurements included height and body weight, which were measured using a portable stadiometer (SECA 213®, Hamburg, Germany) and an electronic scale (Kendall graduated platform scale), respectively. BMI was estimated in kg/m² from the measured body weight and height. WC was measured using inextensible anthropometric tape with the subjects standing erect and relaxed, with their arms at their sides and their feet positioned close together, parallel to the floor. WtHR was calculated as the ratio of WC (cm) to height (cm). The other anthropometric indexes (BRI, ABSI, and CI) were calculated using the following formulas: $BRI = 364.2 - 365.5 (1 - \pi^{-2} WC^2 (m) Height^{-2} (m))^{1/2}$ [15]; $ABSI = WC (m)/(BMI^{2/3}(kg/m^2) Height^{1/2} (m))$ [13]; $CI = 0.109^{-1} WC (m) (Weight (kg)/Height (m))^{-1/2}$ [22].

2.3. Serum Biochemical Examination

After an overnight fast, blood was collected in the morning. Blood samples were centrifuged for 10 min at 3000 rpm, 30 min after sampling. All samples were delivered to a single central laboratory (Dinamica Laboratories, Bogotá, Colombia) for analysis within 24 h. Serum fasting glucose, low-density lipoprotein cholesterol (LDL-C), high-density lipoprotein cholesterol (HDL-C), total cholesterol, and triglycerides (TG) were analyzed using enzymatic colorimetric methods (Olympus AU5200, Melville, NY, USA). Low-density lipoprotein cholesterol (LDL-C) was estimated using the Friedewald equation ((LDL-C) = (Total Cholesterol) − (HDL-C) − ((TG)/5)).

2.4. Blood Pressure Determination

We measured systolic (SBP) and diastolic (DBP) blood pressure levels using an automatic blood pressure monitor (OMRON HEM-705, Omron Healthcare Co., Ltd., Kyoto, Japan), following the recommendations of the American College of Cardiology Foundation/American Heart Association 2011 Expert Consensus Document on Hypertension in the Elderly [23]. Values were recorded after 5 min of rest in the sitting position and three consecutive measures were obtained, waiting for at least 30 s between readings. The average of the three values for each measurement were used in the analysis.

2.5. Diagnostic Criteria of Metabolic Syndrome

MetS was defined according to the most recent Joint Interim Statement of the IDF [6] by adopting the Ethnic Central and South American criteria for WC. Participants were classified as having MetS if they had at least three of following metabolic risk factors or components (MetS-components): abdominal obesity (WC ≥90 cm for Latin-American males and ≥80 cm for Latin-American females), elevated TG (fasting serum TG ≥150 mg/dL or taking medication for abnormal lipid levels), low HDL-C (fasting serum HDL-C <40 mg/dL in males and <50 mg/dL in females, or specific treatment for this lipid abnormality), elevated blood pressure (SBP ≥130 mmHg or DBP ≥85 mmHg or taking hypertension medication), or elevated fasting glucose (serum glucose level ≥100 mg/dL or taking diabetes medication).

2.6. Definition of Cardiometabolic Risk Index

We calculated the CMRI as a continuous score of the MetS risk factors. The CMRI was calculated using sex- and race-specific algorithms for the IDF criteria cut-off values, using the values of the participants' SBP and DBP, TG, HDL-C, fasting glucose, and WC. For each of these variables, a z-score was computed as the number of standard deviation (SD) units from the sample mean after normalization of the variables, that is, z-score = ((value − sample mean)/sample SD)). The HDL-C z-score was multiplied by −1 to indicate higher cardiovascular risk with increasing value. Individuals with a

CMRI ≥ 1 SD above the mean were identified as having increased cardiometabolic risk, and a lower CMRI (<1 SD) being indicative of a healthier risk profile.

2.7. Co-Variables

For lifestyle characteristics, personal habits regarding alcohol intake (participants were categorized as those who do not drink and those who drink less than one day per week, two to six days a week, or every day) and cigarette smoking (participants were categorized as those who do not smoke and those who have never-smoked, those who currently smoke or those who previously smoked) were recorded. A "proxy physical activity" report was conducted by the following questions: (i) "Have you regularly exercised, such as jogging or dancing, or performed rigorous physical activity at least three times a week for the past year?"; (ii) "do you walk at least three times a week between nine and 20 blocks (1.6 km) without resting?"; (iii) "do you walk at least three times a week eight blocks (0.5 km) without resting?". Participants were considered physically active if they responded affirmatively to two of the three questions [24].

Medical information including multimorbidity, as well as chronic conditions adapted from the original SABE study, was assessed by asking the participants if they had been medically diagnosed with hypertension, type 2 diabetes mellitus, chronic obstructive pulmonary disease, CVD (heart attack, angina), stroke, cancer, arthritis, osteoporosis, or sensory impairments (vision and hearing loss).

Race/ethnicity was self-reported and grouped into indigenous (people belonging to various indigenous groups such as Ika, Kankuamo, Emberá, Misak, Nasa, Wayuu, Awuá, and Mokane); black, "mulatto", or Afro-Colombian; white; and other (mestizo, gypsy, etc.).

Socioeconomic status was determined on a scale of one to six based on the housing stratum, with one representing the highest level of poverty and six the greatest wealth. This classification was developed by the National Government of Colombia and considers the physical characteristics of the dwellings as well as their surroundings. Classification into one of the six strata was taken to approximate the hierarchical socioeconomic differences from poverty to wealth.

2.8. Statistical Analysis

Descriptive analyses using the mean ± SD or standard error (SE) for the continuous variables, median and interquartile range for the skewed continuous variables, and the frequency distribution of the categorical variables were used to determine the characteristics of the sample. Data normality was examined using the Kolmogorov–Smirnoff test. Significant differences between men and women were analyzed using Student's t-test, Wilcoxon rank-sum test, or chi-square (χ^2) post-hoc test. To visualize the relationship between CMRI and anthropometric indices, Spearman and Pearson correlation and linear regression analysis were applied to the total sample and individual genders. The linear regression analysis was adjusted by age as a covariate.

The area under receiver operating characteristic (ROC) curves was calculated to evaluate the abilities of the anthropometric indices to predict high CMRI. Cut-off points were proposed after calculation of Youden's Index (sensitivity + specificity − 1) [25]. The DeLong et al. [26] non-parametric approach was used to compare the areas under the ROC curves. Since abdominal obesity is a component of CMRI, we conducted a multicollinearity test for the anthropometric indices that included WC (WtHR, CI, BRI, and ABSI), and the variance inflation factor (VIF) was calculated. Each cardiometabolic risk factor among BMI, WtHR, BRI, ABSI, and CI was determined using analysis of variance without any adjustment and then after adjusting (analysis of covariance, ANCOVA) for ethnicity, socio-economic status, smoking status, alcohol intake, physical activity "proxy", and medical conditions (i.e., presence or absence of osteoporosis, CVD, hypertension, type 2 diabetes, cancer, or respiratory diseases) as covariates, followed by Tukey's test. Collinearity was tested between all anthropometric indexes that included WC; a VFI > 10, was interpreted as high collinearity [27].

Statistical analyses were performed using SPSS v24.0 (IBM, Armonk, NY, USA) and JASP v0.9 (JASP Team, Amsterdam, The Netherlands). Statistical significance was defined as $p < 0.05$.

3. Results

3.1. Baseline Characteristics of the Participants

The participants' characteristics are summarized in Table 1. Of the 1502 older adults studied, 60.3% were women, and the mean age was 70 ± 7.6 years. The prevalence of smoking (9.7%), alcohol intake (12.7%), and a physical activity proxy (17.7%) was relatively low, but significantly higher in CMRI ≥ 1 SD than in CMRI < 1 SD (alcohol: 13.1% vs. 12.6%, $p < 0.001$). The means (SD or range interquartile) of the WtHR, BMI, BRI, ABSI, and CI in the overall sample were 0.59 (0.1), 27.3 (24–30) kg/m^2, 5.2 (4.1–6.3), 0.081 (0.078–0.085), and 22.2 (20.9–23.8), respectively. The overall prevalence of MetS was 58.7%. Significant differences were found between the high/low CMRI status groups for almost all characteristics, with the exception of height, LDL-C and HDL-C levels.

Table 1. Characteristics of study participants according to high (≥ 1 SD) and low (< 1 SD) cardiometabolic risk index (CMRI) status among Colombian older adults.

Characteristics	Total Sample (n = 1502)	High CMRI ≥ 1 SD (n = 397)	Low CMRI < 1 SD (n = 1105)	p-Value
Sex, n (%)				
Men	596 (39.7)	141 (23.7)	455 (76.3)	<0.001
Women	906 (60.3)	254 (28.0)	652 (72.0)	<0.001
Socioeconomic status				
1	456 (30.4)	121 (30.5)	335 (32.1)	<0.001
2	635 (42.3)	176 (44.3)	459 (41.5)	<0.001
3	375 (25.0)	98 (24.7)	277 (25.1)	<0.001
4	29 (1.9)	2 (0.5)	27 (2.4)	<0.001
>5	7 (0.5)	0 (0.0)	7 (0.6)	N.A
Ethnic group				
Indigenous	78 (5.2)	25 (6.3)	53 (4.8)	0.002
Black	119 (7.9)	28 (7.1)	91 (8.2)	<0.001
White	396 (26.4)	106 (26.7)	290 (26.2)	<0.001
Others	909 (60.5)	194 (48.9)	512 (46.3)	<0.001
Smoking status, n (%)				
Yes	145 (9.7)	29 (7.3)	116 (10.5)	<0.001
No	1357 (90.3)	368 (92.7)	989 (89.5)	<0.001
Alcohol intake, n (%)				
Yes	191 (12.7)	52 (13.1)	139 (12.6)	<0.001
No	1310 (87.2)	345 (86.9)	965 (87.3)	<0.001
Physical Activity "proxy", n (%)				
Physically active	266 (17.7)	70 (17.6)	196 (17.7)	0.980
Non-Physically active	1231 (82.0)	323 (81.4)	908 (82.2)	<0.001
Anthropometric measures/indices				
Height (m)	1.55 (1.49–1.62)	1.54 (1.49–1.62)	1.55 (1.49–1.62)	0.170
Weight (kg)	64 (57–72)	71 (63–79)	62 (55–69)	<0.001
Waist circumference (cm)	92 (85–100)	101 (93–107)	89 (83–97)	<0.001
Body mass index (kg/m^2)	27 (24–30)	29.7 (26.7–33)	26.1 (23.3–29)	<0.001
WtHR	0.59 (0.1)	0.64 (0.06)	0.57 (0.06)	<0.001
BRI	5.2 (4.1–6.3)	6.4 (5.3–7.7)	4.8 (3.9–5.9)	<0.001
ABSI (m$^{11/6}$ · kg$^{-2/3}$)	0.081 (0.078–0.085)	0.083 (0.080–0.086)	0.081 (0.077–0.084)	<0.001
CI	22.2 (20.9–23.8)	21.1 (19.8–22.4)	22.6 (21.4–24.1)	<0.001
Metabolic syndrome components, n (%)				
Prevalence of MetS	811 (58.7)	308 (77.6)	503 (45.5)	<0.001
Abdominal obesity	1177 (78.4)	374 (94.2)	803 (72.7)	<0.001
Hypertension	790 (52.6)	304 (76.6)	486 (44.0)	<0.001
High levels of fasting glucose	465 (31.0)	220 (55.4)	245 (22.2)	<0.001
High levels of triglycerides	696 (46.3)	253 (63.7)	443 (40.1)	<0.001
Low levels of HDL-C	821 (54.7)	219 (55.2)	602 (54.5)	0.393

Table 1. em Cont.

Characteristics	Total Sample (n = 1502)	High CMRI ≥ 1 SD (n = 397)	Low CMRI < 1 SD (n = 1105)	p-Value
Cardiometabolic measurements				
SBP (mmHg)	130 (117–145)	142 (130–163)	126 (114–140)	**<0.001**
DBP (mmHg)	72 (65–79)	78 (72–86)	70 (64–77)	**<0.001**
MBP (mmHg)	92 (84–101)	100 (91–111)	89 (81–97)	**<0.001**
Total cholesterol (mg/dL)	193 (166–221)	202 (171–232)	190 (164–216)	**<0.001**
Triglycerides (mg/dL)	144 (105–192)	174 (134–252)	134 (101–180)	**<0.001**
LDL-C (mg/dL)	126 (102–149)	127 (103–152)	125 (102–147)	0.116
HDL-C (mg/dL)	43 (36–53)	43 (36–54)	44 (36–53)	0.740
Glucose (mg/dL)	94 (86–102)	102 (93–121)	91 (84–98)	**<0.001**
CMRI	−0.21 (−1.41–1.07)	2.00 (1.44–2.84)	−0.83 (−1.83–0.05)	**<0.001**
Self-report comorbid chronic diseases, n (%)				
Hypertension	826 (55.0)	249 (62.7)	577 (52.2)	**<0.001**
Diabetes	245 (16.3)	113 (28.5)	132 (11.9)	**<0.001**
Respiratory diseases	165 (11.0)	49 (12.3)	116 (10.5)	**<0.001**
Cardiovascular diseases	213 (14.2)	155 (39.0)	58 (5.2)	**<0.001**
Stroke	70 (4.7)	22 (5.5)	48 (4.3)	**<0.001**
Osteoporosis	184 (12.3)	66 (16.6)	118 (10.7)	**<0.001**
Cancer	80 (5.3)	56 (14.1)	24 (2.2)	**<0.001**
Hearing loss	360 (24.1)	89 (22.4)	271 (24.5)	**<0.001**
Vision loss	851 (56.7)	228 (57.4)	623 (56.4)	**<0.001**

Skewed continuous variables are reported as median and interquartile range (Q3-Q1), for non-skewed continuous variables mean values (standard deviations (SD)) are given, and categorical variables are reported as numbers and percentages in brackets. Significant between-sex differences (Student's t-test, Wilcoxon rank-sum test or χ2). BMI: body mass index; WtHR: waist-to-height ratio; BRI: body roundness index; ABSI: a body shape index; CI: conicity index; LDL-C: low-density lipoprotein cholesterol; HDL-C: high-density lipoprotein cholesterol; CMRI: cardiometabolic risk index. p-values marked in bold are significant.

3.2. Association between Surrogate Anthropometric Indices with CMRI

Linear regression analyses of surrogate anthropometric indices and CMRI on the total sample and also stratified by sex are shown in Figure 1. Overall, we found an acceptable-to-moderate positive correlation of CMRI with WtHR ($r = 0.52$, $p < 0.001$), ABSI ($r = 0.17$, $p < 0.001$), BMI ($r = 0.46$, $p < 0.001$), and BRI ($r = 0.52$, $p < 0.001$), whereas CI was negatively correlated with CMRI ($r = −0.42$, $p < 0.001$). When analyzing by sex, the decreasing order of the correlation coefficients in men was WtHR ($r = 0.50$, $p < 0.001$), BRI ($r = 0.50$, $p < 0.001$), BMI ($r = 0.49$, $p < 0.001$), CI ($r = −0.46$, $p < 0.001$), and ABSI ($r = 0.16$, $p < 0.001$), while in women the decreasing order of the correlation coefficients was WtHR ($r = 0.55$, $p < 0.001$), BRI ($r = 0.54$, $p < 0.001$), BMI ($r = 0.45$, $p < 0.01$), CI ($r = −0.44$, $p < 0.001$), and ABSI ($r = 0.22$, $p < 0.001$).

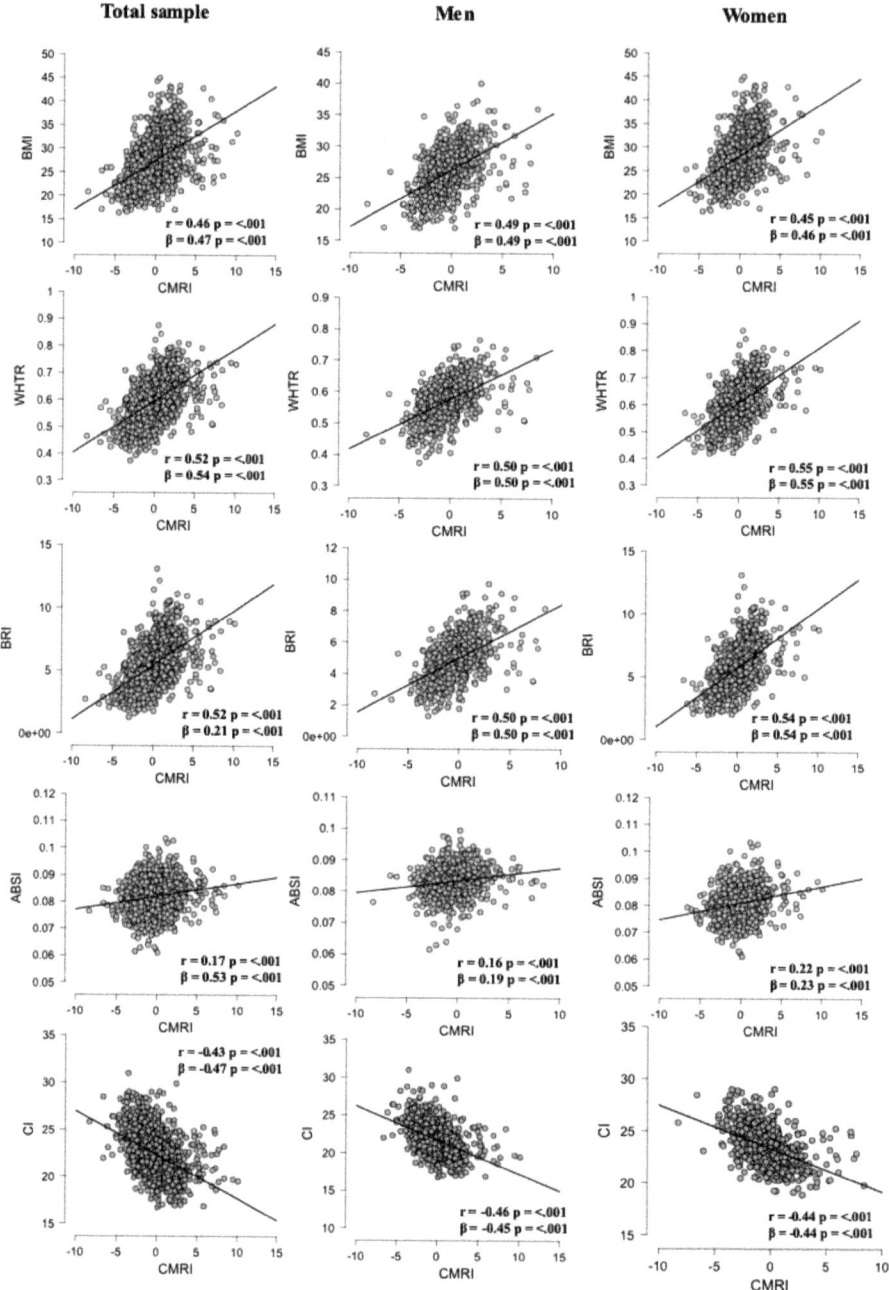

Figure 1. Association between surrogate anthropometric indices and CMRI, on the total sample and stratified by sex. BMI: body mass index; WtHR: waist to height ratio; BRI: body roundness index; ABSI: a body shape index; CI: conicity index; CMRI: cardiometabolic risk index.

3.3. Optimal Cut-Offs for Screening for CMRI by Sex

The ROC curve analyses of the diagnostic performance of BMI, WtHR, BRI, ABSI, and CI in identifying a high cardiometabolic risk are shown in Table 2 and Figure 2. In men, when considering the full sample, the best cut-off vales of BMI, WtHR, BRI, ABSI, and CI for detecting high cardiometabolic risk (CMRI ≥ 1 SD) were 25.2 (area under curve, AUC 0.76, sensitivity 84.4% and specificity 54.7%), 0.56 (AUC 0.77, sensitivity 83.6% and specificity 58.9%), 4.71 (AUC 0.77, sensitivity 83.6% and specificity 58.9%), 0.083 (AUC 0.60, sensitivity 69.5% and specificity 53.6%), and 22.9 (AUC 0.75, sensitivity 72.3% and specificity 65.9%), respectively. For women, the best cut-off values of BMI, WtHR, BRI, ABSI, and CI for detecting high cardiometabolic risk (CMRI ≥ 1 SD) were 28.4 (AUC 0.71, sensitivity 69.5% and specificity 64.1%), 0.63 (AUC 0.77, sensitivity 64.4% and specificity 76.7%), 6.20 (AUC 0.77, sensitivity 65.2% and specificity 76.1%), 0.080 (AUC 0.62, sensitivity 68.7% and specificity 51.6%), and 21.0 (AUC 0.71, sensitivity 63.6% and specificity 70.2%), respectively.

Table 2. Cut-off points, area under curve, sensitivity and specificity for BMI, WtHR, BRI, ABSI, and CI to detect high cardiometabolic risk (CMRI ≥ 1 SD) by sex.

Parameters	BMI		WtHR		BRI		ABSI		CI	
	Men	Women	Men	Women	Men	Women	Men	Women	Men	Women
Area under curve	0.76	0.71	0.77	0.77	0.77	0.77	0.60	0.62	0.75	0.71
p-value	<0.0001	<0.0001	<0.0001	<0.0001	<0.0001	<0.0001	<0.0001	<0.0001	<0.0001	<0.0001
Optimal cut-off	25.2	28.4	0.56	0.63	4.71	6.20	0.083	0.080	22.9	21.0
Youden index J	0.39	0.33	0.42	0.41	0.42	0.41	0.23	0.20	0.38	0.33
Sensitivity (%)	84.4	69.5	83.6	64.4	83.6	65.2	69.5	68.7	72.3	63.6
Specificity (%)	54.7	64.1	58.9	76.7	58.9	76.1	53.6	51.6	65.9	70.2
(+) Likelihood ratio	1.83	1.93	2.00	2.70	2.04	2.74	1.50	1.42	2.12	2.14
(−) Likelihood ratio	0.29	0.48	0.28	0.47	0.28	0.46	0.57	0.60	0.42	0.52

BMI: body mass index; WtHR: waist to height ratio; BRI: body roundness index; ABSI: a body shape index; CI: conicity index.

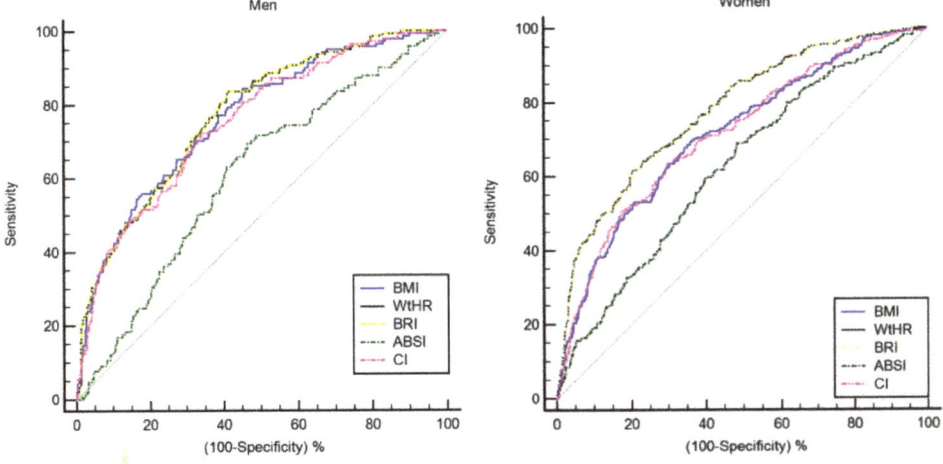

Figure 2. Diagnostic performance of surrogate anthropometric indices to detect high risk of CMRI by gender. BMI: body mass index; WtHR: waist-to-height ratio; BRI: body roundness index; ABSI: a body shape index; CI: conicity index.

The ROC curves were compared using a pairwise comparison method and the differences between the five methods are shown in Table 3. Independently of sex, the ROC-AUC of WtHR did not significantly differ from that of BRI. The results indicated that WtHR and BRI seem to provide the best results in Colombian older adults, owing to their greater precision in identifying subjects with a high cardiometabolic risk.

Table 3. Pairwise comparison for receiver operating characteristic (ROC) curves among Colombian older adults by sex.

Parameters	BMI–WtHR	BMI–BRI	BMI–ABSI	BMI–CI	WtHR–BRI	WtHR–ABSI	WtHR–CI	BRI–ABSI	BRI–CI	ABSI–CI
Men										
Diff. AUC	0.000	0.00	0.15	0.01	0.00	0.16	0.01	0.16	0.02	0.14
SE	0.01	0.01	0.03	0.00	0.00	0.02	0.01	0.02	0.01	0.03
p-value	0.542	0.540	**0.001**	0.220	0.090	**0.001**	0.100	**0.001**	0.090	**0.001**
Women										
Diff. AUC	0.06	0.06	0.08	0.00	0.00	0.15	0.06	0.15	0.06	0.08
SE	0.01	0.01	0.03	0.00	0.00	0.02	0.01	0.02	0.01	0.03
p-value	**0.001**	**0.001**	**0.001**	0.99	0.97	**0.001**	**0.001**	**0.001**	**0.001**	**0.001**

AUC: area under curve; SE: standard error; BMI: body mass index; WtHR: waist to height ratio; BRI: body roundness index; ABSI: a body shape index; CI: conicity index. P-values marked in bold are significant.

3.4. Sex Thresholds for Surrogate Anthropometric Indices to Screen for CMRI

Thresholds were determined for each of the surrogate anthropometric indices for the low/high CMRI in males and females, with corresponding differences in cardiometabolic parameters (Figure 2 and Table 4). In all groups (healthy/unhealthy) thresholds may be used to categorize individuals into one of two risk categories (i.e., low and high), on the combined basis of sex and surrogate anthropometric indices. In both sexes, after adjusting for ethnicity, socioeconomic status, smoking status, alcohol intake, physical activity proxy, and medical conditions (presence or absence of osteoporosis, CVD, hypertension, diabetes, cancer, and respiratory disease), the ANCOVA revealed that there were differences in blood pressure, HDL-C, and glucose in the BMI and CI parameters. By contrast, diagnostic performance results for CMRI without the central obesity component (i.e., WC) revealed lower accuracy (AUC) in all thresholds for surrogate anthropometric indices (Supplementary Material Table S1).

Finally, the collinearity test for all anthropometric indices that included WC in their calculation was found to be negative for BRI (VFI: 9.3), ABSI (VFI: 3.5), and WtHR (VFI: 9.1) and positive for CI (VFI: 10.9).

Table 4. Adjusted thresholds for surrogate anthropometric indices with cardiometabolic measurements among Colombian older adults by sex.

Variables	Cut-Off	BMI Mean (SE)	BMI p-Value	WtHR Mean (SE)	WtHR p-Value	BRI Mean (SE)	BRI p-Value	ABSI Mean (SE)	ABSI p-Value	CI Mean (SE)	CI p-Value
Men											
SBP (mmHg)	healthy	130.1 (1.5)	0.001	131.7 (1.5)	0.107	131.5 (1.4)	0.045	134.7 (2.1)	0.477	131.3 (1.3)	0.005
	unhealthy	136.1 (1.3)		135.0 (1.3)		135.6 (1.4)		133.3 (1.1)		136.6 (1.5)	
DBP (mmHg)	healthy	72.3 (0.8)	0.001	73.8 (0.8)	0.250	73.7 (0.7)	0.131	76.1 (13.4)	0.176	73.1 (0.7)	0.003
	unhealthy	76.3 (0.7)		75.3 (0.7)		75.4 (0.7)		74.1 (0.6)		76.5 (0.8)	
MBP (mmHg)	healthy	91.5 (1.0)	0.001	93.1 (0.9)	0.148	92.9 (0.9)	0.064	95.5 (1.3)	0.282	92.4 (0.8)	0.003
	unhealthy	96.1 (0.8)		95.0 (0.8)		95.4 (0.9)		93.8 (0.7)		96.4 (0.9)	
Total cholesterol (mg/dL)	healthy	189.5 (2.0)	0.011	190.0 (2.5)	0.010	188.0 (2.4)	0.099	186.6 (3.5)	0.947	186.6 (2.2)	0.224
	unhealthy	181.8 (2.2)		181.2 (2.2)		182.4 (2.3)		184.7 (1.9)		183.1 (2.5)	
Triglycerides (mg/dL)	healthy	149.6 (5.7)	0.22	149.4 (5.6)	0.088	151.4 (5.3)	0.176	147.4 (7.8)	00.054	150.7 (4.9)	00.054
	unhealthy	162.7 (4.9)		163.2 (4.9)		162.5 (5.2)		160.0 (4.2)		165.4 (5.6)	
LDL-C (mg/dL)	healthy	123.5 (2.2)	0.055	123.7 (2.1)	0.058	122.5 (2.0)	0.211	119.8 (3.0)	0.511	121.3 (1.9)	0.467
	unhealthy	118.4 (1.8)		118.1 (1.9)		118.8 (1.9)		120.8 (1.6)		119.6 (2.1)	
HDL-C (mg/dL)	healthy	45.1 (0.7)	0.001	44.3 (0.7)	0.001	44.3 (12.4)	0.001	45.4 (1.0)	0.001	43.9 (0.6)	0.001
	unhealthy	39.5 (0.6)		39.6 (0.6)		39.3 (9.5)		40.8 (0.5)		39.2 (0.7)	
Glucose (mg/dL)	healthy	93.7 (1.5)	0.005	93.9 (1.5)	0.009	93.6 (1.4)	0.002	98.0 (2.1)	0.519	95.0 (1.3)	0.028
	unhealthy	99.1 (1.3)		99.0 (1.3)		99.8 (1.4)		96.4 (1.1)		99.0 (1.5)	
CMRI	healthy	−1.09 (0.1)	0.001	−1.05 (0.1)	0.001	−1.05 (0.1)	0.001	−0.66 (0.18)	0.010	−0.87 (0.11)	0.001
	unhealthy	0.36 (0.1)		0.36 (0.1)		0.50 (0.1)		−0.13 (0.09)		0.53 (0.12)	
Women											
SBP (mmHg)	healthy	130.4 (1.1)	0.530	130.6 (1.0)	0.942	130.6 (1.0)	0.935	129.8 (1.2)	0.639	130.4 (1.0)	0.537
	unhealthy	131.1 (1.1)		130.8 (1.3)		130.8 (1.3)		131.4 (1.0)		131.1 (1.2)	
DBP (mmHg)	healthy	70.9 (0.5)	0.021	71.6 (0.5)	0.458	71.6 (0.5)	0.414	72.0 (0.6)	0.993	71.1 (0.5)	0.034
	unhealthy	72.9 (10.5)		72.3 (0.6)		72.3 (0.6)		71.8 (0.5)		73.1 (0.6)	
MBP (mmHg)	healthy	90.6 (0.6)	0.097	91.2 (0.6)	0.721	91.2 (0.6)	0.691	91.2 (0.7)	0.823	90.8 (0.6)	0.139
	unhealthy	92.3 (0.7)		91.7 (0.8)		91.8 (0.8)		91.6 (0.6)		92.4 (0.7)	
Total cholesterol (mg/dL)	healthy	203.7 (1.9)	0.233	204.1 (1.8)	0.098	203.9 (1.8)	0.149	202.0 (2.1)	0.572	203.2 (1.8)	0.376
	unhealthy	200.4 (2.1)		198.8 (2.3)		199.0 (2.4)		202.2 (1.9)		200.5 (2.2)	
Triglycerides (mg/dL)	healthy	161.1 (4.0)	0.111	160.8 (3.7)	0.059	161.2 (3.7)	0.068	157.0 (4.4)	0.044	162.3 (3.8)	0.159
	unhealthy	170.8 (4.3)		173.5 (4.8)		173.4 (4.9)		172.4 (3.9)		170.7 (4.7)	
LDL-C (mg/dL)	healthy	132.3 (1.7)	0.258	132.6 (1.6)	0.164	132.5 (1.5)	0.132	131.1 (37.4)	0.812	132.0 (1.6)	0.381
	unhealthy	129.8 (1.8)		128.8 (2.0)		128.8 (2.1)		131.1 (37.4)		129.9 (2.0)	
HDL-C (mg/dL)	healthy	48.8 (0.6)	0.009	48.8 (0.5)	0.001	48.6 (0.5)	0.007	48.7 (13.9)	0.104	48.5 (0.5)	0.018
	unhealthy	46.1 (0.6)		45.4 (0.7)		45.6 (0.7)		46.9 (12.3)		46.1 (0.7)	
Glucose (mg/dL)	healthy	97.3 (1.1)	0.016	96.8 (1.0)	0.001	96.6 (1.0)	0.001	98.1 (1.2)	0.241	97.0 (1.0)	0.002
	unhealthy	101.2 (1.2)		102.9 (1.3)		103.5 (1.3)		99.9 (1.1)		102.3 (1.3)	
CMRI	healthy	−0.61 (0.09)	0.001	−0.57 (0.08)	0.001	−0.56 (0.08)	0.001	−0.32 (0.10)	0.001	−0.52 (0.08)	0.001
	unhealthy	0.82 (0.09)		1.09 (0.10)		1.16 (0.01)		0.36 (0.09)		0.94 (0.10)	

Data reported as mean and standard error (SE). BMI: body mass index; WtHR: waist-to-height ratio; BRI: body roundness index; ABSI: a body shape index; CI: conicity index; SBP: systolic blood pressure; DBP: diastolic blood pressure; MBP: mean blood pressure. p-value from ANCOVA analysis performed with ethnicity, socio-economic status, smoking status, alcohol intake, physical activity "proxy", and medical conditions (i.e., presence or absence of osteoporosis, cardiovascular diseases, hypertension, diabetes, cancer, or respiratory disease) as covariates. p-values marked in bold are significant.

4. Discussion

Metabolic abnormalities including elevated blood pressure, hypertriglyceridemia, low levels of HDL-C, impaired glucose tolerance and central obesity, have been proposed as cardiometabolic risk factors for CVD and all-cause mortality [28,29]. For this reason, identifying a screening tool for detecting high cardiometabolic risk in older adults is particularly important, as this might facilitate the early implementation of effective strategies to those at high risk. This study investigated multiple anthropometric measurements for predicting cardiometabolic risk in a large population of older Colombian adults. Firstly, we demonstrated that all the surrogate anthropometric indices including BMI, WtHR, BRI, ABSI, and CI significantly correlated with CMRI. Secondly, we showed that WtHR and BRI are the most accurate anthropometric indices for identifying adults at high cardiometabolic risk, supporting the hypothesis that these two indices could effectively predict cardiometabolic risk in the elderly Colombian population.

In the present study, conducted on a representative cohort of older adults, the overall prevalence of MetS was 58.7% according to IDF criteria. These findings differ slightly from the results of Davila et al., who showed that the prevalence of MetS among adults from Medellin (Colombia) aged 25–64 was 41% [30]. Furthermore, the Cardiovascular Risk Factor Multiple Evaluation in Latin America (CARMELA) study estimated a prevalence of 30.1% in men and 48.6% in women, respectively, in the 55–64 age group in Bogotá [31]. The differences in prevalence could be explained by either the MetS cluster used, since the CARMELA study defined MetS according to the National Cholesterol Education Program Adult Treatment Panel III, or the age range of the target populations (55–64 vs. ≥60). Nonetheless, there is a high prevalence of MetS in Latin American populations and, accordingly, there is growing interest in developing accurate tools for identifying subjects at high risk and defining cut-off points for anthropometric indices for detecting high CMRI.

BRI is a novel body index that has recently shown promise for clinical use [15]. We found that BRI has a moderate discriminating power for detecting high cardiometabolic risk in older Colombian adults, supporting the diagnostic potential of this new shape measure. We found that BRI performed better as a predictor of a high CMRI than BMI, the standard measure. Similarly, Tian et al. observed that BRI was suitable for use as a single anthropometric measure for identifying a cluster of cardiometabolic abnormalities, as compared with BMI and WtHR, using data from the 2009 wave of the China Health and Nutrition Survey [32]. Likewise, a recent study assessing the ability of BRI to predict the risk of MetS and its components in Peruvian adults concluded that BRI is a potentially useful clinical predictor of MetS that performs better than BMI [18]. BRI also showed potential for use as an alternative obesity measure in type 2 diabetes mellitus assessment among a rural population from northeastern China, although it performed similarly to BMI [33]. Additionally, Maessen et al. found that BRI could identify both the presence of CVD and cardiovascular risk factors in a population-based study in Nijmegen, the Netherlands, although the authors indicated that its capacity did not exceed that of BMI [19]. The heterogeneity of the population characteristics (ethnicity and age range) might explain the differences between these studies.

We demonstrated that WtHR is also an accurate screening tool for detecting a high cardiometabolic risk in older Colombian adults. Indeed, we found that WtHR was a better predictor of cardiometabolic risk than other anthropometric indices (BMI, CI, and ABSI). Wang et al. [34] also indicated that when evaluating cardiometabolic risk factors among non-obese adults, WtHR functioned as a simple but effective index for Chinese adults and, similarly, Amirabdollahian et al. [35] concluded that WtHR was the best predictor of cardiometabolic risk in a population of young adults from northwestern England. Comparable results were reported in a previous systematic review and meta-analysis involving 300,000 adults from several ethnic groups [36], showing the superiority of WtHR over BMI for detecting cardiometabolic risk factors in both sexes. However, it should be noted that the aforementioned studies did not compare WtHR with ABSI or BRI.

Interestingly, it should be noted that the greatest AUC values were observed for WtHR and BRI in men and women, suggesting that both body indices are capable of detecting a high cardiometabolic risk in the elderly. In addition, the AUC of WtHR did not differ significantly from that of BRI. This highlights the similar diagnostic capabilities of the two anthropometric indices. Furthermore, the AUC value of BRI for identifying metabolic risk factors was very close to that of WtHR in a Chinese population of adults [37]. In fact, Wang et al. concluded that although BRI does not exhibit a significantly better predictive ability than WtHR, it could be used as an alternative body index [34].

Our results showed that ABSI presented the lowest AUC for high cardiometabolic risk in men and women. These observations are consistent with previous studies [18–20,35,37,38]. Tian et al. reported that ABSI had the weakest discriminative power for identifying a cluster of cardiometabolic abnormalities [32]. Similarly, ABSI exhibited the lowest AUC value for identifying cardiometabolic risk factors compared with WtHR and BRI in Chinese adults [37], and a study involving an Iranian population also reported that ABSI was a weak predictor of CVD risk and MetS [38]. In the same line, Stefanescu et al. found that ABSI underperformed against other measures such as BMI and BRI for predicting MetS and its components [18], and Maessen et al. reported that ABSI was incapable of determining the presence of CVD in a Dutch population [19]. Thus, based on both our results and those of previous research, it can be concluded that ABSI does not seem to be a useful anthropometric index for predicting cardiometabolic risk.

The present study has some limitations and strengths that should be mentioned. Firstly, the cross-sectional design of the study meant that causality could not be inferred. Secondly, all of the study participants were of Latin-American ethnicity and resident in Colombia. This may therefore limit the generalizability of our results to other ethnic groups. Further studies involving other populations are therefore warranted. By contrast, the main strength of our study is that we provide gender-specific thresholds for various surrogate anthropometric indices (BMI, WtHR, BRI, ABSI, and CI) with cardiometabolic measurements among older Colombian adults. To our knowledge, no research has previously been published assessing the efficacy of these anthropometric indices for predicting a high CMRI in a Latin-American population. Lastly, the large sample size and the highly standardized procedures of the SABE project, which minimized measurement bias, were also major strengths of this study [39,40].

5. Conclusions

In conclusion, BRI and WtHR have a moderate discriminating power for determining a high cardiometabolic risk in a Colombian population of older adults, supporting the notion that both anthropometric indices should be considered as screening tools for the elderly. Both anthropometric indices were the most accurate among those tested for identifying men and women at a high cardiometabolic risk. In addition, we provide the first BMI, WtHR, BRI, ABSI, and CI thresholds for predicting a high CRMI in older Colombian adults. These data are clinically significant, as anthropometric index reference thresholds can be used to identify those adults who are at high cardiometabolic risk. Further investigation is required to provide reference values applicable to different populations.

Supplementary Materials: The following are available online at http://www.mdpi.com/2072-6643/11/8/1701/s1, Table S1: Area under curve for BMI, WHTR, BRI, ABSI, and CI to detect cardiometabolic risk (without WC) by sex.

Author Contributions: Data curation, R.R.-V. and M.Á.P.-S.; Formal analysis, R.R.-V. and M.Á.P.-S.; Investigation, R.R.-V., C.A.C.-G., J.S.-R., K.G.-R. and M.C.-R.; Methodology, R.R.-V., E.G.-J., J.S.-R., K.G.-R. and M.C.-R.; Project administration, C.A.C.-G.; Resources, C.A.C.-G. and K.G.-R; Supervision, C.A.C.-G. and E.G.-J.; Validation, M.I., K.G.-R. and M.C.-R.; Writing—original draft, R.R.-V., M.Á.P.-S., K.G.-R. and M.C.-R.; Writing—review and editing, R.R.-V., M.I., E.G.-J., J.S.-R. and M.C.-R.

Funding: This study is part of a larger project that has been funded by the Colciencias y Ministerio de Salud y la Protección Social de Colombia (The SABE Study ID 2013, no. 764). Mikel Izquierdo is funded in part by a research grant PI17/01814 of the Ministerio de Economía, Industria y Competitividad (ISCIII, FEDER).

Acknowledgments: We would like to thank the staff, scientists, and participants of the Colombian Health, Well-Being and Aging study (SABE, 2015) Survey for making this work possible.

Conflicts of Interest: The authors declare no conflict of interest.

References

1. Mente, A.; Yusuf, S.; Islam, S.; McQueen, M.J.; Tanomsup, S.; Onen, C.L.; Rangarajan, S.; Gerstein, H.C.; Anand, S.S. INTERHEART Investigators Metabolic Syndrome and Risk of Acute Myocardial Infarction. *J. Am. Coll. Cardiol.* **2010**, *55*, 2390–2398. [CrossRef] [PubMed]
2. Chien, K.-L.; Hsu, H.-C.; Sung, F.-C.; Su, T.-C.; Chen, M.-F.; Lee, Y.-T. Metabolic syndrome as a risk factor for coronary heart disease and stroke: An 11-year prospective cohort in Taiwan community. *Atherosclerosis* **2007**, *194*, 214–221. [CrossRef] [PubMed]
3. Boden-Albala, B.; Sacco, R.L.; Lee, H.-S.; Grahame-Clarke, C.; Rundek, T.; Elkind, M.V.; Wright, C.; Giardina, E.-G.V.; DiTullio, M.R.; Homma, S.; et al. Metabolic Syndrome and Ischemic Stroke Risk. *Stroke* **2008**, *39*, 30–35. [CrossRef] [PubMed]
4. Márquez-Sandoval, F.; Macedo-Ojeda, G.; Viramontes-Hörner, D.; Fernández Ballart, J.; Salas Salvadó, J.; Vizmanos, B. The prevalence of metabolic syndrome in Latin America: A systematic review. *Public Health Nutr.* **2011**, *14*, 1702–1713. [CrossRef] [PubMed]
5. DeBoer, M.D.; Gurka, M.J.; Woo, J.G.; Morrison, J.A. Severity of the metabolic syndrome as a predictor of type 2 diabetes between childhood and adulthood: The Princeton Lipid Research Cohort Study. *Diabetologia* **2015**, *58*, 2745–2752. [CrossRef] [PubMed]
6. Alberti, K.G.M.M.; Eckel, R.H.; Grundy, S.M.; Zimmet, P.Z.; Cleeman, J.I.; Donato, K.A.; Fruchart, J.-C.; James, W.P.T.; Loria, C.M.; Smith, S.C.; et al. Harmonizing the Metabolic Syndrome. *Circulation* **2009**, *120*, 1640–1645. [CrossRef] [PubMed]
7. Correa-Rodríguez, M.; Ramírez-Vélez, R.; Correa-Bautista, J.; Castellanos-Vega, R.; Arias-Coronel, F.; González-Ruíz, K.; Alejandro Carrillo, H.; Schmidt-RioValle, J.; González-Jiménez, E. Association of Muscular Fitness and Body Fatness with Cardiometabolic Risk Factors: The FUPRECOL Study. *Nutrients* **2018**, *10*, 1742. [CrossRef]
8. Ramírez-Vélez, R.; Correa-Bautista, J.; Carrillo, H.; González-Jiménez, E.; Schmidt-RioValle, J.; Correa-Rodríguez, M.; García-Hermoso, A.; González-Ruíz, K. Tri-Ponderal Mass Index vs. Fat Mass/Height3 as a Screening Tool for Metabolic Syndrome Prediction in Colombian Children and Young People. *Nutrients* **2018**, *10*, 412. [CrossRef]
9. Ramírez-Vélez, R.; Correa-Bautista, J.; González-Ruíz, K.; Tordecilla-Sanders, A.; García-Hermoso, A.; Schmidt-RioValle, J.; González-Jiménez, E. The Role of Body Adiposity Index in Determining Body Fat Percentage in Colombian Adults with Overweight or Obesity. *Int. J. Environ. Res. Public Health* **2017**, *14*, 1093. [CrossRef] [PubMed]
10. Knowles, K.M.; Paiva, L.L.; Sanchez, S.E.; Revilla, L.; Lopez, T.; Yasuda, M.B.; Yanez, N.D.; Gelaye, B.; Williams, M.A. Waist Circumference, Body Mass Index, and Other Measures of Adiposity in Predicting Cardiovascular Disease Risk Factors among Peruvian Adults. *Int. J. Hypertens.* **2011**, *2011*. [CrossRef]
11. Browning, L.M.; Hsieh, S.D.; Ashwell, M. A systematic review of waist-to-height ratio as a screening tool for the prediction of cardiovascular disease and diabetes: 0·5 could be a suitable global boundary value. *Nutr. Res. Rev.* **2010**, *23*, 247–269. [CrossRef] [PubMed]
12. Dobbelsteyn, C.; Joffres, M.; MacLean, D.; Flowerdew, G. A comparative evaluation of waist circumference, waist-to-hip ratio and body mass index as indicators of cardiovascular risk factors. The Canadian Heart Health Surveys. *Int. J. Obes.* **2001**, *25*, 652–661. [CrossRef] [PubMed]
13. Krakauer, N.Y.; Krakauer, J.C. A New Body Shape Index Predicts Mortality Hazard Independently of Body Mass Index. *PLoS ONE* **2012**, *7*, e39504. [CrossRef] [PubMed]
14. Mantzoros, C.; Evagelopoulou, K.; Georgiadis, E.; Katsilambros, N. Conicity Index as a Predictor of Blood Pressure Levels, Insulin and Triglyceride Concentrations of Healthy Premenopausal Women. *Horm. Metab. Res.* **1996**, *28*, 32–34. [CrossRef] [PubMed]
15. Thomas, D.M.; Bredlau, C.; Bosy-Westphal, A.; Mueller, M.; Shen, W.; Gallagher, D.; Maeda, Y.; McDougall, A.; Peterson, C.M.; Ravussin, E.; et al. Relationships between body roundness with body fat and visceral adipose tissue emerging from a new geometrical model. *Obesity* **2013**, *21*, 2264–2271. [CrossRef] [PubMed]

16. Li, G.; Wu, H.; Wu, X.; Cao, Z.; Tu, Y.; Ma, Y.; Li, B.; Peng, Q.; Cheng, J.; Wu, B.; et al. The feasibility of two anthropometric indices to identify metabolic syndrome, insulin resistance and inflammatory factors in obese and overweight adults. *Nutrition* **2019**, *57*, 194–201. [CrossRef] [PubMed]
17. Li, G.; Yao, T.; Wu, X.-W.; Cao, Z.; Tu, Y.-C.; Ma, Y.; Li, B.-N.; Peng, Q.-Y.; Wu, B.; Hou, J. Novel and traditional anthropometric indices for identifying arterial stiffness in overweight and obese adults. *Clin. Nutr.* **2019**. [CrossRef] [PubMed]
18. Stefanescu, A.; Revilla, L.; Lopez, T.; Sanchez, S.E.; Williams, M.A.; Gelaye, B. Using A Body Shape Index (ABSI) and Body Roundness Index (BRI) to predict risk of metabolic syndrome in Peruvian adults. *J. Int. Med. Res.* **2019**. [CrossRef]
19. Maessen, M.F.H.; Eijsvogels, T.M.H.; Verheggen, R.J.H.M.; Hopman, M.T.E.; Verbeek, A.L.M.; de Vegt, F. Entering a New Era of Body Indices: The Feasibility of a Body Shape Index and Body Roundness Index to Identify Cardiovascular Health Status. *PLoS ONE* **2014**, *9*, e107212. [CrossRef] [PubMed]
20. Krakauer, N.Y.; Krakauer, J.C. Untangling Waist Circumference and Hip Circumference from Body Mass Index with a Body Shape Index, Hip Index, and Anthropometric Risk Indicator. *Metab. Syndr. Relat. Disord.* **2018**, *16*, 160–165. [CrossRef] [PubMed]
21. Popkin, B.M.; Reardon, T. Obesity and the food system transformation in Latin America. *Obes. Rev.* **2018**, *19*, 1028–1064. [CrossRef] [PubMed]
22. Valdez, R. A simple model-based index of abdominal adiposity. *J. Clin. Epidemiol.* **1991**, *44*, 955–956. [CrossRef]
23. Aronow, W.S.; Banach, M. Ten most important things to learn from the ACCF/AHA 2011 expert consensus document on hypertension in the elderly. *Blood Press.* **2012**, *21*, 3–5. [CrossRef] [PubMed]
24. Ramírez-Vélez, R.; Correa-Bautista, J.E.; García-Hermoso, A.; Cano, C.A.; Izquierdo, M. Reference values for handgrip strength and their association with intrinsic capacity domains among older adults. *J. Cachexia Sarcopenia Muscle* **2019**, *10*, 278–286. [CrossRef] [PubMed]
25. Bewick, V.; Cheek, L.; Ball, J. Statistics review 13: Receiver operating characteristic curves. *Crit. Care* **2004**, *8*, 508–512. [CrossRef] [PubMed]
26. DeLong, E.R.; DeLong, D.M.; Clarke-Pearson, D.L. Comparing the areas under two or more correlated receiver operating characteristic curves: A nonparametric approach. *Biometrics* **1988**, *44*, 837–845. [CrossRef] [PubMed]
27. Kutner, M.H.; Nachtsheim, C.; Neter, J. *Applied Linear Regression Models*; McGraw-Hill/Irwin: New York, NY, USA, 2004; ISBN 0073014664.
28. Tune, J.D.; Goodwill, A.G.; Sassoon, D.J.; Mather, K.J. Cardiovascular consequences of metabolic syndrome. *Transl. Res.* **2017**, *183*, 57–70. [CrossRef] [PubMed]
29. Hamer, M.; Stamatakis, E. Metabolically healthy obesity and risk of all-cause and cardiovascular disease mortality. *J. Clin. Endocrinol. Metab.* **2012**, *97*, 2482–2488. [CrossRef]
30. Davila, E.P.; Quintero, M.A.; Orrego, M.L.; Ford, E.S.; Walke, H.; Arenas, M.M.; Pratt, M. Prevalence and risk factors for metabolic syndrome in Medellin and surrounding municipalities, Colombia, 2008–2010. *Prev. Med.* **2013**, *56*, 30–34. [CrossRef]
31. Escobedo, J.; Schargrodsky, H.; Champagne, B.; Silva, H.; Boissonnet, C.P.; Vinueza, R.; Torres, M.; Hernandez, R.; Wilson, E. Prevalence of the Metabolic Syndrome in Latin America and its association with sub-clinical carotid atherosclerosis: The CARMELA cross sectional study. *Cardiovasc. Diabetol.* **2009**, *8*, 52. [CrossRef]
32. Tian, S.; Zhang, X.; Xu, Y.; Dong, H. Feasibility of body roundness index for identifying a clustering of cardiometabolic abnormalities compared to BMI, waist circumference and other anthropometric indices: The China Health and Nutrition Survey, 2008 to 2009. *Medicine* **2016**, *95*, e4642. [CrossRef] [PubMed]
33. Chang, Y.; Guo, X.; Chen, Y.; Guo, L.; Li, Z.; Yu, S.; Yang, H.; Sun, Y. A body shape index and body roundness index: Two new body indices to identify diabetes mellitus among rural populations in northeast China. *BMC Public Health* **2015**, *15*, 794. [CrossRef] [PubMed]
34. Wang, H.; Liu, A.; Zhao, T.; Gong, X.; Pang, T.; Zhou, Y.; Xiao, Y.; Yan, Y.; Fan, C.; Teng, W.; et al. Comparison of anthropometric indices for predicting the risk of metabolic syndrome and its components in Chinese adults: A prospective, longitudinal study. *BMJ Open* **2017**, *7*, e016062. [CrossRef] [PubMed]

35. Amirabdollahian, F.; Haghighatdoost, F. Anthropometric Indicators of Adiposity Related to Body Weight and Body Shape as Cardiometabolic Risk Predictors in British Young Adults: Superiority of Waist-to-Height Ratio. *J. Obes.* **2018**, *2018*, 8370304. [CrossRef] [PubMed]
36. Ashwell, M.; Gunn, P.; Gibson, S. Waist-to-height ratio is a better screening tool than waist circumference and BMI for adult cardiometabolic risk factors: Systematic review and meta-analysis. *Obes. Rev.* **2012**, *13*, 275–286. [CrossRef] [PubMed]
37. Liu, P.J.; Ma, F.; Lou, H.P.; Zhu, Y.N. Comparison of the ability to identify cardiometabolic risk factors between two new body indices and waist-to-height ratio among Chinese adults with normal BMI and waist circumference. *Public Health Nutr.* **2017**, *20*, 984–991. [CrossRef] [PubMed]
38. Haghighatdoost, F.; Sarrafzadegan, N.; Mohammadifard, N.; Asgary, S.; Boshtam, M.; Azadbakht, L. Assessing body shape index as a risk predictor for cardiovascular diseases and metabolic syndrome among Iranian adults. *Nutrition* **2014**, *30*, 636–644. [CrossRef] [PubMed]
39. Perez-Sousa, M.A.; Venegas-Sanabria, L.C.; Chavarro-Carvajal, D.A.; Cano-Gutierrez, C.A.; Izquierdo, M.; Correa-Bautista, J.E.; Ramírez-Vélez, R. Gait speed as a mediator of the effect of sarcopenia on dependency in activities of daily living. *J. Cachexia Sarcopenia Muscle* **2019**. [CrossRef] [PubMed]
40. Gomez, F.; Corchuelo, J.; Curcio, C.L.; Calzada, M.T.; Mendez, F. SABE Colombia: Survey on Health, Well-Being, and Aging in Colombia-Study Design and Protocol. *Curr. Gerontol. Geriatr. Res.* **2016**, *2016*. [CrossRef]

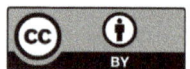

© 2019 by the authors. Licensee MDPI, Basel, Switzerland. This article is an open access article distributed under the terms and conditions of the Creative Commons Attribution (CC BY) license (http://creativecommons.org/licenses/by/4.0/).

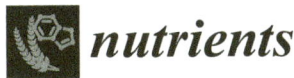 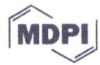

Communication

Assessing and Managing the Metabolic Syndrome in Children and Adolescents

Mark D. DeBoer

Department of Pediatrics, University of Virginia, Charlottesville, VA 22908, USA; deboer@virginia.edu;
Tel.: +1-434-924-9833; Fax: +1-434-924-9181

Received: 29 June 2019; Accepted: 30 July 2019; Published: 2 August 2019

Abstract: The metabolic syndrome (MetS) is a group of cardiovascular risk factors that are associated with insulin resistance and are driven by underlying factors, including visceral obesity, systemic inflammation, and cellular dysfunction. These risks increasingly begin in childhood and adolescence and are associated with a high likelihood of future chronic disease in adulthood. Efforts should be made at both recognition of this metabolic risk, screening for potential associated Type 2 diabetes, and targeting affected individuals for appropriate treatment with an emphasis on lifestyle modification. Effective interventions have been linked to reductions in MetS—and in adults, reductions in the severity of MetS have been linked to reduced diabetes and cardiovascular disease.

Keywords: metabolic syndrome; obesity; insulin resistance; risk; pediatric; adolescent

1. Introduction

The roots of cardiovascular disease—the most common cause of mortality among adults worldwide—begin in childhood [1], underscoring the need to identify and intervene in at-risk children [2]. These issues have become even more important in light of the global obesity epidemic, in which over 100 million children worldwide are obese [3], including in developing areas more commonly associated with food scarcity [4]. One predictor of future risk is the metabolic syndrome (MetS), a cluster of cardiovascular risk factors including central obesity (typically measured by high waist circumference or high BMI), hypertension, high fasting triglycerides, low high density lipoprotein (HDL) cholesterol and high fasting glucose [5]. These individual components of MetS occur together more often than would be expected by chance—as though they are driven by similar underlying processes that lead to insulin resistance, including cellular dysfunction in adipocytes, myocytes, and hepatocytes; oxidative stress; and cellular inflammation [6,7]. In addition to predicting cardiovascular disease (CVD), MetS is also a predictor of future Type 2 diabetes among children [8,9].

This review addresses means of assessing MetS in children and adolescents, the implications of altered metabolic status, and approaches toward intervening among affected children and adolescents.

2. What is MetS?

MetS, at its core, appears to be due to dysregulated cellular metabolism [7], leading to insulin resistance. A central driver appears to be an excess of central obesity, with visceral adipocytes releasing chemo-attractants, contributing to infiltration by macrophages and release of cytokines and an overall increase in systemic inflammation [6]. Further adipocyte dysfunction includes reduced production of the adipokine adiponectin (which appears to be in the causative pathway of insulin resistance) [10] and higher release of free fatty acids [11]. In peripheral tissues, these high levels of free fatty acids and triglycerides alter mitochondrial function and increase the degree of oxidative stress, with an overall effect of reductions in insulin's ability to stimulate glucose transporters to the cell surface [7]. The degree of insulin resistance results in heightened need for insulin production, and glucose levels rise as the resistance exceeds the ability of the pancreatic beta cells to release adequate amounts of insulin, ultimately contributing to risk for Type 2 diabetes [12]. Further downstream effects include hypertension and reduced levels of HDL cholesterol, both of which contribute additional risk to cardiovascular disease [2]. This multifaceted process has made it difficult to adequately target—though, as we will see, weight reduction to decrease the central adiposity and exercise to increase energy utilization have been effective in reducing the metabolic abnormalities.

3. Clinical Measures of MetS

3.1. Evaluation among Adults

The first observations regarding MetS were related to linking distinct abnormalities in the individual components [5], and this approach ultimately led to forming diagnostic criteria that identified individuals with several of these metabolic abnormalities. These criteria were first set for classifying MetS among adults, with the most commonly-used criteria being those of the National Cholesterol Education Program's Adult Treatment Panel III (ATP-III) [13]. Using ATP-III criteria, an individual is categorized as having MetS if they have measured values that are outside the adult normal range for at least three of the individual MetS components (WC, BP, triglycerides, HDL, glucose—with current diabetes qualifying as an abnormal glucose level even in the absence of an elevated value). Other organizations have proposed slightly different criteria; the World Health Organization criteria utilized results from oral glucose tolerance tests [14], while the International Diabetes Federation (IDF) initially required the presence of central obesity for MetS classification (regardless of how many other MetS abnormalities were present) [15]. The IDF criteria (later harmonized to be in line with ATP-III criteria [16]) also allow for use of separate cut-offs for elevated waist circumference by race/ethnicity, based on evidence demonstrating risk in a specific group [15].

Each of these sets of categories above diagnoses MetS on a dichotomous basis (i.e., you either have it or you do not). Among adults, there have been scoring systems that take into account that MetS abnormalities exist on a spectrum. Approaches to this have often consisted of a summation of standardized z-scores for each individual component among a defined population of interest. We formulated a score of MetS severity using confirmatory factor analysis that allowed for a weighted contribution of the individual criteria, with these weights varying by sex and racial/ethnicity based on how these components correlated together in each sex and racial/ethnic subgroup [17]. Because this was done using nationally-representative data, these MetS-z scores can be used to assess risk in other populations without reformulating the scores based on the distribution of abnormalities for the new population. As compared to dichotomous criteria, use of continuous scores such as this can provide improved power for statistical assessment of MetS-related risk [18]. In addition, whereas dichotomous criteria can only be used to follow for the presence or absence of MetS over time [19], continuous scores are also useful to follow for the risks associated with changes in MetS severity over time [20,21] and how an individual responds to intervention [22].

3.2. Evaluation among Children

Whereas assessment of MetS in adults relied on criteria established by national or international agencies, assessment among children and adolescents has not been as clear [23]. Most assessments have relied on adaptations that were based on adult criteria, with cut-off values for the individual components that were altered to reflect the more moderate values for these risk factors among adolescents (Table 1) [24–26]. The IDF proposed a set of criteria for children that was based on the adult IDF criteria, again requiring abnormal waist circumference for MetS classification [27]. Other criteria have acknowledged the gradual shift over the course of adolescence in normal ranges of the individual components, with cut-offs that change with time [28].

Table 1. Pediatric and adolescent metabolic syndrome (MetS) criteria adapted from the National Cholesterol Education Program Adult Treatment Panel III *.

Central Obesity (WC)	High BP (mmHg)	High Triglycerides (mg/dL)	Low HDL (mg/dL)	High Fasting Glucose
WC ≥ 90th percentile [25]	Systolic or diastolic DBP ≥ 90% for age, sex, height [26]	TG ≥ 110 mg/dL (≥1.24 mmol/L)	HDL ≤ 40 mg/dL (<1.03 mmol/L)	≥100 mg/dL (5.6 mmol/L) or known T2DM

* Individuals need to have at least three abnormalities in MetS components to be classified as having MetS.

As with the assessment of MetS-related risk in adults, continuous scores have frequently been used in pediatrics. There have been multiple approaches to this, again with most consisting of summation of z-scores for a particular underlying population [18]. We again used confirmatory factor analysis in a nationally-representative group of US adolescents age 12–19 to produce MetS severity scores that are weighted to how MetS was manifest by sex and racial/ethnic subgroup [29]. These scores appear to reflect the underlying metabolic disarray in correlating closely with markers of the processes underlying MetS, including C-reactive protein (CRP), uric acid, adiponectin, and insulin [29–32].

Continuous scores are also able to overcome a drawback to sets of criteria, namely, their apparent lack of durability, with a high occurrence of adolescents who toggle between having a diagnosis of MetS or not based on having individual components that are just above or below the cut-off [33,34]. The clinical use of these criteria would likely benefit from incorporation into the electronic medical record [35] but at this time remains less certain, and some researchers have lobbied for an approach that simply targets individual component risk factors [36].

4. Epidemiology

The underlying prevalence of MetS in adolescents depends on the set of MetS criteria used, with overall ranges in the US from 1.2%–9.8% using modified ATP-III [31,37] criteria to 4.5%–8.4% using the IDF adolescent criteria [38,39]. Assessments among school-aged children and early adolescents is lower (0.2%–1.2%) [37,40], which is likely because of the strong effects of puberty on insulin resistance. For example, insulin resistance as estimated by measures such as the homeostasis model of insulin resistance—which usually tracks closely with MetS [41]—at age 8 years is half that seen among those at 15 years, consistent with the concept that puberty itself may be involved with the progression of abnormal metabolic processes [42].

In addition to variation by age, the prevalence of MetS also varies significantly by sex, with male adolescents having a greater prevalence than females (Figure 1). Interestingly, there is also variation by race/ethnicity, being more common in whites and Hispanics compared to African Americans (Figure 1). This is surprising, given tight associations of MetS with insulin resistance, diabetes, and CVD mortality—all of which are more common in African Americans [38]. The reason for this appears to be more favorable lipid levels in African Americans, particularly lower triglyceride levels, which appear to have a lower baseline levels but do increase with worsening insulin resistance [43].

Not surprisingly, MetS varies by location, with one meta-analysis estimating a lower prevalence in Europe (2.1%) and the Far East (3.3%) compared to the Americas (4.5%) and the Middle East (6.5%) [44]. Even in the US, prevalence varies by geography, with higher prevalence in the Midwest and South of the US compared to the West and Northeast (Figure 2), with potential implications for allocation of resources by region toward improved lifestyle efforts [45]. While MetS has traditionally been thought of as a problem of developed countries, the increase in pediatric obesity across the globe has made MetS a concern in developing countries as well [46]. The prevalence of MetS in developing areas of the world is likely to worsen with changing diet patterns as calorie-dense foods become increasingly available [46]. Worldwide variation in MetS prevalence is compounded by an apparent increase in susceptibility for obesity and MetS by race/ethnicity [47].

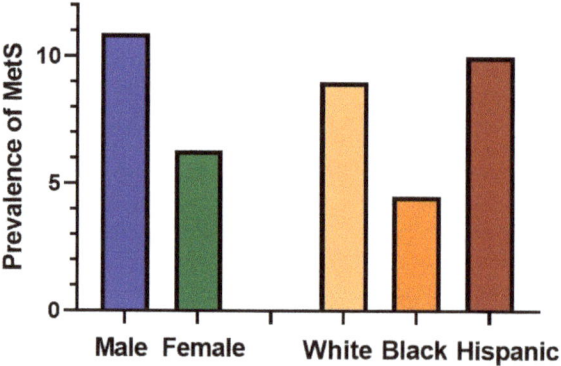

Figure 1. Prevalence of metabolic syndrome in adolescents by sex and race ethnicity. Data are for adolescent participants age 12–19 years from the National Health and Nutrition Examination Survey 1999–2012 as reported in Lee et al. [31].

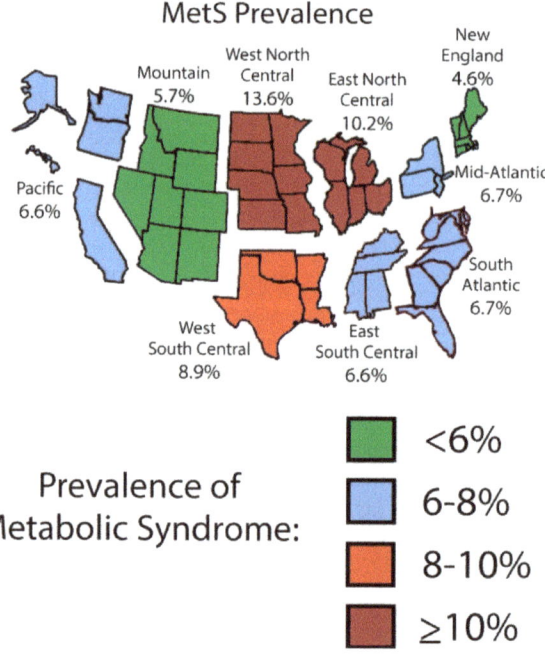

Figure 2. Geographic variation in MetS prevalence among US adolescents. Data are for adolescents age 12–19 years from National Health and Nutrition Examination Survey 1999–2014. (From, DeBoer et al. used with permission.) [45].

The high prevalence of MetS in adolescents coincides with the current obesity levels, and there has not been evidence of a decrease in the prevalence of MetS by classical criteria. However, there has been a recent decrease in the severity of MetS as assessed by a continuous score over time. This is surprising and appears to be due to decreases in triglycerides, potentially from lower consumption of saturated fat [31].

5. Long-Term Risks

The importance of considering MetS in ongoing patient care is driven home by the long-term associations between MetS and future disease. While the downstream sequelae of childhood MetS are usually greater than 10 years in development, studies that followed children for MetS-related characteristics in the 1970s and followed up in the 2000s have demonstrated strong links, with childhood MetS (vs. no MetS) carrying an odds ratio of 2.3–11.5 for future T2DM 14–31 years later [9,48], 2.0 for elevated carotid artery media thickness (a subclinical marker of CVD risk) 14–27 years later [48], and 14.6 for CVD 24–31 years later [8]. In utilizing a MetS Z-score in childhood to assess risk of adult disease 24–31 years later, the odds ratio of increased risk for every 1 standard deviation of the score was 2.7 and 9.8 for future T2DM [49] and CVD [50] (respectively). Moreover, the change in score over time was associated with a further increase in disease risk [49,50], suggesting potential utility in following an adolescent's MetS score during lifestyle modification treatment as a means of following ongoing risks and motivating further improvements.

It is notable that the prevalence of MetS in the 1970s was only 3.9% [9], compared to the prevalence of 9.8% today [31]. This underscores an enormous risk for future T2DM and CVD based on prevalence of risk factors in the current generation of US adolescents. In addition, MetS is also linked to other obesity-related disease processes, including non-alcoholic fatty liver disease (NAFLD) [51] and renal function [52], with implications for chronic kidney disease [53].

6. An Emphasis on Prevention

It should be noted that the best means of reducing the prevalence of MetS in the future is to prevent the occurrence of obesity among children and adolescents. This includes efforts at encouraging an active lifestyle from a young age and preserving of levels of physical activity among younger children (before the usual decline in activity during adolescence [54]). It also includes encouraging families to maintain consumption of fresh foods and avoid energy-dense foods, including as these are increasingly introduced to developed parts of the world [46]. As discussed below, after the development of overweight or obesity, it is difficult to lose excess weight, and stronger efforts should be made at preventing obesity and MetS, including from the standpoint of public policy, including availability of safe spaces for physical activity and healthy nutrition choices in schools [55].

7. Use of Criteria in Clinical Settings

Identify Individuals at Highest Need for Assessment

Given the potential long-term sequelae of MetS, the chief roles of MetS as a concept in pediatric clinical care is in-risk identification and patient motivation. However, while the sets of criteria described above provide a means of categorizing MetS and assessing related factors and long-term risk, there is a sense that these criteria are not commonly used in clinical settings [36]. This may be because of the potentially time-intensive nature of comparing measured values of each component with cut-off values. Clearly, the process would be improved by automatic assessments performed by electronic health record systems [35]—though such tools are not commonly available for assessment of pediatric and adolescent MetS. In all settings, including in developing areas in the world, attention should be given to obtaining accurate height and weight measures and assessing how a child's BMI compares to standardized percentiles for age, such as those of the World Health Organization [56].

Children and adolescents who present with obesity and/or findings associated with MetS should receive extra attention toward reducing long-term risks for future chronic disease. Many of the interventions against MetS (described below) are likely to also have benefits among all overweight children [57]; nevertheless, children classified as having MetS are likely to benefit from additional time and encouragement because of their additional CVD risk factors [36]. In the absence of formal screening for MetS itself (which requires a fasting blood draw and waist circumference measurement), other indicators of insulin resistance and long-term risk for chronic disease may offer alternative means of identifying patients at higher risk. This includes the presence of a strong family history of T2DM [58] or CVD [59] upon questioning or of acanthosis nigricans [60] or hypertension [36] upon physical exam. The presence of these factors in an overweight patient should prompt assessment for potential concurrent Type 2 diabetes, through assessment of symptoms such as polyuria, polydipsia, and unintended weight loss, and through testing HbA1c, with a HbA1c level of 5.7%–6.4% reflective of a pre-diabetes state and a level ≥6.5% consistent with Type 2 diabetes [61].

Discussion regarding how MetS influences a child's or adolescent's risk and how reductions in MetS severity may improve their chances of disease development [22] may assist in motivation toward change [2]. Use of such risk identification as a motivator is a key consideration, as the difficulty in care for adolescents with MetS-related risk for future T2D and CVD is not usually in the identification of at-risk adolescents—using either accepted algorithms or looking at higher-risk groups based on epidemiology—or even in advising interventions but in achieving adherence to these interventions, discussed in the following section.

8. Intervention

Because of the strong connection between MetS and obesity, most interventions for MetS have paralleled those for pediatric obesity in general, namely interventions aimed at altering unhealthy lifestyle factors that likely contributed to the metabolic problems in the first place. This includes diets that are high in saturated fat and carbohydrates (and ultimately an excess of overall calories) [31] and physical activity levels that fall far short of recommendations [54]. In addition, further abnormalities in the components of MetS should be addressed if present. In some cases, this could include, for example, treating hypertension with medication. However, because the predominant "lesion" in MetS is the central obesity, the majority of approaches have focused on lifestyle approaches, as addressed in the following section.

Interventions that have been assessed for efficacy in reducing the proportion of children with MetS have thus focused on altering dietary choices, increasing physical activity, and a combination of both. The goal of these is to thus decrease the ratio of energy ingested vs. energy expended, primarily to reduce the degree of central obesity that drives the metabolic abnormalities. Unfortunately, the unfavorable balance of energy ingested vs. expended has occurred because many children and adolescents have developed suboptimal lifestyle practices due to ease, availability or palatability, and it can be difficult to motivate pediatric patients (and adults as well) to overcome the draw toward these unhealthy lifestyle choices. Effective approaches have included efforts at exploring the motivation of adolescents using techniques such as motivational interviewing, which involves assessments of an individual patient's readiness to change [62]. These approaches are thus tailored to the individual patient and require the time to probe the patient's current food choices and level of physical activity—and a degree of flexibility in working out a treatment plan to which the child/adolescent is willing to commit. This kind of approach is able to increase the adherence rate of adolescents to a treatment plan [62].

8.1. Dietary Changes

The main approach for dietary changes for children and adolescents as recommended by the American Academy of Pediatrics, the American Heart Association, and the World Health Organization has been an increase in vegetable and fruit consumption and a reduced intake of saturated fat in lieu of unsaturated fat (e.g., olive oil and other vegetable oils), as well as a reduction in sugar intake [56]. A meta-analysis of studies that recommended these changes (though usually as part of an approach combined with changes in physical activity, as compared to no change) demonstrated decreases in BMI. One helpful way of achieving these changes has been through implementation of the Mediterranean diet, which incorporates vegetables and olive oil. With respect to MetS itself, a 16-week trial of the

Mediterranean diet among children and adolescents revealed a decrease in MetS prevalence (16% to 5%) among those on the Mediterranean diet compared to no change or worsening in the control group (Velazquez-Lopez). Other studies have supported additional concepts such as that intake of highly-processed food was associated with a 2.5-fold increased risk of MetS [63], and intake of sugar-sweetened beverages (vs. not) is associated with >5-fold risk of MetS [64].While intervention studies assessing effects of eliminating sugar-sweetened beverages on MetS have not been performed, randomized trials have shown some efficacy of sugar-sweetened beverage elimination on improved weight status [55,65], which clearly contributes to risk of MetS. Overall, among patients with MetS, efforts should be made toward reducing consumption of sugar-sweetened beverages, saturated fat, and calorie-dense food (e.g., fast food) and toward increasing consumption of oils and vegetables—likely through negotiating individual changes with adolescents and their families.

8.2. Physical Activity Changes

Increases in physical activity serve to maintain or increase total energy expenditure in the face of reduced caloric intake. The US Center for Disease Control and Prevention and the World Health Organization recommend at least 60 minutes of moderate to vigorous physical activity among school-age children and adolescents [66]—though adolescents do particularly poorly in meeting these goals, with <30% engaging in this much activity [54]. As expected, lower levels of physical activity are associated with a greater risk for MetS, including higher levels of a MetS z-score [67,68]. Physical activity is particularly good at increasing insulin sensitivity [69].

A goal of increasing physical activity in clinical practice has been through incorporating these activities into a child's or adolescent's usual routine. One research group assessed the likelihood of MetS among children and adolescents who rode their bicycle to school (vs. not), finding lower odds of MetS associated with bicycle use [70]. Other approaches have involved providing pedometers to patients and negotiating a daily goal for total steps taken—which the child can document and take personal pride in achieving. Increased walks with family, friends or pets can be a way to ensure continued activity. Finally, participation in sports, either through schools, clubs or regular meetings with friends, can further sustain physical activity and maintain higher energy expenditure. There is a tendency toward declining physical activity with age [54], so encouragement at continuing activity starting at younger ages may be more successful.

8.3. Combined Intervention Approaches

The most effective interventions are likely to include a combined approach incorporating reducing calorie intake while increasing energy expenditure. This is because isolated increased physical activity may lead to a compensatory increase in food intake [71], while isolated caloric restriction results in a lowering of basal metabolic rate [72]—while a combination of these approaches aims to prevent these counterproductive reactions. Combined interventions to reduce MetS have focused on nutritional counselling with specific goals for physical activity—usually consisting of at least three weekly exercise sessions [73,74]. This kind of approach can produce dramatic reductions in MetS over time, with one group reporting a decrease from 27% at baseline to 8.3% after one year of combined nutrition and activity interventions [73].

While it is more difficult among children and adolescents to demonstrate the long-term benefits of approaches like this, we evaluated adults in the Diabetes Prevention Program, revealing that the degree of decrease in MetS severity among adults randomized to intensive lifestyle change (compared to those randomized to usual care) was associated with reductions in further odds of developing diabetes or CVD [22]. This underscores the potential utility in following for MetS changes over time during intervention—potentially as a motivator for patients [2] to track changes in future risk.

Thus, in most clinical intervention care, the medical team makes recommendations for improvements in dietary choices and physical activity concurrently [75] with follow-up to encourage ongoing adherence [76]. Success rates in clinical settings have not always been stellar [77], but children and adolescents who make these changes are likely to improve their metabolic status, with likely long-term health benefits.

9. Conclusions

Overall, the high prevalence that we see of MetS currently and the strong associations of MetS with future diabetes and CVD is a great cause of concern that should alarm practitioners who care for children and adolescents. This is particularly true with worsening obesity prevalence worldwide, including in developing areas. Prevention of childhood obesity is critical to reducing future MetS. Screening for obesity and MetS should be incorporated in multiple aspects of pediatric clinical care. Finally, recognizing the presence of MetS and intervening with targeted lifestyle recommendations—with repeated follow-up to encourage adherence—is likely to improve the future health of these children.

Author Contributions: M.D.D. researched and wrote the paper.

Funding: This research received no external funding.

Conflicts of Interest: I have no conflicts of interest to report.

References

1. Berenson, G.S.; Srinivasan, S.R.; Bao, W.; Newman, W.P.; Wattigney, W.A. Association between multiple cardiovascular risk factors and atherosclerosis in children and young adults. The Bogalusa Heart Study. *N. Engl. J. Med.* **1998**, *338*, 1650–1656. [CrossRef] [PubMed]
2. DeBoer, M.D. Obesity, systemic inflammation, and increased risk for cardiovascular disease and diabetes among adolescents: A need for screening tools to target interventions. *Nutrition* **2013**, *29*, 379–386. [CrossRef] [PubMed]
3. Afshin, A.; Forouzanfar, M.H.; Reitsma, M.B.; Sur, P.; Estep, K.; Lee, A.; Marczak, L.; Mokdad, A.H.; Moradi-Lakeh, M.; Naghavi, M.; et al. Health Effects of Overweight and Obesity in 195 Countries over 25 Years. *N. Engl. J. Med.* **2017**, *377*, 13–27.
4. Kelishadi, R. Childhood overweight, obesity, and the metabolic syndrome in developing countries. *Epidemiol. Rev.* **2007**, *29*, 62–76. [CrossRef] [PubMed]
5. Reaven, G.M. Banting lecture 1988. Role of insulin resistance in human disease. *Diabetes* **1988**, *37*, 1595–1607. [CrossRef]
6. Tilg, H.; Moschen, A.R. Inflammatory mechanisms in the regulation of insulin resistance. *Mol. Med.* **2008**, *14*, 222–231. [CrossRef] [PubMed]
7. Shulman, G.I. Ectopic fat in insulin resistance, dyslipidemia, and cardiometabolic disease. *N. Engl. J. Med.* **2014**, *371*, 2237–2238. [CrossRef]
8. Morrison, J.A.; Friedman, L.A.; Gray-McGuire, C. Metabolic syndrome in childhood predicts adult cardiovascular disease 25 years later: The Princeton Lipid Research Clinics follow-up study. *Pediatrics* **2007**, *120*, 340–345. [CrossRef]
9. Morrison, J.A.; Friedman, L.A.; Wang, P.; Glueck, C.J. Metabolic syndrome in childhood predicts adult metabolic syndrome and type 2 diabetes mellitus 25 to 30 years later. *J. Pediatr.* **2008**, *152*, 201–206. [CrossRef]
10. Kadowaki, T.; Yamauchi, T.; Kubota, N.; Hara, K.; Ueki, K.; Tobe, K. Adiponectin and adiponectin receptors in insulin resistance, diabetes, and the metabolic syndrome. *J. Clin. Investig.* **2006**, *116*, 1784–1792. [CrossRef]
11. de Ferranti, S.; Mozaffarian, D. The perfect storm: Obesity, adipocyte dysfunction, and metabolic consequences. *Clin. Chem.* **2008**, *54*, 945–955. [CrossRef] [PubMed]
12. Defronzo, R.A. Banting Lecture. From the triumvirate to the ominous octet: A new paradigm for the treatment of type 2 diabetes mellitus. *Diabetes* **2009**, *58*, 773–795. [CrossRef] [PubMed]
13. Grundy, S.M.; Cleeman, J.I.; Daniels, S.R.; Donato, K.A.; Eckel, R.H.; Franklin, B.A.; Gordon, D.J.; Krauss, R.M.; Savage, P.J.; Smith, S.C.J.; et al. Diagnosis and management of the metabolic syndrome—An American Heart Association/National Heart, Lung, and Blood Institute Scientific Statement. *Circulation* **2005**, *112*, 2735–2752. [CrossRef] [PubMed]

14. Alberti, K.G.; Zimmet, P.Z. Definition, diagnosis and classification of diabetes mellitus and its complications. Part 1: Diagnosis and classification of diabetes mellitus provisional report of a WHO consultation. *Diabet. Med.* **1998**, *15*, 539–553. [CrossRef]
15. Alberti, K.G.; Zimmet, P.; Shaw, J. Metabolic syndrome-a new world-wide definition. A Consensus Statement from the International Diabetes Federation. *Diabet. Med.* **2006**, *23*, 469–480. [CrossRef] [PubMed]
16. Alberti, K.G.; Eckel, R.H.; Grundy, S.M.; Zimmet, P.Z.; Cleeman, J.I.; Donato, K.A.; Fruchart, J.C.; James, W.P.T.; Loria, C.M.; Smith, S.C.J. Harmonizing the metabolic syndrome: A joint interim statement of the International Diabetes Federation Task Force on Epidemiology and Prevention; National Heart, Lung, and Blood Institute; American Heart Association; World Heart Federation; International Atherosclerosis Society; and International Association for the Study of Obesity. *Circulation* **2009**, *120*, 1640–1645. [PubMed]
17. Gurka, M.J.; Lilly, C.L.; Norman, O.M.; DeBoer, M.D. An Examination of Sex and Racial/Ethnic Differences in the Metabolic Syndrome among Adults: A Confirmatory Factor Analysis and a Resulting Continuous Severity Score. *Metabolism* **2014**, *63*, 218–225. [CrossRef]
18. Eisenmann, J.C. On the use of a continuous metabolic syndrome score in pediatric research. *Cardiovasc. Diabetol.* **2008**, *7*, 17. [CrossRef]
19. Vishnu, A.; Gurka, M.J.; DeBoer, M.D. The severity of the metabolic syndrome increases over time within individuals, independent of baseline metabolic syndrome status and medication use: The Atherosclerosis Risk in Communities Study. *Atherosclerosis* **2015**, *243*, 278–285. [CrossRef]
20. DeBoer, M.D.; Gurka, M.J.; Golden, S.H.; Musani, S.K.; Sims, M.; Vishnu, A.; Guo, Y.; Cardel, M.; Pearson, T.A. Independent Associations between Metabolic Syndrome Severity & Future Coronary Heart Disease by Sex and Race. *J. Am. Coll. Card.* **2017**, *69*, 1204–1205.
21. Gurka, M.J.; Golden, S.H.; Musani, S.K.; Sims, M.; Vishnu, A.; Guo, Y.; Cardel, M.; Pearson, T.A.; DeBoer, M.D. Independent associations between a metabolic syndrome severity score and future diabetes by sex and race: The Atherosclerosis Risk in Communities Study and Jackson Heart Study. *Diabetologia* **2017**, *60*, 1261–1270. [CrossRef] [PubMed]
22. DeBoer, M.D.; Filipp, S.L.; Gurka, M.J. Use of a Metabolic Syndrome Severity Z Score to Track Risk During Treatment of Prediabetes: An Analysis of the Diabetes Prevention Program. *Diabetes Care* **2018**, *41*, 2421–2430. [CrossRef] [PubMed]
23. Reinehr, T.; de Sousa, G.; Toschke, A.M.; Andler, W. Comparison of metabolic syndrome prevalence using eight different definitions: A critical approach. *Arch. Dis. Child.* **2007**, *92*, 1067–1072. [CrossRef] [PubMed]
24. Ford, E.S.; Li, C.; Cook, S.; Choi, H.K. Serum concentrations of uric acid and the metabolic syndrome among US children and adolescents. *Circulation* **2007**, *115*, 2526–2532. [CrossRef] [PubMed]
25. Fernandez, J.R.; Redden, D.T.; Pietrobelli, A.; Allison, D.B. Waist circumference percentiles in nationally representative samples of African-American, European-American, and Mexican-American children and adolescents. *J. Pediatr.* **2004**, *145*, 439–444. [CrossRef] [PubMed]
26. National High Blood Pressure Education Program Working Group. The fourth report on the diagnosis, evaluation, and treatment of high blood pressure in children and adolescents. *Pediatrics* **2004**, *114*, 555–576. [CrossRef]
27. Zimmet, P.; Alberti, K.G.M.; Kaufman, F.; Tajima, N.; Silink, M.; Arslanian, S.; Wong, G.; Bennett, P.; Shaw, J.; Caprio, S.; et al. The metabolic syndrome in children and adolescents—An IDF consensus report. *Pediatr. Diabetes* **2007**, *8*, 299–306. [CrossRef]
28. Jolliffe, C.J.; Janssen, I. Development of age-specific adolescent metabolic syndrome criteria that are linked to the Adult Treatment Panel III and International Diabetes Federation criteria. *J. Am. Coll. Cardiol.* **2007**, *49*, 891–898. [CrossRef]
29. Gurka, M.J.; Ice, C.L.; Sun, S.S.; DeBoer, M.D. A confirmatory factor analysis of the metabolic syndrome in adolescents: An examination of sex and racial/ethnic differences. *Cardiovasc. Diabetol.* **2012**, *11*, 128. [CrossRef]
30. DeBoer, M.D.; Gurka, M.J.; Morrison, J.A.; Woo, J.G. Inter-relationships between the severity of metabolic syndrome, insulin and adiponectin and their relationship to future type 2 diabetes and cardiovascular disease. *Int. J. Obes.* **2016**, *40*, 1353–1359. [CrossRef]
31. Lee, A.M.; Gurka, M.J.; DeBoer, M.D. Trends in Metabolic Syndrome Severity and Lifestyle Factors Among Adolescents. *Pediatrics* **2016**, *137*, 1–9. [CrossRef] [PubMed]

32. Lee, A.M.; Fermin, C.R.; Filipp, S.L.; Gurka, M.J.; DeBoer, M.D. Examining trends in prediabetes and its relationship with the metabolic syndrome in US adolescents, 1999–2014. *Acta Diabetol.* **2017**, *54*, 373–381. [CrossRef] [PubMed]
33. Gustafson, J.K.; Yanoff, L.B.; Easter, B.D.; Brady, S.M.; Keil, M.F.; Roberts, M.D.; Sebring, N.G.; Han, J.C.; Yanovski, S.Z.; Hubbard, V.S.; et al. The Stability of Metabolic Syndrome in Children and Adolescents. *J. Clin. Endocrinol. Metab.* **2009**, *94*, 4828–4834. [CrossRef] [PubMed]
34. Li, C.; Ford, E.S.; Huang, T.T.-K.; Sun, S.S.; Goodman, E. Patterns of change in cardiometabolic risk factors associated with the metabolic syndrome among children and adolescents: The Fels Longitudinal Study. *J. Pediatr.* **2009**, *155*, S5.e9–S5.e16. [CrossRef] [PubMed]
35. Scheitel, M.R.; Kessler, M.E.; Shellum, J.L.; Peters, S.G.; Milliner, D.S.; Liu, H.; Elayavilli, R.K.; Poterack, K.A.; Miksch, T.A.; Boysen, J.J.; et al. Effect of a Novel Clinical Decision Support Tool on the Efficiency and Accuracy of Treatment Recommendations for Cholesterol Management. *Appl. Clin. Inform.* **2017**, *8*, 124–136. [CrossRef] [PubMed]
36. Magge, S.N.; Goodman, E.; Armstrong, S.C. The Metabolic Syndrome in Children and Adolescents: Shifting the Focus to Cardiometabolic Risk Factor Clustering. *Pediatrics* **2017**, *140*, e20171603. [CrossRef] [PubMed]
37. Messiah, S.E.; Arheart, K.L.; Luke, B.; Lipshultz, S.E.; Miller, T.L. Relationship between body mass index and metabolic syndrome risk factors among US 8-to 14-year-olds, 1999 to 2002. *J. Pediatr.* **2008**, *153*, 215–221. [CrossRef] [PubMed]
38. Walker, S.E.; Gurka, M.J.; Oliver, M.N.; Johns, D.W.; DeBoer, M.D. Racial/ethnic discrepancies in the metabolic syndrome begin in childhood and persist after adjustment for environmental factors. *Nutr. Metab. Cardiovasc. Dis.* **2012**, *22*, 141–148. [CrossRef] [PubMed]
39. Ford, E.S.; Li, C.; Zhao, G.; Pearson, W.S.; Mokdad, A.H. Prevalence of the metabolic syndrome among U.S. adolescents using the definition from the International Diabetes Federation. *Diabetes Care* **2008**, *31*, 587–589. [CrossRef] [PubMed]
40. Morrison, J.A.; Friedman, L.A.; Harlan, W.R.; Harlan, L.C.; Barton, B.A.; Schreiber, G.B.; Klein, D.J. Development of the metabolic syndrome in black and white adolescent girls: A longitudinal assessment. *Pediatrics* **2005**, *116*, 1178–1182. [CrossRef] [PubMed]
41. DeBoer, M.D.; Gurka, M.J. Ability among adolescents for the metabolic syndrome to predict elevations in factors associated with type 2 diabetes and cardiovascular disease: Data from the national health and nutrition examination survey 1999-2006. *Metab. Syndr. Relat. Disord.* **2010**, *8*, 343–353. [CrossRef] [PubMed]
42. Aradillas-García, C.; Rodríguez-Morán, M.; Garay-Sevilla, M.E.; Malacara, J.M.; Rascon-Pacheco, R.A.; Guerrero-Romero, F. Distribution of the homeostasis model assessment of insulin resistance in Mexican children and adolescents. *Eur. J. Endocrinol.* **2012**, *166*, 301–306. [CrossRef] [PubMed]
43. DeBoer, M.D. Underdiagnosis of Metabolic Syndrome in Non-Hispanic Black Adolescents: A Call for Ethnic-Specific Criteria. *Curr. Cardiovasc. Risk Rep.* **2010**, *4*, 302–310. [CrossRef] [PubMed]
44. Friend, A.; Craig, L.; Turner, S. The prevalence of metabolic syndrome in children: A systematic review of the literature. *Metab. Syndr. Relat. Disord.* **2013**, *11*, 71–80. [CrossRef] [PubMed]
45. DeBoer, M.D.; Filipp, S.L.; Gurka, M.J. Geographical variation in the prevalence of obesity and metabolic syndrome among US adolescents. *Pediatr. Obes.* **2019**, *14*, e12483. [CrossRef] [PubMed]
46. Gupta, N.; Goel, K.; Shah, P.; Misra, A. Childhood obesity in developing countries: Epidemiology, determinants, and prevention. *Endocr. Rev.* **2012**, *33*, 48–70. [CrossRef] [PubMed]
47. Cossrow, N.; Falkner, B. Race/ethnic issues in obesity and obesity-related comorbidities. *J. Clin. Endocrinol. Metab.* **2004**, *89*, 2590–2594. [CrossRef]
48. Magnussen, C.G.; Koskinen, J.; Chen, W.; Thomson, R.; Schmidt, M.D.; Srinivasan, S.R.; Kivimaki, M.; Mattsson, N.; Kähönen, M.; Laitinen, T.; et al. Pediatric metabolic syndrome predicts adulthood metabolic syndrome, subclinical atherosclerosis, and type 2 diabetes mellitus but is no better than body mass index alone: The Bogalusa Heart Study and the Cardiovascular Risk in Young Finns Study. *Circulation* **2010**, *122*, 1604–1611. [CrossRef]
49. DeBoer, M.D.; Gurka, M.J.; Woo, J.G.; Morrison, J.A. Severity of the metabolic syndrome as a predictor of type 2 diabetes between childhood and adulthood: The Princeton Lipid Research Cohort Study. *Diabetologia* **2015**, *58*, 2745–2752. [CrossRef]

50. DeBoer, M.D.; Gurka, M.J.; Woo, J.G.; Morrison, J.A. Severity of Metabolic Syndrome as a Predictor of Cardiovascular Disease Between Childhood and Adulthood: The Princeton Lipid Research Cohort Study. *J. Amer. Coll. Card.* **2015**, *66*, 755–757. [CrossRef]
51. Deboer, M.D.; Wiener, R.C.; Barnes, B.H.; Gurka, M.J. Ethnic differences in the link between insulin resistance and elevated ALT. *Pediatrics* **2013**, *132*, e718–e726. [CrossRef] [PubMed]
52. Lee, A.M.; Charlton, J.R.; Carmody, J.B.; Gurka, M.J.; DeBoer, M.D. Metabolic risk factors in nondiabetic adolescents with glomerular hyperfiltration. *Nephrol. Dial. Transpl.* **2016**, *32*, 1517–1524. [CrossRef] [PubMed]
53. DeBoer, M.D.; Filipp, S.L.; Musani, S.K.; Sims, M.; Okusa, M.D.; Gurka, M.J. Metabolic Syndrome Severity and Risk of CKD and Worsened GFR: The Jackson Heart Study. *Kidney Blood Press. Res.* **2018**, *43*, 555–567. [CrossRef] [PubMed]
54. Nader, P.R.; Bradley, R.H.; Houts, R.M.; McRitchie, S.L.; O'Brien, M. Moderate-to-vigorous physical activity from ages 9 to 15 years. *JAMA* **2008**, *300*, 295–305. [CrossRef] [PubMed]
55. Scharf, R.J.; DeBoer, M.D. Sugar-Sweetened Beverages and Children's Health. *Annu. Rev. Public Health* **2016**, *37*, 273–293. [CrossRef] [PubMed]
56. World Health Organization. *Interim Report of the Commission on Ending Childhood Obesity*; World Health Organization: Geneva, Switzerland, 2015.
57. O'Connor, E.A.; Evans, C.V.; Burda, B.U.; Walsh, E.S.; Eder, M.; Lozano, P. Screening for Obesity and Intervention for Weight Management in Children and Adolescents: Evidence Report and Systematic Review for the US Preventive Services Task Force. *JAMA* **2017**, *317*, 2427–2444. [CrossRef] [PubMed]
58. Morrison, J.A.; Glueck, C.J.; Horn, P.S.; Wang, P. Childhood predictors of adult type 2 diabetes at 9 and 26-year follow-ups. *Arch. Pediatr. Adolesc. Med.* **2010**, *164*, 53–60. [CrossRef] [PubMed]
59. Daniels, S.R.; Greer, F.R. Lipid screening and cardiovascular health in childhood. *Pediatrics* **2008**, *122*, 198–208. [CrossRef] [PubMed]
60. Brickman, W.J.; Huang, J.; Silverman, B.L.; Metzger, B.E. Acanthosis nigricans identifies youth at high risk for metabolic abnormalities. *J. Pediatr.* **2010**, *156*, 87–92. [CrossRef]
61. American Diabetes Association. 2. Classification and Diagnosis of Diabetes. *Diabetes Care* **2018**, *41*, S13–S27. [CrossRef]
62. Bean, M.K.; Powell, P.; Quinoy, A.; Ingersoll, K.; Wickham, E.P., III; Mazzeo, S.E. Motivational interviewing targeting diet and physical activity improves adherence to paediatric obesity treatment: Results from the MI Values randomized controlled trial. *Pediatr. Obes.* **2015**, *10*, 118–125. [CrossRef] [PubMed]
63. Tavares, L.F.; Fonseca, S.C.; Garcia Rosa, M.L.; Yokoo, E.M. Relationship between ultra-processed foods and metabolic syndrome in adolescents from a Brazilian Family Doctor Program. *Public Health Nutr.* **2012**, *15*, 82–87. [CrossRef] [PubMed]
64. Chan, T.-F.; Lin, W.-T.; Huang, H.-L.; Lee, C.-Y.; Wu, P.-W.; Chiu, Y.-W.; Huang, C.-C.; Tsai, S.; Lin, C.-L.; Lee, C.-H. Consumption of sugar-sweetened beverages is associated with components of the metabolic syndrome in adolescents. *Nutrients* **2014**, *6*, 2088–2103. [CrossRef] [PubMed]
65. Ebbeling, C.B.; Ludwig, D.S. Sugar-sweetened beverages, genetic risk, and obesity. *N. Engl. J. Med.* **2013**, *368*, 287. [PubMed]
66. CDC. 2008 Physical Activity Guidelines Americans. Available online: https://health.gov/paguidelines/pdf/paguide.pdf (accessed on 1 August 2019).
67. Ekelund, U.; Anderssen, S.A.; Froberg, K.; Sardinha, L.B.; Andersen, L.B.; Brage, S. Independent associations of physical activity and cardiorespiratory fitness with metabolic risk factors in children: The European youth heart study. *Diabetologia* **2007**, *50*, 1832–1840. [CrossRef] [PubMed]
68. Stabelini Neto, A.; de Campos, W.; Dos Santos, G.C.; Junior, O.M. Metabolic syndrome risk score and time expended in moderate to vigorous physical activity in adolescents. *BMC Pediatr.* **2014**, *14*, 42. [CrossRef] [PubMed]
69. Guinhouya, B.C.; Samouda, H.; Zitouni, D.; Vilhelm, C.; Hubert, H. Evidence of the influence of physical activity on the metabolic syndrome and/or on insulin resistance in pediatric populations: A systematic review. *Int. J. Pediatr. Obes.* **2011**, *6*, 361–388. [CrossRef] [PubMed]
70. Ramírez-Vélez, R.; García-Hermoso, A.; Agostinis-Sobrinho, C.A.; Mota, J.; Santos, R.; Correa-Bautista, J.E.; Amaya-Tambo, D.C.; Villa-González, E. Cycling to School and Body Composition, Physical Fitness, and Metabolic Syndrome in Children and Adolescents. *J. Pediatr.* **2017**, *188*, 57–63. [CrossRef] [PubMed]

71. Blundell, J.E.; Stubbs, R.J.; Hughes, D.A.; Whybrow, S.; King, N.A. Cross talk between physical activity and appetite control: Does physical activity stimulate appetite? *Proc. Nutr. Soc.* **2003**, *62*, 651–661. [CrossRef]
72. Martin, C.K.; Heilbronn, L.K.; De Jonge, L.; Delany, J.P.; Volaufova, J.; Anton, S.D.; Redman, L.M.; Smith, S.R.; Ravussin, E.; Jonge, L. Effect of calorie restriction on resting metabolic rate and spontaneous physical activity. *Obesity* **2007**, *15*, 2964–2973. [CrossRef]
73. Caranti, D.A.; De Mello, M.T.; Prado, W.L.; Tock, L.; Siqueira, K.O.; De Piano, A.; Lofrano, M.C.; Cristofalo, D.M.; Lederman, H.; Tufik, S.; et al. Short and long-term beneficial effects of a multidisciplinary therapy for the control of metabolic syndrome in obese adolescents. *Metabolism* **2007**, *56*, 1293–1300. [CrossRef]
74. Leite, N.; Milano, G.; Cieslak, F.; Lopes, W.; Rodacki, A.; Radominski, R. Effects of physical exercise and nutritional guidance on metabolic syndrome in obese adolescents. *Braz. J. Phys. Ther.* **2009**, *12*, 73–81. [CrossRef]
75. WHO. Global Strategy on Diet, Physical Activity and Health. Available online: http://www.who.int/dietphysicalactivity/factsheet_young_people/en/ (accessed on 1 August 2019).
76. Walker, S.E.; Smolkin, M.E.; O'Leary, M.L.; Cluett, S.B.; Norwood, V.F.; DeBoer, M.D.; Gurka, M.J. Predictors of Retention and BMI Loss or Stabilization in Obese Youth Enrolled in a Weight Loss Intervention. *Obes. Res. Clin. Pract.* **2012**, *6*, e330–e339. [CrossRef]
77. Wu, T.; Gao, X.; Chen, M.; Van Dam, R.M. Long-term effectiveness of diet-plus-exercise interventions vs. diet-only interventions for weight loss: A meta-analysis. *Obes. Rev.* **2009**, *10*, 313–323. [CrossRef]

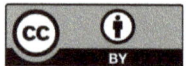

© 2019 by the author. Licensee MDPI, Basel, Switzerland. This article is an open access article distributed under the terms and conditions of the Creative Commons Attribution (CC BY) license (http://creativecommons.org/licenses/by/4.0/).

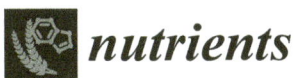

Communication

Ethnicity and Metabolic Syndrome: Implications for Assessment, Management and Prevention

Scott A. Lear [1,2,*] and Danijela Gasevic [3,4]

1. Faculty of Health Sciences, Simon Fraser University, Burnaby, BC V5A 1S6, Canada
2. Division of Cardiology, Providence Health Care, Vancouver, BC V6Z 1Y6, Canada
3. School of Public Health and Preventive Medicine, Monash University, Melbourne, VIC 3004, Australia; danijela.gasevic@monash.edu
4. Usher Institute, University of Edinburgh, Edinburgh EH8 9AG, UK
* Correspondence: slear@providencehealth.bc.ca; Tel.: +1-604-682-2344 (ext. 62778)

Received: 25 November 2019; Accepted: 17 December 2019; Published: 19 December 2019

Abstract: The metabolic syndrome (MetS) is a constellation of cardiometabolic risk factors that identifies people at increased risk for type 2 diabetes and cardiovascular disease. While the global prevalence is 20%–25% of the adult population, the prevalence varies across different racial/ethnic populations. In this narrative review, evidence is reviewed regarding the assessment, management and prevention of MetS among people of different racial/ethnic groups. The most popular definition of MetS considers race/ethnicity for assessing waist circumference given differences in visceral adipose tissue and cardiometabolic risk. However, defining race/ethnicity may pose challenges in the clinical setting. Despite 80% of the world's population being of non-European descent, the majority of research on management and prevention has focused on European-derived populations. In these studies, lifestyle management has proven an effective therapy for reversal of MetS, and randomised studies are underway in specific racial/ethnic groups. Given the large number of people at risk for MetS, prevention efforts need to focus at community and population levels. Community-based interventions have begun to show promise, and efforts to improve lifestyle behaviours through alterations in the built environment may be another avenue. However, careful consideration needs to be given to take into account the unique cultural context of the target race/ethnic group.

Keywords: metabolic syndrome; ethnicity; prevention; lifestyle; cardiometabolic

1. Introduction

The metabolic syndrome (MetS) is a constellation of cardiometabolic risk factors that results in an increased risk for type 2 diabetes (T2D), cardiovascular disease and premature mortality [1]. At its foundation is insulin resistance, in which the actions of insulin decrease, resulting in hyperinsulinemia. Left unchecked, insulin resistance can progress to MetS and prediabetes, and further to T2D. MetS is defined as the presence of at least three of the following five common clinical measures, which occur in people with insulin resistance: elevated triglycerides (TG), low high-density lipoprotein cholesterol (HDL-C), elevated blood sugar, elevated blood pressure (BP) and elevated waist circumference (WC) (Table 1, Table 2) [2]. Within primary care and other front-line care environments, the MetS is a simple tool with which to identify people with insulin resistance and prediabetes, and therefore, at early risk for T2D and cardiovascular disease. As a result, it provides an opportune time for primary care providers to intervene and prevent progression to overt disease.

Table 1. Criteria of the metabolic syndrome defined as three of more of the five measures.

Measure	Threshold
Elevated triglycerides	≥1.70 mmol/L *
Reduced HDL-C	≤1.00 mmol/L (males) * ≤1.30 mmol/L (females) *
Elevated blood pressure	Systolic ≥ 130 mmHg and/or Diastolic ≥ 85 mmHg *
Elevated fasting glucose	≥5.6 mmol/L *
Elevated waist circumference	See population-specific thresholds in Table 2

* Or appropriate drug treatment. HDL-C = high-density lipoprotein cholesterol.

Table 2. Population-specific waist circumference thresholds [2].

Population	Men	Women
Central/South American, Chinese, Japanese, South Asian	≥90 cm	≥80 cm
Mediterranean, Middle East, Sub-Saharan African	≥94 cm	≥80 cm
Europid (includes Canada, Europe and United States) *	≥102 cm (≥94 cm)	≥88 cm (≥88 cm)

* While thresholds of ≥94 cm for men and ≥80 cm for women are more common in research, the thresholds of ≥102 for men and ≥88 for women are used more commonly in clinical practice.

Despite the ease of assessment, the worldwide prevalence of MetS is not known [3,4], in part due to MetS not being a common clinical indicator, such as T2D, and thus not widely assessed. Further complicating estimates is the variation in definitions used in countries before, and even since [5], the MetS definition was harmonised in 2009 [2]. However, estimates suggest the worldwide prevalence of MetS to be 20%–25% of the population, based on a presumed prevalence threefold higher than T2D [4]. As the prevalence of obesity and T2D is expected to rise, so too is the prevalence of MetS. In countries where prevalence data do exist, it is clear that it differs by country. For example, the estimated prevalence of MetS in the United States is 33.4% [6], while in China, it is 14.4% [7].

The difference in MetS prevalence across countries is likely the result of different governmental, institutional and sociocultural factors at the population level, which can affect a range of upstream determinants including, but not limited to, the type of available foods and access, health care policies, education, employment and the physical environment. This is in addition to individual factors such as biology/genetics and sociocultural aspects, which are also likely relevant to the different prevalence of MetS between countries. These latter aspects may be collectively referred to as ethnic or racial differences, as many of these characteristics often cluster in specific and identifiable populations. Even within the same country, in the same local environment, the prevalence of MetS differs along certain predefined racial/ethnic groups. For example, in the United States, the prevalence of MetS is highest in Hispanics and lowest in African-Americans, with the prevalence of MetS in whites in between the two [8]. (It is important to recognise that the term "white" does not describe an ethnicity or ethnic group. The use of the term "white" in this article is only used when the authors of the original article that has been cited have used this term to describe one of their study populations without providing additional information on that group's ethnic origins.) While recent national level data in Canada have not been reported, an earlier study reported MetS to be highest in people of Indigenous ancestry, followed by South Asians, Europeans and East Asians [9]. In Singapore, MetS is highest in South Asians, followed by Malays and then people of Chinese background [10]. Understanding the influence race/ethnicity has with respect to MetS is important for its proper assessment, treatment and prevention.

Ethnicity and race are fluid constructs that have no clear-cut definition, which are often (and incorrectly) used interchangeably. Despite these challenges, ethnicity and race are still used in medical literature as a means to differentiate between populations and recognise such differences in health management and disease prevention. Furthernore, ethnic and racial groupings often differ across the medical literature based on the research purpose, methods of data collection and even the lens of the researchers themselves. While individuals may ascribe their ethnicity within sociocultural aspects, medical guidelines such as those for the MetS attempt to define ethnicity primarily on common biomedical (whether biological or genetic) and/or geographical aspects. These are generally broad classifications, which often group multiple ethnic and racial groups into one. Sometimes this is based exclusively on geographical origins (for example, "Asian" or "European") without recognising the ethnic or racial heterogeneity within these groupings and thus incorrectly inferring that the populations are homogeneous. While some biomedical characteristics align with certain ethnic and racial groups, this should not be interpreted that ethnicity and race are biomedical constructs, nor should ethnic and racial classifications be interpreted to reflect genetic variation.

It should also be noted that ethnicity and race are not the same. Race infers some biological foundations for differences among groups, while ethnicity views populations from a more social/cultural lens. However, these terms may be used in medical literature as if they are the same. Across the many papers cited in this review, some authors grouped study participants into categories they termed "race", while others used groupings termed "ethnicity", commonly without defining the terms or the categories. This lack of consistency makes it challenging to compare and contrast across the various studies. As a result, for the sake of this review, the terms are combined (albeit not ideally) into one called "race/ethnicity", and when citing research, we have used the same race/ethnicity group names as the original authors.

2. Assessment

Of the five cardiometabolic risk factors, four of the definition thresholds apply to all race/ethnic groups. The fifth, WC, entails different threshold values based on race/ethnic background (Table 2). These differing thresholds are based on evidence that the association between WC, an indicator of abdominal obesity, and risk of cardiometabolic diseases differs by race/ethnicity. For example, at a similar WC, people of Chinese and South Asian background have higher values of total cholesterol and other cardiometabolic risk factors compared with people of European background [11–13]. If the goal is to identify people at the same level of cardiometabolic risk, lower WC thresholds for people of Asian background were created.

The requirement for lower WC thresholds in some racial/ethnic groups has its foundation in the differences in visceral adipose tissue (VAT). In particular, people of Asian backgrounds (South Asian, East Asian, Southeast Asian) have higher amounts of VAT at a given body size and WC [14]. For South Asians, this higher amount of VAT accounts for much of their elevated cardiometabolic risk compared with European-derived populations [15]. In African-Americans, VAT tends to be lower than whites at a similar body size [16]. Despite a higher prevalence of obesity and T2D [17,18], levels of VAT in North American Indigenous populations appear to be similar to that of Europeans of the same size [14,19].

While the use of race/ethnic-specific WC thresholds is reflective of the differing risk in different racial/ethnic groups, it can pose a challenge during assessment of MetS. This is reflected in the above biological foundations for having different WC thresholds for MetS. It must be acknowledged that the MetS uses a broad definition of race/ethnicity and population grouping based on geographical location, which does not reflect the many varying races and ethnicities within those groupings. There is even limited agreement in how race/ethnicity is defined [20]; however, it is probably best defined by self-report, meaning, each individual is likely to provide the most "accurate" identification of their own race/ethnicity.

In predominantly homogeneous populations found in many parts of Asia, the use of race/ethnic-specific WC thresholds should not pose a challenge [21]. However, in diverse populations such as in Europe and the Americas, determining the race/ethnicity of a patient can be challenging [22]. While self-identification may be the best indicator of race/ethnicity, this may be a conversation in which health care professionals may feel uncomfortable engaging. In addition, people who descend from a different geographical or race/ethnic region from where they currently live may identify more with the local context than their ancestral one. This may result in a conflict between how an individual identifies his/herself and how race/ethnicity is defined in the health system. In many locations, people may also identify with more than one race/ethnicity. Guessing on the part of the health care professional may be no better. The increasingly common prevalence of offspring from mixed ethnic partnerships can further complicate the matter [23], as there are no studies on how to apply the race/ethnic-specific WC thresholds to these individuals.

3. Treatment

As MetS allows for the presence of overt risk factors such as hypercholesterolemia, hypertension and T2D, when present, these should be treated as per local clinical guidelines. For patients with MetS but without overt risk factors, treatment through lifestyle therapy is effective at reversing MetS. In the Diabetes Prevention Program (55% white, 20% African-American, 16% Hispanic, 5% Native American and 4% Asian in the original trial [24], no analysis by race/ethnicity), the combined intervention of physical activity and diet resulted in a more than twofold reversal of the MetS compared with the placebo group and a 65% greater reversal rate than the metformin group [25]. A subsequent meta-analysis of combined physical activity and diet interventions found a twofold greater rate of MetS reversal compared with control interventions [26].

In isolation, regular aerobic physical activity of low-to-moderate intensity has resulted in reversal of the MetS in postmenopausal women (65% white, 30% African-American and 6% other in original trial [27], no analysis by race/ethnicity) [28] and reduction in MetS severity in a workplace setting using a wrist-worn activity monitor and smartphone app designed to enhance physical activity (conducted in Germany, race/ethnicity not reported) [29]. In addition to aerobic exercise interventions, a 12-week resistance training program was effective in reversing MetS in older women (race/ethnicity not reported) [30]. However, aerobic physical activity alone in men and women (56% white, 44% African-American) or a combination of aerobic and resistance physical activity may be superior to resistance training alone [31]. A randomised trial in Norwegian men and women focused on differing intensities of exercise on reversing the MetS is currently underway [32].

A secondary analysis in the PREDIMED randomised trial of participants with the MetS (approximately 97% European) at the study's onset reported the Mediterranean diet resulted in an approximately 28%–35% reversal of MetS compared with the control diet [33]. However, due to later concerns with the PREDIMED methods [34] and republication with a smaller sample attesting to similar conclusions [35], the exact effect of the intervention may not be accurately reflected in this analysis.

Despite more than 80% of the world's population being of non-European descent, the overwhelming majority of research on MetS is limited by the predominant focus on European-derived populations and a lack of race/ethnic-specific analyses. In terms of the benefits of interventions aimed at reducing or reversing MetS in other race/ethnic groups, few studies exist. Short-term diet studies have reported reversal of MetS in Iranians [36], South Asians [37] and people of Asian descent living in the United States [38]. A combined lifestyle intervention in Arabs living in Saudi Arabia reported a greater reduction in MetS compared with the group receiving general advice [39]. One randomised trial currently underway is investigating a combined lifestyle intervention of physical activity, nutrition improvement and weight loss in a diverse population in the United Kingdom [40], while another exercise-focused trial in African-American women with MetS is also in progress [41].

3.1. Comprehensive Lifestyle Interventions

Much information on reversing MetS may also be gleaned from randomised intervention studies that target individual components of the MetS or prevention/treatment of T2D. A small randomised study of Japanese men with MetS reported that a three-month intervention of diet and physical activity reduced WC and glycated haemoglobin, along with a nonsignificant reduction in MetS prevalence compared to control [42]. In African-Americans with T2D, a lifestyle weight loss intervention of 12 weeks resulted in lower weight, improved BP and glycaemic control compared with usual care after six months [43]. Similarly, a six-month weight loss program in African-Americans in the Southern United States resulted in reduction of WC and BP [44]. The Da Qing Diabetes Prevention Study in China reported reduced incidence of T2D by 45% following six years of a diet and physical activity intervention in people with glucose intolerance [45]. In Hispanic obese women, a community implementation of the Diabetes Prevention Program resulted in a greater decrease in WC and improved glycaemic control compared with metformin or standard care after 12 months [46]. In Brazil, a randomised intervention of lifestyle counselling resulted in improvements in WC and BP [47]. A nonrandomised study of translation of the Diabetes Prevention Program in Aboriginal people in the United States showed promise in reducing risk for T2D [48]. In Jewish and Bedouin women with post-gestational diabetes, a lifestyle counselling intervention resulted in reduction in glucose [49]. In South Asians living in the United Kingdom, compared with control, a diet and physical activity intervention resulted in improved WC but not glucose and BP after two years [50].

3.2. Nutritional Interventions

A wide variety of nutritional interventions ranging from macronutrient comparisons to supplementation with single foods or supplements have been carried out in a number of racial/ethnic groups. The most common dietary interventions are those focused on energy restriction in order to target weight loss, which generally improves cardiometabolic risk factors [51–53]. More recent attention has focused on the macronutrient combinations, and in particular, low-carbohydrate diets. A number of small randomised studies have indicated low-carbohydrate diets to result in more favourable improvements to glucose, insulin sensitivity, triglycerides and HDL-C [54], which may be independent of weight loss, suggesting a specific mechanism by which carbohydrates may promote cardiometabolic risk [55]. However, not all studies are in agreement and a meta-analysis of 23 randomised trials reported no difference in cardiometabolic risk factors between low-carbohydrate and low-fat diets [56].

In non-European-derived populations, diets with an emphasis on fruits and vegetables, healthy proteins and sodium reduction (such as the DASH diet) have demonstrated reductions in BP among African-Americans [57,58], East Asians [59,60] and South Asians [61,62]. For people with T2D, dietary interventions consisting of nutrition counselling following local guidelines for T2D care have resulted in improved glycaemic control, lipids and anthropometric measures in Arabs [63] and African-Americans [64]. Overweight and obese Malaysian adults undergoing a six-month trial of a high-protein, high-fibre diet had improvements to WC and glucose metabolism compared with control [65]. Studies in South Asians focusing on healthy protein, whether through meal replacement or nut supplementation, have reported reductions in glucose and WC, along with increases in HDL-C [61,62,66]. In Chinese men and women, a number of different randomised dietary interventions (high-protein, low-carbohydrate diets) have resulted in reductions in WC and lipid measures [67,68]. Diet supplemented with whole grain oats over six months reduced WC in Chinese men and women compared with control [69]. Very few studies have investigated interventions in Indigenous populations. A randomised study of flaxseed supplementation in Native Americans resulted in lowering low-density lipoprotein cholesterol (LDL-C) but did not affect HDL-C or TG [70], while a high-protein diet in Maori in New Zealand resulted in a greater decrease in WC compared with a low-fat or control diet [71].

3.3. Physical Activity Interventions

Numerous studies of various forms of physical activity have been conducted in a range of populations. In randomised trials, exercise interventions have demonstrated improvements in one or more of the components of MetS in South Asians [72–74] and East Asians [75,76]. In Chinese men, an intervention of Tai Chi was effective at reducing BP and TG [77]. Less is known about how similar interventions may be effective in African-American, Hispanic and Aboriginal/Indigenous populations. However, higher levels of physical activity and fitness have been reported to be associated with a lower prevalence of MetS in African-Americans [78], Hispanics [79] and Aboriginals [80].

To complement physical activity interventions, consideration should be given to interventions to limit sedentary behaviour such as sitting. Prospective studies have reported extended sedentary time to be positively associated with increased risk for type 2 diabetes, cardiovascular disease and premature mortality [81]. These associations occur even independently of physical activity levels. Cross-sectional studies in Americans [82], Brazilians [83] and Koreans [84] have reported positive associations between sedentary time and MetS. Randomised interventions aimed at reducing sedentary time have proven successful in increasing physical activity [85,86].

4. Prevention

Given the overall numbers of people with, and at risk for, MetS in most countries, individual-based prevention approaches are unlikely to be efficient and feasible. Instead, prevention strategies should be targeted to populations at the community level [87] and must be culturally tailored, as what works in one race/ethnic group may not necessarily work in another. These can vary from upstream, high-level policy initiatives to downstream, on the ground programs targeted at high-risk groups.

Policies such as the introduction of a sugar tax show promise. A high consumption of sugar, and sugar-sweetened beverages in particular, has been associated with a higher prevalence of MetS in a number of countries [88,89]. Countries and regions that have implemented a sugar tax have reported reductions in the consumption of sugar-sweetened beverages [90–92]. However, at present, there is no evidence to indicate this translates into a reduction in the incidence of MetS or its components, most likely because these policies are relatively new and may need more time for a downstream effect to be realised.

Another area influenced by policy at the local level is the built environment, which comprises the human-made infrastructure in which we live. This consists of such things as the street network, the placement of stores, community centres and residential areas, as well as the presence of sidewalks. Aspects of the built environment are associated with both physical activity and diet [93] and may be an upstream determinant for MetS.

People living in areas that are considered walkable (such as those with high street connectivity, mixed land use, and sidewalks) have higher physical activity levels and are at lower risk for T2D compared with those living in nonwalkable areas [94]. Similarly, living in an area with a high proportion of fast food restaurants and limited opportunities to buy healthy foods is associated with a greater prevalence of obesity [95]. These findings are consistent with a systematic review, which found cross-sectional associations of the built environment with obesity, hypertension and MetS, such that areas considered more walkable had a lower prevalence of these conditions [96]. Being cross-sectional, these studies cannot provide insight into causal relations or address the possible numerous confounders such as socioeconomic status (SES) and that some people are able to choose their neighbourhood based on their preferred lifestyle, while others may be limited in opportunities of residential movement as a result of their SES and race/ethnic minority status due to historical segregation. A limited number of longitudinal studies have reported that changes in the built environment associated with more walkability have corresponded with increased walking [97,98].

While some studies have indicated that the local food environment is associated with diets of nearby residents [99,100], not all studies have [101]. Similarly, the association of the food environment with risk factors is less clear. Some studies reported a positive association between fast food restaurants and obesity [95,102], a negative association between supermarkets and obesity [103], while others observed no association between food stores and obesity [104]. However, it appears these associations may depend on socioeconomic strata, which in heterogeneous populations often aligns along race/ethnicity, as the positive relationship between fast food restaurants and obesity was strongest in those with the lowest income [100,105]. Whether interventions to change the local food environment affect risk for the MetS is not known. Introduction of a supermarket in an area previously absent of any had a modest effect on diet quality, such as reduced sugar consumption in nearby residents compared with a control neighbourhood [106]. However, dietary assessment was conducted less than a year after the supermarket opened, and it may take a longer time, and more supermarkets, to change food purchasing behaviours.

Of importance is that many people in high- and middle-income countries who are at high risk for MetS are also among those with the lowest SES [107,108]. In addition, in countries with a diverse population, racial/ethnic minorities tend to be the most marginalised in that society. In lower SES communities, there are fewer opportunities for physical activity (such as green areas and community centres), less access to grocery stores and supermarkets (which sell healthy foods) and a higher proportion of fast food restaurants [109,110]. Targeted built environment interventions in these high-risk communities may be worthwhile to improve lifestyle behaviours known to protect against MetS.

While built environment initiatives affect the whole population, targeting interventions in high-risk communities by bringing prevention strategies to places where people gather have demonstrated substantial promise. These types of programs are needed, as access to health services for prevention and treatment (whether physical or cultural) is often worse for those of lower SES and/or of a minority racial/ethnic status [111]. In African-American communities in the United States, this has taken on the form of BP interventions at local barbershops. Both encouragement of lifestyle modification by their barber and integration with onsite pharmacists resulted in significant BP reductions, with the latter intervention being significantly better than barber encouragement alone [112]. Similar intervention studies are ongoing in faith-based communities and places of worship [113].

Success has also been reported using workplace interventions, which have resulted in improvements in activity and nutrition compared with control [114]. In Delhi, a multifactorial six-month worksite intervention focusing on education resulted in improvements in HDL-C, TG and WC compared with control groups [115]. Others have looked at translating successful interventions in European-derived populations to different racial/ethnic groups and delivering them in local communities. These studies have demonstrated significant reduction in MetS risk factors in African-Americans, [116] Hispanics [117,118] and South Asians living in India, Pakistan and the United Kingdom [119–121]. Community initiatives have also worked in increasing physical activity through walking programs in Hispanic neighbourhoods [122] and improving nutrition through local dietary counselling in African-American neighbourhoods [123]. Other community-based interventions have reported improvements in HDL-C, BP and WC compared with control in Taiwan [124]. A cluster-randomised study of communes in Vietnam found a six-month physical activity and nutrition intervention also improved cardiometabolic risk factors and a slightly better reduction in prevalence of MetS compared with an educational intervention [125]. In Iran, community-based educational programs have been successful in reducing the incidence of MetS compared with nonintervention controls [126,127].

Another area of promise for individual interventions but on a population scale is the use of consumer technology devices such as tablets, smartphones and wearables. A number of randomised studies have reported on experimental interventions that have improved lifestyle behaviours and/or cardiometabolic risk factors related to MetS, whether through wearable technology, smartphone apps or simple text messaging [29,128,129]. With the increasing ubiquity of global ownership of these devices, the opportunity to leverage these technologies to intervene on a population level has grown.

Recent studies have demonstrated the possible effectiveness of large-scale interventions [130] and the feasibility of reach in pragmatic trials [131].

5. Other Considerations

While both physical activity and dietary interventions are likely to be efficacious treatments for MetS, the intervention that is effective in one racial/ethnic group may not be effective in a different racial/ethnic group. This can be due to not only different cultural contexts of physical activity and diet but also due to structural barriers and policies, which cater to the majority population and may pose barriers to maintaining health and disease prevention for minority populations. Various cultures also view physical activity in different lights. For example, South Asians have lower physical activity levels compared with other populations [132,133], which may be rooted in cultural context [134]. In addition, adherence to and enjoyment of exercise may be based on the physical activity type, which also may have cultural relevance, such as Bhangra dance in South Asians [73] or Tai Chi in East Asians [135].

Similarly, food is strongly rooted in culture, and availability and cost may differ from place to place. Therefore, interventions need to consider what foods target groups have access to, the cultural meaning of food and the financial opportunity of the individuals. If interventions are not designed taking cultural preferences into account, they are unlikely to be engaged by the population and be successful [136]. In addition to cultural differences, in many high-income countries, many racial/ethnic groups comprise a minority population and are commonly marginalised in society, creating further barriers for treatment. To be effective, interventions must also address real and perceived structural barriers and policies present within each racial/ethnic group. For example, as a result of residential schools in Canada, there is distrust between people of Aboriginal background and government-funded health care [137]. Therefore, trust in the health care system and health care professionals, who may not be from the same community, is needed before effective prevention and intervention can begin [138].

6. Future Directions and Conclusions

Despite more than 80% of the world's population being of non-European descent, the overwhelming majority of research on MetS, from prevalence to treatment, is in predominantly European-derived populations. This is a critical gap in knowledge given that cardiometabolic risk may differ along racial/ethnic lines. Indeed, the recognised different WC thresholds reflect the nuances of race/ethnicity when assessing MetS. Current evidence in prevention and treatment of MetS suggests lifestyle interventions proved in European-derived populations can be effective at treating and reversing MetS; however, they need to be translated into the local cultural context to ensure success. For widespread prevention of MetS, interventions targeted at the population level are likely to be most successful. In order to grow our knowledge of MetS in different populations around the world, we need to conduct more rigorous cohort and randomised trials in populations beyond those of European descent. In addition, studies in countries with significant diversity should include unrepresented racial/ethnic groups as well as analyses stratified by race/ethnicity.

Author Contributions: S.A.L. conceptualised and wrote the manuscript. D.G. reviewed and revised the manuscript. All authors have read and agreed to the published version of the manuscript.

Funding: This research received no external funding.

Acknowledgments: S.A.L. holds the Pfizer/Heart and Stroke Foundation Chair in Cardiovascular Prevention Research at St. Paul's Hospital.

Conflicts of Interest: The authors have no conflict of interest to declare.

References

1. Ballantyne, C.M.; Hoogeveen, R.C.; McNeill, A.M.; Heiss, G.; Schmidt, M.I.; Duncan, B.B.; Pankow, J.S. Metabolic syndrome risk for cardiovascular disease and diabetes in the ARIC study. *Int. J. Obes. (Lond.)* **2008**, *32* (Suppl. S2), S21–S24. [CrossRef] [PubMed]
2. Alberti, K.G.; Eckel, R.H.; Grundy, S.M.; Zimmet, P.Z.; Cleeman, J.I.; Donato, K.A.; Fruchart, J.C.; James, W.P.; Loria, C.M.; Smith, S.C., Jr. Harmonizing the metabolic syndrome: A joint interim statement of the International Diabetes Federation Task Force on Epidemiology and Prevention; National Heart, Lung, and Blood Institute; American Heart Association; World Heart Federation; International Atherosclerosis Society; and International Association for the Study of Obesity. *Circulation* **2009**, *120*, 1640–1645. [CrossRef] [PubMed]
3. Nolan, P.B.; Carrick-Ranson, G.; Stinear, J.W.; Reading, S.A.; Dalleck, L.C. Prevalence of metabolic syndrome and metabolic syndrome components in young adults: A pooled analysis. *Prev. Med. Rep.* **2017**, *7*, 211–215. [CrossRef] [PubMed]
4. Saklayen, M.G. The Global Epidemic of the Metabolic Syndrome. *Curr. Hypertens. Rep.* **2018**, *20*, 12. [CrossRef]
5. O'Neill, S.; O'Driscoll, L. Metabolic syndrome: A closer look at the growing epidemic and its associated pathologies. *Obes. Rev.* **2015**, *16*, 1–12. [CrossRef]
6. Moore, J.X.; Chaudhary, N.; Akinyemiju, T. Metabolic Syndrome Prevalence by Race/Ethnicity and Sex in the United States, National Health and Nutrition Examination Survey, 1988–2012. *Prev. Chronic Dis.* **2017**, *14*, E24. [CrossRef]
7. Lan, Y.; Mai, Z.; Zhou, S.; Liu, Y.; Li, S.; Zhao, Z.; Duan, X.; Cai, C.; Deng, T.; Zhu, W.; et al. Prevalence of metabolic syndrome in China: An up-dated cross-sectional study. *PLoS ONE* **2018**, *13*, e0196012. [CrossRef]
8. Aguilar, M.; Bhuket, T.; Torres, S.; Liu, B.; Wong, R.J. Prevalence of the metabolic syndrome in the United States, 2003–2012. *JAMA* **2015**, *313*, 1973–1974. [CrossRef]
9. Anand, S.S.; Yi, Q.; Gerstein, H.; Lonn, E.; Jacobs, R.; Vuksan, V.; Teo, K.; Davis, B.; Montague, P.; Yusuf, S. Relationship of metabolic syndrome and fibrinolytic dysfunction to cardiovascular disease. *Circulation* **2003**, *108*, 420–425. [CrossRef]
10. Tan, C.E.; Ma, S.; Wai, D.; Chew, S.K.; Tai, E.S. Can we apply the National Cholesterol Education Program Adult Treatment Panel definition of the metabolic syndrome to Asians? *Diabetes Care* **2004**, *27*, 1182–1186. [CrossRef]
11. Lear, S.A.; Chen, M.M.; Birmingham, C.L.; Frohlich, J.J. The relationship between simple anthropometric indices and c-reactive protein: Ethnic and gender differences. *Metabolism* **2003**, *52*, 1542–1546. [CrossRef] [PubMed]
12. Lear, S.A.; Chen, M.M.; Frohlich, J.J.; Birmingham, C.L. The relationship between waist circumference and metabolic risk factors: Cohorts of European and Chinese descent. *Metabolism* **2002**, *51*, 1427–1432. [CrossRef] [PubMed]
13. Lear, S.A.; Toma, M.; Birmingham, C.L.; Frohlich, J.J. Modification of the relationship between simple anthropometric indices and risk factors by ethnic background. *Metabolism* **2003**, *52*, 1295–1301. [CrossRef]
14. Lear, S.A.; Humphries, K.H.; Kohli, S.; Chockalingam, A.; Frohlich, J.J.; Birmingham, C.L. Visceral adipose tissue accumulation differs according to ethnic background: Results of the Multicultural Community Health Assessment Trial (M-CHAT). *Am. J. Clin. Nutr.* **2007**, *86*, 353–359. [CrossRef] [PubMed]
15. Lear, S.A.; Chockalingam, A.; Kohli, S.; Richardson, C.G.; Humphries, K.H. Elevation in cardiovascular disease risk in South Asians is mediated by differences in visceral adipose tissue. *Obesity (Silver Spring)* **2012**, *20*, 1293–1300. [CrossRef] [PubMed]
16. Hoffman, D.J.; Wang, Z.; Gallagher, D.; Heymsfield, S.B. Comparison of visceral adipose tissue mass in adult African Americans and whites. *Obes. Res.* **2005**, *13*, 66–74. [CrossRef]
17. Katzmarzyk, P.T. Obesity and physical activity among Aboriginal Canadians. *Obesity (Silver Spring)* **2008**, *16*, 184–190. [CrossRef]
18. Turin, T.C.; Saad, N.; Jun, M.; Tonelli, M.; Ma, Z.; Barnabe, C.C.M.; Manns, B.; Hemmelgarn, B. Lifetime risk of diabetes among First Nations and non-First Nations people. *CMAJ* **2016**, *188*, 1147–1153. [CrossRef]
19. Gautier, J.F.; Milner, M.R.; Elam, E.; Chen, K.; Ravussin, E.; Pratley, R.E. Visceral adipose tissue is not increased in Pima Indians compared with equally obese Caucasians and is not related to insulin action or secretion. *Diabetologia* **1999**, *42*, 28–34. [CrossRef]

20. Gasevic, D.; Kohli, S.; Khan, N.; Lear, S.A. Abdominal Adipose Tissue and Insulin Resistance: The Role of Ethnicity. In *Nutrition in the Prevention and Treatment of Abdominal Obesity*; Academic Press; Elsevier, Inc.: Waltham, MA, USA, 2014; pp. 125–140.
21. Lear, S.A.; James, P.T.; Ko, G.T.; Kumanyika, S. Appropriateness of waist circumference and waist-to-hip ratio cutoffs for different ethnic groups. *Eur. J. Clin. Nutr.* **2010**, *64*, 42–61. [CrossRef]
22. Kaneshiro, B.; Geling, O.; Gellert, K.; Millar, L. The challenges of collecting data on race and ethnicity in a diverse, multiethnic state. *Hawaii Med. J.* **2011**, *70*, 168–171. [PubMed]
23. Aspinall, P.J. Concepts, terminology and classifications for the "mixed" ethnic or racial group in the United Kingdom. *J. Epidemiol. Community Health* **2010**, *64*, 557–560. [CrossRef] [PubMed]
24. Knowler, W.C.; Barrett-Connor, E.; Fowler, S.E.; Hamman, R.F.; Lachin, J.M.; Walker, E.A.; Nathan, D.M. Reduction in the incidence of type 2 diabetes with lifestyle intervention or metformin. *N. Engl. J. Med.* **2002**, *346*, 393–403. [CrossRef] [PubMed]
25. Orchard, T.J.; Temprosa, M.; Goldberg, R.; Haffner, S.; Ratner, R.; Marcovina, S.; Fowler, S. The effect of metformin and intensive lifestyle intervention on the metabolic syndrome: The Diabetes Prevention Program randomized trial. *Ann. Intern. Med.* **2005**, *142*, 611–619. [CrossRef]
26. Yamaoka, K.; Tango, T. Effects of lifestyle modification on metabolic syndrome: A systematic review and meta-analysis. *BMC Med.* **2012**, *10*, 138. [CrossRef]
27. Church, T.S.; Earnest, C.P.; Skinner, J.S.; Blair, S.N. Effects of different doses of physical activity on cardiorespiratory fitness among sedentary, overweight or obese postmenopausal women with elevated blood pressure: A randomized controlled trial. *JAMA* **2007**, *297*, 2081–2091. [CrossRef]
28. Earnest, C.P.; Johannsen, N.M.; Swift, D.L.; Lavie, C.J.; Blair, S.N.; Church, T.S. Dose effect of cardiorespiratory exercise on metabolic syndrome in postmenopausal women. *Am. J. Cardiol.* **2013**, *111*, 1805–1811. [CrossRef]
29. Haufe, S.; Kerling, A.; Protte, G.; Bayerle, P.; Stenner, H.T.; Rolff, S.; Sundermeier, T.; Kuck, M.; Ensslen, R.; Nachbar, L.; et al. Telemonitoring-supported exercise training, metabolic syndrome severity, and work ability in company employees: A randomised controlled trial. *Lancet Public Health* **2019**, *4*, e343–e352. [CrossRef]
30. Tomeleri, C.M.; Souza, M.F.; Burini, R.C.; Cavaglieri, C.R.; Ribeiro, A.S.; Antunes, M.; Nunes, J.P.; Venturini, D.; Barbosa, D.S.; Sardinha, L.B.; et al. Resistance training reduces metabolic syndrome and inflammatory markers in older women: A randomized controlled trial. *J. Diabetes* **2018**, *10*, 328–337. [CrossRef]
31. Earnest, C.P.; Johannsen, N.M.; Swift, D.L.; Gillison, F.B.; Mikus, C.R.; Lucia, A.; Kramer, K.; Lavie, C.J.; Church, T.S. Aerobic and strength training in concomitant metabolic syndrome and type 2 diabetes. *Med. Sci. Sports Exerc.* **2014**, *46*, 1293–1301. [CrossRef]
32. Tjonna, A.E.; Ramos, J.S.; Pressler, A.; Halle, M.; Jungbluth, K.; Ermacora, E.; Salvesen, O.; Rodrigues, J.; Bueno, C.R., Jr.; Munk, P.S.; et al. EX-MET study: Exercise in prevention on of metabolic syndrome—A randomized multicenter trial: Rational and design. *BMC Public Health* **2018**, *18*, 437. [CrossRef] [PubMed]
33. Babio, N.; Toledo, E.; Estruch, R.; Ros, E.; Martinez-Gonzalez, M.A.; Castaner, O.; Bullo, M.; Corella, D.; Aros, F.; Gomez-Gracia, E.; et al. Mediterranean diets and metabolic syndrome status in the PREDIMED randomized trial. *CMAJ* **2014**, *186*, E649–E657. [CrossRef] [PubMed]
34. Agarwal, A.; Ioannidis, J.P.A. PREDIMED trial of Mediterranean diet: Retracted, republished, still trusted? *BMJ* **2019**, *364*, l341. [CrossRef] [PubMed]
35. Estruch, R.; Ros, E.; Salas-Salvado, J.; Covas, M.I.; Corella, D.; Aros, F.; Gomez-Gracia, E.; Ruiz-Gutierrez, V.; Fiol, M.; Lapetra, J.; et al. Retraction and Republication: Primary Prevention of Cardiovascular Disease with a Mediterranean Diet. *N. Engl. J. Med.* **2018**, *378*, 2441–2442. [CrossRef] [PubMed]
36. Ehteshami, M.; Shakerhosseini, R.; Sedaghat, F.; Hedayati, M.; Eini-Zinab, H.; Hekmatdoost, A. The Effect of Gluten Free Diet on Components of Metabolic Syndrome: A Randomized Clinical Trial. *Asian Pac. J. Cancer Prev. APJCP* **2018**, *19*, 2979–2984. [CrossRef] [PubMed]
37. Gupta Jain, S.; Puri, S.; Misra, A.; Gulati, S.; Mani, K. Effect of oral cinnamon intervention on metabolic profile and body composition of Asian Indians with metabolic syndrome: A randomized double -blind control trial. *Lipids Health Dis.* **2017**, *16*, 113. [CrossRef]
38. Wu, H.; Pan, A.; Yu, Z.; Qi, Q.; Lu, L.; Zhang, G.; Yu, D.; Zong, G.; Zhou, Y.; Chen, X.; et al. Lifestyle counseling and supplementation with flaxseed or walnuts influence the management of metabolic syndrome. *J. Nutr.* **2010**, *140*, 1937–1942. [CrossRef]

39. Alfawaz, H.A.; Wani, K.; Alnaami, A.M.; Al-Saleh, Y.; Aljohani, N.J.; Al-Attas, O.S.; Alokail, M.S.; Kumar, S.; Al-Daghri, N.M. Effects of Different Dietary and Lifestyle Modification Therapies on Metabolic Syndrome in Prediabetic Arab Patients: A 12-Month Longitudinal Study. *Nutrients* **2018**, *10*, 383. [CrossRef]
40. Dunkley, A.J.; Davies, M.J.; Stone, M.A.; Taub, N.A.; Troughton, J.; Yates, T.; Khunti, K. The Reversal Intervention for Metabolic Syndrome (TRIMS) study: Rationale, design, and baseline data. *Trials* **2011**, *12*, 107. [CrossRef]
41. Dash, C.; Makambi, K.; Wallington, S.F.; Sheppard, V.; Taylor, T.R.; Hicks, J.S.; Adams-Campbell, L.L. An exercise trial targeting African-American women with metabolic syndrome and at high risk for breast cancer: Rationale, design, and methods. *Contemp. Clin. Trials* **2015**, *43*, 33–38. [CrossRef]
42. Nanri, A.; Tomita, K.; Matsushita, Y.; Ichikawa, F.; Yamamoto, M.; Nagafuchi, Y.; Kakumoto, Y.; Mizoue, T. Effect of six months lifestyle intervention in Japanese men with metabolic syndrome: Randomized controlled trial. *J. Occup. Health* **2012**, *54*, 215–222. [CrossRef] [PubMed]
43. Agurs-Collins, T.D.; Kumanyika, S.K.; Ten Have, T.R.; Adams-Campbell, L.L. A randomized controlled trial of weight reduction and exercise for diabetes management in older African-American subjects. *Diabetes Care* **1997**, *20*, 1503–1511. [CrossRef] [PubMed]
44. Ard, J.D.; Carson, T.L.; Shikany, J.M.; Li, Y.; Hardy, C.M.; Robinson, J.C.; Williams, A.G.; Baskin, M.L. Weight loss and improved metabolic outcomes amongst rural African American women in the Deep South: Six-month outcomes from a community-based randomized trial. *J. Intern. Med.* **2017**, *282*, 102–113. [CrossRef] [PubMed]
45. Li, G.; Zhang, P.; Wang, J.; An, Y.; Gong, Q.; Gregg, E.W.; Yang, W.; Zhang, B.; Shuai, Y.; Hong, J.; et al. Cardiovascular mortality, all-cause mortality, and diabetes incidence after lifestyle intervention for people with impaired glucose tolerance in the Da Qing Diabetes Prevention Study: A 23-year follow-up study. *Lancet Diabetes Endocrinol.* **2014**, *2*, 474–480. [CrossRef]
46. O'Brien, M.J.; Perez, A.; Scanlan, A.B.; Alos, V.A.; Whitaker, R.C.; Foster, G.D.; Ackermann, R.T.; Ciolino, J.D.; Homko, C. PREVENT-DM Comparative Effectiveness Trial of Lifestyle Intervention and Metformin. *Am. J. Prev. Med.* **2017**, *52*, 788–797. [CrossRef]
47. Saboya, P.P.; Bodanese, L.C.; Zimmermann, P.R.; Gustavo, A.D.; Macagnan, F.E.; Feoli, A.P.; Oliveira, M.D. Lifestyle Intervention on Metabolic Syndrome and its Impact on Quality of Life: A Randomized Controlled Trial. *Arq. Bras. Cardiol.* **2017**, *108*, 60–69. [CrossRef]
48. Jiang, L.; Manson, S.M.; Beals, J.; Henderson, W.G.; Huang, H.; Acton, K.J.; Roubideaux, Y. Translating the Diabetes Prevention Program into American Indian and Alaska Native communities: Results from the Special Diabetes Program for Indians Diabetes Prevention demonstration project. *Diabetes Care* **2013**, *36*, 2027–2034. [CrossRef]
49. Zilberman-Kravits, D.; Meyerstein, N.; Abu-Rabia, Y.; Wiznitzer, A.; Harman-Boehm, I. The Impact of a Cultural Lifestyle Intervention on Metabolic Parameters After Gestational Diabetes Mellitus A Randomized Controlled Trial. *Matern. Child Health J.* **2018**, *22*, 803–811. [CrossRef]
50. Bhopal, R.S.; Douglas, A.; Wallia, S.; Forbes, J.F.; Lean, M.E.; Gill, J.M.; McKnight, J.A.; Sattar, N.; Sheikh, A.; Wild, S.H.; et al. Effect of a lifestyle intervention on weight change in south Asian individuals in the UK at high risk of type 2 diabetes: A family-cluster randomised controlled trial. *Lancet Diabetes Endocrinol.* **2014**, *2*, 218–227. [CrossRef]
51. Bajerska, J.; Chmurzynska, A.; Muzsik, A.; Krzyzanowska, P.; Madry, E.; Malinowska, A.M.; Walkowiak, J. Weight loss and metabolic health effects from energy-restricted Mediterranean and Central-European diets in postmenopausal women: A randomized controlled trial. *Sci. Rep.* **2018**, *8*, 11170. [CrossRef]
52. Harvie, M.N.; Pegington, M.; Mattson, M.P.; Frystyk, J.; Dillon, B.; Evans, G.; Cuzick, J.; Jebb, S.A.; Martin, B.; Cutler, R.G.; et al. The effects of intermittent or continuous energy restriction on weight loss and metabolic disease risk markers: A randomized trial in young overweight women. *Int. J. Obes. (Lond.)* **2011**, *35*, 714–727. [CrossRef] [PubMed]
53. Sundfor, T.M.; Svendsen, M.; Tonstad, S. Effect of intermittent versus continuous energy restriction on weight loss, maintenance and cardiometabolic risk: A randomized 1-year trial. *Nutr. Metab. Cardiovasc. Dis.* **2018**, *28*, 698–706. [CrossRef] [PubMed]
54. Volek, J.S.; Phinney, S.D.; Forsythe, C.E.; Quann, E.E.; Wood, R.J.; Puglisi, M.J.; Kraemer, W.J.; Bibus, D.M.; Fernandez, M.L.; Feinman, R.D. Carbohydrate restriction has a more favorable impact on the metabolic syndrome than a low fat diet. *Lipids* **2009**, *44*, 297–309. [CrossRef] [PubMed]

55. Hyde, P.N.; Sapper, T.N.; Crabtree, C.D.; LaFountain, R.A.; Bowling, M.L.; Buga, A.; Fell, B.; McSwiney, F.T.; Dickerson, R.M.; Miller, V.J.; et al. Dietary carbohydrate restriction improves metabolic syndrome independent of weight loss. *JCI Insight* **2019**, *4*. [CrossRef]
56. Hu, T.; Mills, K.T.; Yao, L.; Demanelis, K.; Eloustaz, M.; Yancy, W.S., Jr.; Kelly, T.N.; He, J.; Bazzano, L.A. Effects of low-carbohydrate diets versus low-fat diets on metabolic risk factors: A meta-analysis of randomized controlled clinical trials. *Am. J. Epidemiol.* **2012**, *176* (Suppl. S7), S44–S54. [CrossRef]
57. Svetkey, L.P.; Erlinger, T.P.; Vollmer, W.M.; Feldstein, A.; Cooper, L.S.; Appel, L.J.; Ard, J.D.; Elmer, P.J.; Harsha, D.; Stevens, V.J. Effect of lifestyle modifications on blood pressure by race, sex, hypertension status, and age. *J. Hum. Hypertens.* **2005**, *19*, 21–31. [CrossRef]
58. Svetkey, L.P.; Simons-Morton, D.; Vollmer, W.M.; Appel, L.J.; Conlin, P.R.; Ryan, D.H.; Ard, J.; Kennedy, B.M. Effects of dietary patterns on blood pressure: Subgroup analysis of the Dietary Approaches to Stop Hypertension (DASH) randomized clinical trial. *Arch. Intern. Med.* **1999**, *159*, 285–293. [CrossRef]
59. Schroeder, N.; Park, Y.H.; Kang, M.S.; Kim, Y.; Ha, G.K.; Kim, H.R.; Yates, A.A.; Caballero, B. A randomized trial on the effects of 2010 Dietary Guidelines for Americans and Korean diet patterns on cardiovascular risk factors in overweight and obese adults. *J. Acad. Nutr. Diet.* **2015**, *115*, 1083–1092. [CrossRef]
60. Zhao, X.; Yin, X.; Li, X.; Yan, L.L.; Lam, C.T.; Li, S.; He, F.; Xie, W.; Sang, B.; Luobu, G.; et al. Using a low-sodium, high-potassium salt substitute to reduce blood pressure among Tibetans with high blood pressure: A patient-blinded randomized controlled trial. *PLoS ONE* **2014**, *9*, e110131. [CrossRef]
61. Gulati, S.; Misra, A.; Pandey, R.M.; Bhatt, S.P.; Saluja, S. Effects of pistachio nuts on body composition, metabolic, inflammatory and oxidative stress parameters in Asian Indians with metabolic syndrome: A 24-wk, randomized control trial. *Nutrition* **2014**, *30*, 192–197. [CrossRef]
62. Mohan, V.; Gayathri, R.; Jaacks, L.M.; Lakshmipriya, N.; Anjana, R.M.; Spiegelman, D.; Jeevan, R.G.; Balasubramaniam, K.K.; Shobana, S.; Jayanthan, M.; et al. Cashew Nut Consumption Increases HDL Cholesterol and Reduces Systolic Blood Pressure in Asian Indians with Type 2 Diabetes: A 12-Week Randomized Controlled Trial. *J. Nutr.* **2018**, *148*, 63–69. [CrossRef] [PubMed]
63. Al-Shookri, A.; Khor, G.L.; Chan, Y.M.; Loke, S.C.; Al-Maskari, M. Effectiveness of medical nutrition treatment delivered by dietitians on glycaemic outcomes and lipid profiles of Arab, Omani patients with Type 2 diabetes. *Diabet Med.* **2012**, *29*, 236–244. [CrossRef] [PubMed]
64. Ziemer, D.C.; Berkowitz, K.J.; Panayioto, R.M.; El-Kebbi, I.M.; Musey, V.C.; Anderson, L.A.; Wanko, N.S.; Fowke, M.L.; Brazier, C.W.; Dunbar, V.G.; et al. A simple meal plan emphasizing healthy food choices is as effective as an exchange-based meal plan for urban African Americans with type 2 diabetes. *Diabetes Care* **2003**, *26*, 1719–1724. [CrossRef] [PubMed]
65. Mitra, S.R.; Tan, P.Y. Effect of an individualised high-protein, energy-restricted diet on anthropometric and cardio-metabolic parameters in overweight and obese Malaysian adults: A 6-month randomised controlled study. *Br. J. Nutr.* **2019**, *121*, 1002–1017. [CrossRef]
66. Gulati, S.; Misra, A.; Tiwari, R.; Sharma, M.; Pandey, R.M.; Yadav, C.P. Effect of high-protein meal replacement on weight and cardiometabolic profile in overweight/obese Asian Indians in North India. *Br. J. Nutr.* **2017**, *117*, 1531–1540. [CrossRef]
67. Chen, W.; Liu, Y.; Yang, Q.; Li, X.; Yang, J.; Wang, J.; Shi, L.; Chen, Y.; Zhu, S. The Effect of Protein-Enriched Meal Replacement on Waist Circumference Reduction among Overweight and Obese Chinese with Hyperlipidemia. *J. Am. Coll. Nutr.* **2016**, *35*, 236–244. [CrossRef]
68. Liu, X.; Zhang, G.; Ye, X.; Li, H.; Chen, X.; Tang, L.; Feng, Y.; Shai, I.; Stampfer, M.J.; Hu, F.B.; et al. Effects of a low-carbohydrate diet on weight loss and cardiometabolic profile in Chinese women: A randomised controlled feeding trial. *Br. J. Nutr.* **2013**, *110*, 1444–1453. [CrossRef]
69. Zhang, J.; Li, L.; Song, P.; Wang, C.; Man, Q.; Meng, L.; Cai, J.; Kurilich, A. Randomized controlled trial of oatmeal consumption versus noodle consumption on blood lipids of urban Chinese adults with hypercholesterolemia. *Nutr. J.* **2012**, *11*, 54. [CrossRef]
70. Patade, A.; Devareddy, L.; Lucas, E.A.; Korlagunta, K.; Daggy, B.P.; Arjmandi, B.H. Flaxseed reduces total and LDL cholesterol concentrations in Native American postmenopausal women. *J. Womens Health (2002)* **2008**, *17*, 355–366. [CrossRef]
71. Brooking, L.A.; Williams, S.M.; Mann, J.I. Effects of macronutrient composition of the diet on body fat in indigenous people at high risk of type 2 diabetes. *Diabetes Res. Clin. Pract.* **2012**, *96*, 40–46. [CrossRef]

72. Andersen, E.; Hostmark, A.T.; Anderssen, S.A. Effect of a physical activity intervention on the metabolic syndrome in Pakistani immigrant men: A randomized controlled trial. *J. Immigr. Minor. Health* **2012**, *14*, 738–746. [CrossRef] [PubMed]
73. Lesser, I.A.; Singer, J.; Hoogbruin, A.; Mackey, D.C.; Katzmarzyk, P.T.; Sohal, P.; Leipsic, J.; Lear, S.A. Effectiveness of Exercise on Visceral Adipose Tissue in Older South Asian Women. *Med. Sci. Sports Exerc.* **2016**, *48*, 1371–1378. [CrossRef] [PubMed]
74. Martin, C.A.; Gowda, U.; Smith, B.J.; Renzaho, A.M.N. Systematic Review of the Effect of Lifestyle Interventions on the Components of the Metabolic Syndrome in South Asian Migrants. *J. Immigr. Minor. Health* **2018**, *20*, 231–244. [CrossRef] [PubMed]
75. Igarashi, Y.; Akazawa, N.; Maeda, S. Regular aerobic exercise and blood pressure in East Asians: A meta-analysis of randomized controlled trials. *Clin. Exp. Hypertens. (NY 1993)* **2018**, *40*, 378–389. [CrossRef]
76. Matsuo, T.; So, R.; Shimojo, N.; Tanaka, K. Effect of aerobic exercise training followed by a low-calorie diet on metabolic syndrome risk factors in men. *Nutr. Metab. Cardiovasc. Dis.* **2015**, *25*, 832–838. [CrossRef]
77. Choi, Y.S.; Song, R.; Ku, B.J. Effects of a T'ai Chi-Based Health Promotion Program on Metabolic Syndrome Markers, Health Behaviors, and Quality of Life in Middle-Aged Male Office Workers: A Randomized Trial. *J. Altern. Complement. Med.* **2017**, *23*, 949–956. [CrossRef]
78. Adams-Campbell, L.L.; Dash, C.; Kim, B.H.; Hicks, J.; Makambi, K.; Hagberg, J. Cardiorespiratory Fitness and Metabolic Syndrome in Postmenopausal African-American Women. *Int. J. Sports Med.* **2016**, *37*, 261–266. [CrossRef]
79. Vella, C.A.; Zubia, R.Y.; Ontiveros, D.; Cruz, M.L. Physical activity, cardiorespiratory fitness, and metabolic syndrome in young Mexican and Mexican-American women. *Appl. Physiol. Nutr. Metab.* **2009**, *34*, 10–17. [CrossRef]
80. Liu, J.; Young, T.K.; Zinman, B.; Harris, S.B.; Connelly, P.W.; Hanley, A.J. Lifestyle variables, non-traditional cardiovascular risk factors, and the metabolic syndrome in an Aboriginal Canadian population. *Obesity (Silver Spring)* **2006**, *14*, 500–508. [CrossRef]
81. Biswas, A.; Oh, P.I.; Faulkner, G.E.; Bajaj, R.R.; Silver, M.A.; Mitchell, M.S.; Alter, D.A. Sedentary time and its association with risk for disease incidence, mortality, and hospitalization in adults: A systematic review and meta-analysis. *Ann. Intern. Med.* **2015**, *162*, 123–132. [CrossRef]
82. Bankoski, A.; Harris, T.B.; McClain, J.J.; Brychta, R.J.; Caserotti, P.; Chen, K.Y.; Berrigan, D.; Troiano, R.P.; Koster, A. Sedentary activity associated with metabolic syndrome independent of physical activity. *Diabetes Care* **2011**, *34*, 497–503. [CrossRef] [PubMed]
83. Lemes, I.R.; Sui, X.; Fernandes, R.A.; Blair, S.N.; Turi-Lynch, B.C.; Codogno, J.S.; Monteiro, H.L. Association of sedentary behavior and metabolic syndrome. *Public Health* **2019**, *167*, 96–102. [CrossRef] [PubMed]
84. Nam, J.Y.; Kim, J.; Cho, K.H.; Choi, Y.; Choi, J.; Shin, J.; Park, E.C. Associations of sitting time and occupation with metabolic syndrome in South Korean adults: A cross-sectional study. *BMC Public Health* **2016**, *16*, 943. [CrossRef] [PubMed]
85. Compernolle, S.; DeSmet, A.; Poppe, L.; Crombez, G.; De Bourdeaudhuij, I.; Cardon, G.; van der Ploeg, H.P.; Van Dyck, D. Effectiveness of interventions using self-monitoring to reduce sedentary behavior in adults: A systematic review and meta-analysis. *Int. J. Behav. Nutr. Phys. Act.* **2019**, *16*, 63. [CrossRef]
86. Balducci, S.; D'Errico, V.; Haxhi, J.; Sacchetti, M.; Orlando, G.; Cardelli, P.; Vitale, M.; Bollanti, L.; Conti, F.; Zanuso, S.; et al. Effect of a Behavioral Intervention Strategy on Sustained Change in Physical Activity and Sedentary Behavior in Patients With Type 2 Diabetes: The IDES_2 Randomized Clinical Trial. *JAMA* **2019**, *321*, 880–890. [CrossRef]
87. Pandit, K.; Goswami, S.; Ghosh, S.; Mukhopadhyay, P.; Chowdhury, S. Metabolic syndrome in South Asians. *Indian J. Endocrinol. Metab.* **2012**, *16*, 44–55. [CrossRef]
88. Malik, V.S.; Popkin, B.M.; Bray, G.A.; Despres, J.P.; Willett, W.C.; Hu, F.B. Sugar-sweetened beverages and risk of metabolic syndrome and type 2 diabetes: A meta-analysis. *Diabetes Care* **2010**, *33*, 2477–2483. [CrossRef]
89. Seo, E.H.; Kim, H.; Kwon, O. Association between Total Sugar Intake and Metabolic Syndrome in Middle-Aged Korean Men and Women. *Nutrients* **2019**, *11*, 2042. [CrossRef]
90. Colchero, M.A.; Rivera-Dommarco, J.; Popkin, B.M.; Ng, S.W. In Mexico, Evidence Of Sustained Consumer Response Two Years After Implementing A Sugar-Sweetened Beverage Tax. *Health Aff. (Proj. Hope)* **2017**, *36*, 564–571. [CrossRef]

91. Lee, M.M.; Falbe, J.; Schillinger, D.; Basu, S.; McCulloch, C.E.; Madsen, K.A. Sugar-Sweetened Beverage Consumption 3 Years After the Berkeley, California, Sugar-Sweetened Beverage Tax. *Am. J. Public Health* **2019**, *109*, 637–639. [CrossRef]
92. Nakamura, R.; Mirelman, A.J.; Cuadrado, C.; Silva-Illanes, N.; Dunstan, J.; Suhrcke, M. Evaluating the 2014 sugar-sweetened beverage tax in Chile: An observational study in urban areas. *PLoS Med.* **2018**, *15*, e1002596. [CrossRef] [PubMed]
93. Papas, M.A.; Alberg, A.J.; Ewing, R.; Helzlsouer, K.J.; Gary, T.L.; Klassen, A.C. The built environment and obesity. *Epidemiol. Rev.* **2007**, *29*, 129–143. [CrossRef] [PubMed]
94. Booth, G.L.; Creatore, M.I.; Luo, J.; Fazli, G.S.; Johns, A.; Rosella, L.C.; Glazier, R.H.; Moineddin, R.; Gozdyra, P.; Austin, P.C. Neighbourhood walkability and the incidence of diabetes: An inverse probability of treatment weighting analysis. *J. Epidemiol. Community Health* **2019**, *73*, 287–294. [CrossRef]
95. Li, F.; Harmer, P.; Cardinal, B.J.; Bosworth, M.; Johnson-Shelton, D. Obesity and the built environment: Does the density of neighborhood fast-food outlets matter? *Am. J. Health Promot.* **2009**, *23*, 203–209. [CrossRef] [PubMed]
96. Malambo, P.; Kengne, A.P.; De Villiers, A.; Lambert, E.V.; Puoane, T. Built Environment, Selected Risk Factors and Major Cardiovascular Disease Outcomes: A Systematic Review. *PLoS ONE* **2016**, *11*, e0166846. [CrossRef] [PubMed]
97. Hirsch, J.A.; Moore, K.A.; Clarke, P.J.; Rodriguez, D.A.; Evenson, K.R.; Brines, S.J.; Zagorski, M.A.; Diez Roux, A.V. Changes in the built environment and changes in the amount of walking over time: Longitudinal results from the multi-ethnic study of atherosclerosis. *Am. J. Epidemiol.* **2014**, *180*, 799–809. [CrossRef]
98. Sun, G.; Oreskovic, N.M.; Lin, H. How do changes to the built environment influence walking behaviors? A longitudinal study within a university campus in Hong Kong. *Int. J. Health Geogr.* **2014**, *13*, 28. [CrossRef]
99. Morland, K.; Wing, S.; Diez Roux, A. The contextual effect of the local food environment on residents' diets: The atherosclerosis risk in communities study. *Am. J. Public Health* **2002**, *92*, 1761–1767. [CrossRef]
100. Mackenbach, J.D.; Burgoine, T.; Lakerveld, J.; Forouhi, N.G.; Griffin, S.J.; Wareham, N.J.; Monsivais, P. Accessibility and Affordability of Supermarkets: Associations With the DASH Diet. *Am. J. Prev. Med.* **2017**, *53*, 55–62. [CrossRef]
101. Jiao, J.; Moudon, A.V.; Kim, S.Y.; Hurvitz, P.M.; Drewnowski, A. Health Implications of Adults' Eating at and Living near Fast Food or Quick Service Restaurants. *Nutr. Diabetes* **2015**, *5*, e171. [CrossRef]
102. Inagami, S.; Cohen, D.A.; Brown, A.F.; Asch, S.M. Body mass index, neighborhood fast food and restaurant concentration, and car ownership. *J. Urban Health* **2009**, *86*, 683–695. [CrossRef] [PubMed]
103. Drewnowski, A.; Aggarwal, A.; Hurvitz, P.M.; Monsivais, P.; Moudon, A.V. Obesity and supermarket access: Proximity or price? *Am. J. Public Health* **2012**, *102*, e74–e80. [CrossRef] [PubMed]
104. Mazidi, M.; Speakman, J.R. Higher densities of fast-food and full-service restaurants are not associated with obesity prevalence. *Am. J. Clin. Nutr.* **2017**, *106*, 603–613. [CrossRef] [PubMed]
105. Burgoine, T.; Forouhi, N.G.; Griffin, S.J.; Brage, S.; Wareham, N.J.; Monsivais, P. Does neighborhood fast-food outlet exposure amplify inequalities in diet and obesity? A cross-sectional study. *Am. J. Clin. Nutr.* **2016**, *103*, 1540–1547. [CrossRef] [PubMed]
106. Dubowitz, T.; Ghosh-Dastidar, M.; Cohen, D.A.; Beckman, R.; Steiner, E.D.; Hunter, G.P.; Florez, K.R.; Huang, C.; Vaughan, C.A.; Sloan, J.C.; et al. Diet And Perceptions Change With Supermarket Introduction In A Food Desert, But Not Because Of Supermarket Use. *Health Aff. (Proj. Hope)* **2015**, *34*, 1858–1868. [CrossRef]
107. Karlamangla, A.S.; Merkin, S.S.; Crimmins, E.M.; Seeman, T.E. Socioeconomic and ethnic disparities in cardiovascular risk in the United States, 2001–2006. *Ann. Epidemiol.* **2010**, *20*, 617–628. [CrossRef]
108. Zhan, Y.; Yu, J.; Chen, R.; Gao, J.; Ding, R.; Fu, Y.; Zhang, L.; Hu, D. Socioeconomic status and metabolic syndrome in the general population of China: A cross-sectional study. *BMC Public Health* **2012**, *12*, 921. [CrossRef]
109. Block, J.P.; Scribner, R.A.; DeSalvo, K.B. Fast food, race/ethnicity, and income: A geographic analysis. *Am. J. Prev. Med.* **2004**, *27*, 211–217.
110. Burgoine, T.; Sarkar, C.; Webster, C.J.; Monsivais, P. Examining the interaction of fast-food outlet exposure and income on diet and obesity: Evidence from 51,361 UK Biobank participants. *Int. J. Behav. Nutr. Phys. Act.* **2018**, *15*, 71. [CrossRef]
111. Palafox, B.; McKee, M.; Balabanova, D.; AlHabib, K.F.; Avezum, A.J.; Bahonar, A.; Ismail, N.; Chifamba, J.; Chow, C.K.; Corsi, D.J.; et al. Wealth and cardiovascular health: A cross-sectional study of wealth-related

112. Victor, R.G.; Lynch, K.; Li, N.; Blyler, C.; Muhammad, E.; Handler, J.; Brettler, J.; Rashid, M.; Hsu, B.; Foxx-Drew, D.; et al. A Cluster-Randomized Trial of Blood-Pressure Reduction in Black Barbershops. *N. Engl. J. Med.* **2018**, *378*, 1291–1301. [CrossRef] [PubMed]
113. Carter-Edwards, L.; Lindquist, R.; Redmond, N.; Turner, C.M.; Harding, C.; Oliver, J.; West, L.B.; Ravenell, J.; Shikany, J.M. Designing Faith-Based Blood Pressure Interventions to Reach Young Black Men. *Am. J. Prev. Med.* **2018**, *55*, S49–S58. [CrossRef] [PubMed]
114. Smith, M.L.; Wilson, M.G.; Robertson, M.M.; Padilla, H.M.; Zuercher, H.; Vandenberg, R.; Corso, P.; Lorig, K.; Laurent, D.D.; DeJoy, D.M. Impact of a Translated Disease Self-Management Program on Employee Health and Productivity: Six-Month Findings from a Randomized Controlled Trial. *Int. J. Environ. Res. Public Health* **2018**, *15*, 851. [CrossRef] [PubMed]
115. Shrivastava, U.; Fatma, M.; Mohan, S.; Singh, P.; Misra, A. Randomized Control Trial for Reduction of Body Weight, Body Fat Patterning, and Cardiometabolic Risk Factors in Overweight Worksite Employees in Delhi, India. *J. Diabetes Res.* **2017**, *2017*, 7254174. [CrossRef]
116. Parra-Medina, D.; Wilcox, S.; Salinas, J.; Addy, C.; Fore, E.; Poston, M.; Wilson, D.K. Results of the Heart Healthy and Ethnically Relevant Lifestyle trial: A cardiovascular risk reduction intervention for African American women attending community health centers. *Am. J. Public Health* **2011**, *101*, 1914–1921. [CrossRef]
117. McCurley, J.L.; Gutierrez, A.P.; Gallo, L.C. Diabetes Prevention in U.S. Hispanic Adults: A Systematic Review of Culturally Tailored Interventions. *Am. J. Prev. Med.* **2017**, *52*, 519–529. [CrossRef]
118. Vincent, D.; McEwen, M.M.; Hepworth, J.T.; Stump, C.S. The effects of a community-based, culturally tailored diabetes prevention intervention for high-risk adults of Mexican descent. *Diabetes Educ.* **2014**, *40*, 202–213. [CrossRef]
119. Kandula, N.R.; Dave, S.; De Chavez, P.J.; Bharucha, H.; Patel, Y.; Seguil, P.; Kumar, S.; Baker, D.W.; Spring, B.; Siddique, J. Translating a heart disease lifestyle intervention into the community: The South Asian Heart Lifestyle Intervention (SAHELI) study; a randomized control trial. *BMC Public Health* **2015**, *15*, 1064. [CrossRef]
120. Telle-Hjellset, V.; Raberg Kjollesdal, M.K.; Bjorge, B.; Holmboe-Ottesen, G.; Wandel, M.; Birkeland, K.I.; Eriksen, H.R.; Hostmark, A.T. The InnvaDiab-DE-PLAN study: A randomised controlled trial with a culturally adapted education programme improved the risk profile for type 2 diabetes in Pakistani immigrant women. *Br. J. Nutr.* **2013**, *109*, 529–538. [CrossRef]
121. Wijesuriya, M.; Fountoulakis, N.; Guess, N.; Banneheka, S.; Vasantharajah, L.; Gulliford, M.; Viberti, G.; Gnudi, L.; Karalliedde, J. A pragmatic lifestyle modification programme reduces the incidence of predictors of cardio-metabolic disease and dysglycaemia in a young healthy urban South Asian population: A randomised controlled trial. *BMC Med.* **2017**, *15*, 146. [CrossRef]
122. Schulz, A.J.; Israel, B.A.; Mentz, G.B.; Bernal, C.; Caver, D.; DeMajo, R.; Diaz, G.; Gamboa, C.; Gaines, C.; Hoston, B.; et al. Effectiveness of a walking group intervention to promote physical activity and cardiovascular health in predominantly non-Hispanic black and Hispanic urban neighborhoods: Findings from the walk your heart to health intervention. *Health Educ. Behav.* **2015**, *42*, 380–392. [CrossRef] [PubMed]
123. Miller, E.R., 3rd; Cooper, L.A.; Carson, K.A.; Wang, N.Y.; Appel, L.J.; Gayles, D.; Charleston, J.; White, K.; You, N.; Weng, Y.; et al. A Dietary Intervention in Urban African Americans: Results of the "Five Plus Nuts and Beans" Randomized Trial. *Am. J. Prev. Med.* **2016**, *50*, 87–95. [CrossRef] [PubMed]
124. Chang, S.H.; Chen, M.C.; Chien, N.H.; Lin, H.F. Effectiveness of community-based exercise intervention programme in obese adults with metabolic syndrome. *J. Clin. Nurs.* **2016**, *25*, 2579–2589. [CrossRef] [PubMed]
125. Tran, V.D.; James, A.P.; Lee, A.H.; Jancey, J.; Howat, P.A.; Thi Phuong Mai, L. Effectiveness of a Community-Based Physical Activity and Nutrition Behavior Intervention on Features of the Metabolic Syndrome: A Cluster-Randomized Controlled Trial. *Metab. Syndr. Relat. Disord.* **2017**, *15*, 63–71. [CrossRef] [PubMed]
126. Azizi, F.; Mirmiran, P.; Momenan, A.A.; Hadaegh, F.; Habibi Moeini, A.; Hosseini, F.; Zahediasl, S.; Ghanbarian, A.; Hosseinpanah, F. The effect of community-based education for lifestyle intervention on the prevalence of metabolic syndrome and its components: Tehran lipid and glucose study. *Int. J. Endocrinol. Metab.* **2013**, *11*, 145–153. [CrossRef] [PubMed]

127. Khalili, D.; Asgari, S.; Lotfaliany, M.; Zafari, N.; Hadaegh, F.; Momenan, A.A.; Nowroozpoor, A.; Hosseini-Esfahani, F.; Mirmiran, P.; Amiri, P.; et al. Long-Term Effectiveness of a Lifestyle Intervention: A Pragmatic Community Trial to Prevent Metabolic Syndrome. *Am. J. Prev. Med.* **2019**, *56*, 437–446. [CrossRef]
128. Shariful Islam, S.M.; Farmer, A.J.; Bobrow, K.; Maddison, R.; Whittaker, R.; Pfaeffli Dale, L.A.; Lechner, A.; Lear, S.; Eapen, Z.; Niessen, L.W.; et al. Mobile phone text-messaging interventions aimed to prevent cardiovascular diseases (Text2PreventCVD): Systematic review and individual patient data meta-analysis. *Open Heart* **2019**, *6*, e001017. [CrossRef]
129. Kim, E.K.; Kwak, S.H.; Jung, H.S.; Koo, B.K.; Moon, M.K.; Lim, S.; Jang, H.C.; Park, K.S.; Cho, Y.M. The Effect of a Smartphone-Based, Patient-Centered Diabetes Care System in Patients With Type 2 Diabetes: A Randomized, Controlled Trial for 24 Weeks. *Diabetes Care* **2019**, *42*, 3–9. [CrossRef]
130. Ganesan, A.N.; Louise, J.; Horsfall, M.; Bilsborough, S.A.; Hendriks, J.; McGavigan, A.D.; Selvanayagam, J.B.; Chew, D.P. International Mobile-Health Intervention on Physical Activity, Sitting, and Weight: The Stepathlon Cardiovascular Health Study. *J. Am. Coll. Cardiol.* **2016**, *67*, 2453–2463. [CrossRef]
131. Perez, M.V.; Mahaffey, K.W.; Hedlin, H.; Rumsfeld, J.S.; Garcia, A.; Ferris, T.; Balasubramanian, V.; Russo, A.M.; Rajmane, A.; Cheung, L.; et al. Large-Scale Assessment of a Smartwatch to Identify Atrial Fibrillation. *N. Engl. J. Med.* **2019**, *381*, 1909–1917. [CrossRef]
132. Liu, R.; So, L.; Mohan, S.; Khan, N.; King, K.; Quan, H. Cardiovascular risk factors in ethnic populations within Canada: Results from national cross-sectional surveys. *Open Med.* **2010**, *4*, e143–e153. [PubMed]
133. Williams, E.D.; Stamatakis, E.; Chandola, T.; Hamer, M. Physical activity behaviour and coronary heart disease mortality among South Asian people in the UK: An observational longitudinal study. *Heart* **2011**, *97*, 655–659. [CrossRef] [PubMed]
134. Lucas, A.; Murray, E.; Kinra, S. Heath beliefs of UK South Asians related to lifestyle diseases: A review of qualitative literature. *J. Obes.* **2013**, *2013*, 827674. [CrossRef] [PubMed]
135. Huston, P.; McFarlane, B. Health benefits of tai chi: What is the evidence? *Can. Fam. Physician* **2016**, *62*, 881–890. [PubMed]
136. Vlaar, E.M.A.; Nierkens, V.; Nicolaou, M.; Middelkoop, B.J.C.; Busschers, W.B.; Stronks, K.; van Valkengoed, I.G.M. Effectiveness of a targeted lifestyle intervention in primary care on diet and physical activity among South Asians at risk for diabetes: 2-year results of a randomised controlled trial in the Netherlands. *BMJ Open* **2017**, *7*, e012221. [CrossRef] [PubMed]
137. Vogel, L. Broken trust drives native health disparities. *CMAJ* **2015**, *187*, E9–E10. [CrossRef]
138. Kirkendoll, K.; Clark, P.C.; Grossniklaus, D.; Igho-Pemu, P.; Mullis, R.; Dunbar, S.B. Metabolic syndrome in African Americans: Views on making lifestyle changes. *J. Transcult. Nurs.* **2010**, *21*, 104–113. [CrossRef]

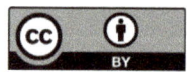

© 2019 by the authors. Licensee MDPI, Basel, Switzerland. This article is an open access article distributed under the terms and conditions of the Creative Commons Attribution (CC BY) license (http://creativecommons.org/licenses/by/4.0/).

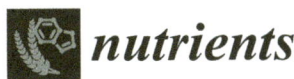

Discussion

Metabolic Syndrome—Role of Dietary Fat Type and Quantity

Peter Clifton

School of Pharmacy and Medical Sciences, University of South Australia, Adelaide SA 5000, Australia; peter.clifton@unisa.edu.au

Received: 27 May 2019; Accepted: 24 June 2019; Published: 26 June 2019

Abstract: Background: Metabolic syndrome increases the risk of cardiovascular disease (CVD) over and above that related to type 2 diabetes. The optimal diet for the treatment of metabolic syndrome is not clear. Materials and Methods: A review of dietary interventions in volunteers with metabolic syndrome as well as studies examining the impact of dietary fat on the separate components of metabolic syndrome was undertaken using only recent meta-analyses, if available. Results: Most of the data suggest that replacing carbohydrates with any fat, but particularly polyunsaturated fat, will lower triglyceride(TG), increase high density lipoprotein (HDL) cholesterol, and lower blood pressure, but have no effects on fasting glucose in normal volunteers or insulin sensitivity, as assessed by euglycemic hyperinsulinemic clamps. Fasting insulin may be lowered by fat. Monounsaturated fat (MUFA) is preferable to polyunsaturated fat (PUFA) for fasting insulin and glucose lowering. The addition of 3–4 g of N3 fats will lower TG and blood pressure (BP) and reduce the proportion of subjects with metabolic syndrome. Dairy fat (50% saturated fat) is also related to a lower incidence of metabolic syndrome in cohort studies.

Keywords: carbohydrate; polyunsaturated fat; monounsaturated fat; saturated fat; fish oil; meta-analyses; lipids; glucose; blood pressure; insulin resistance

---

1. Introduction

The metabolic syndrome is associated with an increased risk of cardiovascular disease and type 2 diabetes and enhances the risk of CVD in people with diabetes [1]. There are currently four definitions of metabolic syndrome, three of which require insulin resistance, as evidenced by central obesity, or fasting hyperinsulinemia or a disturbance in glucose homeostasis, plus two other abnormalities [2]. The National Cholesterol Education Program Adult Treatment Panel (NCEP ATP-III (revision 2005) guidelines does not require this, but demands 3 of 5 possible abnormalities—central obesity, impaired fasting glucose, hypertriglyceridemia, low HDL cholesterol, and blood pressure (>130 systolic or >85 diastolic). The other criteria vary with different levels of blood pressure (140/90), with a combination of high TG and low HDL as one criterion, and varying levels of fasting TG—either 1.7 or 2 mmol/L—and varying levels of HDL cholesterol. This review will focus on the components of the metabolic syndrome and where there are data on the presence or absence of metabolic syndrome, the criterion used will be mentioned. The aim of this review is to systematically examine meta-analyses that summarise the evidence from interventions on fat amount and type in metabolic syndrome or its separate components. Some evidence from individual trials that are illustrative will be included.

2. Aim

To systematically review meta-analyses of interventions that replace carbohydrates with fat in people with metabolic syndrome and interventions that examine these effects on the individual components of the syndrome.

3. Methods

Pubmed was searched (all years available) with the terms "meta-analysis AND dietary fat AND carbohydrate AND intervention AND (TG, OR, HDL, OR blood pressure, OR glucose, OR weight)". We reviewed 102 titles.

4. Results

4.1. Lipids

A large amount of evidence has accumulated that replacing carbohydrates (usually quality unspecified) with fat of any sort will lower fasting triglyceride and increase HDL cholesterol. A meta-analysis by Mensink and Katan [3] found that a 1% increase in fat calories in place of carbohydrates led to a fall in TG of 0.026 mmol/L (95% confidence intervals: 0.020–0.031) with polyunsaturated fat, 0.021 (0.015–0.027) with saturated fat, and 0.019 (0.014–0.024) with monounsaturated fat from 100 studies with 45 diets. For HDL cholesterol the same diets led to an increase in HDL cholesterol of 0.006 (0.003–0.009) mmol/L, 0.010 (0.007–0.013), and 0.008 (0.005–0.011), respectively. Overall saturated fat is about 30% more effective than the other two fats in the combined lowering of TG and HDL cholesterol. However, differences in HDL cholesterol from genetic variance have not been associated with differences in coronary heart disease (CHD) risk [4], whereas TG lowering genetically has been associated with CVD reduction, with the same degree of benefit per mg/dL apoB lowering as a reduction in LDL cholesterol [5]. Thus, PUFA is preferred to other fat types for carbohydrate replacement. In a small study of 39 men with metabolic syndrome, PUFA produced greater TG lowering than MUFA (both 5–30% of energy). Overall, 25% (4 of 16) assigned to PUFA and 13% (3 of 23) to MUFA did not have metabolic syndrome after the intervention [6]. Metabolic syndrome in this study was based on NCEP-III (2001). A high total dairy intake (and, presumably, a lower carbohydrate diet) is associated with a 6% reduced risk of metabolic syndrome per additional serving of dairy [7]. Most studies in this meta-analysis of 16 case-control/cross-sectional studies used the NCEP-III criteria.

The relationship between carbohydrate intake and TG has been controversial for many years with arguments about the persistence of the TG elevation effect [8,9], with the moderating or even nullifying effect of fibre on TG elevation [10], the contrasting effects of higher versus lower sugar with sugars replacing starch [11,12], and the absence of TG elevation in Pima Indians with type 2 diabetes mellitus (DM) with increased carbohydrates [13]. Just when the landscape was reasonably predictable from interventions, the TOSCA.IT showed in 18,785 people with type 2 DM that increasing fat intake from <25% to >35% increased TG, while increasing carbohydrate intake from <45% to >65% decreased TG [14]. TG was lower in the highest tertile of the relative Mediterranean diet score, which had lower added sugars, more fibre, but less fat and more carbohydrates. [15]. However, the TOSCA-IT is a large cohort study and its results may well be confounded as they do not match the results from dietary intervention studies in people with type 2 DM. The Qian meta-analysis [16] of 24 studies with 1460 participants showed that fasting TG was reduced by 0.31 mmol/L (95% confidence interval −0.44, −0.18) with replacement of carbohydrates with MUFA. A high fibre intake is associated with a 30% lowering in the risk of metabolic syndrome [17].

In a meta-analysis of high-fat versus low-fat diets in people with obesity, but no overt metabolic disturbance, Lu et al. (2018) [18] found a significantly higher level of TG (WMD: 11.68 mg/dL (0.13 mmol/l), 95 % CI 5.90, 17.45; $p < 0.001$) and a lower level of HDL-cholesterol (WMD: −2.57 mg/dL (−0.07 mmol/l); 95 % CI −3.85, −1.28; $p < 0.001$) after the low-fat diets, compared with high-fat diets in 20 studies with 2016 participants.

4.2. Fish Oil Fatty Acids

Guo et al. [19] performed a meta-analysis of seven case-control and 20 cross-sectional studies and found that a higher level of plasma/serum n-3 PUFAs was associated with a lower metabolic syndrome risk (pooled OR = 0.63, 95% CI: 0.49, 0.81). The plasma/serum n-3 PUFAs in controls were significantly higher than in metabolic syndrome cases (WMD: 0.24; 95% CI: 0.04, 0.43), especially docosapentaenoic acid and docosahexaenoic acid.

The addition of fish oil fatty acids of at least 1 g/day lowers fasting TG and a metanalysis performed by Eslick et al. [20] of 47 studies showed that taking fish oils (weighted average daily intake of 3.25 g of EPA and/or DHA) produced a clinically significant reduction of TG (−0.34 mmol/L, 95% CI: −0.41 to −0.27), with a very slight increase in HDL (0.01 mmol/L, 95% CI: 0.00 to 0.02) and LDL cholesterol (0.06 mmol/L, 95% CI: 0.03 to 0.09). The reduction of TG correlated with EPA plus DHA intake and initial TG level.

4.3. Glucose

Fasting glucose lowering by reducing carbohydrate and replacing it with fat is far more controversial. A recent meta-analysis by Wanders et al. [21] showed no effect in normal subjects of replacing carbohydrate with polyunsaturated fat, even though fasting insulin was reduced. A 5% increase in energy from PUFA significantly reduced insulin by 5.8 pmol/L (95% CI −10.2 to −1.3 pmol/L), but not glucose (change −0.07, 95% CI −0.17 to 0.04 mmol/L) and even in the group with the highest intake of PUFA, glucose was still not significant (−0.09, 95% CI −0.18 to 0.01 mmol/L). Imamura et al. [22] found that replacing 5% energy from carbohydrates with SFA had no significant effect on fasting glucose (+0.02 mmol/L, 95% CI = −0.01, +0.04; n trials = 99), but lowered fasting insulin (−1.1 pmol/L; −1.7, −0.5; n = 90). Replacing saturated fat with PUFA lowered fasting glucose (0.04mmol/L; 0.01, 0.07). Thus, PUFA is clearly the better fat for replacing carbohydrates in normal people. In people with type 2 diabetes [16], high MUFA diets compared with high carbohydrate diets lowered fasting plasma glucose (WMD −0.57 mmol/L [95% CI −0.76, −0.39]) in 24 studies containing 1460 participants. HDL cholesterol was increased by 0.06 mmol/L (0.02, 0.10) [16]. Surprisingly, in this study, replacing PUFA with MUFA lowered fasting glucose by a large amount (−0.87 mmol/L (−1.67, −0.07)) but the data are much less reliable, taken from only four studies and 44 participants.

4.4. Blood Pressure

There are much less data on blood pressure and carbohydrate replacement with fat in non-diabetics and the effects are relatively small. A meta-analysis performed by Shah et al. [23] found that diets rich in carbohydrates resulted in significantly higher systolic blood pressure (difference: 2.6 (95% CI: 0.4, 4.7) mm Hg; p = 0.02) and diastolic blood pressure (1.8 (0.01, 3.6) mm Hg; p = 0.05) than did diets rich in cis-monounsaturated fat. Huntress et al. [24] examined low carbohydrate diets in people with type 2 diabetes from data at one year. Eighteen trials were included in the meta-analysis, which found that the low carbohydrate diet lowered systolic blood pressure (estimated effect = −2.74 mmHg, 95% CI −5.27 to −0.20), but diastolic BP was not significant. In the meta-analysis from Qian et al. [16], MUFA lowered systolic blood pressure (−2.31 mmHg (−4.13, −0.49)) when it replaced carbohydrates.

4.5. Diet Composition During Weight Loss and Lipid Changes

Mansoor et al. [25] performed a meta-analysis of 11 weight loss trials with 1369 participants with a low carbohydrate level being defined as <20% carbohydrates. Compared with participants on low fat diets, participants on low carbohydrate diets experienced a greater reduction in body weight (weighted mean difference [WMD] −2.17 kg; 95% CI −3.36, −0.99) and TG (WMD −0.26 mmol/L; 95% CI −0.37, −0.15), but a greater increase in HDL-cholesterol (WMD 0·14 mmol/l; 95% CI 0.09, 0.19) and LDL-cholesterol (WMD 0·16 mmol/L; 95% CI 0.003, 0.33). Most of the low carbohydrate diets followed an Atkins style diet with an increase in saturated fat, which accounted for the rise in LDL cholesterol. If carbohydrates are replaced by unsaturated fat and not saturated fat, no rise in LDL cholesterol is seen in either six months [26], or one- [27] or two-year follow ups [28].

4.6. Insulin Resistance

Insulin resistance is a key and essential element of the metabolic syndrome (except the NCEP111 criteria), usually assumed on the basis of central adiposity. As noted by Wanders et al. [21], replacing carbohydrates with PUFA led to a lowering of fasting insulin, as did saturated fat, suggesting reduced insulin resistance, at least in the liver. There have been a small number of formal hyperinsulemic euglycemic clamp studies, but no meta-analysis. Tardy et al. [29] compared high dairy and industrial trans fatty acids with low trans fat diets in 63 healthy women with abdominal obesity. After four weeks of 60 g low-TFA lipids/day (0.54 g/day; $n = 21$), ruminant TFA-rich lipids (4.86 g/day; $n = 21$), or industrial TFA-rich lipids (5.58 g/day; $n = 21$), no changes in peripheral insulin sensitivity were seen. Bendtsen et al. [30] found no effect either of 15 g/day of trans fat in partially hydrogenated soybean oil for 16 weeks in 52 overweight postmenopausal women. Fasching et al. [31] found no effect of exchanging 200 g of carbohydrates with 90 g of PUFA, MUFA, or saturated fat for one week in a randomised crossover study in eight men with insulin sensitivity, assessed with a euglycemic hyperinsulinemic clamp. Borkmann et al. [32] found no effect of substituting saturated fat for carbohydrates on insulin sensitivity in eight non-diabetic subjects, despite large changes in LDL and TG (the latter down 33%.) The KANWU study [33] showed that a high MUFA diet for three months reduced insulin resistance, compared with a high saturated fat diet in 162 healthy subjects, but carbohydrate levels were not examined. Fish oil had no effect and the effect of MUFA was lost when fat intake was >37% of energy. In a very small study in patients with fatty liver disease, a high MUFA Mediterranean diet improved insulin sensitivity, compared with a high carbohydrate diet ($p = 0.03$) accompanied by a reduction in liver fat [34]

A contrary result was found in the Lipgene study [35] where 472 volunteers with metabolic syndrome were randomised to one diet for 12 weeks: High MUFA or high saturated fat diets or high carbohydrate diets with and without fish oil (1.2 g/day). In the highest HOMA-IR tertile, MUFA and n3 fats lowered insulin significantly, compared with saturated fat. In the lowest HOMA-IR tertile, insulin and glucose rose with all diets, but it rose less with MUFA and N3 fats compared with saturated fat. There is regression to the mean in both these tertiles and there is no statistical contrast between the effect of diets in the different tertiles, so we don't actually know if there is a tertile/diet interaction. Triglycerides fell with N3 fats in tertiles 1 and 2, but surprisingly, not in the highest tertile with the highest TG level. Replacing carbohydrates with MUFA or saturated fat had no effect on TG in any tertile, which is contrary to the much bigger meta-analysis of Mensink et al. (3) and there is no good explanation other than strong time-related changes.

In another report from the same study, in 337 volunteers [36], the prevalence of metabolic syndrome (NECP-III) fell by 20.5% after the n-3 diet (blood pressure and TG fell), compared with the high saturated fat diet (10.6%), high MUFA diet (12%) diet, and high carbohydrate diet (10.4%) ($p < 0.028$).

5. Conclusions

Most meta-analyses show that replacement of carbohydrates with fat lowers fasting TG and glucose and blood pressure, and increases HDL cholesterol with some differences, depending on whether the population has type 2 diabetes or not. There are some large intervention and cohort studies that show the opposite results, but these are in the minority. PUFA is probably superior to MUFA, while fish oil is superior to both.

Conflicts of Interest: The author declares no conflict of interest.

References

1. Reaven, G.M. Banting lecture 1988. Role of insulin resistance in human disease. *Diabetes* **1988**, *37*, 1595–1607. [CrossRef] [PubMed]

2. Kassi, E.; Pervanidou, P.; Kaltsas, G.; Chrousos, G. Metabolic syndrome: Definitions and controversies. *BMC Med.* **2011**, *9*, 48. [CrossRef] [PubMed]
3. Mensink, R.P.; Zock, P.L.; Kester, A.D.; Katan, M.B. Effects of dietary fatty acids and carbohydrates on the ratio of serum total to HDL cholesterol and on serum lipids and apolipoproteins: A meta-analysis of 60 controlled trials. *Am. J. Clin. Nutr.* **2003**, *77*, 1146–1155. [CrossRef] [PubMed]
4. Vitali, C.; Khetarpal, S.A.; Rader, D.J. Cholesterol Metabolism and the Risk of CHD: New Insights from Human Genetics. *Curr. Cardiol. Rep.* **2017**, *19*, 132. [CrossRef] [PubMed]
5. Ference, B.A.; Kastelein, J.J.P.; Ray, K.K.; Ginsberg, H.N.; Chapman, M.J.; Packard, C.J.; Laufs, U.; Oliver-Williams, C.; Wood, A.M.; Butterworth, A.S.; et al. Association of Triglyceride-Lowering LPL Variants and LDL-C-Lowering LDLR Variants with Risk of Coronary Heart Disease. *JAMA* **2019**, *321*, 364–373. [CrossRef] [PubMed]
6. Miller, M.; Sorkin, J.D.; Mastella, L.; Sutherland, A.; Rhyne, J.; Donnelly, P.; Simpson, K.; Goldberg, A.P. Poly is more effective than monounsaturated fat for dietary management in the metabolic syndrome: The muffin study. *J. Clin. Lipidol.* **2016**, *10*, 996–1003. [CrossRef] [PubMed]
7. Chen, G.C.; Szeto, I.M.; Chen, L.H.; Han, S.F.; Li, Y.J.; van Hekezen, R.; Qin, L.Q. Dairy products consumption and metabolic syndrome in adults: Systematic review and meta-analysis of observational studies. *Sci. Rep.* **2015**, *5*, 14606. [CrossRef]
8. Coulston, A.M.; Hollenbeck, C.B.; Reaven, G.M.; Swislocki, A.L.M. Persistence of Hypertriglyceridemic Effect of Low-Fat High-Carbohydrate Diets in NIDDM Patients. *Diabetes Care* **1989**, *12*, 94–101. [CrossRef]
9. Hollenbeck, C.B.; Coulston, A.M. Effects of dietary carbohydrate and fat intake on glucose and lipoprotein metabolism in individuals with diabetes mellitus. *Diabetes Care* **1991**, *14*, 774–785. [CrossRef]
10. Riccardi, G.; Rivellese, A.A.; Mokdad, A.H.; Ford, E.S.; Bowman, B.A.; Nelson, D.E.; Engelgau, M.M.; Vinicor, F.; Marks, J.S. Effects of Dietary Fiber and Carbohydrate on Glucose and Lipoprotein Metabolism in Diabetic Patients. *Diabetes Care* **1991**, *14*, 1115–1125. [CrossRef]
11. Te Morenga, L.A.; Howatson, A.J.; Jones, R.M.; Mann, J. Dietary sugars and cardiometabolic risk: Systematic review and meta-analyses of randomized controlled trials of the effects on blood pressure and lipids. *Am. J. Clin. Nutr.* **2014**, *100*, 65–79. [CrossRef] [PubMed]
12. Gibson, S.; Gunn, P.; Wittekind, A.; Cottrell, R. The Effects of Sucrose on Metabolic Health: A Systematic Review of Human Intervention Studies in Healthy Adults. *Crit. Rev. Food Sci. Nutr.* **2013**, *53*, 591–614. [CrossRef] [PubMed]
13. Howard, B.V.; Abbott, W.G.; A Swinburn, B. Evaluation of Metabolic Effects of Substitution of Complex Carbohydrates for Saturated Fat in Individuals with Obesity and NIDDM. *Diabetes Care* **1991**, *14*, 786–795. [CrossRef] [PubMed]
14. Vitale, M.; Masulli, M.; Rivellese, A.A.; Babini, A.C.; Boemi, M.; Bonora, E.; Buzzetti, R.; Ciano, O.; Cignarelli, M.; Cigolini, M.; et al. Influence of dietary fat and carbohydrates proportions on plasma lipids, glucose control and low-grade inflammation in patients with type 2 diabetes-The TOSCA.IT Study. *Eur. J. Nutr.* **2016**, *55*, 1645–1651. [CrossRef] [PubMed]
15. Vitale, M.; Masulli, M.; Calabrese, I.; Rivellese, A.A.; Bonora, E.; Signorini, S.; Perriello, G.; Squatrito, S.; Buzzetti, R.; Sartore, G.; et al. Impact of a Mediterranean Dietary Pattern and Its Components on Cardiovascular Risk Factors, Glucose Control, and Body Weight in People with Type 2 Diabetes: A Real-Life Study. *Nutrients* **2018**, *10*, 1067. [CrossRef]
16. Qian, F.; Korat, A.A.; Malik, V.; Hu, F.B. Metabolic Effects of Monounsaturated Fatty Acid–Enriched Diets Compared with Carbohydrate or Polyunsaturated Fatty Acid–Enriched Diets in Patients with Type 2 Diabetes: A Systematic Review and Meta-analysis of Randomized Controlled Trials. *Diabetes Care* **2016**, *39*, 1448–1457. [CrossRef]
17. Chen, J.P.; Chen, G.C.; Wang, X.P.; Qin, L.; Bai, Y. Dietary Fiber and Metabolic Syndrome: A Meta-Analysis and Review of Related Mechanisms. *Nutrients* **2017**, *10*, 24. [CrossRef]
18. Lu, M.; Wan, Y.; Yang, B.; Huggins, C.E.; Li, D. Effects of low-fat compared with high-fat diet on cardiometabolic indicators in people with overweight and obesity without overt metabolic disturbance: A systematic review and meta-analysis of randomised controlled trials. *Br. J. Nutr.* **2018**, *119*, 96–108. [CrossRef]

19. Guo, X.F.; Li, X.; Shi, M.; Li, D. n-3 Polyunsaturated Fatty Acids and Metabolic Syndrome Risk: A Meta-Analysis. *Nutrients* **2017**, *9*, 703. [CrossRef]
20. Eslick, G.D.; Howe, P.R.; Smith, C.; Priest, R.; Bensoussan, A. Benefits of fish oil supplementation in hyperlipidemia: A systematic review and meta-analysis. *Int. J. Cardiol.* **2009**, *136*, 4–16. [CrossRef]
21. Wanders, A.J.; Blom, W.A.M.; Zock, P.L.; Geleijnse, J.M.; A Brouwer, I.; Alssema, M. Plant-derived polyunsaturated fatty acids and markers of glucose metabolism and insulin resistance: A meta-analysis of randomized controlled feeding trials. *BMJ Open Diabetes Res. Care* **2019**, *7*, e000585. [CrossRef] [PubMed]
22. Imamura, F.; Micha, R.; Wu, J.H.; de Oliveira Otto, M.C.; Otite, F.O.; Abioye, A.I.; Mozaffarian, D. Effects of Saturated Fat, Polyunsaturated Fat, Monounsaturated Fat, and Carbohydrate on Glucose-Insulin Homeostasis: A Systematic Review and Meta-analysis of Randomised Controlled Feeding Trials. *PLoS Med.* **2016**, *13*, e1002087. [CrossRef] [PubMed]
23. Shah, M.; Adams-Huet, B.; Garg, A. Effect of high-carbohydrate or high-cis-monounsaturated fat diets on blood pressure: A meta-analysis of intervention trials. *Am. J. Clin. Nutr.* **2007**, *85*, 1251–1256. [CrossRef] [PubMed]
24. Huntriss, R.; Campbell, M.; Bedwell, C. The interpretation and effect of a low-carbohydrate diet in the management of type 2 diabetes: A systematic review and meta-analysis of randomised controlled trials. *Eur. J. Clin. Nutr.* **2018**, *72*, 311–325. [CrossRef] [PubMed]
25. Mansoor, N.; Vinknes, K.J.; Veierød, M.B.; Retterstøl, K. Effects of low-carbohydrate diets v. low-fat diets on body weight and cardiovascular risk factors: A meta-analysis of randomised controlled trials. *Br. J. Nutr.* **2016**, *115*, 466–479. [CrossRef]
26. Luscombe-Marsh, N.D.; Noakes, M.; Buckley, J.; Wittert, G.A.; Yancy, W.S.; Brinkworth, G.D.; Tay, J.; Thompson, C.H. A Very Low-Carbohydrate, Low–Saturated Fat Diet for Type 2 Diabetes Management: A Randomized Trial. *Diabetes Care* **2014**, *37*, 2909–2918. [CrossRef]
27. Tay, J.; Luscombe-Marsh, N.D.; Thompson, C.H.; Noakes, M.; Buckley, J.; Wittert, G.A.; Yancy, W.S., Jr.; Brinkworth, G.D. Comparison of low- and high-carbohydrate diets for type 2 diabetes management: A randomized trial. *Am. J. Clin. Nutr.* **2015**, *102*, 780–790. [CrossRef]
28. Tay, J.; Thompson, C.H.; Luscombe-Marsh, N.D.; Wycherley, T.P.; Noakes, M.; Buckley, J.D.; Wittert, G.A.; Yancy, W.S., Jr.; Brinkworth, G.D. Effects of an energy-restricted low-carbohydrate, high unsaturated fat/low saturated fat diet versus a high-carbohydrate, low-fat diet in type 2 diabetes: A 2-year randomized clinical trial. *Diabetes Obes. Metab.* **2018**, *20*, 858–871. [CrossRef]
29. Tardy, A.L.; Lambert-Porcheron, S.; Malpuech-Brugère, C.; Giraudet, C.; Rigaudière, J.P.; Laillet, B.; Leruyet, P.; Peyraud, J.L.; Boirie, Y.; Laville, M.; et al. Dairy and industrial sources of trans fat do not impair peripheral insulin sensitivity in overweight women. *Am. J. Clin. Nutr.* **2009**, *90*, 88–94. [CrossRef]
30. Bendsen, N.T.; Haugaard, S.B.; Larsen, T.M.; Chabanova, E.; Stender, S.; Astrup, A. Effect of trans-fatty acid intake on insulin sensitivity and intramuscular lipids–a randomized trial in overweight postmenopausal women. *Metabolism* **2011**, *60*, 906–913. [CrossRef]
31. Fasching, P.; Ratheiser, K.; Schneeweiss, B.; Rohac, M.; Nowotny, P.; Waldhäusl, W. No effect of short-term dietary supplementation of saturated and poly-and monounsaturated fatty acids on insulin secretion and sensitivity in healthy men. *Ann. Nutr. Metab.* **1996**, *40*, 116–122. [CrossRef] [PubMed]
32. Borkman, M.; Campbell, L.V.; Chisholm, D.J.; Storlien, L.H. Comparison of the effects on insulin sensitivity of high carbohydrate and high fat diets in normal subjects. *J. Clin. Endocrinol. Metab.* **1991**, *72*, 432–437. [CrossRef] [PubMed]
33. Vessby, B.; Uusitupa, M.; Hermansen, K.; Riccardi, G.; Rivellese, A.A.; Tapsell, L.C.; Nälsén, C.; Berglund, L.; Louheranta, A.; Rasmussen, B.M.; et al. Substituting dietary saturated for monounsaturated fat impairs insulin sensitivity in healthy men and women: The KANWU Study. *Diabetologia* **2001**, *44*, 312–319. [CrossRef] [PubMed]
34. Ryan, M.C.; Itsiopoulos, C.; Thodis, T.; Ward, G.; Trost, N.; Hofferberth, S.; O'Dea, K.; Desmond, P.V.; Johnson, N.A.; Wilson, A.M. The Mediterranean diet improves hepatic steatosis and insulin sensitivity in individuals with non-alcoholic fatty liver disease. *J. Hepatol.* **2013**, *59*, 138–143. [CrossRef] [PubMed]

35. Yubero-Serrano, E.M.; Delgado-Lista, J.; Tierney, A.C.; Perez-Martinez, P.; Garcia-Rios, A.; Alcala-Diaz, J.F.; Castaño, J.P.; Tinahones, F.J.; A Drevon, C.; Defoort, C.; et al. Insulin resistance determines a differential response to changes in dietary fat modification on metabolic syndrome risk factors: The LIPGENE study. *Am. J. Clin. Nutr.* **2015**, *102*, 1509–1517. [CrossRef] [PubMed]
36. Paniagua, J.A.; Pérez-Martinez, P.; Gjelstad, I.M.; Tierney, A.C.; Delgado-Lista, J.; Defoort, C.; Blaak, E.E.; Risérus, U.; Drevon, C.A.; Kiec-Wilk, B.; et al. A low-fat high-carbohydrate diet supplemented with long-chain n-3 PUFA reduces the risk of the metabolic syndrome. *Atherosclerosis* **2011**, *218*, 443–450. [CrossRef] [PubMed]

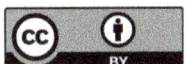

© 2019 by the author. Licensee MDPI, Basel, Switzerland. This article is an open access article distributed under the terms and conditions of the Creative Commons Attribution (CC BY) license (http://creativecommons.org/licenses/by/4.0/).

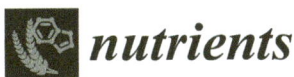

Article

Linseed Components Are More Effective Than Whole Linseed in Reversing Diet-Induced Metabolic Syndrome in Rats

Siti Raihanah Shafie [1,†], Stephen Wanyonyi [1], Sunil K. Panchal [1] and Lindsay Brown [1,2,*]

1. Functional Foods Research Group, University of Southern Queensland, Toowoomba, QLD 4350, Australia
2. School of Health and Wellbeing, University of Southern Queensland, Toowoomba, QLD 4350, Australia
* Correspondence: Lindsay.Brown@usq.edu.au; Tel.: +61-7-4631-1319
† Current Address: Department of Nutrition and Dietetics, Faculty of Medicine and Health Sciences, Universiti Putra Malaysia, 43000 UPM Serdang, Selangor, Malaysia.

Received: 21 June 2019; Accepted: 19 July 2019; Published: 22 July 2019

Abstract: Linseed is a dietary source of plant-based ω–3 fatty acids along with fiber as well as lignans including secoisolariciresinol diglucoside (SDG). We investigated the reversal of signs of metabolic syndrome following addition of whole linseed (5%), defatted linseed (3%), or SDG (0.03%) to either a high-carbohydrate, high-fat or corn starch diet for rats for the final eight weeks of a 16–week protocol. All interventions reduced plasma insulin, systolic blood pressure, inflammatory cell infiltration in heart, ventricular collagen deposition, and diastolic stiffness but had no effect on plasma total cholesterol, nonesterified fatty acids, or triglycerides. Whole linseed did not change the body weight or abdominal fat in obese rats while SDG and defatted linseed decreased abdominal fat and defatted linseed increased lean mass. Defatted linseed and SDG, but not whole linseed, improved heart and liver structure, decreased fat vacuoles in liver, and decreased plasma leptin concentrations. These results show that the individual components of linseed produce greater potential therapeutic responses in rats with metabolic syndrome than whole linseed. We suggest that the reduced responses indicate reduced oral bioavailability of the whole seeds compared to the components.

Keywords: linseed; secoisolariciresinol diglucoside; obesity; blood pressure; high-carbohydrate; high-fat diet

1. Introduction

Linseed or flax (*Linum usitatissimum* L.) has widely reported health benefits from studies with many forms including whole or ground seeds, oil, defatted meal, and mucilage extracts [1,2]. Linseed and its components, especially α–linolenic acid (ALA, C18:3n–3) and the lignan, secoisolariciresinol diglucoside (SDG), may protect against metabolic syndrome and cardiovascular disease by lowering blood pressure, reducing blood glucose concentrations, delaying postprandial glucose absorption, and decreasing oxidative stress and inflammation [3–5]. However, the health benefits of introducing linseed into the diet have not been fully defined [6]. In addition, processing including dehusking, crushing, milling, and defatting may increase bioavailability of individual components such as lignans and ALA [7–9]. Furthermore, no studies have compared physiological responses to whole linseed or linseed components using the same animal model or humans.

Linseed has a hard outer layer which may allow the seeds to pass unchanged through the gut and reduce absorption of useful nutrients by the body [10]. Thus, it may be more beneficial to consume ground linseeds over whole linseeds. This implied difference in oral bioavailability could markedly alter the choice of linseed preparations as functional foods, since both whole linseeds and ground linseed flour are readily available. In humans fed muffins with either 30 g whole or ground linseed, or flaxseed oil with 6 g ALA, plasma ALA concentrations were 0.024 mg/mL with whole linseed (not significantly different from control) but increased to 0.031 mg/mL with ground linseed and 0.055 mg/mL with linseed oil, suggesting reduced absorption from whole linseeds [11]. In a randomized, crossover study involving 12 healthy subjects, the bioavailability of enterolignans formed as lignan metabolites in the liver more than tripled after feeding on crushed linseed relative to whole linseed and further increased with milled linseed [8]. In rats following oral administration, SDG was metabolized in the gastrointestinal tract and not absorbed while the oral bioavailability of secoisolariciresinol was about 25% with a half–life within the body following intravenous administration of 4 h [12].

In this study, we evaluated the cardiovascular, liver, and metabolic responses of whole linseed, and two of its components, defatted ground linseed, and SDG–enriched fraction, by using an established model of high-carbohydrate, high-fat diet-fed rats mimicking the human metabolic syndrome [13]. We have compared these results with our earlier study on 3% linseed oil containing ALA, which normalized systolic blood pressure, and improved heart function and glucose tolerance [14]. Measurements included body weight, systolic blood pressure, oral glucose tolerance test, left ventricular diastolic stiffness, histology of the heart and liver, and plasma biochemistry. Doses of the linseed components were chosen so as to be similar to the proportion in whole linseed. Our hypothesis was that whole linseeds and the isolated components would improve cardiovascular, metabolic, and liver changes in diet-induced metabolic syndrome in rats.

2. Materials and Methods

2.1. Rats and Diet

All experimental protocols were approved by the University of Southern Queensland Animal Ethics Committee under the guidelines of the National Health and Medical Research Council of Australia. Male Wistar rats were purchased from Animal Resource Centre, Murdoch, WA, Australia. Rats were housed individually in temperature-controlled, 12 h light/dark conditions in the animal house facility of the University of Southern Queensland. The rats were acclimatized and given free access to water and standard rat powdered food prior to initiation of the protocol diets.

Rats (8–9 weeks old, weighing 330–340 g, $n = 96$) were randomly divided into 8 experimental groups: corn starch diet-fed rats (C; $n = 12$), corn starch diet-fed rats treated with 5% whole linseed in food (CW; $n = 12$), corn starch diet-fed rats treated with 3% defatted ground linseed in food (CD; $n = 12$), corn starch diet-fed rats treated with 0.03% SDG in food (CS; $n = 12$), high-carbohydrate, high-fat diet-fed rats (H; $n = 12$), high-carbohydrate, high-fat diet-fed rats treated with 5% whole linseed in food (HW; $n = 12$), high-carbohydrate, high-fat diet-fed rats treated with 3% defatted ground linseed in food (HD; $n = 12$), and high-carbohydrate, high-fat diet-fed rats treated with 0.03% SDG in food (HS; $n = 12$). Preparation of C and H diets has been described previously [13]. The energy densities of C and H diets were 11.23 kJ/g and 17.83 kJ/g, respectively, with an additional 3.85 kJ/mL in drinking water for fructose intake in high-carbohydrate, high-fat diet-fed rats [13].

Whole linseed- and defatted linseed–supplemented diets were prepared by replacing 5% water with 5% whole linseed (not ground) and 3% water with 3% defatted linseed, respectively, in C and H diets. The whole linseed dose replicated our previous study which used 5% chia seeds in food [15], as the oil composition of chia seed and linseed are similar. Since the oil content of linseed is about 40% [16], the non-oil component, defined here as defatted linseed, is 60% so defatted linseed flour was added at 3% in the food. The SDG-supplemented diets were prepared by adding 0.03% SDG (0.3 g of SDG/kg food) in C and H diets.

The whole linseed, defatted linseed, and SDG diets were administered for 8 weeks starting 8 weeks after the initiation of C or H diet. H, HW, HD, and HS groups were given 25% fructose in drinking water along with the diets for the 16-week duration of the study. Normal drinking water without any supplementation was given to C, CW, CD, and CS rats. Rats were monitored daily for body weight and food and water intakes. Energy intake and food conversion efficiency were calculated based on the food intake and body weight gain [14,15].

Whole linseed was a gift from AustGrains (Moree, NSW, Australia) and was also ground and extracted with *n*-hexane to produce defatted linseed. SDG (40% purity) was a gift from the Archer Daniels Midland Company (Chicago, IL, USA). The analysis of SDG content was conducted by St. Boniface Hospital Research, Winnipeg, MB, Canada. Total gross energy content of whole linseed, defatted linseed, and SDG samples were measured by bomb calorimetry (XRY-1A Oxygen Bomb calorimeter, Shanghai Changji Geological Instrument Co. Ltd., Shanghai, China) in triplicate. One gram of whole linseed, defatted linseed, or SDG were burnt in compressed oxygen (25 kg/cm^2) in the calorimetric bomb immersed in water. The energy densities for whole linseed, defatted linseed, and SDG were 23.76 kJ/g, 16.98 kJ/g, and 17.48 kJ/g, respectively.

2.2. Measurements in Live Rats

Systolic blood pressure was measured at the end of the protocol under light sedation by intraperitoneal injection with Zoletil (tiletamine 10 mg/kg, zolazepam 10 mg/kg; Virbac, Peakhurst, NSW, Australia). Measurements were performed using an MLT1010 Piezo-Electric Pulse Transducer (ADInstruments, Sydney, NSW, Australia) and an inflatable tail-cuff connected to an MLT844 Physiological Pressure Transducer (ADInstruments) connected to a PowerLab data acquisition unit (ADInstruments) [13].

Oral glucose tolerance tests were performed at the end of the protocol on rats after overnight (12 h) food deprivation. During this time, fructose-supplemented drinking water in H, HW, HD, and HS rats was replaced with tap water. Basal blood glucose concentrations were determined in tail vein blood using Medisense Precision Q.I.D. glucometer (Abbott Laboratories, Bedford, MA, USA). The rats were given 2 g/kg body weight of glucose as a 40% (w/v) aqueous glucose solution via oral gavage. Tail vein blood samples were taken at 30, 60, 90, and 120 min following glucose administration [13].

Dual-energy X-ray absorptiometry (DXA) was performed on all rats after 16 weeks of feeding using a Norland XR36 DXA instrument (Norland Corp., Fort Atkinson, WI, USA). Rats were anesthetized using intraperitoneal injection of Zoletil (tiletamine 10 mg/kg and zolazepam 10 mg/kg) and Ilium Xylazil (xylazine 6 mg/kg; Troy Laboratories, Smithfield, NSW, Australia). Scans were analyzed using the manufacturer's recommended software for use in laboratory animals (Small Subject Analysis Software, version 2.5.3/1.3.1; Norland Corp.) [13]. Visceral adiposity index (%) was calculated based on the abdominal fat content obtained during terminal experiments [15].

2.3. Measurements after Euthanasia

Terminal euthanasia was induced by intraperitoneal injection of Lethabarb (pentobarbitone sodium, 100 mg/kg; Virbac) and ~6 mL blood was immediately drawn from the abdominal aorta, collected into heparinized tubes, and centrifuged for plasma [13]. Hearts ($n = 8$–10) were separated into right ventricle and left ventricle with septum for weighing. Liver and abdominal fat pads (retroperitoneal, epididymal, and omental) were isolated and weighed ($n = 8$–10). Organ weights were normalized to the tibial length and presented in mg of tissue/mm of tibial length [13].

A portion of the heart, liver, small intestine, and large intestine was collected and fixed in 10% neutral buffered formalin for 3 days. Standard histological procedures were followed to process tissues for staining with hematoxylin and eosin or picrosirius red staining [13]. Two slides were prepared per tissue specimen and two random, non-overlapping fields per slide were taken to avoid biased analysis. To examine collagen distribution in the heart, the tissue was stained with picrosirius red stain and imaged using EVOS FL Color Imaging System (version 1.4 (Rev 26059); Advanced Microscopy Group, Bothwell, WA, USA) [14]. Small and large intestine sections were stained with periodic acid-Schiff stain to identify goblet cells [17]. Left ventricular collagen deposition was estimated by analysis with NIH ImageJ software (https://imagej.nih.gov/ij/).

Plasma samples collected during terminal experiments were used to test plasma activities of alanine transaminase and aspartate transaminase, and plasma concentrations of total cholesterol, triglycerides, and nonesterified fatty acids [13].

2.4. Statistical Analysis

All data are presented as mean ± standard error of the mean (SEM). Group data were tested for variance using Bartlett's test. Variables that were not normally distributed were transformed (using log 10 function) prior to statistical analysis. Groups were tested for effects of diet, treatment, and their interactions using two-way analysis of variance. When interaction and/or the main effects were significant, means were compared using Newman-Keuls multiple-comparison post hoc test. All statistical analyses were performed using Prism version 6.00 for Windows (GraphPad Software, San Diego, CA, USA). *p*-value of < 0.05 was considered as statistically significant.

3. Results

3.1. Dietary Intakes

Food and water intakes were lower in H rats than in C rats but energy intakes were higher in H rats than in C rats (Table 1). There were no differences between food intakes of C, CW, CD, and CS or between H, HW, HD, and HS groups (Table 1). Water intake was unchanged among C, CW, CD, and CS groups and there was no difference in water intake among H, HW, HD, and HS rats (Table 1). Doses of SDG were 31.9 ± 1.3 mg/kg/day and 15.9 ± 0.3 mg/kg/day for CS and HS rats, respectively. Intakes of whole linseed were 4.36 ± 0.14 g/kg/day and 2.51 ± 0.16 g/kg/day for CW and HW rats, respectively, while intakes of defatted linseed were 2.64 ± 0.09 g/kg/day and 1.57 ± 0.04 g/kg/day for CD and HD rats, respectively.

3.2. Body Composition and Organ Weights

Body weight was higher in H rats than in C rats and whole linseed, defatted linseed and SDG did not change body weight in HW, HD, and HS rats, whereas the body weight was higher in CW rats than in C rats, and CS and CD rats had intermediate body weights to C and CW rats (Figure 1A and Table 1). Body weight gain was lower in HS rats compared to H, HW, and HD rats, whereas body weight gain was in the order C=CS>CD>CW among the C diet groups (Table 1). Feed conversion efficiency was higher in H rats than in C rats. Interventions did not change feed conversion efficiency in H diet-fed rats (HW, HD, and HS rats), whereas whole linseed increased the feed conversion efficiency in CW rats with no change in CS and CD rats (Table 1). Bone mineral content was higher in H rats than in C rats. None of the interventions changed bone mineral content in C diet groups (CW, CD, and CS), whereas HD rats showed reduction in this parameter compared to H, HW, and HS rats (Table 1). Lean mass did not differ between C and H rats. CW, CD, and HD rats had higher lean mass; CS, H, and HS rats had lower lean mass, whereas C and HW had intermediate lean mass (Table 1). H rats had higher fat mass compared to all C diet groups (C, CW, CD, and CS rats). HD rats had lower fat mass compared to H and HW rats, whereas HS rats had fat mass intermediate to H and HD rats (Table 1). Abdominal circumference and visceral adiposity index were unchanged in CW, CD, and CS rats compared to C rats, whereas these parameters were increased in H rats compared to C rats (Table 1). HD rats had lower abdominal circumference compared to H and HW rats, whereas visceral adiposity index was higher in HW rats compared to HS and HD rats (Table 1).

Table 1. Dietary intakes, body composition, and organ wet weights.

Variables	C	CW	CD	CS	H	HW	HD	HS	Diet	Treatment	Interaction
Food intake, g/day	35.0 ± 0.6 a	34.6 ± 1.2 a	33.9 ± 1.2 a	35.5 ± 0.8 a	25.2 ± 0.6 b	23.4 ± 0.6 b	24.4 ± 0.4 b	26.3 ± 0.4 b	<0.0001	0.06	0.59
Water intake, mL/day	28.7 ± 1.8 a	30.7 ± 2.1 a	32.7 ± 0.9 a	30.4 ± 2.7 a	25.6 ± 1.0 b	26.9 ± 0.4 ab	25.7 ± 1.1 b	25.2 ± 1.0 b	<0.0001	0.54	0.61
Energy intake, kJ/day	392 ± 7 b	433 ± 14 b	397 ± 14 b	420 ± 13 b	552 ± 13 a	561 ± 14 a	542 ± 9 a	555 ± 8 a	<0.0001	0.11	0.37
Body weight gained (week 8–16), %	7.4 ± 1.0 d	18.2 ± 0.8 b	13.2 ± 1.6 c	9.1 ± 1.7 d	23.3 ± 0.9 a	23.4 ± 0.6 a	22.7 ± 1.4 a	18.9 ± 1.3 b	<0.0001	<0.0001	0.0006
Final body weight (week 16)	375 ± 4 a	432 ± 6 b	400 ± 5 a	392 ± 10 a	526 ± 10 c	539 ± 10 c	521 ± 8 c	519 ± 11 c	<0.0001	0.0004	0.06
Feed conversion efficiency, %	1.8 ± 0.2 c	4.9 ± 0.3 b	3.2 ± 0.4 c	2.6 ± 0.5 c	9.6 ± 0.6 a	9.2 ± 0.6 a	9.0 ± 0.6 a	8.1 ± 0.7 a	<0.0001	0.004	0.005
Bone mineral content, g	12.0 ± 0.4 c	12.1 ± 0.2 c	11.9 ± 0.2 c	13.2 ± 0.6 c	16.5 ± 0.4 a	17.3 ± 0.7 a	15.3 ± 0.6 b	16.8 ± 0.4 a	<0.0001	0.024	0.20
Total fat mass, g	98 ± 16 c	103 ± 7 c	77 ± 6 c	122 ± 16 c	256 ± 21 a	253 ± 21 a	189 ± 22 b	227 ± 7 ab	<0.0001	0.014	0.25
Total lean mass, g	276 ± 14 ab	317 ± 7 a	309 ± 5 a	267 ± 9 b	268 ± 14 b	277 ± 11 ab	312 ± 15 a	246 ± 7 b	0.035	<0.0001	0.24
Abdominal circumference, cm	18.4 ± 0.2 c	19.1 ± 0.2 c	19.1 ± 0.1 c	18.9 ± 0.2 c	23.0 ± 0.2 a	23.6 ± 0.4 a	21.2 ± 0.2 b	22.7 ± 0.2 a	<0.0001	0.016	0.19
Visceral adiposity index, %	4.9 ± 0.4 d	4.7 ± 0.3 d	4.2 ± 0.1 d	4.8 ± 0.6 d	9.6 ± 0.7 ab	10.4 ± 0.9 a	7.3 ± 0.5 c	8.5 ± 0.4 bc	<0.0001	0.007	0.09
Retroperitoneal fat, mg/mm *	189 ± 18 c	179 ± 18 c	151 ± 20 c	194 ± 31 c	531 ± 41 a	554 ± 59 a	407 ± 31 b	469 ± 31 ab	<0.0001	0.55	0.34
Epididymal fat, mg/mm *	89 ± 10 d	98 ± 8 d	74 ± 5 d	112 ± 20 cd	259 ± 17 a	278 ± 28 a	154 ± 16 c	211 ± 11 b	<0.0001	0.29	0.037
Omental fat, mg/mm *	114 ± 15 c	124 ± 9 c	102 ± 7 c	102 ± 13 c	240 ± 25 ab	280 ± 18 a	198 ± 14 b	207 ± 8 b	<0.0001	0.013	0.26
Total abdominal fat, mg/mm *	392 ± 39 d	401 ± 35 d	308 ± 36 d	408 ± 63 d	1031 ± 79 ab	1113 ± 105 a	663 ± 92 c	887 ± 45 b	<0.0001	0.23	0.18
Liver, mg/mm *	201 ± 5 b	213 ± 12 b	216 ± 7 b	213 ± 8 b	327 ± 12 a	337 ± 15 a	310 ± 8 a	306 ± 9 a	<0.0001	0.32	0.22

Values are expressed as mean ± SEM, n = 8–12. Means with different superscripts (a, b, c, or d) differ, $p < 0.05$. C, corn starch diet-fed rats; CW, corn starch diet-fed rats treated with whole linseed; CD, corn starch diet-fed rats treated with defatted linseed; CS, corn starch diet-fed rats treated with secoisolariciresinol diglucoside (SDG); H, high-carbohydrate, high-fat diet-fed rats; HW, high-carbohydrate, high-fat diet-fed rats treated with whole linseed; HD, high-carbohydrate, high-fat diet-fed rats treated with defatted linseed; and HS, high-carbohydrate, high-fat diet-fed rats treated with SDG. * Denotes the values that were normalized against tibial length and presented as tissue weight in mg/mm of tibial length.

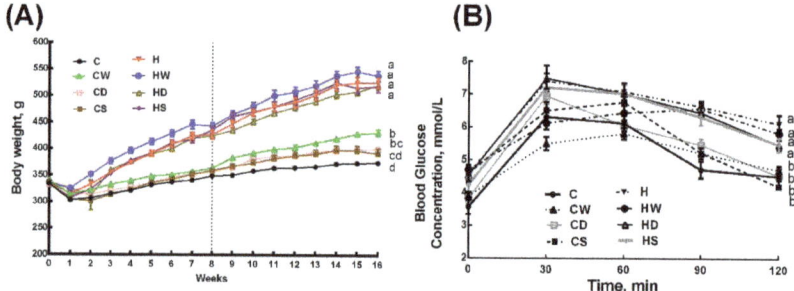

Figure 1. Effects of whole linseed, defatted linseed, and secoisolariciresinol diglucoside (SDG) on (**A**) body weight and (**B**) oral glucose tolerance test. The vertical dotted grid line in (**A**) at week 8 represents the start of treatment for rats. Data are presented as mean ± SEM, n = 10–12. End-point means with different letters (a, b, c, or d) are significantly different, $p < 0.05$. C, corn starch diet-fed rats; CW, corn starch diet-fed rats treated with whole linseed; CD, corn starch diet-fed rats treated with defatted linseed; CS, corn starch diet-fed rats treated with SDG; H, high-carbohydrate, high-fat diet-fed rats; HW, high-carbohydrate, high-fat diet-fed rats treated with whole linseed; HD, high-carbohydrate, high-fat diet-fed rats treated with defatted linseed; HS, high-carbohydrate, high-fat diet-fed rats treated with SDG.

Retroperitoneal, epididymal, and omental fat pads were higher in H rats than in C rats. CW, CD, and CS rats had no difference in these fat pads and total abdominal fat compared to C rats. SDG decreased epididymal fat in HS rats, whereas retroperitoneal, omental, and total abdominal fats were unchanged compared to H rats. Whole linseed did not change the individual fat pads in HW rats compared to H rats, whereas defatted linseed lowered retroperitoneal, epididymal, and total abdominal fat in HD rats compared to H rats (Table 1). Liver wet weights were higher in H rats than in C rats. Whole linseed, defatted linseed, and SDG treatment did not change liver wet weight compared to C or H rats (Table 1).

3.3. Metabolic Parameters

During oral glucose tolerance test, H rats showed higher basal blood glucose concentrations than C rats. Similarly, H rats showed higher 120 min glucose concentration (Figure 1B). Area under the curve for glucose tolerance test was higher in H rats compared to C, CW, CD, and CS rats. HW, HD, and HS rats were similar to H rats in area under the curve for glucose tolerance test (Table 2). Plasma total cholesterol concentrations were not different among all groups (Table 2). Plasma nonesterified fatty acids and triglyceride concentrations were higher in H rats compared to C rats, and these were unchanged with whole linseed, defatted linseed, or SDG treatment in any of the groups compared to their diet respective controls (Table 2). Plasma insulin concentrations were higher in H rats compared to C rats. HW, HD, and HS rats had lower plasma insulin concentrations compared to H rats, whereas plasma insulin concentrations were higher in CW, CD, and CS rats compared to C rats (Table 2). Plasma leptin concentrations were higher in H rats compared to C rats. CW, CD, and CS rats had no change in plasma leptin concentrations compared to C rats. Whole linseed did not change plasma leptin concentrations, whereas both SDG and defatted linseed decreased plasma leptin concentrations (Table 2).

Table 2. Metabolic, cardiovascular, and liver parameters.

Variables	C	CW	CD	CS	H	HW	HD	HS	p Value Diet	p Value Treatment	p Value Interaction
Area under the curve, mmol/L×min	636 ± 19 bc	625 ± 14 c	680 ± 14 b	687 ± 20 b	794 ± 13 a	735 ± 17 ab	770 ± 17 a	765 ± 25 a	<0.0001	0.037	0.09
Plasma total cholesterol, mmol/L	1.5 ± 0.05 a	1.3 ± 0.10 a	1.4 ± 0.10 a	1.6 ± 0.06 a	1.6 ± 0.04 a	1.5 ± 0.10 a	1.6 ± 0.10 a	1.6 ± 0.06 a	0.09	0.023	0.39
Plasma nonesterified fatty acids, mmol/L	0.9 ± 0.2 b	1.5 ± 0.2 b	1.5 ± 0.2 b	1.4 ± 0.2 b	4.3 ± 0.6 a	4.0 ± 0.3 a	3.7 ± 0.4 a	3.7 ± 0.5 a	<0.0001	0.86	0.31
Plasma triglycerides, mmol/L	0.4 ± 0.06 b	0.4 ± 0.10 b	0.5 ± 0.01 b	0.4 ± 0.06 b	1.6 ± 0.30 a	1.5 ± 0.20 a	1.3 ± 0.20 a	1.3 ± 0.20 a	<0.0001	0.68	0.68
Plasma insulin, μmol/L	1.3 ± 0.01 e	2.9 ± 0.05 c	1.7 ± 0.05 d	1.7 ± 0.01 d	7.7 ± 0.09 a	5.9 ± 0.12 b	5.8 ± 0.04 b	6.0 ± 0.11 b	<0.0001	<0.0001	<0.0001
Plasma leptin, μmol/L	3.2 ± 0.40 d	4.2 ± 0.06 d	3.9 ± 0.03 d	2.1 ± 0.62 d	12.3 ± 1.54 a	13.1 ± 0.03 a	10.2 ± 0.08 b	6.3 ± 0.97 c	<0.0001	<0.0001	0.005
Heart, mg/mm *	22.0 ± 1.0 c	25.4 ± 0.7 bc	25.3 ± 0.9 bc	21.5 ± 0.4 c	26.8 ± 1.1 b	31.5 ± 2.1 a	26.9 ± 0.9 b	23.6 ± 0.9 bc	<0.0001	<0.0001	0.18
Left ventricle + septum, mg/mm *	18.1 ± 0.7 b	21.6 ± 0.6 b	20.8 ± 0.8 b	17.2 ± 0.3 b	20.8 ± 0.8 b	27.1 ± 1.8 a	22.3 ± 0.8 b	18.5 ± 0.8 b	0.0002	<0.0001	0.09
Right ventricle, mg/mm *	4.0 ± 0.4	4.5 ± 0.4	4.5 ± 0.3	4.4 ± 0.2	6.3 ± 1.7	5.8 ± 0.4	4.7 ± 0.2	5.0 ± 0.1	0.03	0.79	0.53
Systolic blood pressure, mmHg	128 ± 3 bc	129 ± 2 bc	120 ± 3 c	133 ± 2 b	148 ± 2 a	134 ± 2 b	129 ± 5 bc	133 ± 3 b	<0.0001	0.026	0.0004
Diastolic stiffness constant (κ)	23.0 ± 0.4 bc	24.2 ± 0.7 abc	21.9 ± 0.3 c	23.0 ± 0.8 bc	26.6 ± 0.9 a	25.1 ± 0.5 ab	23.7 ± 1.3 bc	22.0 ± 0.5 c	0.034	0.001	0.004
Plasma alanine transaminase, U/L	26.8 ± 2.5 b	30.9 ± 3.8 b	28.3 ± 2.0 b	23.2 ± 1.6 b	33.7 ± 1.5 a	27.8 ± 2.5 ab	33.8 ± 1.5 a	33.6 ± 1.7 a	0.017	0.74	0.017
Plasma aspartate transaminase, U/L	64.6 ± 4.6 a	66.4 ± 5.9 a	66.3 ± 2.8 a	61.6 ± 1.8 a	68.8 ± 2.6 a	61.6 ± 3.7 a	67.5 ± 2.9 a	69.6 ± 6.8 a	0.52	0.84	0.38
Left ventricle collagen deposition, %	6.51 ± 1.0 b	6.57 ± 1.1 b	5.29 ± 0.2 b	4.96 ± 0.5 b	16.1 ± 3.7 a	13.9 ± 1.3 a	8.2 ± 0.5 b	8.3 ± 1.0 b	<0.0001	<0.0001	<0.0001
Left ventricle inflammatory cells, n	9.0 ± 2.5 b	7.5 ± 1.2 b	10.5 ± 1.6 b	12.3 ± 1.1 b	60.0 ± 4.0 a	10.8 ± 1.4 b	12.3 ± 1.1 b	10.8 ± 1.1 b	<0.0001	<0.0001	<0.0001
Liver fat vacuoles, n	4.0 ± 0.6 c	10.8 ± 1.6 c	4.0 ± 1.2 c	3.5 ± 1.0 c	75.0 ± 4.6 a	39.7 ± 4.4 b	3.5 ± 1.0 c	1.5 ± 0.9 c	<0.0001	<0.0001	<0.0001
Ileum goblet cells, n	91.5 ± 6.0 c	82.3 ± 6.1 d	107.3 ± 2.1 abc	100.3 ± 2.5 cd	124.3 ± 3.4 ab	118.3 ± 8.6 ab	94.8 ± 3.4 bc	110.8 ± 4.4 ab	0.0005	0.3224	0.0004
Colon goblet cells, n	97.5 ± 2.9 c	42 ± 5.1 d	84.5 ± 2.6 c	90.8 ± 5.2 c	78.8 ± 3.9 c	135.3 ± 2.3 b	203.8 ± 14.5 a	131.3 ± 7.3 b	<0.0001	<0.0001	<0.0001

Values are expressed as mean ± SEM, n = 8–12. Means with different superscripts (a, b, c, d, or e) differ, p < 0.05. C, corn starch diet-fed rats; CW, corn starch diet-fed rats treated with whole linseed; CD, corn starch diet-fed rats treated with defatted linseed; CS, corn starch diet-fed rats treated with secoisolariciresinol diglucoside (SDG); H, high-carbohydrate, high-fat diet-fed rats; HW, high-carbohydrate, high-fat diet-fed rats treated with whole linseed; HD, high-carbohydrate, high-fat diet-fed rats treated with defatted linseed; and HS, high-carbohydrate, high-fat diet-fed rats treated with SDG. For histological scoring, values are expressed as mean ± SEM, n = 4. * Denotes the values that were normalized against tibial length and presented as tissue weight in mg/mm of tibial length.

3.4. Cardiovascular, Liver, and Gut Parameters

Heart wet weights were higher in H rats compared to C rats. CW, CD, and CS rats showed no difference in heart weight compared to C rats. HW rats had higher heart weight compared to H rats, whereas HS and HD rats had similar heart weight to H rats (Table 2). H rats had higher systolic blood pressure than C rats. Whole linseed, defatted linseed, and SDG reduced blood pressure in HW, HD, and HS rats, respectively, compared to H rats, whereas these interventions did not change systolic blood pressure in CW, CD, and CS rats compared to C rats (Table 2). H rats had higher ventricular diastolic stiffness than C rats. SDG and defatted linseed reduced diastolic stiffness in HS and HD rats, respectively, compared to H rats, whereas none of the interventions reduced diastolic stiffness in CW, CD, or CS rats compared to C rats (Table 2).

H rats showed increased infiltration of inflammatory cells (Figure 2E) and greater interstitial collagen deposition (Figure 3E) as compared to other groups (Figure 2; Figure 3; Table 2). HW, HD, and HS rats had reduced infiltration of inflammatory cells (Figure 2F–H) and ventricular collagen deposition (Figure 3F–H; Table 2) compared to H rats.

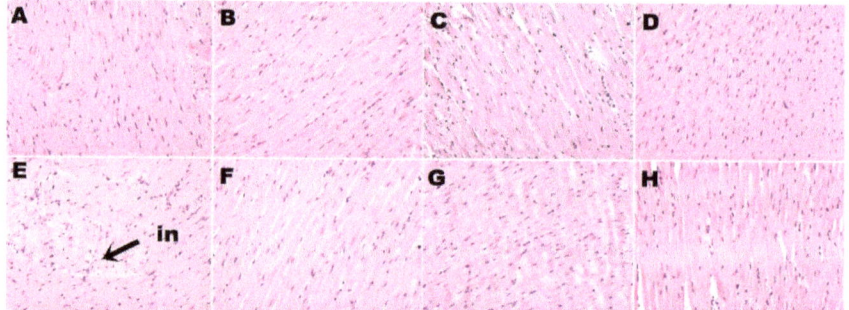

Figure 2. Hematoxylin and eosin staining of left ventricle showing infiltration of inflammatory cells (magnification ×20; shown by arrow) in rats fed corn starch diet-fed rats (**A**), corn starch diet-fed rats treated with whole linseed (**B**), corn starch diet-fed rats treated with defatted linseed (**C**), corn starch diet-fed rats treated with SDG (**D**), high-carbohydrate, high-fat diet-fed rats (**E**), high-carbohydrate, high-fat diet-fed rats treated with whole linseed (**F**), high-carbohydrate, high-fat diet-fed rats treated with defatted linseed (**G**), and high-carbohydrate, high-fat diet-fed rats treated with SDG (**H**). Inflammatory cells are marked as "in".

H rats had higher plasma alanine transaminase activity than C rats. None of the treatments in this study changed the plasma activities of alanine transaminase or aspartate transaminase (Table 2). Staining of liver sections showed increased lipid deposition and inflammatory cell infiltration in H rats (Figure 4E) compared to C rats (Figure 4A). HW (Figure 4F), HD (Figure 4G), and HS (Figure 4H) rats showed decreased inflammatory cell infiltration compared to H rats. HW rats showed some reduction in liver lipid deposition (Figure 4F), whereas HD (Figure 4G) and HS (Figure 4H) rats showed minimal lipid deposition (Table 2). CW (Figure 4B), CS (Figure 4C), and CD (Figure 4D) rats showed no changes in the liver in inflammatory cell infiltration and lipid deposition compared to C rats (Figure 4A; Table 2).

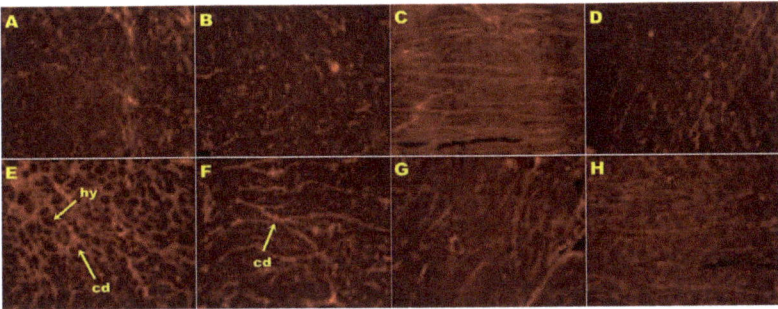

Figure 3. Picrosirius red staining of left ventricular interstitial collagen deposition (magnification ×20; shown by arrows) in rats fed corn starch diet-fed rats (**A**), corn starch diet-fed rats treated with whole linseed (**B**), corn starch diet-fed rats treated with defatted linseed (**C**), corn starch diet-fed rats treated with SDG (**D**), high-carbohydrate, high-fat diet-fed rats (**E**), high-carbohydrate, high-fat diet-fed rats treated with whole linseed (**F**), high-carbohydrate, high-fat diet-fed rats treated with defatted linseed (**G**), and high-carbohydrate, high-fat diet-fed rats treated with SDG (**H**). Collagen deposition is marked as "cd" and hypertrophied cardiomyocytes are marked as "hy".

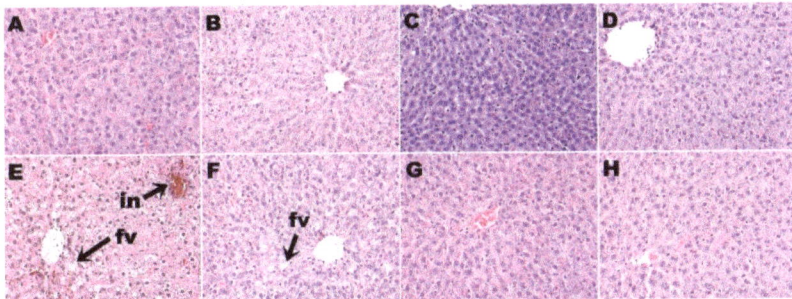

Figure 4. Hematoxylin and eosin staining of liver showing fat vacuoles and infiltration of inflammatory cells (magnification ×20; shown by arrows) in corn starch diet-fed rats (**A**), corn starch diet-fed rats treated with whole linseed (**B**), corn starch diet-fed rats treated with defatted linseed (**C**), corn starch diet-fed rats treated with SDG (**D**), high-carbohydrate, high-fat diet-fed rats (**E**), high-carbohydrate, high-fat diet-fed rats treated with whole linseed (**F**), high-carbohydrate, high-fat diet-fed rats treated with defatted linseed (**G**), and high-carbohydrate, high-fat diet-fed rats treated with SDG (**H**). Fat vacuoles are marked as "fv" and inflammatory cells are marked as "in".

Histological analyses of small intestine showed more goblet cells in H rats (Figure 5E) compared to C rats (Figure 5A; Table 2). HW (Figure 5F) and HS (Figure 5H) rats showed no change in the number of goblet cells in the small intestine, whereas HD rats (Figure 5G) showed reduction in the number of goblet cells (Table 2) compared to H rats (Figure 5E). Colon from C rats (Figure 6A) and H rats (Figure 6E) showed no difference in the number of goblet cells (Table 2). HW (Figure 6F), HD (Figure 6G), and HS (Figure 6H) rats showed an increase in the number of goblet cells in colons compared to H rats (Figure 6E; Table 2).

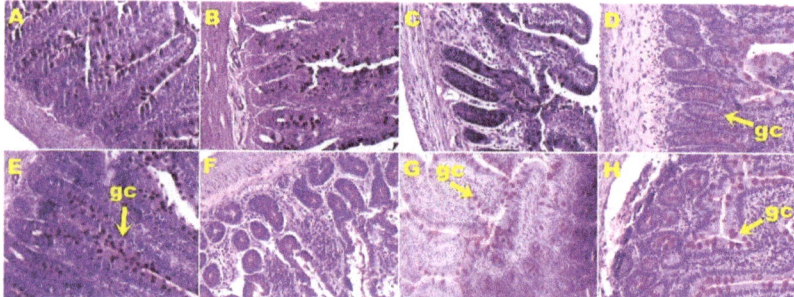

Figure 5. Periodic acid-Schiff staining of ileum showing goblet cells (magnification ×20; shown by arrows) in corn starch diet-fed rats (**A**), corn starch diet-fed rats treated with whole linseed (**B**), corn starch diet-fed rats treated with defatted linseed (**C**), corn starch diet-fed rats treated with SDG (**D**), high-carbohydrate, high-fat diet-fed rats (**E**), high-carbohydrate, high-fat diet-fed rats treated with whole linseed (**F**), high-carbohydrate, high-fat diet-fed rats treated with defatted linseed (**G**), and high-carbohydrate, high-fat diet-fed rats treated with SDG (**H**). Goblet cells are marked as "gc".

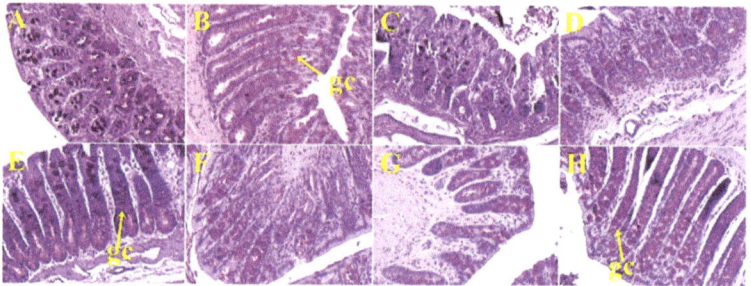

Figure 6. Periodic acid-Schiff staining of colon showing goblet cells (magnification ×20; shown by arrows) in corn starch diet-fed rats (**A**), corn starch diet-fed rats treated with whole linseed (**B**), corn starch diet-fed rats treated with defatted linseed (**C**), corn starch diet-fed rats treated with SDG (**D**), high-carbohydrate, high-fat diet-fed rats (**E**), high-carbohydrate, high-fat diet-fed rats treated with whole linseed (**F**), high-carbohydrate, high-fat diet-fed rats treated with defatted linseed (**G**), and high-carbohydrate, high-fat diet-fed rats treated with SDG (**H**). Goblet cells are marked as "gc".

4. Discussion

Metabolic syndrome, including obesity, hypertension, impaired glucose tolerance, insulin resistance, dyslipidemia, and fatty liver, is a major risk factor for cardiovascular disease and type 2 diabetes, and may be attenuated by functional foods [18]. Many trials have been conducted to determine the responses to linseed and its components in humans with obesity, hypertension, or diabetes [19,20]. However, few trials have compared responses to individual components of linseed in patients with metabolic syndrome or in appropriate rat models. Rats fed a diet with increased content of fructose, sucrose, and saturated and *trans* fatty acids developed signs of metabolic syndrome in humans, especially abdominal obesity, hypertension, impaired glucose and leptin, dyslipidemia, and diminished cardiac function [13–15]. Using this rat model of diet-induced metabolic syndrome, we have now compared responses to whole linseed, defatted linseed flour, and SDG and included comparison with an earlier study on ALA from linseed oil with the same rat model [14].

Our results show that addition of defatted linseed or SDG improved metabolic parameters and the structure and function of the heart and liver, as we previously showed with linseed oil [14]. In contrast, the only metabolic parameter to be improved by whole linseed was plasma insulin concentration, while body weight, abdominal fat pads, and liver parameters were unchanged. Although whole linseed decreased systolic blood pressure, left ventricular diastolic stiffness, infiltration of inflammatory cells, and collagen deposition in the heart, these changes were to a lesser extent than defatted linseed, showing reduced or absent responses in cardiovascular, hepatic structure and function, adiposity, lipid, and glucose parameters. We suggest that the reason for these reduced responses to whole linseed is that the oral bioavailability of ALA, fiber, and SDG when presented as whole linseed is reduced, leading to reduced responses to the whole seeds, even though the components are effective when given individually. This could be tested in further studies by measurement of the pharmacokinetics of linseed components such as ALA, fiber, or SDG in rats fed an obesogenic diet.

In this study with whole linseeds and their components in rats, we were unable to show decreases in body weight or abdominal circumference with whole linseed treatment in diet-induced obese rats. In contrast, we showed decreased total fat and abdominal fat in rats treated with defatted linseed or SDG. We have previously shown that ALA from linseed decreased obesity in the same diet-induced rat model of metabolic syndrome [14]. Other studies also showed decreased obesity with linseed products: young rats fed a linseed flour intervention for the first 90 days showed higher lean mass, lower fat mas, and a smaller adipocyte area [21] and linseed dietary fiber reduced apparent energy and fat digestibility leading to decreased abdominal fat and body weight [22]. Linseed contains 20 to 30% globulin-rich proteins with a high content of arginine [23,24] which has been associated with increases in lean mass [25,26] thereby providing a possible mechanism for lean mass increase as well as fat mass decrease [27]. In high-fat diet-fed mice, SDG decreased abdominal fat and body weight by inducing adiponectin expression at a much higher dose of 0.5 or 1% in diet [28] and inhibiting adipogenesis at a dose of 50 mg/kg/day [29]. Furthermore, the SDG metabolites, enterolactone and enterodiol, induced adiponectin expression, adipogenesis, and lipid uptake in 3T3-L1 adipocytes [28,30]. We are not aware of any studies with whole linseeds in obese rats, but freshly ground flaxseed did not change body weight or blood pressure in non-obese WKY or SHR rats and in cyclosporine-induced hypertensive rats [31,32].

These rodent results translate to some extent to humans. Linseed products reduced human obesity in randomized controlled trials, shown by a meta-analysis of 45 of these trials with 2561 subjects aged 25.6–67.0 years including 21 trials on milled or ground linseed, one on defatted linseed, 18 on linseed oil, and five on linseed lignan but none on whole linseeds [19]. This meta-analysis showed that supplementation of linseed products for more than 12 weeks in individuals with a body mass index higher than 27 kg/m^2 reduced body weight by an average of 0.99 kg, body mass index by an average of 0.30 kg/m^2, and waist circumference by an average of 0.80 cm [19]. These changes are relatively small, approximating 1% of these parameters in a 1.80 m tall person weighing 88 kg to give a body mass index of 27 kg/m^2 fitting the definition of obesity with waist circumference more than 94 cm. Differences of around 1% as in the above meta-analysis on human trials would not be statistically significant in our group of 12 rats treated for eight weeks. In addition, data from the US National Health and Nutrition Examination Survey 2001-10 provided epidemiological evidence that urinary enterolactone is inversely associated with obesity in adult males [33].

Linseed products also reduced blood pressure in rodents. Both linseed oil and SDG prevented the increase in systolic blood pressure in rats with metabolic syndrome induced by feeding with 30% fructose, likely due to decreased oxidative stress [34]. In deoxycorticosterone acetate (DOCA)-salt hypertensive rats, linseed lignan concentrate lowered blood pressure, and improved antioxidant status, serum electrolytes, and lipid profiles [35]. A lignan-enriched linseed powder reduced blood pressure, body weight, and fat accumulation, and improved lipid profiles in rats fed a high-fat and high-fructose diet [36]. In humans with peripheral artery disease, ground linseed (30 g/day) for 12 months decreased central systolic and diastolic blood pressure by 10 and 6 mmHg, respectively, with corresponding changes in plasma oxylipins [37]. Meta-analysis of 15 randomized controlled trials with linseed components on hypertension have shown reductions in both systolic and diastolic blood pressure of 3.10 and 2.62 mmHg, respectively, in a subset of trials of 12 weeks or longer, but there were no effects with linseed oil or SDG on systolic blood pressure [20].

Hyperlipidemia is a key component of metabolic syndrome. In rats fed a high-fat diet, a lignan-enriched linseed powder improved the plasma lipid profile as well as decreasing body weight, visceral fat accumulation, and blood pressure [36]. In rats fed with lard and cholic acid, treatment with powdered linseed or defatted linseed for eight weeks did not change plasma cholesterol, low-density lipoproteins (LDL) cholesterol, or triglyceride concentrations but decreased liver fat and cholesterol and increased bacterial glycolytic activity in the distal intestine [38]. Intervention with linseed powder (30 g/day for 40 days) produced small but significant decreases in body weight and decreased plasma cholesterol, LDL, and triglyceride concentrations in 35 hyperlipidemic subjects [39]. Furthermore, linseed may reduce plasma concentrations of the inflammatory marker, C-reactive protein, in subjects with a body mass index (BMI) > 30 kg/m^2 [40]; this meta-analysis included trials on ground linseed, flour, oil, and ALA-enriched products, but there were no studies on whole linseeds.

The combination of ALA, dietary fiber, and lignans in linseed may be useful in preventing and treating diabetes, especially in rodent models [41]. SDG and its enteric metabolite enterodiol affected glucose transport and adipogenesis by regulating the transcription of adiponectin, leptin, and peroxisome proliferator-activated receptor gamma (PPARγ) genes [28]. By altering the expression profile of adiponectin and leptin, SDG may increase rates of fatty acid oxidation and mediate an insulin-sensitizing effect [42]. Although these findings are consistent with the decrease in plasma insulin and leptin observed in our study, it is not clear why glucose tolerance was only improved in the whole linseed group.

Thus, our results are broadly consistent with both rodent and human studies on individual signs of metabolic syndrome and individual components of linseeds. However, these literature studies do not compare results in the range of signs in metabolic syndrome in the same subject groups or rodent models, nor allow comparison of linseed components. Furthermore, no study has administered whole linseeds, so the comparison between whole linseeds and components has not been previously made.

Gastrointestinal changes could play a role in the metabolic responses to ground or defatted linseed, but studies on whole linseeds have not been reported. Linseed is a rich source of dietary fiber (35–45%) consisting of soluble and insoluble fiber in ratios that vary between 1:4 and 2:3 [43]. Rats on a control diet fed 10% dietary fiber from linseeds showed decreased body weight with decreased fat digestibility, which was greater when the proportion of viscous dietary fiber was increased [22]. In obese rats fed a high-fat diet with cholic acid, ground linseed prevented an increase in intestinal glucosidase activity while defatted ground linseed increased mucosal disaccharidase activities; both forms decreased fat absorption but only the defatted product decreased liver expression of PPARα, showing important differences between defatted and whole ground linseed [38]. Fermentation of dietary fiber by colonic microflora generates short-chain fatty acids such as acetate, propionate, and butyrate which decrease signs of metabolic syndrome and other gastrointestinal disorders [44]. High-fermentable fiber of milled whole linseed led to increased *Enterobacteriaceae* diversity in mice which was associated with an increased body weight compared to milled defatted linseed [45]. In healthy, non-obese adult men given 0.3 g/kg/day ground linseed for one week, enterolignan production was increased, but there were no changes in fecal metabolome or dominant bacterial communities [46]. Thus, the responses to defatted linseed in contrast to whole linseed could be produced by the increased bioavailable fiber content acting on the colonic microflora and liver, and possibly on goblet cell function. Goblet cells in the gastrointestinal tract are responsible for secretion of mucus, but the location of the goblet cells determines whether secretion is continuous or upon stimulation to form the protective inner colonic mucosal layer [47]. Mice fed a high-fat diet showed increased goblet cells in the duodenum [48]. Dietary intervention with whole ground linseed increased goblet cells, mucus secretion, and concentrations of short-chain fatty acids in healthy male mice which should be beneficial [49]. This increase could be due to an increase in fiber [50], consistent with our results in rats fed defatted linseed. However, the intervention with whole ground linseed worsened the damage by dextran sodium sulfate suggesting a role for context in interventions [49], but similar studies in high-fat diet-fed rats are not available. The different results in rats fed whole linseed, SDG, and defatted linseed suggest that these components of linseed produce different responses in goblet cells in the colon, possibly due to different types of goblet cells, requiring detailed research to define adequately.

The marked differences in responses between whole linseeds and the components of linseeds could be due to toxic compounds present in the whole linseed, such as the cyanogenic glycosides, leading to cyanide production by the activity of bacterial glucosidases in the large intestine [51]. However, ingestion of 30 g linseed by humans produced small and transient increases in plasma thiocyanate concentrations, indicating a low bioavailability of the cyanide from cyanogenic glycosides such as linustatin [52]. Thus, we suggest that a more likely explanation for the lower responses in whole linseeds is a markedly reduced oral bioavailability of the bioactive components when whole linseeds are given.

5. Conclusions

This study has highlighted the importance of using a single animal model to investigate the bioactivities of individual functional foods contained in linseed. We hypothesized that whole linseeds and the isolated components would improve cardiovascular, metabolic, and liver changes. We showed that the responses to the whole linseeds were reduced compared to defatted linseed, SDG, and ALA. We suggest that a markedly reduced bioavailability of these components from the whole linseeds underlies the reduced responses. Thus, our hypothesis was substantiated by measurements of physiological responses to the components of linseeds. However, ALA, defatted linseed, or SDG are likely to be better therapeutic agents in metabolic syndrome than whole linseeds.

Author Contributions: Conceptualization, S.K.P. and L.B.; Formal analysis, S.R.S. and S.W.; Investigation, S.R.S. and S.W.; Methodology, S.R.S., S.W., and S.K.P.; Project administration, S.K.P.; Resources, L.B.; Supervision, S.K.P. and L.B. All authors read and approved the final manuscript.

Funding: We thank the University of Southern Queensland Research & Innovation Division for the Strategic Research Funds required for this study.

Acknowledgments: We thank Brian Bynon (School of Veterinary Science, The University of Queensland, Gatton, QLD, Australia) for helping with plasma analyses for this study. SDG (40% purity) was a gift from Archer Daniels Midland Company (Chicago, IL, USA). We thank St. Boniface Hospital Research (Winnipeg, MB, Canada) for providing SDG and its analysis. We also thank AustGrains (Moree, NSW, Australia) for providing linseed for this study.

Conflicts of Interest: The authors declare no conflict of interest.

References

1. Goyal, A.; Sharma, V.; Upadhyay, N.; Gill, S.; Sihag, M. Flax and flaxseed oil: An ancient medicine & modern functional food. *J. Food Sci. Technol.* **2014**, *51*, 1633–1653. [CrossRef]
2. Shim, Y.Y.; Gui, B.; Arnison, P.G.; Wang, Y.; Reaney, M.J.T. Flaxseed (*Linum usitatissimum* L.) bioactive compounds and peptide nomenclature: A review. *Trends Food Sci. Technol.* **2014**, *38*, 5–20. [CrossRef]
3. Parikh, M.; Netticadan, T.; Pierce, G.N. Flaxseed: Its bioactive components and their cardiovascular benefits. *Am. J. Physiol. Heart Circ. Physiol.* **2018**, *314*, H146–H159. [CrossRef]
4. Shafie, S.R.; Poudyal, H.; Panchal, S.K.; Brown, L. Linseed as a functional food for the management of obesity. In *Omega-3 Fatty Acids: Keys to Nutritional Health*; Hegde, M.V., Zanwar, A.A., Adekar, S.P., Eds.; Springer International Publishing: Cham, Switzerland, 2016; pp. 173–187.
5. Imran, M.; Ahmad, N.; Anjum, F.M.; Khan, M.K.; Mushtaq, Z.; Nadeem, M.; Hussain, S. Potential protective properties of flax lignan secoisolariciresinol diglucoside. *Nutr. J.* **2015**, *14*, 71. [CrossRef]
6. Parikh, M.; Pierce, G.N. Dietary flaxseed: What we know and don't know about its effects on cardiovascular disease. *Can. J. Physiol. Pharmacol.* **2018**, *97*, 75–81. [CrossRef]
7. Oomah, B.D.; Mazza, G. Effect of dehulling on chemical composition and physical properties of flaxseed. *LWT—Food Sci. Technol.* **1997**, *30*, 135–140. [CrossRef]
8. Kuijsten, A.; Arts, I.C.W.; van't Veer, P.; Hollman, P.C.H. The relative bioavailability of enterolignans in humans is enhanced by milling and crushing of flaxseed. *J. Nutr.* **2005**, *135*, 2812–2816. [CrossRef]

9. Waszkowiak, K.; Gliszczynska-Swiglo, A.; Barthet, V.; Skrety, J. Effect of extraction method on the phenolic and cyanogenic glucoside profile of flaxseed extracts and their antioxidant capacity. *J. Am. Oil Chem. Soc.* **2015**, *92*, 1609–1619. [CrossRef]
10. Kajla, P.; Sharma, A.; Sood, D.R. Flaxseed-a potential functional food source. *J. Food Sci. Technol.* **2015**, *52*, 1857–1871. [CrossRef]
11. Austria, J.A.; Richard, M.N.; Chahine, M.N.; Edel, A.L.; Malcolmson, L.J.; Dupasquier, C.M.; Pierce, G.N. Bioavailability of *a*-linolenic acid in subjects after ingestion of three different forms of flaxseed. *J. Am. Coll. Nutr.* **2008**, *27*, 214–221. [CrossRef]
12. Mukker, J.K.; Singh, R.S.; Muir, A.D.; Krol, E.S.; Alcorn, J. Comparative pharmacokinetics of purified flaxseed and associated mammalian lignans in male Wistar rats. *Br. J. Nutr.* **2015**, *113*, 749–757. [CrossRef] [PubMed]
13. Panchal, S.K.; Poudyal, H.; Iyer, A.; Nazer, R.; Alam, M.A.; Diwan, V.; Kauter, K.; Sernia, C.; Campbell, F.; Ward, L.; et al. High-carbohydrate, high-fat diet-induced metabolic syndrome and cardiovascular remodeling in rats. *J. Cardiovasc. Pharmacol.* **2011**, *57*, 611–624. [CrossRef] [PubMed]
14. Poudyal, H.; Kumar, S.A.; Iyer, A.; Waanders, J.; Ward, L.C.; Brown, L. Responses to oleic, linoleic and *a*-linolenic acids in high-carbohydrate, high-fat diet-induced metabolic syndrome in rats. *J. Nutr. Biochem.* **2013**, *24*, 1381–1392. [CrossRef] [PubMed]
15. Poudyal, H.; Panchal, S.K.; Waanders, J.; Ward, L.; Brown, L. Lipid redistribution by *a*-linolenic acid-rich chia seed inhibits stearoyl-CoA desaturase-1 and induces cardiac and hepatic protection in diet-induced obese rats. *J. Nutr. Biochem.* **2012**, *23*, 153–162. [CrossRef] [PubMed]
16. Khattab, R.Y.; Zeitoun, M.A. Quality evaluation of flaxseed oil obtained by different extraction techniques. *LWT—Food Sci. Technol.* **2013**, *53*, 338–345. [CrossRef]
17. Ghattamaneni, N.K.R.; Panchal, S.K.; Brown, L. An improved rat model for chronic inflammatory bowel disease. *Pharmacol. Rep.* **2018**, *71*, 149–155. [CrossRef] [PubMed]
18. Brown, L.; Poudyal, H.; Panchal, S.K. Functional foods as potential therapeutic options for metabolic syndrome. *Obes. Rev.* **2015**, *16*, 914–941. [CrossRef] [PubMed]
19. Mohammadi-Sartang, M.; Mazloom, Z.; Raeisi-Dehkordi, H.; Barati-Boldaji, R.; Bellissimo, N.; Totosy de Zepetnek, J.O. The effect of flaxseed supplementation on body weight and body composition: A systematic review and meta-analysis of 45 randomized placebo-controlled trials. *Obes. Rev.* **2017**, *18*, 1096–1107. [CrossRef]
20. Ursoniu, S.; Sahebkar, A.; Andrica, F.; Serban, C.; Banach, M. Effects of flaxseed supplements on blood pressure: A systematic review and meta-analysis of controlled clinical trial. *Clin. Nutr.* **2016**, *35*, 615–625. [CrossRef]
21. Da Costa, C.A.; da Silva, P.C.; Ribeiro, D.C.; Pereira, A.D.; dos Santos Ade, S.; de Abreu, M.D.; Pessoa, L.R.; Boueri, B.F.; Pessanha, C.R.; do Nascimento-Saba, C.C.; et al. Effects of diet containing flaxseed flour (*Linum usitatissimum*) on body adiposity and bone health in young male rats. *Food Funct.* **2016**, *7*, 698–703. [CrossRef]
22. Kristensen, M.; Knudsen, K.E.; Jorgensen, H.; Oomah, D.; Bugel, S.; Toubro, S.; Tetens, I.; Astrup, A. Linseed dietary fibers reduce apparent digestibility of energy and fat and weight gain in growing rats. *Nutrients* **2013**, *5*, 3287–3298. [CrossRef] [PubMed]
23. Sammour, R.H. Proteins of linseed (*Linum usitatissimum* L.), extraction and characterization by electrophoresis. *Bot. Bull. Acad. Sin.* **1999**, *40*, 121–126.
24. Chung, M.W.Y.; Lei, B.; Li-Chan, E.C.Y. Isolation and structural characterization of the major protein fraction from NorMan flaxseed (*Linum usitatissimum* L.). *Food Chem.* **2005**, *90*, 271–279. [CrossRef]
25. Borsheim, E.; Bui, Q.U.; Tissier, S.; Kobayashi, H.; Ferrando, A.A.; Wolfe, R.R. Effect of amino acid supplementation on muscle mass, strength and physical function in elderly. *Clin. Nutr.* **2008**, *27*, 189–195. [CrossRef] [PubMed]
26. Pahlavani, N.; Entezari, M.H.; Nasiri, M.; Miri, A.; Rezaie, M.; Bagheri-Bidakhavidi, M.; Sadeghi, O. The effect of L-arginine supplementation on body composition and performance in male athletes: A double-blinded randomized clinical trial. *Eur. J. Clin. Nutr.* **2017**, *71*, 544–548. [CrossRef] [PubMed]
27. Alam, M.A.; Kauter, K.; Withers, K.; Sernia, C.; Brown, L. Chronic L-arginine treatment improves metabolic, cardiovascular and liver complications in diet-induced obesity in rats. *Food Funct.* **2013**, *4*, 83–91. [CrossRef] [PubMed]

28. Fukumitsu, S.; Aida, K.; Ueno, N.; Ozawa, S.; Takahashi, Y.; Kobori, M. Flaxseed lignan attenuates high-fat diet-induced fat accumulation and induces adiponectin expression in mice. *Br. J. Nutr.* **2008**, *100*, 669–676. [CrossRef] [PubMed]
29. Kang, J.; Park, J.; Kim, H.L.; Jung, Y.; Youn, D.H.; Lim, S.; Song, G.; Park, H.; Jin, J.S.; Kwak, H.J.; et al. Secoisolariciresinol diglucoside inhibits adipogenesis through the AMPK pathway. *Eur. J. Pharmacol.* **2018**, *820*, 235–244. [CrossRef] [PubMed]
30. Biasiotto, G.; Zanella, I.; Predolini, F.; Archetti, I.; Cadei, M.; Monti, E.; Luzzani, M.; Pacchetti, B.; Mozzoni, P.; Andreoli, R.; et al. 7-Hydroxymatairesinol improves body weight, fat and sugar metabolism in C57BJ/6 mice on a high-fat diet. *Br. J. Nutr.* **2018**, *120*, 751–762. [CrossRef] [PubMed]
31. Talom, R.T.; Judd, S.A.; McIntosh, D.D.; McNeill, J.R. High flaxseed (linseed) diet restores endothelial function in the mesenteric arterial bed of spontaneously hypertensive rats. *Life Sci.* **1999**, *64*, 1415–1425. [CrossRef]
32. Al-Bishri, W.M. Favorable effects of flaxseed supplemented diet on liver and kidney functions in hypertensive Wistar rats. *J. Oleo Sci.* **2013**, *62*, 709–715. [CrossRef] [PubMed]
33. Xu, C.; Liu, Q.; Zhang, Q.; Gu, A.; Jiang, Z.Y. Urinary enterolactone is associated with obesity and metabolic alteration in men in the US National Health and Nutrition Examination Survey 2001-10. *Br. J. Nutr.* **2015**, *113*, 683–690. [CrossRef] [PubMed]
34. Pilar, B.; Gullich, A.; Oliveira, P.; Stroher, D.; Piccoli, J.; Manfredini, V. Protective role of flaxseed oil and flaxseed lignan secoisolariciresinol diglucoside against oxidative stress in rats with metabolic syndrome. *J. Food Sci.* **2017**, *82*, 3029–3036. [CrossRef] [PubMed]
35. Sawant, S.H.; Bodhankar, S.L. Flax lignan concentrate reverses alterations in blood pressure, left ventricular functions, lipid profile and antioxidant status in DOCA-salt induced renal hypertension in rats. *Ren. Fail.* **2016**, *38*, 411–423. [CrossRef] [PubMed]
36. Park, J.B.; Velasquez, M.T. Potential effects of lignan-enriched flaxseed powder on bodyweight, visceral fat, lipid profile, and blood pressure in rats. *Fitoterapia* **2012**, *83*, 941–946. [CrossRef] [PubMed]
37. Caligiuri, S.P.; Rodriguez-Leyva, D.; Aukema, H.M.; Ravandi, A.; Weighell, W.; Guzman, R.; Pierce, G.N. Dietary flaxseed reduces central aortic blood pressure without cardiac involvement but through changes in plasma oxylipins. *Hypertension* **2016**, *68*, 1031–1038. [CrossRef] [PubMed]
38. Opyd, P.M.; Jurgonski, A.; Juskiewicz, J.; Fotschki, B.; Koza, J. Comparative effects of native and defatted flaxseeds on intestinal enzyme activity and lipid metabolism in rats fed a high-fat diet containing cholic acid. *Nutrients* **2018**, *10*, 1181. [CrossRef]
39. Torkan, M.; Entezari, M.H.; Siavash, M. Effect of flaxseed on blood lipid level in hyperlipidemic patients. *Rev. Recent Clin. Trials* **2015**, *10*, 61–67. [CrossRef]
40. Ren, G.Y.; Chen, C.Y.; Chen, G.C.; Chen, W.G.; Pan, A.; Pan, C.W.; Zhang, Y.H.; Qin, L.Q.; Chen, L.H. Effect of flaxseed intervention on inflammatory marker C-reactive protein: A systematic review and meta-analysis of randomized controlled trials. *Nutrients* **2016**, *8*, 136. [CrossRef]
41. Kailash, P.; Arti, D. Flaxseed and diabetes. *Curr. Pharm. Des.* **2016**, *22*, 141–144. [CrossRef]
42. Dyck, D.J.; Heigenhauser, G.J.; Bruce, C.R. The role of adipokines as regulators of skeletal muscle fatty acid metabolism and insulin sensitivity. *Acta Physiol.* **2006**, *186*, 5–16. [CrossRef] [PubMed]
43. Singh, K.K.; Mridula, D.; Rehal, J.; Barnwal, P. Flaxseed: A potential source of food, feed and fiber. *Crit. Rev. Food Sci. Nutr.* **2011**, *51*, 210–222. [CrossRef] [PubMed]
44. Requena, T.; Martínez-Cuesta, M.C.; Peláez, C. Diet and microbiota linked in health and disease. *Food Funct.* **2018**, *9*, 688–704. [CrossRef] [PubMed]
45. Pulkrabek, M.; Rhee, Y.; Gibbs, P.; Hall, C. Flaxseed- and buckwheat-supplemented diets altered *Enterobacteriaceae* diversity and prevalence in the cecum and feces of obese mice. *J. Diet. Suppl.* **2017**, *14*, 667–678. [CrossRef] [PubMed]
46. Lagkouvardos, I.; Kläring, K.; Heinzmann, S.S.; Platz, S.; Scholz, B.; Engel, K.-H.; Schmitt-Kopplin, P.; Haller, D.; Rohn, S.; Skurk, T.; et al. Gut metabolites and bacterial community networks during a pilot intervention study with flaxseeds in healthy adult men. *Mol. Nutr. Food Res.* **2015**, *59*, 1614–1628. [CrossRef] [PubMed]
47. Birchenough, G.M.; Johansson, M.E.; Gustafsson, J.K.; Bergstrom, J.H.; Hansson, G.C. New developments in goblet cell mucus secretion and function. *Mucosal Immunol.* **2015**, *8*, 712–719. [CrossRef] [PubMed]

48. Lecomte, M.; Couedelo, L.; Meugnier, E.; Plaisancie, P.; Letisse, M.; Benoit, B.; Gabert, L.; Penhoat, A.; Durand, A.; Pineau, G.; et al. Dietary emulsifiers from milk and soybean differently impact adiposity and inflammation in association with modulation of colonic goblet cells in high-fat fed mice. *Mol. Nutr. Food Res.* **2016**, *60*, 609–620. [CrossRef] [PubMed]
49. Power, K.A.; Lepp, D.; Zarepoor, L.; Monk, J.M.; Wu, W.; Tsao, R.; Liu, R. Dietary flaxseed modulates the colonic microenvironment in healthy C57Bl/6 male mice which may alter susceptibility to gut-associated diseases. *J. Nutr. Biochem.* **2016**, *28*, 61–69. [CrossRef] [PubMed]
50. Tanabe, H.; Ito, H.; Sugiyama, K.; Kiriyama, S.; Morita, T. Dietary indigestible components exert different regional effects on luminal mucin secretion through their bulk-forming property and fermentability. *Biosci. Biotechnol. Biochem.* **2006**, *70*, 1188–1194. [CrossRef]
51. Cressey, P.; Reeve, J. Metabolism of cyanogenic glycosides: A review. *Food Chem. Toxicol.* **2019**, *125*, 225–232. [CrossRef]
52. Schulz, V.; Loffler, A.; Gheorghiu, T. Resorption of hydrocyanic acid from linseed. *Leber Magen Darm* **1983**, *13*, 10–14.

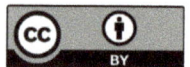

© 2019 by the authors. Licensee MDPI, Basel, Switzerland. This article is an open access article distributed under the terms and conditions of the Creative Commons Attribution (CC BY) license (http://creativecommons.org/licenses/by/4.0/).

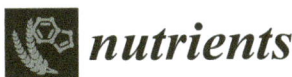 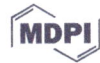

Review

Negative Energy Balance Induced by Exercise or Diet: Effects on Visceral Adipose Tissue and Liver Fat

Robert Ross *, Simrat Soni and Sarah Houle

School of Kinesiology and Health Studies, Department of Endocrinology and Metabolism, Queen's University, Kingston, ON K7L 3N6, Canada; s.soni@queensu.ca (S.S.); sarah.houle@queensu.ca (S.H.)
* Correspondence: rossr@queensu.ca; Tel.: +(613)-533-6583

Received: 18 February 2020; Accepted: 17 March 2020; Published: 25 March 2020

Abstract: The indisputable association between visceral adipose tissue (VAT) and cardiometabolic risk makes it a primary target for lifestyle-based strategies designed to prevent or manage health risk. Substantive evidence also confirms that liver fat (LF) is positively associated with increased health risk and that reduction is associated with an improved metabolic profile. The independent associations between reductions in VAT, LF, and cardiometabolic risk is less clear. In this narrative review, we summarize the evidence indicating whether a negative energy balance induced by either an increase in energy expenditure (aerobic exercise) or a decrease in energy intake (hypocaloric diet) are effective strategies for reducing both VAT and LF. Consideration will be given to whether a dose-response relationship exists between the negative energy balance induced by exercise or diet and reduction in either VAT or LF. We conclude with recommendations that will help fill gaps in knowledge with respect to lifestyle-based strategies designed to reduce VAT and LF.

Keywords: exercise; abdominal obesity; energy balance; caloric restriction; non-alcoholic fatty liver disease; physical activity

1. Introduction

Decades of evidence have firmly established that VAT is associated with cardiometabolic risk factors beyond obesity per se [1]. There is no dispute that VAT represents a primary treatment target for strategies designed to prevent or manage the health risks associated with abdominal obesity. The findings from systematic reviews confirm that a negative energy balance induced by exercise or diet is associated with significant reductions in VAT and associated cardiometabolic risk factors [2,3]. Routine exercise consistent with current guidelines, in combination with a balanced diet, is associated with significant reductions in VAT. Whether exercise or a hypocaloric diet is associated with VAT reduction in a dose-response manner remains unclear. It is also unclear whether exercise intensity is positively associated with VAT reduction. What is clear, however, is that exercise or diet is associated with a reduction in VAT and associated cardiometabolic risk factors with minimal or no weight loss [4]. This is good news for practitioners who seek treatment options for their patients/clients.

Non-alcoholic fatty liver disease (NAFLD), an umbrella term that encompasses the deposition of lipid in the liver to more progressive steatosis and associated hepatitis, fibrosis, and cirrhosis, is recognized as an ectopic site of fat deposition that has serious health consequences [5]. Although LF accumulation is positively associated with VAT, there is evidence to suggest that LF is associated with cardiometabolic risk factors independent of VAT [6]. Thus, LF represents another target for strategies designed to reduce obesity-related health risk. In adults with or without NAFLD, exercise induced-negative energy balance consistent with current guidelines is associated with a marked reduction in LF.

In this narrative review, we summarize the evidence indicating whether a negative energy balance induced by either an increase in energy expenditure (aerobic exercise), or a decrease in energy intake (hypocaloric diet), are effective strategies for reducing both VAT and LF. The primary focus of this review was to report on findings from randomized trials with supervised aerobic exercise and monitoredhypocaloric diet interventions. Consideration was given to whether a dose-response relationship exists between the negative energy balance induced by exercise or diet and reduction in either VAT or LF. We conclude with recommendations that will help fill gaps in knowledge with respect to lifestyle-based strategies designed to reduce VAT and LF.

2. Visceral Adipose Tissue (VAT)

2.1. Measurement of VAT

Several methodologies for assessing VAT volume and distribution have been established. The criterion methods, which provide direct measurement of partial or total volumes, include magnetic resonance imaging (MRI) and computed tomography (CT) [4]. More recently, dual energy X-ray absorptiometry (DXA) has been identified as a reference method for assessing body composition [7]. However, due to high cost and feasibility issues, indirect estimates of VAT are often performed using anthropometric measures, including waist circumference, sagittal diameter, and bioelectrical impedance analysis [4]. When using MRI or CT to determine the effects of exercise or diet on VAT, it is important to note that change in VAT determined using a single image (e.g., a single image obtained at the level of the L4-L5 intervertebral space) is not materially different from the corresponding reduction in VAT derived using a multiple-image protocol [8]. Thus, when accessible, a single MRI or CT image can be used to accurately determine VAT distribution and/or reduction throughout the abdomen.

2.2. Is VAT Reduced in Response to Chronic Exercise or Hypocaloric Diets?

Evidence from a systematic review and meta-analysis clearly established that an increase in energy expenditure (aerobic exercise), or a decrease in energy intake (hypocaloric diet), are both associated with significant reductions in VAT, measured using gold standard methods [2]. Ross and colleagues were the first to investigate whether differences in VAT reduction were observed in response to equivalent diet- versus exercise-induced weight loss in either men [9] or women [10]. These RCTs were characterized by control of both energy expenditure (supervised exercise) and energy intake (self-reported intake every day). VAT was quantified using MRI. In these trials, participants in the exercise group did not increase or decrease their energy intake throughout the intervention, whereas those in the hypocaloric diet group did not increase physical activity levels. The primary finding from these trials revealed that when the diet- and exercise-induced weight loss was carefully matched, reductions in abdominal obesity and VAT in response to 12–14 weeks of exercise or diet were similar. Regardless of biological sex, a ~7% weight loss was associated with a ~25% reduction in VAT in response to diet or exercise[1]. These observations are consistent with the recent systematic review of Verheggen et al., wherein the results from eight studies in adults revealed that diet or exercise is associated with similar reductions in VAT when the negative energy balance and duration of intervention is matched [2]. Additionally, in response to an 18-month diet and exercise-based intervention among 278 sedentary adults with abdominal obesity, Gepner and colleagues reported that diet combined with exercise results in greater reductions in VAT than diet alone, assessed using MRI [11]. In summary, regardless of age or biological sex, a negative energy balance induced by diet or exercise is associated with marked reductions in VAT that are not materially different.

2.2.1. Exercise Amount and VAT

While the evidence reviewed clearly establishes that regular exercise combined with a healthful diet is associated with a marked reduction in VAT, independent of age and biological sex, the separate effects of exercise amount and intensity on VAT are less clear. The findings from a systematic review suggest that a dose-response relationship exists between exercise amount, defined by the metabolic equivalent of task (MET-hours/week), and reductions in VAT in individuals without metabolic disorder [12]. All 16 studies included in the review measured VAT using CT or MRI.

The findings from the few randomized trials specifically designed to examine the independent contributions of exercise amount on VAT suggested that increasing exercise amount (caloric expenditure) is not positively associated with VAT reduction. Keating et al. randomized inactive, obese adults to eight weeks of either; (i) low to moderate intensity, high amount aerobic exercise (50% VO_2 peak, 60 min); (ii) high intensity, low amount aerobic exercise (70% VO_2 peak, 45 min); (iii) low to moderate intensity, low amount aerobic exercise (50% VO_2 peak, 45 min); or iv) control [13]. The authors' primary observation was that exercise conditions varying in amount (minutes) resulted in MRI-measured VAT reductions of a similar magnitude. Similarly, Slentz et al. randomized 175 sedentary, overweight adults to a control group, or for eight months, to one of three exercise groups: (i) low amount, moderate intensity, equivalent to walking 12 miles/week (19.2 km/week) at 40%–55% of VO_2 peak; (ii) low amount, vigorous intensity, equivalent to jogging 12 miles/week at 65%–80% of VO_2 peak; or (iii) high amount, vigorous intensity, equivalent to jogging 20 miles/week (32.0 km) [14]. Despite substantial differences in the amount (caloric expenditure) of exercise performed between groups, the primary finding was that there was no difference in CT-measured VAT reduction [12]. More recently, Cowan et al. randomized 103 previously sedentary, abdominally obese adults to one of four groups: (i) control; (ii) low amount, low-intensity exercise (180 kcal/session (women) and 300 kcal/session (men) at 50% VO_2 peak); (iii) high-amount, low-intensity exercise (HALI; 360 kcal/session (women) and 600 kcal/session (men) at 50% VO_2 peak); or (iv) high-amount, high-intensity exercise (HAHI; 360 kcal/session (women) and 600 kcal/session (men) at 75% VO_2 peak) for 24 weeks [15]. Consistent with prior findings, MRI-measured VAT was reduced by 15% to 20% by comparison to controls across exercise groups, despite substantial differences in exercise-induced energy expenditure between groups. Analysis of daily self-reported diet records suggested that change in dietary intake did not differ between groups. Similarly, reduction in body weight did not differ between exercise groups. Thus, increasing exercise amount (kilocalories) without changes in energy intake for six months was not associated with greater VAT reduction in adults with abdominal obesity.

2.2.2. Exercise Intensity and VAT

Whether exercise intensity is associated with VAT reduction independent of exercise amount is unclear. A systematic review that compared exercise groups that varied in exercise intensity from 14 studies suggests that exercise intensity should be at least moderate to vigorous if VAT reduction is the objective [16]. It is important to note, however, that this observation did not account for possible variation in exercise amount performed between studies. Indeed, with few exceptions, preliminary findings from randomized trials specifically designed to determine the effect of exercise intensity on VAT reduction suggest that the intensity of exercise performed is not a primary determinant of change in VAT [13–15,17]. Irving et al. reported that while VAT reduction was not significantly different between high intensity and low intensity exercise groups, significant within-group VAT changes by comparison to control were only observed in the high intensity group [17]. Similar to the observations for exercise amount described above, Keating et al. [13] and Slentz et al. [14] reported no effect of increasing exercise intensity on VAT reduction when measured using criterion methods. These observations were confirmed by Cowan et al. who reported that the reduction in VAT was not different independent of exercise intensity ranging from 50% to 70% of VO_2 peak performed for 24 weeks (Figure 1) [15].

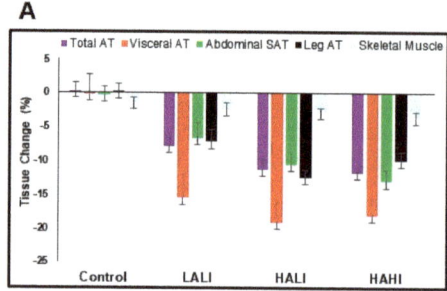 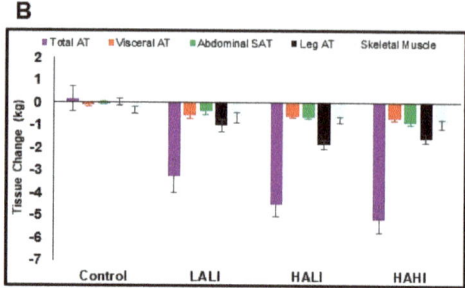

LALI = low amount, low intensity
HALI = high amount, low intensity
HAHI = high amount, high intensity

Figure 1. Illustration of relative (%, Panel **A**) and absolute (kg, Panel **B**) response of adipose and skeletal muscle tissues to variations in exercise dose. Taken from Reference [14]. Used with permission from Obesity. Absolute (left) and relative (right) changes in AT and skeletal muscle depots. With the exception of skeletal muscle, all AT depot changes (absolute and relative) were significantly different from control ($p < 0.008$; both panels). Relative change in VAT was greater than all other AT and skeletal muscle depots ($p < 0.01$; right panel). AT, adipose tissue; HAHI, high amount, high intensity; HALI, high amount, low intensity; LALI, low amount, low intensity.

These observations regarding the effects of exercise intensity on CT-measured VAT differ from a recently completed trial wherein 220 abdominally obese Chinese adults were randomized to either a high- or moderate-intensity exercise group for 12 months [18]. The primary finding was that vigorous-moderate exercise is associated with greater reductions in VAT compared to moderate exercise. However, it is important to note that in this trial, the vigorous exercise group performed supervised exercise for the entire 12 months, whereas the moderate exercise group self-reported their exercise behaviour. Self-reported physical activity behaviour is notoriously unreliable, thus confounds interpretation [19]. Self-reported physical activity can be under- or overestimated [19].

Emerging evidence has considered whether high intensity interval training (HITT) is associated with change in VAT. HITT is characterized by brief, intermittent bursts of exercise completed at a high intensity. High intensity exercise bouts are separated by brief recovery periods of inactivity or low-intensity exercise. Although there is no consensus established for the optimal durations of exercise and rest periods for HITT protocols, active bouts may be performed from 10 s to 5 min at 70–90% of VO_2 peak or 85%–95% of peak heart rate. Recovery periods range from 30 s to 3 min. Zhang et al. randomized 47 participants to a 12-week HIIT or moderate-intensity continuous training (MICT) intervention using a cycle ergometer three times a week [20]. Participants in the HIIT group performed cycles of 4-min high intensity bouts at 90% $VO_{2\,max}$, followed by 3 min of recovery until the targeted energy expenditure (300 kJ) was achieved. The MICT group performed continuous exercise until the matched energy expenditure target was reached (300 kJ). Similar reductions in VAT were observed regardless of exercise intervention. Winding et al. randomized 29 participants to an 11-week HIIT or MICT cycling intervention involving 10 1-min intervals (95% peak workload) with 1-min recovery or 40 min (50% peak workload), respectively [21]. Despite a lower exercise-induced energy expenditure, HIIT showed similar reductions in DXA-measured VAT compared to MICT. In both studies, participants were instructed to maintain their dietary intake throughout the intervention.

In summary, aerobic exercise combined with a balanced diet, wherein the participant does not increase energy intake, is associated with a robust reduction in VAT independent of amount or intensity. A 7% weight loss resulting from a lifestyle-based strategy consistent with current recommendations is likely to result in a 25% reduction in VAT. These observations provide treatment options for practitioners who target VAT reduction as part of a comprehensive lifestyle-based strategy designed to reduce health risk.

2.2.3. Individual Variability in VAT Response to Standardized Exercise

Since all adults acquire and inherit characteristics that vary substantially, their response to a treatment designed to change a given trait will vary substantially. Although increasing exercise is a primary determinant of improvement in numerous traits (e.g., cardiorespiratory fitness) at the group level, there is a growing body of evidence that the response to regular exercise varies substantially among individuals [22]. The extent to which individual variability in VAT response to a standard dose of exercise has only recently been considered. Brennan et al. performed a study to determine the effect of exercise amount and intensity on the proportion of individuals for whom the MRI-measured VAT response was above the minimal clinically important difference, defined as a reduction in VAT greater than 0.28 kg or 9%, and whether clinically meaningful changes in waist circumference, defined as greater than 2 cm, reflect individual VAT responses that are above the minimal clinically important difference [23]. Abdominally obese men and women were randomized to (i) control ($n = 20$); (ii) low amount, low intensity ($n = 24$); (iii) high amount, low intensity ($n = 30$); or (iv) high amount, high intensity ($n = 29$) treadmill exercise for 24 weeks.

Inspection of the individual responses to standardized exercise illustrated in Figure 2 clearly document the extraordinary variability in VAT response to exercise independent of exercise amount or intensity. The observation that most adults reduce VAT regardless of exercise strategy and that clinically important reductions in VAT can be determined by corresponding reductions in waist circumference that exceed 2 cm is encouraging (Figure 2). These observations underscore the value of routinely measuring waist circumference to determine the efficacy of treatment designed to reduce VAT and that, for some adults, substantial reduction in VAT may require altering the exercise dose by increasing either the amount and/or intensity of exercise. Whether some adults are resistant to reduction in VAT regardless of exercise dose is unknown and should be the subject of future investigations.

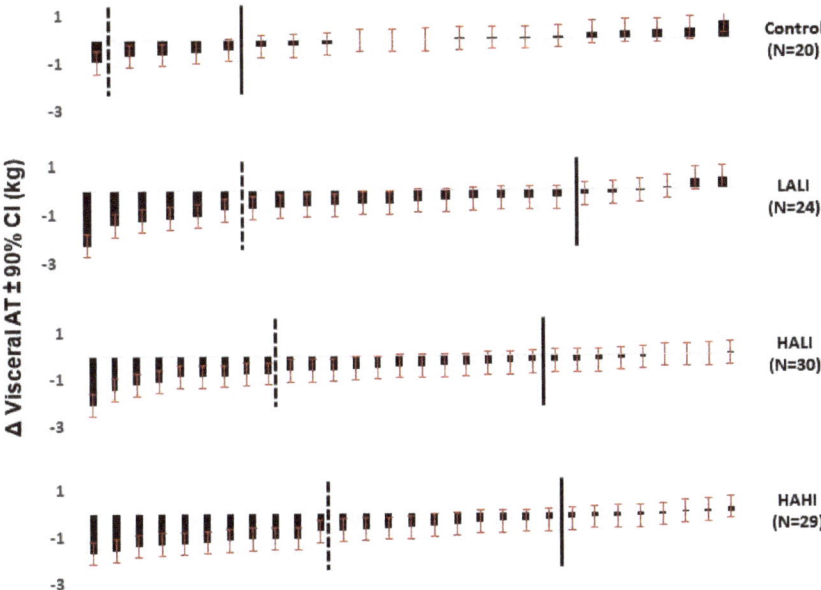

Figure 2. Variability of visceral adipose tissue (VAT) response to standardized exercise. Taken from Reference [19]. Used with permission from MSSE. Distribution of individual responses for change in VAT (kg) ± 90% CI in the control and intervention groups. The solid black line distinguishes participants whose observed response exceeds the MCID (e.g., those participants to the left of the solid line reduced visceral AT by < 0.28 kg). The dashed black line distinguishes participants whose observed response ± 90% CI exceeds the MCID (e.g., those participants to the left of the dashed line have CI where the top range is < 0.28 kg). LALI (low amount (~30 min), low intensity (50% VO_2 peak)), HALI (high amount (~60 min), low intensity (50% VO_2 peak)), HAHI (High amount (~40 min), high intensity (75% VO_2 peak)).

3. Liver Fat (LF)

3.1. Measurements of LF

Liver biopsy is an established method to assess liver fat and diagnose the severity of NAFLD with precision [6]. However, the invasive nature, cost, sampling error, and morbidity associated with the procedure are acknowledged limitations [6]. CT is a technique that estimates steatosis by quantitatively measuring liver density. However, the sensitivity and specificity of CT are clinically unacceptable at mild steatosis levels [6,16]. MRI is a technique that uses quantitative and qualitative information to assess intrahepatic fat content. The heterogeneity of the magnetic field, time demanding nature, low sensitivity, and poor image quality when disturbed are limitations of this technique [6]. Ultrasound is a common technique that is used to assess LF because of the low cost, vast availability and noninvasive nature [6]. Ultrasonography is limited as a single diagnostic tool because of the lack of sufficient sensitivity [6,24,25]. Accuracy of an ultrasound decreases with increasing body mass index [26–28]. Magnetic resonance spectroscopy (MRS) is cited as the gold standard MR technique to quantify LF. There is a high level of accuracy and reproducibility with this method, however, it is limited in availability because of the high degree of skill and specialized software required. Similar to liver biopsies, only a portion of the liver is analyzed, and so, sampling errors may occur [26].

3.2. Is Liver Fat Reduced in Response to Chronic Exercise or a Hypocaloric Diet?

As with VAT, evidence from systematic reviews and meta-analyses confirm that exercise or a hypocaloric diet is associated with a reduction in LF in previously sedentary, overweight and obese men and women [3,29].

3.3. Exercise and Liver Fat

Evidence from observational studies have established that adults with elevated levels of LF or NAFLD are physically inactive by comparison to those without NAFLD. Kistler and colleagues performed a retrospective analysis on 813 adults with biopsy-proven NAFLD, enrolled in the Nonalcoholic Steatohepatitis Clinical Research Network (NASH CRN) [30]. Physical activity levels were derived from self-reported responses to a questionnaire. The principle finding of this cross-sectional study was that neither moderate-intensity exercise nor total exercise per week was associated with NASH. However, vigorous exercise was associated with a decreased risk of having NASH (odds ratio (OR): 0.65 (0.43–0.98)). Thus, exercise intensity may be an important consideration when prescribing exercise to reduce LF. A limitation of this study was that exercise behaviour was assessed by self-report, which is notably unreliable [19].

Based on data derived from the National Health and Nutrition Examination Survey (NHANES) 2003–2006, Gerber and colleagues evaluated the associations between levels of physical activity and NAFLD in a large subsample of adults from this database [31]. NAFLD was defined as a fatty liver index >60 in the absence of other chronic liver diseases. The fatty liver index of hepatic steatosis is calculated based on measures of triglycerides, body mass index, waist circumference, and gamma-glutamyl transpeptidase. Physical activity levels were measured objectively over seven days using accelerometry.

Counter to the findings of Kistler et al. [30], Gerber and colleagues observed that adults with NAFLD (n = 1263), who were older and had a higher body mass index, perform less physical activity at any intensity level compared to adults without NAFLD (n = 1793) [31]. Thus, from initial epidemiological evidence, adults with NAFLD were physically inactive by comparison to adults without NAFLD, suggesting that exercise may be an important strategy for reducing LF. Physical activity was reported using accelerometers, which objectivity measure physical activity frequency and duration in a minimally invasive manner. However, accelerometers are limited in detecting non-ambulatory activities [19].

Evidence from controlled trials confirm the potential of exercise as a strategy to manage LF. Keating and colleagues reported that, in pooled data from six studies (156 overweight and abdominally obese adults), aerobic type exercise alone (no hypocaloric diet) ranging from two to 24 weeks at intensities between 45% and 85%, resulted in modest, yet significant reductions in LF (effect size 0.37) [29].

Keating et al. randomized 48 inactive overweight or obese adults to one of four groups varying in exercise amounts and intensities that are generally consistent with current exercise guidelines for 8 weeks [13]. LF was measured by MRS. The major finding was that LF was reduced by 1% to 3% compared to controls independent of exercise amount or intensity. The authors noted that, while the reductions in LF were modest, they were observed in association with minimal or no change in body weight.

In a much larger trial, Zhang et al. randomized 220 adults with NAFLD to 150 min per week for 12 months of either brisk walking (moderate intensity exercise) or jogging (moderate-vigorous intensity exercise) [18]. In this study, LF was assessed using MRS. All participants were asked not to change their diet during the trial. The principle finding was a decrease in LF that approximated 6% compared to controls, with no difference between exercise groups—thus, exercise intensity was not associated with LF reduction. In this trial, after controlling for the exercise-induced weight loss (3%–6%), the net changes in LF content were reduced and became nonsignificant between the exercise and control groups. Thus, the benefit of exercise was explained in large measure by the ability to induce weight loss.

Few studies have evaluated the association between cardiorespiratory fitness and LF. Pälve and colleagues found that in 463 adults, participants with fatty liver had lower cardiorespiratory fitness levels compared to participants without fatty liver ($VO_{2\ peak}$ 27.2 mL· kg^{-1}·min^{-1} and 31.6 mL·kg^{-1}·min^{-1}, p < 0.0001) [32]. LF was assessed using ultrasound. This relationship remained significant when adjusted for physical activity, adiposity, smoking, alcohol consumption, serum lipids, insulin, glucose, and C-reactive protein. Participants with abdominal obesity (waist circumference > 80 cm in women and >94 cm in men) with higher fitness levels (higher than age- and sex-specific median of $VO_{2\ Peak}$) had lower prevalence of fatty liver than participants who were obese and unfit (below median), (11.7% vs. 34.8%, p = 0.0003). In a longitudinal study (nine months of follow up), Kantartzis et al. found that cardiorespiratory fitness (VO_2 peak) at baseline was a strong predictor of change in MRS-measured LF in response to an exercise intervention. Independent of total fat, visceral fat, subcutaneous fat or exercise intensity, cardiorespiratory fitness was negatively associated with LF at baseline [33].

Exercise-induced reductions in intrahepatic fat are observed independent of weight change [34]. A systematic review by Hashida and colleagues showed a 20-30% relative risk reduction in LF with exercise in the absence of weight loss [35]. Sullivan and colleagues found that the effect of MRS-measured LF following an exercise intervention, according to the physical activity guidelines (150–300 min of moderate intensity exercise), were independent of weight loss [36]. In previously sedentary adults, body weight, body fat mass, and fat-free mass did not change after the intervention. However, there was a decrease (10.3% ± 4.6%) in LF in the exercise group compared with the control group (p = 0.04). Interestingly, obese individuals who consumed moderate to excessive amounts of alcohol underwent a 12-week exercise intervention. In this randomized trial, exercise induced reductions in both subcutaneous and visceral fat, however, there was no reduction of MRI-measured LF. This finding suggests that moderate to excessive amounts of alcohol consumption may attenuate the beneficial effects of exercise on NAFLD [37].

Qiu and colleagues conducted a meta-analysis and observed that the amount of physical activity in men was inversely associated with the risk of NAFLD in a dose-dependent manner [38]. The authors report that 500 MET-minutes/week (approximately 150 minutes/week) of physical activity was associated with an 18% risk reduction of NALFD (RR = 0.82, 95% CI 0.73–0.91). Further increases in physical activity (1000 MET-minutes/week) were associated with a 33% risk reduction in NAFLD (RR = 0.67, 95% CI 0.54–0.83). These findings are consistent with those of Li and colleagues who reported that moderate- and vigorous-intensity physical activity effectively reduced the risk of NAFLD independent of energy intake and sedentary time (>684 MET-minutes/week compared to none: OR 0.58, 95% CI 0.40 to 0.86, vigorous-intensity physical activity: >960 MET-min/week compared to none: OR 0.63, 95% CI 0.41 to 0.95) [39]. Li et al. used ultrasound measurements to assess LF. Kwak et al. also found an inverse dose-response relationship between the amount of self-reported physical activity and the prevalence of NAFLD, independent of insulin resistance and VAT in 3718 adult men and women [40]. However, self-reported physical activity behaviour is notoriously unreliable, thus confounding interpretation [19].

Emerging evidence has also considered whether HITT is associated with change in LF. Hallworth and colleagues randomized participants to 12 weeks of HITT on a cycle ergometer three times a week. Participants were instructed to perform 5 intervals of cycling at 16–17 on the Borg scale for 3 min followed by 3 min of recovery [39]. Abdelbasset et al. randomized participants to an eight-week cycling protocol. Participants completed three sets of 4-min cycling at 80 to 85% of VO_2 max with 2-min recovery, three days a week [40]. In both studies, participants were instructed to make no modifications to their diets. Several authors have observed reductions in LF after HIIT compared to controls [41,42]. The change in LF was measured using MRI and/or ultrasonography. When HITT and moderate intensity exercise were matched for energy expenditure, there were no differences in LF reduction [41–43].

3.4. Hypocaloric Diet and LF

It is well established that diet-induced weight loss is a cornerstone of treatment for persons with NAFLD. In 2003, Tiikkainen and colleagues reported that LF, as measured by MRS, was reduced by about 39% in premenopausal women consequent to an 8% weight loss achieved within three to six months [43]. Of note, the authors reported that the reduction in LF was directly related to baseline levels. Larson-Meyer et al. reported results from the CALERIE study wherein a loss of body weight approximating 10% via hypocaloric diet or diet and exercise combined, was associated with a 29% to 40% reduction in MRS-measured LF in overweight adults. As with exercise-induced weight loss, diet-induced weight loss is associated with a marked reduction in MRI-measured LF [11]. Very low-calorie diets also resulted in significant reductions of LF, however, very low-calorie diets cannot be maintained long term [44–46].

Thoma and colleagues performed a systematic review of the literature to evaluate the effects of various lifestyle-based interventions on LF [3]. For diet only interventions, the authors uncovered 10 studies wherein 11 groups totaling 322 participants were prescribed a hypocaloric diet varying in composition and negative energy balance. Only two studies included control groups. The duration of the diet interventions ranged from one to six months. The mean weight loss across the studies ranged from 4% to 14% and the relative reduction in LF, as measured by MRS, ranged from 42% to 81%. No clear relationship between diet composition and LF reduction was reported. However, consistent with the evidence cited above, the reduction in LF was strongly associated with weight loss.

3.5. Exercise and Hypocaloric Diet Combined

Lifestyle interventions that include a hypocaloric diet and an exercise intervention have been considered in several systematic reviews. The reviews investigate if a combination of diet and exercise is more effective than exercise or diet alone to decrease LF [3,29,47–49]. Keating and colleagues did not find a significant pooled effect of combined interventions of diet and exercise; however, the authors discuss being limited by a low sample size and statistical power [29]. Thoma et al. reported on seven studies that conducted lifestyle modification interventions to decrease energy intake and increase physical activity or exercise over 3–12 months [3].The authors concluded that lifestyle modifications consistently resulted in LF reduction. Similarly, other systematic reviews conducted by Hens and colleagues, as well as Whitsett and colleagues, found that lifestyle modification can reduce LF [48,49]. Golabi et al. found that exercise alone and a combination of diet and exercise both significantly decrease LF [47].

4. Anthropometric Markers of VAT and LF

Criterion measurement of both VAT and LF requires sophisticated radiological techniques (e.g., magnetic resonance imaging or computed tomography) that are not readily accessible in most clinical settings. LF can also be determined using biopsy methods, but this too is invasive and presents a burden to the patient. Accordingly, the validity of simple anthropometric methods has been considered as an alternative, pragmatic option. There is general agreement that waist circumference represents the single best anthropometric marker of VAT [1,50]. However, due in large measure to the inter-individual variability between the quantity of abdominal subcutaneous and VAT [51], the variance explained in VAT change by waist circumference is modest, ranging from 25% to 75%[1]. At present, there is no universally accepted method for the measurement of waist circumference. The two most often used protocols are at the level of the iliac crest and the mid-point between the iliac crest and last rib [52]. Whether the associations between these two WC methods provide different values for VAT across sex, age, and ethnicity is unclear.

In 2006, Bedogni et al. derived a simple index (Fatty Liver Index) of hepatic steatosis that was calculated based on the measures of triglycerides, body mass index, waist circumference and gamma-glutamyl transpeptidase (GGT) [53]. Fatty liver index has a very good discriminative ability to predict fatty liver in both Asian and Western adult populations [54,55]. Motamed et al. recently validated the discriminative ability of the Fatty Liver Index to predict fatty liver in a sample of 5052 adults [56]. Fatty liver or NAFLD was determined by ultrasound. Interestingly, although the Fatty Liver Index showed good discriminative ability for the diagnosis of NAFLD (AUC = 0.87 (95%CI: 0.85–0.88), there was no significant difference in the discriminative ability determined by waist circumference alone (AUC = 0.85, 95%CI: 0.84–0.86). Thus, on a population basis, waist circumference alone may be a useful measure of both VAT and LF. However, the utility of either waist circumference or Fatty Liver Index to predict VAT and LF, respectively, on an individual basis is unknown.

5. Summary

It is now firmly established that both regular aerobic exercise and the consumption of a hypocaloric diet are associated with a substantial reduction in VAT and LF independent of age, biological sex, or ethnicity. Whereas exercise is associated with VAT reduction with or without weight loss, reductions in LF are positively associated with weight, independent of the strategy to induce weight loss. Despite decades of research into the associations between lifestyle-based interventions and VAT reduction, the threshold of VAT reduction that is required for health benefit remains unclear. Similarly, while it is clear that weight loss is associated with LF reduction, optimal levels of weight loss for attenuating LF are unclear. Nevertheless, it is extremely encouraging that regular exercise (4–6 months) consistent with consensus recommendations (30–60 min per day at moderate-to-vigorous intensity; e.g., brisk walking or jogging) combined with a balanced, healthful diet is associated with substantial reductions in VAT (15%–20%). Similarly, weight loss of 5% to 10% can be achieved by 4–6 months with reasonable reductions in caloric intake with or without exercise. Thus, practitioners in health care settings have options when counselling adults regarding the utility of lifestyle-based interventions designed to reduce both VAT and LF. The objective of this review was assessing strategies for reducing VAT and LF. The focus was on a negative energy balance induced aerobic exercise and a decrease in energy intake. Future research is required to determine if some adults are resistant to reductions in VAT and LF regardless of exercise dose.

Direct measurement of VAT or LF in most health care settings is not feasible. Waist circumference remains the single best anthropometric marker of change in VAT. While precise measurement of change in VAT using waist circumference on an individual basis is unlikely, it is extremely likely that reductions in waist circumference (e.g., greater than 2 cm) are associated with a corresponding reduction in VAT. While initial results suggest that waist circumference may be as useful as the LF Index to follow change in LF, additional evidence from large scale studies in diverse populations is required. Nevertheless, these observations are encouraging and reinforce the importance of measuring waist circumference in all health care settings.

Author Contributions: R.R. conceptualized the manuscript. S.H. and S.S. reviewed and assisted in writing the manuscript. All authors have read and agreed to the published version of the manuscript.

Funding: This research received funding in part from a Project Grant awarded to Dr. Ross from the Canadian Institutes of Health Research.

Conflicts of Interest: The authors declare no conflicts of interest.

References

1. Neeland, I.J.; Ross, R.; Després, J.-P.; Matsuzawa, Y.; Yamashita, S.; Shai, I.; Seidell, J.; Magni, P.; Santos, R.D.; Arsenault, B.; et al. International Atherosclerosis Society; International Chair on Cardiometabolic Risk Working Group on Visceral Obesity. Visceral and Ectopic Fat, Atherosclerosis, and Cardiometabolic Disease: A Position Statement. *Lancet Diabetes Endocrinol.* **2019**, *7*, 715–725. [CrossRef]
2. Verheggen, R.J.H.M.; Maessen, M.F.H.; Green, D.J.; Hermus, A.R.M.M.; Hopman, M.T.E.; Thijssen, D.H.T. A Systematic Review and Meta-Analysis on the Effects of Exercise Training versus Hypocaloric Diet: Distinct Effects on Body Weight and Visceral Adipose Tissue. *Obes. Rev.* **2016**, *17*, 664–690. [CrossRef]
3. Thoma, C.; Day, C.P.; Trenell, M.I. Lifestyle Interventions for the Treatment of Non-Alcoholic Fatty Liver Disease in Adults: A Systematic Review. *J. Hepatol.* **2012**, *56*, 255–266. [CrossRef]
4. Shuster, A.; Patlas, M.; Pinthus, J.H.; Mourtzakis, M. The Clinical Importance of Visceral Adiposity: A Critical Review of Methods for Visceral Adipose Tissue Analysis. *Br. J. Radiol.* **2012**, *85*, 1–10. [CrossRef]
5. Targher, G.; Day, C.P.; Bonora, E. Risk of Cardiovascular Disease in Patients with Nonalcoholic Fatty Liver Disease. *N. Engl. J. Med.* **2010**, *363*, 1341–1350. [CrossRef]
6. Fabbrini, E.; Magkos, F.; Mohammed, B.S.; Pietka, T.; Abumrad, N.A.; Patterson, B.W.; Okunade, A.; Klein, S. Intrahepatic Fat, not Visceral Fat, Is Linked with Metabolic Complications of Obesity. *Proc. Natl. Acad. Sci. USA* **2009**, *106*, 15430–15435. [CrossRef]
7. Heymsfield, S.B.; Wang, Z.; Baumgartner, R.N.; Ross, R. Human Body Composition: Advances in Models and Methods. *Annu. Rev. Nutr.* **1997**, *17*, 527–558. [CrossRef]
8. Ross, R.; Rissanen, J.; Pedwell, H.; Clifford, J.; Shragge, P. Influence of Diet and Exercise on Skeletal Muscle and Visceral Adipose Tissue in Men. *J. Appl. Physiol.* **1996**, *81*, 2445–2455. [CrossRef]
9. Ross, R.; Dagnone, D.; Jones, P.J.; Smith, H.; Paddags, A.; Hudson, R.; Janssen, I. Reduction in Obesity and Related Comorbid Conditions after Diet-Induced Weight Loss or Exercise-Induced Weight Loss in Men. A Randomized, Controlled Trial. *Ann. Intern. Med.* **2000**, *133*, 92–103. [CrossRef]
10. Ross, R.; Janssen, I.; Dawson, J.; Kungl, A.-M.; Kuk, J.L.; Wong, S.L.; Nguyen-Duy, T.-B.; Lee, S.; Kilpatrick, K.; Hudson, R. Exercise-Induced Reduction in Obesity and Insulin Resistance in Women: A Randomized Controlled Trial. *Obes. Res.* **2004**, *12*, 789–798. [CrossRef]
11. Gepner, Y.; Shelef, I.; Schwarzfuchs, D.; Zelicha, H.; Tene, L.; Yaskolka Meir, A.; Tsaban, G.; Cohen, N.; Bril, N.; Rein, M.; et al. Effect of Distinct Lifestyle Interventions on Mobilization of Fat Storage Pools: Central Magnetic Resonance Imaging Randomized Controlled Trial. *Circulation* **2018**, *137*, 1143–1157. [CrossRef]
12. Ohkawara, K.; Tanaka, S.; Miyachi, M.; Ishikawa-Takata, K.; Tabata, I. A Dose-Response Relation between Aerobic Exercise and Visceral Fat Reduction: Systematic Review of Clinical Trials. *Int. J. Obes. (Lond.)* **2007**, *31*, 1786–1797. [CrossRef]

13. Keating, S.E.; Hackett, D.A.; Parker, H.M.; O'Connor, H.T.; Gerofi, J.A.; Sainsbury, A.; Baker, M.K.; Chuter, V.H.; Caterson, I.D.; George, J.; et al. Effect of Aerobic Exercise Training Dose on Liver Fat and Visceral Adiposity. *J. Hepatol.* **2015**, *63*, 174–182. [CrossRef]
14. Slentz, C.A.; Aiken, L.B.; Houmard, J.A.; Bales, C.W.; Johnson, J.L.; Tanner, C.J.; Duscha, B.D.; Kraus, W.E. Inactivity, Exercise, and Visceral Fat. STRRIDE: A Randomized, Controlled Study of Exercise Intensity and Amount. *J. Appl. Physiol.* **2005**, *99*, 1613–1618. [CrossRef]
15. Cowan, T.E.; Brennan, A.M.; Stotz, P.J.; Clarke, J.; Lamarche, B.; Ross, R. Separate Effects of Exercise Amount and Intensity on Adipose Tissue and Skeletal Muscle Mass in Adults with Abdominal Obesity. *Obesity (Silver Spring)* **2018**, *26*, 1696–1703. [CrossRef]
16. Vissers, D.; Hens, W.; Taeymans, J.; Baeyens, J.-P.; Poortmans, J.; Van Gaal, L. The Effect of Exercise on Visceral Adipose Tissue in Overweight Adults: A Systematic Review and Meta-Analysis. *PLoS ONE* **2013**, *8*, e56415. [CrossRef]
17. Irving, B.A.; Davis, C.K.; Brock, D.W.; Weltman, J.Y.; Swift, D.; Barrett, E.J.; Gaesser, G.A.; Weltman, A. Effect of Exercise Training Intensity on Abdominal Visceral Fat and Body Composition. *Med. Sci. Sports Exerc.* **2008**, *40*, 1863–1872. [CrossRef]
18. Zhang, H.-J.; He, J.; Pan, L.-L.; Ma, Z.-M.; Han, C.-K.; Chen, C.-S.; Chen, Z.; Han, H.-W.; Chen, S.; Sun, Q.; et al. Effects of Moderate and Vigorous Exercise on Nonalcoholic Fatty Liver Disease: A Randomized Clinical Trial. *JAMA Intern. Med.* **2016**, *176*, 1074–1082. [CrossRef]
19. Ainsworth, B.; Cahalin, L.; Buman, M.; Ross, R. The Current State of Physical Activity Assessment Tools. *Prog. Cardiovasc. Dis.* **2015**, *57*, 387–395. [CrossRef]
20. Zhang, H.; Tong, T.K.; Qiu, W.; Zhang, X.; Zhou, S.; Liu, Y.; He, Y. Comparable Effects of High-Intensity Interval Training and Prolonged Continuous Exercise Training on Abdominal Visceral Fat Reduction in Obese Young Women. Available online: https://www.hindawi.com/journals/jdr/2017/5071740/ (accessed on 14 March 2020).
21. Winding, K.M.; Munch, G.W.; Iepsen, U.W.; Van Hall, G.; Pedersen, B.K.; Mortensen, S.P. The Effect on Glycaemic Control of Low-Volume High-Intensity Interval Training versus Endurance Training in Individuals with Type 2 Diabetes. *Diabetes Obes. Metab.* **2018**, *20*, 1131–1139. [CrossRef]
22. Ross, R.; Goodpaster, B.H.; Koch, L.G.; Sarzynski, M.A.; Kohrt, W.M.; Johannsen, N.M.; Skinner, J.S.; Castro, A.; Irving, B.A.; Noland, R.C.; et al. Precision Exercise Medicine: Understanding Exercise Response Variability. *Br. J. Sports Med.* **2019**, *53*, 1141–1153. [CrossRef]
23. Brennan, A.M.; Day, A.G.; Cowan, T.E.; Clarke, G.J.; Lamarche, B.; Ross, R. Individual Response to Standardized Exercise: Total and Abdominal Adipose Tissue. *Med. Sci. Sports Exerc.* **2019**. [CrossRef]
24. Lv, S.; Jiang, S.; Liu, S.; Dong, Q.; Xin, Y.; Xuan, S. Noninvasive Quantitative Detection Methods of Liver Fat Content in Nonalcoholic Fatty Liver Disease. *J. Clin. Transl. Hepatol.* **2018**, *6*, 217–221. [CrossRef]
25. Kramer, H.; Pickhardt, P.J.; Kliewer, M.A.; Hernando, D.; Chen, G.-H.; Zagzebski, J.A.; Reeder, S.B. Accuracy of Liver Fat Quantification with Advanced CT, MRI, and Ultrasound Techniques: Prospective Comparison with MR Spectroscopy. *AJR Am. J. Roentgenol.* **2017**, *208*, 92–100. [CrossRef] [PubMed]
26. Chartampilas, E. Imaging of Nonalcoholic Fatty Liver Disease and Its Clinical Utility. *Hormones* **2018**, *17*, 69–81. [CrossRef]
27. Bohte, A.E.; van Werven, J.R.; Bipat, S.; Stoker, J. The Diagnostic Accuracy of US, CT, MRI and 1H-MRS for the Evaluation of Hepatic Steatosis Compared with Liver Biopsy: A Meta-Analysis. *Eur. Radiol.* **2011**, *21*, 87–97. [CrossRef]
28. Fitzpatrick, E.; Dhawan, A. Noninvasive Biomarkers in Non-Alcoholic Fatty Liver Disease: Current Status and a Glimpse of the Future. *World J. Gastroenterol.* **2014**, *20*, 10851–10863. [CrossRef]
29. Keating, S.E.; Hackett, D.A.; George, J.; Johnson, N.A. Exercise and Non-Alcoholic Fatty Liver Disease: A Systematic Review and Meta-Analysis. *J. Hepatol.* **2012**, *57*, 157–166. [CrossRef]
30. Kistler, K.D.; Brunt, E.M.; Clark, J.M.; Diehl, A.M.; Sallis, J.F.; Schwimmer, J.B.; NASH CRN Research Group. Physical Activity Recommendations, Exercise Intensity, and Histological Severity of Nonalcoholic Fatty Liver Disease. *Am. J. Gastroenterol.* **2011**, *106*, 460–468. [CrossRef]
31. Gerber, L.; Otgonsuren, M.; Mishra, A.; Escheik, C.; Birerdinc, A.; Stepanova, M.; Younossi, Z.M. Non-Alcoholic Fatty Liver Disease (NAFLD) Is Associated with Low Level of Physical Activity: A Population-Based Study. *Aliment. Pharmacol. Ther.* **2012**, *36*, 772–781. [CrossRef]

32. Pälve, K.S.; Pahkala, K.; Suomela, E.; Aatola, H.; Hulkkonen, J.; Juonala, M.; Lehtimäki, T.; Rönnemaa, T.; Viikari, J.S.A.; Kähönen, M.; et al. Cardiorespiratory Fitness and Risk of Fatty Liver: The Young Finns Study. *Med. Sci. Sports Exerc.* **2017**, *49*, 1834–1841. [CrossRef]
33. Kantartzis, K.; Thamer, C.; Peter, A.; Machann, J.; Schick, F.; Schraml, C.; Königsrainer, A.; Königsrainer, I.; Kröber, S.; Niess, A.; et al. High Cardiorespiratory Fitness Is an Independent Predictor of the Reduction in Liver Fat during a Lifestyle Intervention in Non-Alcoholic Fatty Liver Disease. *Gut* **2009**, *58*, 1281–1288. [CrossRef]
34. Katsagoni, C.N.; Georgoulis, M.; Papatheodoridis, G.V.; Panagiotakos, D.B.; Kontogianni, M.D. Effects of Lifestyle Interventions on Clinical Characteristics of Patients with Non-Alcoholic Fatty Liver Disease: A Meta-Analysis. *Metab. Clin. Exp.* **2017**, *68*, 119–132. [CrossRef]
35. Hashida, R.; Kawaguchi, T.; Bekki, M.; Omoto, M.; Matsuse, H.; Nago, T.; Takano, Y.; Ueno, T.; Koga, H.; George, J.; et al. Aerobic vs. Resistance Exercise in Non-Alcoholic Fatty Liver Disease: A Systematic Review. *J. Hepatol.* **2017**, *66*, 142–152. [CrossRef]
36. Sullivan, S.; Kirk, E.P.; Mittendorfer, B.; Patterson, B.W.; Klein, S. Randomized Trial of Exercise Effect on Intrahepatic Triglyceride Content and Lipid Kinetics in Nonalcoholic Fatty Liver Disease. *Hepatology* **2012**, *55*, 1738–1745. [CrossRef]
37. Houghton, D.; Hallsworth, K.; Thoma, C.; Cassidy, S.; Hardy, T.; Heaps, S.; Hollingsworth, K.G.; Taylor, R.; Day, C.P.; Masson, S.; et al. Effects of Exercise on Liver Fat and Metabolism in Alcohol Drinkers. *Clin. Gastroenterol. Hepatol.* **2017**, *15*, 1596–1603.e3. [CrossRef]
38. Qiu, S.; Cai, X.; Sun, Z.; Li, L.; Zügel, M.; Steinacker, J.M.; Schumann, U. Association between Physical Activity and Risk of Nonalcoholic Fatty Liver Disease: A Meta-Analysis. *Therap. Adv. Gastroenterol.* **2017**, *10*, 701–713. [CrossRef]
39. Li, Y.; He, F.; He, Y.; Pan, X.; Wu, Y.; Hu, Z.; Lin, X.; Xu, S.; Peng, X.-E. Dose-Response Association between Physical Activity and Non-Alcoholic Fatty Liver Disease: A Case-Control Study in a Chinese Population. *BMJ Open* **2019**, *9*, e026854. [CrossRef]
40. Kwak, M.-S.; Kim, D.; Chung, G.E.; Kim, W.; Kim, Y.J.; Yoon, J.-H. Role of Physical Activity in Nonalcoholic Fatty Liver Disease in Terms of Visceral Obesity and Insulin Resistance. *Liver Int.* **2015**, *35*, 944–952. [CrossRef]
41. Hallsworth, K.; Thoma, C.; Hollingsworth, K.G.; Cassidy, S.; Anstee, Q.M.; Day, C.P.; Trenell, M.I. Modified High-Intensity Interval Training Reduces Liver Fat and Improves Cardiac Function in Non-Alcoholic Fatty Liver Disease: A Randomized Controlled Trial. *Clin. Sci.* **2015**, *129*, 1097–1105. [CrossRef]
42. Abdelbasset, W.K.; Tantawy, S.A.; Kamel, D.M.; Alqahtani, B.A.; Soliman, G.S. A Randomized Controlled Trial on the Effectiveness of 8-Week High-Intensity Interval Exercise on Intrahepatic Triglycerides, Visceral Lipids, and Health-Related Quality of Life in Diabetic Obese Patients with Nonalcoholic Fatty Liver Disease. *Medicine (Baltim.)* **2019**, *98*, e14918. [CrossRef]
43. Tiikkainen, M.; Bergholm, R.; Vehkavaara, S.; Rissanen, A.; Häkkinen, A.-M.; Tamminen, M.; Teramo, K.; Yki-Järvinen, H. Effects of Identical Weight Loss on Body Composition and Features of Insulin Resistance in Obese Women with High and Low Liver Fat Content. *Diabetes* **2003**, *52*, 701–707. [CrossRef]
44. Lewis, M.C.; Phillips, M.L.; Slavotinek, J.P.; Kow, L.; Thompson, C.H.; Toouli, J. Change in Liver Size and Fat Content after Treatment with Optifast Very Low Calorie Diet. *Obes. Surg.* **2006**, *16*, 697–701. [CrossRef]
45. Gu, Y.; Yu, H.; Li, Y.; Ma, X.; Lu, J.; Yu, W.; Xiao, Y.; Bao, Y.; Jia, W. Beneficial Effects of an 8-Week, Very Low Carbohydrate Diet Intervention on Obese Subjects. *Evid. Based Complement Altern. Med.* **2013**, *2013*. [CrossRef]
46. Lim, E.L.; Hollingsworth, K.G.; Aribisala, B.S.; Chen, M.J.; Mathers, J.C.; Taylor, R. Reversal of Type 2 Diabetes: Normalisation of Beta Cell Function in Association with Decreased Pancreas and Liver Triacylglycerol. *Diabetologia* **2011**, *54*, 2506–2514. [CrossRef]
47. Golabi, P.; Locklear, C.T.; Austin, P.; Afdhal, S.; Byrns, M.; Gerber, L.; Younossi, Z.M. Effectiveness of Exercise in Hepatic Fat Mobilization in Non-Alcoholic Fatty Liver Disease: Systematic Review. *World J. Gastroenterol.* **2016**, *22*, 6318–6327. [CrossRef]
48. Hens, W.; Taeymans, J.; Cornelis, J.; Gielen, J.; Gaal, L.V.; Vissers, D. The Effect of Lifestyle Interventions on Excess Ectopic Fat Deposition Measured by Noninvasive Techniques in Overweight and Obese Adults: A Systematic Review and Meta-Analysis. *J. Phys. Act. Health* **2016**, *13*, 671–694. [CrossRef]

49. Whitsett, M.; VanWagner, L.B. Physical Activity as a Treatment of Non-Alcoholic Fatty Liver Disease: A Systematic Review. *World J. Hepatol.* **2015**, *7*, 2041–2052. [CrossRef]
50. Ross, R.; Neeland, I.J.; Yamashita, S.; Shai, I.; Seidell, J.; Magni, P.; Santos, R.D.; Arsenault, B.; Cuevas, A.; Hu, F.B.; et al. Waist Circumference as a Vital Sign in Clinical Practice: A Consensus Statement from the IAS and ICCR Working Group on Visceral Obesity. *Nat. Rev. Endocrinol.* **2020**, *16*, 177–189. [CrossRef]
51. Lee, S.; Janssen, I.; Ross, R. Interindividual Variation in Abdominal Subcutaneous and Visceral Adipose Tissue: Influence of Measurement Site. *J. Appl. Physiol.* **2004**, *97*, 948–954. [CrossRef]
52. Ross, R.; Berentzen, T.; Bradshaw, A.J.; Janssen, I.; Kahn, H.S.; Katzmarzyk, P.T.; Kuk, J.L.; Seidell, J.C.; Snijder, M.B.; Sørensen, T.I.A.; et al. Does the Relationship between Waist Circumference, Morbidity and Mortality Depend on Measurement Protocol for Waist Circumference? *Obes. Rev.* **2008**, *9*, 312–325. [CrossRef]
53. Bedogni, G.; Bellentani, S.; Miglioli, L.; Masutti, F.; Passalacqua, M.; Castiglione, A.; Tiribelli, C. The Fatty Liver Index: A Simple and Accurate Predictor of Hepatic Steatosis in the General Population. *BMC Gastroenterol.* **2006**, *6*, 33. [CrossRef]
54. Yang, B.-L.; Wu, W.-C.; Fang, K.-C.; Wang, Y.-C.; Huo, T.-I.; Huang, Y.-H.; Yang, H.-I.; Su, C.-W.; Lin, H.-C.; Lee, F.-Y.; et al. External Validation of Fatty Liver Index for Identifying Ultrasonographic Fatty Liver in a Large-Scale Cross-Sectional Study in Taiwan. *PLoS ONE* **2015**, *10*, e0120443. [CrossRef]
55. Koehler, E.M.; Schouten, J.N.L.; Hansen, B.E.; Hofman, A.; Stricker, B.H.; Janssen, H.L.A. External Validation of the Fatty Liver Index for Identifying Nonalcoholic Fatty Liver Disease in a Population-Based Study. *Clin. Gastroenterol. Hepatol.* **2013**, *11*, 1201–1204. [CrossRef]
56. Motamed, N.; Sohrabi, M.; Ajdarkosh, H.; Hemmasi, G.; Maadi, M.; Sayeedian, F.S.; Pirzad, R.; Abedi, K.; Aghapour, S.; Fallahnezhad, M.; et al. Fatty Liver Index vs. Waist Circumference for Predicting Non-Alcoholic Fatty Liver Disease. *World J. Gastroenterol.* **2016**, *22*, 3023–3030. [CrossRef]

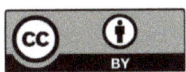

© 2020 by the authors. Licensee MDPI, Basel, Switzerland. This article is an open access article distributed under the terms and conditions of the Creative Commons Attribution (CC BY) license (http://creativecommons.org/licenses/by/4.0/).

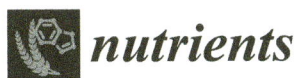

Review

Physical Activity, Cardiorespiratory Fitness, and the Metabolic Syndrome

Jonathan Myers [1,*], Peter Kokkinos [2] and Eric Nyelin [3]

1. Cardiology Division, Veterans Affairs Palo Alto Health Care System and Stanford University, Stanford, CA 94304, USA
2. Cardiology Division, Washington DC Veterans Affairs Medical Center and Rutgers University, Washington, DC 20422, USA
3. Endocrinology Division, Washington DC Veterans Affairs Medical Center, Washington, DC 20422, USA
* Correspondence: drj993@aol.com; Tel.: +1-(650)-493-5000 (ext. 64661)

Received: 27 May 2019; Accepted: 17 July 2019; Published: 19 July 2019

Abstract: Both observational and interventional studies suggest an important role for physical activity and higher fitness in mitigating the metabolic syndrome. Each component of the metabolic syndrome is, to a certain extent, favorably influenced by interventions that include physical activity. Given that the prevalence of the metabolic syndrome and its individual components (particularly obesity and insulin resistance) has increased significantly in recent decades, guidelines from various professional organizations have called for greater efforts to reduce the incidence of this condition and its components. While physical activity interventions that lead to improved fitness cannot be expected to normalize insulin resistance, lipid disorders, or obesity, the combined effect of increasing activity on these risk markers, an improvement in fitness, or both, has been shown to have a major impact on health outcomes related to the metabolic syndrome. Exercise therapy is a cost-effective intervention to both prevent and mitigate the impact of the metabolic syndrome, but it remains underutilized. In the current article, an overview of the effects of physical activity and higher fitness on the metabolic syndrome is provided, along with a discussion of the mechanisms underlying the benefits of being more fit or more physically active in the prevention and treatment of the metabolic syndrome.

Keywords: metabolic syndrome; cardiorespiratory fitness; insulin resistance; cardiovascular disease; exercise training

1. Overview

Chronic, non-communicable diseases currently represent the predominant challenge to global health. In a recent global status report on chronic disease, the World Health Organization stated that non-communicable conditions, including cardiovascular disease (CVD), diabetes and obesity, now account for roughly two-thirds of deaths worldwide [1]. The prevalence of many of the components of the "metabolic syndrome", particularly obesity and diabetes, has grown considerably throughout the Western World since this term was initially suggested by Haller in 1977 [2]. Given that the metabolic syndrome is an important precursor to CVD and other chronic conditions [3–7], guidelines from various professional organizations have called for greater efforts to reduce the incidence of this condition and its components [3,4]. A notable parallel over the last 4 decades is the fact that numerous surveys and cohort studies have consistently reported that Western societies are significantly less physically active than past generations [7–11]. Moreover, a growing number of studies has reported that higher cardiorespiratory fitness (CRF; which is defined as the maximal capacity of the cardiovascular and respiratory systems to supply oxygen to the skeletal muscles during exercise) is inversely related to the development of the metabolic syndrome [12,13]. These studies, along with recent intervention trials [14,15], suggest a compelling link between impaired CRF, low physical activity patterns (defined as movement that requires energy), exercise (defined as planned, structured, repetitive, intentional movement intended to improve CRF), and the metabolic syndrome.

Although the metabolic syndrome is complex and has been defined differently by different organizations, the clustering of risk factors that define it (high waist circumference, dyslipidemia, hypertension, and insulin resistance) are, to a certain extent, commonly associated with sedentary lifestyles. Indeed, numerous studies in recent decades have shown that increasing amounts of physical activity and higher CRF have a favorable impact on each of the components of the metabolic syndrome [12–16]. While physical activity interventions alone cannot be expected to normalize insulin resistance, lipid disorders, or obesity, the combined effect of increasing activity on these risk markers, an improvement in CRF, or both, can have a major impact on health outcomes related to the metabolic syndrome. However, physical activity as a treatment for metabolic disease remains underutilized. In fact, physical activity interventions are often dismissed in favor of pharmacologic treatments or other interventions that tend to be more economically driven [8,17–19]. Although physical activity counseling is now mandated by many health care systems, the fact remains that activity counseling rarely occurs as part of clinical encounters [20,21]. The lack of attention paid to physical activity is unfortunate given the strength of exercise interventions on health outcomes among individuals with metabolic disorders [12–16].

In the following, an overview of the effects of physical activity and CRF on the metabolic syndrome is provided, along with a discussion of the mechanisms underlying the benefits of being more fit or more physically active in the prevention and treatment of the metabolic syndrome.

2. Physical Activity and the Metabolic Syndrome

Collectively, studies on the impact of being more physically active, whether studied in a cross-sectional cohort or as a result of a structured exercise intervention, have been shown to have an important impact on cardiometabolic risk. Regular exercise can help to reduce weight, reduce blood pressure, and improve lipid disorders, including raising HDL and lowering triglycerides [7,16–22]. Among the physiological systems that respond favorably to physical activity, it has been argued that one of the most demonstrable effects of regular exercise is its impact on insulin resistance [23,24]. A summary of key studies is shown in Table 1; notably, these studies are categorically consistent in demonstrating the benefits of being more physically active in terms of reducing risk for the metabolic syndrome.

Table 1. Sampling of studies assessing the impact of physical activity patterns or exercise intervention on the metabolic syndrome.

Observational Studies			
Author, Year; (Reference)	N (Men/Women), Mean Age	Assessment	Key Results
Thune, 1998; [25]	5220/5869 34.4 and 33.7 years, respectively	PA self-report	Higher PA associated with better lipid profile, overall metabolic risk profile over 7 years
Laaksonen, 2002; [26]	612 men 51.4 years	Assessment of LTPA over previous 12 months among high risk men; followed for 4 years	>3 h/week moderate to vigorous LTPA half as likely as sedentary men to have MetSyn Men in top 33% VO_2max 75% less likely than unfit men to develop MetSyn over 4 years
Sisson, 2010; [27]	697/749 47.5 years	Accelerometry	MetS prevalence decreased as steps/day increased; odds of having MetSyn were 10% lower for each additional 1000 steps/day

Table 1. Cont.

Observational Studies			
Author, Year; (Reference)	N (Men/Women), Mean Age	Assessment	Key Results
Healy, 2008; [28]	67/102 53.4 years	Accelerometer evaluation of time spent in sedentary, light, moderate-to-vigorous, and mean activity intensity in participants with diabetes and obesity	Moderate-to-vigorous activity associated with lower triglycerides. Sedentary time, light-intensity time, and exercise intensity associated with waist circumference and clustered metabolic risk
Ekelund, 2007; [29]	103/155 40.8 years	Accelerometry, exercise test, biometric measures on adults with a family history of type 2 diabetes	Total body movement inversely associated with triglycerides, insulin, HDL and clustered metabolic risk; moderate-and vigorous-intensity PA inversely associated with clustered metabolic risk
Exercise Intervention Studies			
Author, Year	N	Intervention	Key Results
Look AHEAD, 2013; [30]	3063/2082 58.8 years	Subjects with type 2 diabetes randomly assigned to intensive lifestyle intervention or diabetes support and education	Intervention group had greater reductions in weight loss, glycated hemoglobin and greater initial improvements in exercise capacity and all cardiovascular risk factors (except LDL)
Stewart, 2004; [31]	53/62 63.6 years	6 months of exercise training in subjects with or at high risk for MetSyn	Exercise group improved peak VO$_2$, muscle strength, and lean body mass; reductions in total and abdominal fat related to improved CVD risk
Katzmarzyk, 2003; [32]	288/333 31.6	20 weeks of supervised aerobic exercise training	Of 105 patients with MetSyn, 30.5% were no longer classified as having metabolic syndrome after exercise training
Balducci, 2008; [33]	329/234	Twice weekly aerobic & resistance training for 1 year	Exercise group improved fitness, HbA1c, and CVD risk profile
Diabetes Prevention Program Research Group, 2002; [34]	3234 50.6	Lifestyle intervention (150 min/week PA and nutritional counseling) vs. Metformin vs. placebo	Lifestyle intervention group achieved a 38% reversal of MetSyn and a 41% reduction of new onset MetSyn.

PA—physical activity; LTPA—leisure time physical activity; MetSyn—metabolic syndrome; HDL—high density lipoprotein; LDL—high density lipoprotein; CVD—cardiovascular disease; HbA1c—glycated hemoglobin.

2.1. Observational Studies Associating Physical Activity Patterns with Metabolic Risk

Observational or cross-sectional studies are inherently limited because they do not demonstrate cause and effect. In the current context, the weaknesses of these studies include the fact that intrinsically healthier individuals may be more likely to engage in physical activity, or that they may be genetically more fit irrespective of lifestyle or behavioral factors. Nevertheless, these studies have provided valuable information regarding patterns between physical activity habits, metabolic risk, and related conditions. Collectively, these studies suggest that more active individuals exhibit either a lower prevalence of risk factors for the metabolic syndrome, have a lower incidence of developing the metabolic syndrome over a given follow-up period, or both. While the levels of activity have been quantified and defined in different ways, these data support the concept that meeting the minimal guidelines on activity (i.e., 150 minutes per week of moderate intensity activity) is associated with a lower prevalence of the metabolic syndrome. In the following, a sampling of some of the key observational studies related to physical activity and the metabolic syndrome are outlined.

As part of the TROMSO study in Norway, Thune and colleagues [25] studied 5220 men and 5869 women who completed two physical activity surveys approximately 7 years apart. BMI and detailed lipid profiles were determined at both evaluations. There was a dose–response relationship between improved serum lipid levels, BMI, and higher levels of physical activity in both genders after adjustments for potential confounders. Differences in BMI and serum lipid levels between sedentary and sustained exercising groups were consistently more pronounced after 7 years than at baseline, especially in the oldest age group. The most dramatic differences in metabolic risk profiles occurred between the most active subjects compared to the least active subjects. An increase in leisure time activity over the 7 years improved metabolic profiles, whereas a decrease worsened them in both genders.

In a cross-sectional evaluation of physical activity and metabolic risk among individuals with a family history of Type 2 diabetes, Ekelund et al. [29] measured total body movement and five other subcomponents of physical activity by accelerometry in 258 at-risk adults. Body composition was determined using bioimpedance and waist circumference, and blood pressure, fasting triglycerides, HDL, glucose, and insulin were determined. In addition, continuously distributed clustered risk was calculated. Total body movement (counts/day) was significantly and independently associated with three of six risk factors (fasting triglycerides, insulin, and HDL) and with clustered metabolic risk after adjustment for age, gender, and obesity. Time spent at moderate- and vigorous-intensity physical activity was independently associated with clustered metabolic risk. Short (5- and 10-minute) bouts of activity, time spent sedentary, and time spent at light-intensity activity were not significantly related with clustered risk after adjustment for confounding factors. The association between total body movement and intermediary phenotypic risk factors for cardiovascular and metabolic disease along with clustered metabolic risk was independent of aerobic fitness and obesity. These investigators suggested that increasing the total amount of physical activity in sedentary and overweight individuals has beneficial effects on metabolic risk.

Laaksonen and colleagues [26] assessed 12-month leisure time physical activity (LTPA), VO_2max, and cardiovascular and metabolic risk factors among 612 middle-aged men without the metabolic syndrome at baseline. After 4 years of follow-up, 107 men had metabolic syndrome (using the WHO definition). Men engaging in 3 h/week of moderate or vigorous LTPA were half as likely as sedentary men to have the metabolic syndrome after adjustment for major confounders (age, BMI, smoking, alcohol, and socioeconomic status) or potentially mediating factors (insulin, glucose, lipids, and blood pressure). Vigorous LTPA had an even stronger inverse association with incidence of the metabolic syndrome among men who were unfit at baseline. Men in the upper tertile of VO_2max were 75% less likely than unfit men to develop the metabolic syndrome, even after adjustment for major confounders. Associations of LTPA and VO_2max with development of the metabolic syndrome were qualitatively similar. These results suggest that high-risk men engaging in commonly recommended levels of physical activity were less likely to develop the metabolic syndrome than sedentary men. CRF was also strongly protective, although possibly not independent of mediating factors.

2.2. Exercise Intervention Studies and the Metabolic Syndrome

Relative to cross-sectional studies, exercise and lifestyle intervention studies can provide more direct information on the cause and effect impact of physical activity, CRF, or both, on risk of the metabolic syndrome. While there is a lengthy history of studies applying exercise interventions to assess the effects of training on individual components of the metabolic syndrome (e.g., insulin resistance, blood pressure, abdominal adiposity), fewer studies have been specifically designed to examine the efficacy of exercise training on the clinical diagnosis or reversal of the metabolic syndrome. In recent years, a growing number of groups have conducted large, multicenter randomized trials of exercise training along with other lifestyle interventions among individuals with or at high risk for the metabolic syndrome.

Two large lifestyle intervention trials, the Finnish Diabetes Prevention Study (DPS) [35], and the US Diabetes Prevention Program (DPP) [36], were designed to either prevent type 2 diabetes in impaired glucose-tolerant subjects or reduce the prevalence of metabolic syndrome through changes in diet and physical activity. The DPS observed a 58% reduction in risk for the development of type 2 diabetes with lifestyle intervention, and the DPP demonstrated a reduced prevalence of the metabolic syndrome in the intervention group. Weight loss appeared to be a major determinant of both improvements in glucose tolerance and the reduction in metabolic syndrome prevalence, whereas physical activity and dietary composition contributed independently. A third trial performed in the Netherlands involved a lifestyle intervention designed to assess the impact of diet and physical activity intervention on glucose tolerance in impaired glucose-tolerant subjects (termed the Study of Lifestyle intervention and Impaired glucose tolerance Maastricht [SLIM] study) [37]. The SLIM study similarly reported a 58% reduction in diabetes risk after 3 years and a 47% reduction at the end of the intervention, despite a relatively modest weight reduction. A follow-up to the SLIM trial determined the effects of the exercise and lifestyle intervention on the incidence and prevalence of the metabolic syndrome during the active intervention and four years thereafter [38]. They observed that the prevalence of the metabolic syndrome was significantly lower in the intervention group (52.6%) compared to the control group (74.6%). In addition, among participants without the metabolic syndrome at baseline, cumulative incidence of the metabolic syndrome was 18.2% in the intervention group at the end of active intervention, compared to 73.7% in the control group. Four years after stopping active intervention, the reduced incidence of metabolic syndrome was maintained.

A landmark multicenter trial performed in the US, termed Action for Health in Diabetes (Look AHEAD) [30], assessed whether an intensive lifestyle intervention for weight loss would decrease cardiovascular morbidity and mortality in patients with Type 2 diabetes. In 16 study centers in the US, 5145 overweight or obese patients with type 2 diabetes were randomly assigned to participate in an intensive lifestyle intervention that promoted weight loss through decreased caloric intake and increased physical activity (intervention group) or to receive diabetes support and education (control group). The primary outcome was a composite of death from cardiovascular causes, nonfatal myocardial infarction, nonfatal stroke, or hospitalization for angina during a maximum follow-up of 13.5 years. The trial was stopped early on the basis of a futility analysis at a median follow-up of 9.6 years. Weight loss was greater in the intervention group than in the control group throughout the study (8.6% vs. 0.7% at 1 year; 6.0% vs. 3.5% at study end). The intensive lifestyle intervention also produced greater reductions in HbA1c and greater initial improvements in fitness and all cardiovascular risk factors, except for LDL cholesterol. The primary outcome occurred in 403 patients in the intervention group and in 418 in the control group (1.83 and 1.92 events per 100 person-years, respectively); these differences were not significant ($p = 0.51$).

While the Look AHEAD study did not reduce the rate of cardiovascular events in overweight or obese adults with type 2 diabetes, there were many notable benefits among subjects in the intervention group. These included the fact that modest weight loss occurred and was maintained over 10 years, clinically meaningful improvements in HbA1c which were greatest during the first year but were at least partly sustained throughout follow-up, fewer subjects needing treatment with insulin, partial remission of diabetes during the first 4 years of the trial vs. control subjects, reduced sleep apnea and depression, and improvements in quality of life, physical functioning, and mobility.

There are also numerous notable single-center trials that have assessed the impact of exercise intervention on metabolic risk. Stewart et al. [31] studied 51 men and 53 women with or at elevated risk for metabolic syndrome who underwent either a 6-month supervised exercise program or usual care. Exercise significantly increased aerobic and muscle fitness, lean mass, and HDL, and reduced total and abdominal fat. Reductions in total body and abdominal fat and increases in leanness, largely independent of weight loss, were associated with improved systolic and diastolic blood pressure, total cholesterol, very low-density lipoprotein cholesterol, triglycerides, lipoprotein(a), and insulin sensitivity. At baseline, 42.3% of participants had metabolic syndrome. At 6 months, nine exercisers (17.7%) and eight controls (15.1%) no longer had metabolic syndrome, whereas four controls (7.6%) and no exercisers developed it.

Katzmarzyk, et al. [32] studied the efficacy of exercise training in treating the metabolic syndrome among 621 participants from the HERITAGE Family Study, identified at baseline as sedentary but apparently healthy. Subjects underwent a 20-week program of exercise training consisting of 3 sessions/week of supervised cycle ergometer training. The presence of the metabolic syndrome and the cluster of associated risk factors were determined before and after the study period. Exercise training resulted in marked improvements in the metabolic profile of the participants, including triglycerides, HDL cholesterol, blood pressure, fasting plasma glucose, and waist circumference. Of the 105 participants with the metabolic syndrome at baseline, 30.5% (32 participants) were no longer classified as having the metabolic syndrome after training. There were no sex or race differences in the efficacy of exercise in treating the metabolic syndrome.

2.3. Meta-Analyses of Exercise and Cardiometabolic Risk

There have been many individual trials in the context of physical activity and the metabolic syndrome, and many have lacked adequate sample sizes. The metabolic syndrome is more complex than many other conditions because it involves the clustering of several risk factors, and has been defined in different ways. Some studies have reported a significant effect on one or several risk factors but a minimal effect on another. Meta-analyses have been particularly helpful in this area by combining results from different studies to obtain a better estimate of the overall effect of a particular intervention. There have been several notable meta-analyses in the area of physical activity and metabolic syndrome which are discussed in the following.

Wewege et al. [39] recently performed a meta-analysis examining the effect of aerobic, resistance and combined (aerobic and resistance) exercise on cardiovascular risk factors among individuals with the metabolic syndrome, but without a diagnosis of diabetes. Interestingly, this is an understudied group, yet it represents the majority of the metabolic syndrome population. Randomized controlled trials >4 weeks in duration that compared an exercise intervention to non-exercise control groups in patients with metabolic syndrome without diabetes were included. Eleven studies with 16 interventions were analyzed (12 aerobic, 4 resistance). Aerobic exercise significantly improved waist circumference, fasting glucose, HDL cholesterol, triglycerides, diastolic blood pressure, and cardiorespiratory fitness (by 4.2 mL/kg/min, $p < 0.01$), among other outcomes. No significant effects were determined following resistance exercise possibly due to limited data. Sub-analyses suggested that aerobic exercise that progressed to vigorous intensity, and conducted 3 days/week for ≥12 weeks, offered larger and more widespread improvements. While these results strongly support the use of aerobic exercise for patients with the metabolic syndrome who have not yet developed diabetes, they also suggest that more studies on resistance/combined exercise programs are required to improve the quality of evidence.

Naci and Ioannidis [40] performed a recent meta-analysis among 14,716 subjects randomized to either a physical activity intervention or usual care. While the analysis did not address metabolic syndrome per se, the results are remarkable in that they provided a direct comparison between exercise and drug therapies for diabetes and CVD risk. Among 57 trials comparing the effects of drug and physical activity interventions on health outcomes compared to usual care, they observed that exercise intervention was similar to drug interventions for the secondary prevention of prediabetes, cardiovascular disease (CVD) and mortality. Importantly, physical activity was markedly superior to drug treatment among patients with stroke. The extent to which standard pharmacologic treatment would complement exercise interventions in treating or preventing diabetes or other health outcomes is unknown since there are so few data on comparative effectiveness involving exercise. These results are striking given the investments made in drug interventions relative to the comparatively meager investments devoted to exercise and other preventive strategies.

Ostman and colleagues [41] performed a meta-analysis that included 16 studies with 23 intervention groups and a total of 77,000 patient-hours of exercise training. All studies included subjects with a clinical diagnosis of the metabolic syndrome at baseline, an intervention involving exercise vs. sedentary controls, and all studies included incidence of mortality and hospitalization. Exercise training duration ranged between 8 weeks and 1 year. In analyses comparing aerobic exercise training versus control groups, there were reductions in BMI, waist circumference, systolic blood pressure and diastolic blood pressure, fasting blood glucose, triglycerides and low-density lipoprotein. Peak VO_2 was significantly improved among those randomized to exercise (mean difference 3.0 mL/kg/min, $p < 0.001$). Similar changes were observed for studies using combined aerobic and resistance exercise.

2.4. Synopsis—Physical Activity and the Metabolic Syndrome

Higher levels of physical activity, whether through observational studies or as part of formal exercise intervention trials, generally have a favorable impact on the metabolic syndrome and its components. In some studies, the proportion of participants who meet the criteria for the metabolic syndrome is reduced with exercise intervention. In longitudinal studies, more active individuals have a lower incidence of the metabolic syndrome. In a limited number of studies in which the dose–response relationship has been assessed, the most active subjects tend to have the greatest reductions in metabolic risk. Although the dose of physical activity has varied in the different studies, achieving the minimal physical activity guidelines (at least 150 minutes per week of moderate-intensity activity or 75 minutes per week of vigorous intensity activity) has been consistently demonstrated to have significant benefits on metabolic risk. While there are comparatively few studies on the impact of strength training on cardiometabolic risk, higher levels of muscular strength are associated with lower risk for developing the metabolic syndrome. Thus, in addition to aerobic exercise, individuals should strive to achieve the minimal recommendations of at least 2 days per week of resistance training.

3. Cardiorespiratory Fitness and the Metabolic Syndrome

Some of the inconsistencies between metabolic syndrome incidence and self-reported physical activity status [26,42] may be explained by the subjectivity and inaccuracy of self-reported physical activity assessments [43]. In this regard, directly measured or estimated VO_2 max based on a standardized exercise treadmill or cycle ergometer represents an objective assessment of CRF, as subject bias in reporting physical activity is removed. Overall, such studies have been consistent in reporting a lower prevalence of metabolic syndrome in those with higher CRF among both men and women regardless of race and after adjustment for relevant confounders [44–48]. An overview of some of the key studies is provided in Table 2.

Table 2. Sampling of studies assessing the association between cardiorespiratory fitness and the metabolic syndrome.

Author, Year; (Reference)	N (Men/Women)	Key Results
Carnethon, 2003; [49]	4487 (2029/2458)	Only men and women in the highest 40% of maximal treadmill performance were protected against developing MetSyn.
Franks, 2004; [50]	847 men	A strong inverse association between physical activity and MetSyn. The magnitude of the association between physical activity and the MetSyn was >3-fold greater than for VO_2max.
LaMonte, 2005; [46]	10,498 (9007/1491)	An independent and progressive decline in the risk of developing MetSyn with higher CRF for men and women. Also, 20% to 26% lower risks occurred among participants with moderate CRF and 53% to 63% lower risks observed in highest CRF categories vs. the lowest CRF category.

Table 2. *Cont.*

Author, Year; (Reference)	N (Men/Women)	Key Results
Hassinen, 2008; [44]	1347 (671/676)	Men and women in the lowest third of VO_2max had 10.2 times (men) and 10.8 times (women) higher risk of having MetSyn than those in the highest VO_2max category.
Hassinen, 2010; [48]	1226 (589/637)	Risk of developing MetSyn within 2 years of follow-up was 44% lower for each 1-SD increase in VO_2 max. Each 1-SD higher VO_2 max from baseline resulted in 1.8 times higher likelihood to resolve MetSyn during 2 years of follow-up.
Earnest, 2013; [51]	38,659 (30,927/7732)	CRF demonstrated a strong inverse relationship with MetSyn in both genders. The association was strongest in those with lower waist circumference and fasting glucose, in both genders.
Adams-Campbell, 2016; [47]	170 women	CRF was inversely related to the prevalence of the metabolic syndrome in overweight/obese African-American postmenopausal women.
Ingle, 2017; [52]	9666 men	The likelihood of developing MetSyn was approximately 50% lower in fit men compared to unfit, independent of BMI particularly in men <50 years.
Kelly, 2018; [45]	3636 (2007/1629)	Significant, inverse and graded association between VO_2max and MetSyn. Highest fit had >20 times lower risk of having MetSyn compared to least-fit individuals. The difference in VO_2max between those with MetSyn and those without was ≈ 2.5 METs.

CRF—cardiorespiratory fitness; BMI—body mass index; MetSyn—metabolic syndrome; METS—metabolic equivalents.

In Finland, men and women in the lowest tertile of VO_2max had 10.2 and 10.8 times, respectively, higher risks of having metabolic syndrome than those in the highest VO_2max category [44]. Similar findings were reported by Kelley et al. [45] in middle-aged men and women in the US. Importantly, an inverse and graded association between CRF and the incidence of metabolic syndrome has been observed with relatively small changes in CRF (e.g., 2.5 metabolic equivalents) yielding significant reductions in risk. The risk of metabolic syndrome prevalence was more than 20 times less likely for individuals in the highest fit category compared to the least-fit individuals. Similarly, the risk of developing metabolic syndrome within 2 years of follow-up was reported to be 44% lower for each 1-SD increase in VO_2 max [48]. Individuals in the highest sex-specific fitness category were 68% less likely to develop metabolic syndrome. In a more recent Finnish study, each 1-SD higher change in VO_2 max from baseline was associated with a 1.8-fold higher likelihood of resolving metabolic syndrome during 2 years of follow-up [48].

An interaction between CRF risk of and metabolic syndrome has also been suggested by the Australian National Health Survey. An inverse association between CRF and the metabolic syndrome was observed in those with lower waist circumference and fasting glucose in both men and women [51]. However, the impact of CRF on metabolic syndrome was independent of obesity as defined by body mass index among 9666 middle-aged (48.7 ± 8.4 years) asymptomatic men [52]. The likelihood of developing metabolic syndrome was approximately 50% lower in fit men compared to unfit men (OR = 0.51, 95% CI 0.46 to 0.57), independent of BMI, particularly in men <50 years. There is also evidence to suggest that objectively measured energy expenditure is a stronger deterrent for the metabolic syndrome than measured VO_2 max. Franks and colleagues [50] reported that the magnitude of the association between physical activity and the metabolic syndrome was >3-fold greater than for VO_2max, suggesting that the risk of metabolic syndrome can be modulated by higher intensity activities as well as lower intensity aerobic activities (below the threshold required to increase aerobic capacity).

Some evidence also suggests that the CRF-metabolic syndrome risk association may be gender-specific. Hassinen et al. [48] observed that each 1-SD higher VO_2 max (6.1 mL/kg/min in men; 4.8 mL/kg/min in women) resulted in 56% and 35% decreased risks of developing metabolic syndrome over two years of follow-up in men and women, respectively. In men, a 4.8 mL/kg/min increase in VO_2 max resulted in a 56% decrease in risk [48]. However, gender differences in the association between CRF and incidence of metabolic syndrome were not supported by the same group in their previous study [44].

There are also indications that only high CRF may offer protection against the development of metabolic syndrome. Laaksonen et al. [26] reported 47% and 75% lower odds of developing metabolic syndrome among men in the middle and highest tertiles of measured VO_2max, respectively, compared to men in the lowest tertile. However, this association was no longer significant after adjustment for baseline metabolic risk factors. Similarly, Carnethon et al. [49] reported that only men and women in the highest 40% of maximal treadmill performance were protected against developing metabolic syndrome. In contrast, LaMonte et al. [46] reported an independent and progressive decline in the risk of developing metabolic syndrome with increased CRF for men and women. Specifically, they reported 20% to 26% lower risks among participants with moderate CRF levels and 53% to 63% lower risks in the highest CRF categories, when compared to those in the lowest CRF category.

Finally, in the Diabetes Prevention Program trial, 3234 subjects (53% with metabolic syndrome) at high risk for diabetes were randomized to a lifestyle intervention group or usual care [34]. Those in the lifestyle intervention group (aerobic exercise 150 minutes per week and nutritional counseling) achieved a 38% reversal of the metabolic syndrome and a 41% reduction of new onset of metabolic syndrome. In contrast, treatment with metformin only reduced new cases of metabolic syndrome by 17%. To prevent one case of diabetes during a period of three years, 6.9 persons would have had to participate in the lifestyle-intervention program, and 13.9 would have had to receive metformin. These findings suggest that a healthy lifestyle may be more effective in preventing metabolic syndrome than the anti-hyperglycemic agent metformin.

Synopsis—Cardiorespiratory Fitness and the Metabolic Syndrome

Although physical activity and CRF are often used interchangeably, it is important to recognize that they are different; physical activity is a behavior and CRF is an attribute. CRF is improved by activity, but it is influenced by other factors, including genetics. Nevertheless, most sedentary individuals will improve CRF by following the widely-recognized minimal guidelines on physical activity. Both CRF levels from observational studies and changes in CRF as a result of 3–12-month exercise interventions have consistently been shown to improve cardiometabolic risk. In some studies, a proportion of a study sample no longer meets the criteria for metabolic syndrome after an exercise intervention that increases CRF. Taken together, cross-sectional studies demonstrate that subjects in the highest-fit categories exhibit between 5- and 20-fold lower likelihood of having the metabolic syndrome vs. subjects in the least-fit groups. Longitudinally, subjects in the highest fit groups exhibit ≈40% to as much as 20-fold lower risks of developing the metabolic syndrome. Efforts to improve CRF should be part of standard therapy for individuals with or at high risk for the metabolic syndrome.

4. Mechanisms Underlying the Metabolic Syndrome and Implications for Physical Activity and Fitness

4.1. Pathophysiology of Metabolic Syndrome

The underlying cause(s) of the metabolic syndrome are unknown, but it is significantly influenced by the twin epidemics of diabetes and obesity. Indeed, metabolic syndrome shares diabetes-related insulin resistance (IR) and dysfunctional adipose fuel handling and central obesity as its core. However, despite the commonality of traits, many subjects with metabolic syndrome do not display IR [53] nor do all obese individuals have metabolic syndrome [54,55]. Thus, neither IR nor central obesity fully explains the pathophysiological features of metabolic syndrome and other factors implicated include inflammation, genetics, epigenetics, and circadian abnormalities. As will be discussed further, enhanced CRF modulates the negative impact of these causative drivers of metabolic syndrome.

4.2. Insulin Resistance

The concept of IR was introduced by Himmsworth in 1936 who showed that diabetes could be subdivided into two categories—insulin-sensitive and insulin-insensitive types [56]—and this was later confirmed by Yalow and Berson with the novel measurement of insulin itself [57]. Once clamp techniques were developed, it was established that IR predominated in type 2 diabetes [58,59] and that hyperinsulinemia was the best predictor of the development of type 2 diabetes in nondiabetic individuals [60]. Reaven coined the term Syndrome X, later renamed by others to metabolic syndrome, to describe the role of IR (i.e., hyperinsulinemia or impaired glucose tolerance) as the driver of atherosclerotic dyslipidemia, type 2 diabetes, and hypertension [61]. Indeed, elevations of insulin concentration were shown to prospectively precede the development of these metabolic disorders [62] and the role of IR in metabolic syndrome was shown to be related to low insulin sensitivity [63]. With an increasing degree of metabolic syndrome components (i.e., metabolic syndrome score), there is an increase in fasting glucose, insulin levels, and HOMA IR [64].

During physiological conditions, insulin binds to its receptor leading to tyrosine phosphorylation of downstream substrates including activation of the phosphoinositide 3-kinase (PI3K) pathway resulting in recruitment of GLUT4 to mediate glucose transport into muscle and adipose tissue where it is phosphorylated and either stored as glycogen or metabolized to produce ATP. However, when a state of compensatory hyperinsulinemia occurs in IR subjects, due to changes in insulin secretion and/or insulin clearance [65], the ensuing response includes mild forms of glucose intolerance, dyslipidemia (high triglycerides, low HDL, small dense LDL), and hypertension which is the pathophysiological construct of the insulin resistance syndrome developed by Reaven leading to increased risk of CVD, as well conditions such as stroke, polycystic ovary syndrome, non-alcoholic fatty liver disease, cancer, and sleep apnea [66]. Importantly, according to Reaven, the individual components of the IR syndrome can occur without IR, and the presence of IR does not have to lead to any of the components of the syndrome. Interestingly, although IR has been considered the central driver of type 2 diabetes and metabolic syndrome, an alternative argument places IR as an adaptive biomarker of poor metabolic health and insulin hyperresponsivness as the root cause [67].

The reason why IR leads to atherogenesis has been attributed to the activation by insulin of the mitogen activated protein (MAP) kinase pathway which, as opposed to the muted PI3K pathway, functions normally in IR. Subnormal PI3K-Akt activity leads to a reduction in endothelial nitric oxide formation and endothelial dysfunction, reduction in GLUT4 translocation, and decreased skeletal muscle and fat glucose uptake [68]. Concurrently, the persistence of MAP kinase activity results in augmented expression of endothelin-1 and endothelial adhesion molecules with vascular smooth muscle cell mitogenesis which leads to vascular abnormalities and increased atherosclerosis risk.

The skeletal muscle mass comprises approximately 40% of total body mass and is the primary source of insulin-mediated glucose uptake and fatty acid oxidation. The exposure to exercise evokes adaptation in skeletal muscle in a multitude of signaling pathways, the functional response to which is determined by training volume, mode of training, intensity and frequency. With persistent exercise exposure, there is mitochondrial biogenesis, fast-to-slow fiber-type transformation, changes in substrate metabolism, and angiogenesis. Moreover, a host of myokines are released from active muscles providing communication throughout the body. Enhanced fitness is associated with high levels of insulin sensitivity/insulin action. While glucose homeostasis at rest is insulin-sensitive, exercise with muscle contractions increases glucose uptake from the circulation that is not reliant on insulin. Indeed, GLUT-4 is responsive to both insulin and muscle contraction independently.

Whatever the role of IR, it is known that exercise augments insulin signaling independent of PI3K and when skeletal muscles are stimulated by contraction combined with insulin, glucose transport and GLUT4 translocation are enhanced. Thus, exercise provides a potent means to avert metabolic syndrome supported by the results of the Diabetes Prevention Program study [36], where exercise intervention decreased metabolic syndrome prevalence significantly compared to the control group throughout the intervention. Interestingly, although both aerobic and resistance training increase glucose transport and are often additive, these metabolic responses appear to be mediated by different mechanisms. In at least one study among nonobese young women, the investigators reported that insulin sensitivity increases in both aerobically-trained and resistance-trained women. However, when data were expressed per kg of free-fat mass (FFM) the improvement in glucose disposal persisted in endurance-trained women, whereas no significant change was noted in resistance-trained subjects or controls. This led to the conclusion that the increased glucose disposal associated with resistance exercise was the result of the increase in the quantity of lean body mass, without altering the intrinsic capacity of the muscle to respond to insulin. On the other hand, endurance training enhanced glucose disposal independent of changes in lean body mass or VO_2max, suggestive of an intrinsic change in the ability of the muscle to metabolize glucose [69].

4.3. Adipose Fuel Metabolism

The metabolic consequences related to an unhealthy lifestyle were proposed in 1923 by Kylin consisting of a syndrome of hypertension, hyperglycemia, hyperuricemia, and obesity [70]. "Androgenic obesity" contributing to diabetes and CVD was proposed later by Vague in 1940 [71]. The upper-body or abdominal obesity type with hyperinsulinemia, in particular, was proposed as the primary factor leading to metabolic syndrome and CVD independent of overall obesity [72–74]. Being a multifunctional organ providing cross-talk between various systems, including the immune and the cardiovascular systems, this type of abdominal obesity, being the most common manifestation of metabolic syndrome, has been viewed as a cellular biomarker of dysfunctional adipose tissue [55] or adiposopathy [75].

Insulin is the major regulator of fuel metabolism in adipocytes and is adversely impacted by excess caloric intake and inactivity. Hyperinsulinemia is well documented in individuals with obesity with or without IR and is related to increases in insulin secretion and decreases in insulin clearance rate [76]. It has been known for some time that insulin insensitivity can cause a distinct biochemical syndrome with elevated free fatty acids [77] and in metabolic syndrome-prone subjects, relative tissue hypoinsulinemia results in release of excess free fatty acids, mainly from visceral depots, resulting in increased liver synthesis VLDL, elevated triglycerides, increased HDL clearance and small dense LDL. Increased free fatty acid release also causes IR in the liver resulting in increased gluconeogenesis and hyperglycemia. These metabolic events result in adipocyte fuel malfunction manifested as adipocyte hypertrophy and ectopic lipid deposition in vital organs such as the liver, pancreas, muscle and heart. In the pancreas, lipid excess can lead to lipotoxicity which can promote endoplasmic reticulum stress-mediated β-cell death [78].

Adipose tissue also harbors fat-derived mesenchymal stem cells which experimentally have the capacity to modify mRNA expression contributing to IR [79]. Moreover, abdominal fat and fat-derived mesenchymal stem cells are responsive to physical activity; both high-intensity aerobic and resistance training decrease visceral fat effectively [80] while the molecular expression of fat-derived mesenchymal stem cells is significantly altered with exercise preventing adipogenesis [81].

4.4. Inflammation

Systemic inflammation has been strongly linked to CVD via multiple immune system biomarkers, factors also associated with metabolic syndrome. Thus, metabolic syndrome is associated with pro-inflammatory cytokines such as TNF, IL-beta, and is characterized by chronic systemic low-grade inflammation manifested by elevated CRP [82]. Chronic inflammation links metabolic syndrome to IR [83,84] and to CVD via promotion of vascular dysfunction [85]. Adipocyte hypertrophy, abnormal local blood flow, hypoxia, altered adipokine expression, and local infiltration of immune cells all conspire to adiposopathy which is infiltrated by macrophages, with elevated TNF and IL-6. Moreover, these macrophage-associated adipocytes are undergoing necrosis. A recent finding showed that the use of the anti-inflammatory agent colchicine significantly improved obesity-associated inflammatory variables in metabolic syndrome and appeared to be safe [86].

The degree of cardiorespiratory fitness in metabolic syndrome subjects has been shown to have inverse associations with CRP, IL-6, and IL-18, partially explained by the degree of abdominal obesity [87]. Using IL-18 as a biomarker of inflammation, aerobic exercise reduced inflammation which was not observed with resistance exercise despite a similar degree of loss of fat mass in metabolic syndrome subjects [88].

4.5. Genetics/Epigenetics

Inheritance plays a role in metabolic syndrome and its influence may range from 10% to 30% being strongest between waist circumference and IR, which has also been documented in twin studies [89]. Techniques such as linkage analysis, candidate gene approach, and genome-wide association (GWAS) studies have been applied to detect gene variants for metabolic syndrome focusing on loci for individual components such as obesity, dyslipidemia, hypertension, and diabetes [90]. For example, eight single nucleotide polymorphisms (SNPs) were associated with the dyslipidemia in metabolic syndrome [91]. In other studies, GWAS associations have shown that transcription factor 7-like 2 (TCF7L2), which is part of the Wnt signaling pathway, mediates metabolic syndrome trait susceptibility towards developing diabetes and dyslipidemia [92]. Another example is the caveolin-1 gene (CAV1) variant associated with IR which is also associated with metabolic syndrome, especially in non-obese subjects [93].

The concept of epigenetics, originally accredited to Waddington, has evolved to specify how gene activation or silencing influence gene expression without changing the DNA sequence itself and the epigenome include DNA methylation, histone modification, and various RNA-mediated processes. The epigenetic expression can be altered during development, during varying nutritional conditions, and by physical activity. One of the epigenetic mechanisms involves DNA methylation which results in a methyl group being attached to a cytosine pyrimidine ring and thereby influence gene expression especially when located in promotor regions. A burgeoning area of inquiry involves DNA methylation which has been reported to be related to several components of the metabolic syndrome [94] including an inverse association between levels of methylation and worsening of the metabolic syndrome [95]. Studies assessing global DNA methylation and also assessing methylation at specific genes related to lipid metabolism appear to be related to causation of the metabolic syndrome [96]. Epigenetic methylation changes related to physical activity have been reported to occur in the regions regulating peroxisome proliferator-activated receptor-1α, the master regulator of exercise-muscle activity, and also impact the adipose tissue response [97–99].

4.6. Circadian Disruption and Metabolic Syndrome

Disrupted diurnal rhythms due to excessive light or shift work can have profound and disruptive whole-body metabolic effects impacting most hormones that are normally governed by circadian rhythmicity so it is not surprising that these perturbations can lead to metabolic syndrome conditions with IR and obesity. Clock genes are expressed in adipose tissue and correlate to metabolic syndrome parameters [100]. A shortened sleep duration less than 6 hours has been associated with increased risk of metabolic syndrome and CVD [101] and meta analyses support these associations between sleep deprivation and risk for metabolic syndrome [102,103]. Moreover, the relationship of shortened sleep and metabolic syndrome may be dose related [104]. However, a normal sleep pattern decreases the risk of metabolic syndrome, albeit prolonged sleep appears to be neutral in this regard [105]. Regular exercise can re-set clock genes and have a salutary impact on clock time which might be another way to inhibit the metabolic syndrome [106,107]. A complementary medical strategy may be the use of a sympatholytic dopamine D2 receptor agonist to combat the circadian disruption and improve metabolic syndrome [108].

5. Summary

Both single center trials and recent meta-analyses suggest that exercise training, higher CRF, or both, improve factors that underlie the metabolic syndrome. Among subjects who meet the criteria for the metabolic syndrome, health outcomes are significantly improved by aerobic or resistance training, or their combination. In some individuals, an exercise program has been demonstrated to improve risk markers to an extent that they no longer meet the criteria for the metabolic syndrome. There are numerous physiological, lifestyle, and genetic factors that account for these salutary effects of physical activity or formal exercise programs. These include the impact of exercise on insulin resistance, adipose fuel metabolism, inflammation, and epigenetic factors. Physical activity interventions clearly have a favorable impact on metabolic disease and the burden it places not only on individuals but also on health care systems. Incorporating physical activity as an integral part of treatment strategies for the metabolic syndrome would appear to go a long way toward reducing the adverse health impact of this condition.

Funding: This research received no external funding.

Conflicts of Interest: The authors declare no conflict of interest.

References

1. Riley, L.; Guthold, R.; Cowan, M.; Savin, S.; Bhatti, L.; Armstrong, T.; Bonita, R. The World Health Organization STEPwise Approach to Noncommunicable Disease Risk-Factor Surveillance: Methods, Challenges, and Opportunities. *Am. J. Public Health* **2016**, *106*, 74–78. [CrossRef] [PubMed]
2. Haller, H. Epidemiology and associated risk factors of hyperlipoproteinemia. *Zeitschrift für Sie Gesamte Innere Medizin und Ihre Grenzgebiete* **1977**, *32*, 124–128.
3. Grundy, S.M.; Cleeman, J.I.; Daniels, S.R.; Donato, K.A.; Eckel, R.H.; Franklin, B.A.; Gordon, D.J.; Krauss, R.M.; Savage, P.J.; Smith, S.C., Jr.; et al. American Heart Association; National Heart, Lung, and Blood Institute. Diagnosis and management of the metabolic syndrome: An American Heart Association/National Heart, Lung, and Blood Institute Scientific Statement. *Circulation* **2005**, *112*, 2735–2752. [CrossRef] [PubMed]
4. Sperling, L.S.; Mechanick, J.I.; Neeland, I.J.; Herrick, C.J.; Després, J.P.; Ndumele, C.E.; Vijayaraghavan, K.; Handelsman, Y.; Puckrein, G.A.; Araneta, M.R.; et al. The CardioMetabolic Health Alliance: Working toward a new care model for the metabolic syndrome. *J. Am. Coll. Cardiol.* **2015**, *66*, 1050–1067. [CrossRef] [PubMed]
5. Mottillo, S.; Filion, K.B.; Genest, J.; Joseph, L.; Pilote, L.; Poirier, P.; Rinfret, S.; Schiffrin, E.L.; Eisenberg, M.J. The metabolic syndrome and cardiovascular risk. A systematic review and meta-analysis. *J. Am. Coll. Cardiol.* **2010**, *56*, 1113–1132. [CrossRef] [PubMed]
6. DeBoer, M.D.; Filipp, S.L.; Gurka, M.J. Use of a metabolic syndrome severity z score to track risk during treatment of prediabetes: An analysis of the diabetes prevention program. *Diabetes Care* **2018**, *41*, dc181079. [CrossRef] [PubMed]
7. Pucci, G. Sex- and gender-related prevalence, cardiovascular risk and therapeutic approach in metabolic syndrome: A review of the literature. *Pharmacol. Res.* **2017**, *120*, 34–42. [CrossRef] [PubMed]
8. Myers, J.; McAuley, P.; Lavie, C.; Despres, J.P.; Arena, R.; Kokkinos, P. Physical activity and cardiorespiratory fitness as major markers of cardiovascular risk: Their independent and interwoven importance to health status. *Prog. Cardiovasc. Dis.* **2015**, *57*, 306–314. [CrossRef]
9. US Department of Health and Human Services. Physical Activity: Facts and Statistics. Available online: https://www.hhs.gov/fitness/resource-center/facts-and-statistics/index.html (accessed on 27 January 2019).
10. Chau, J.; Chey, T.; Burks-Young, S.; Engelen, L.; Bauman, A. Trends in prevalence of leisure time physical activity and inactivity: Results from Australian National Health Surveys 1989 to 2011. *Aust. N. Z. J. Public Health* **2017**, *41*, 617–624. [CrossRef]
11. Hallal, P.C.; Andersen, L.B.; Bull, F.C.; Guthold, R.; Haskell, W.; Ekelund, U. Global physical activity levels: Surveillance progress, pitfalls, and prospects. *Lancet* **2012**, *380*, 247–257. [CrossRef]
12. Duncan, G.E. Exercise, fitness, and cardiovascular disease risk in type 2 diabetes and the metabolic syndrome. *Curr. Diab. Rep.* **2006**, *6*, 29–35. [CrossRef] [PubMed]

13. Church, T. Exercise in obesity, metabolic syndrome, and diabetes. *Prog. Cardiovasc. Dis.* **2011**, *53*, 412–418. [CrossRef] [PubMed]
14. Zhang, D.; Liu, X.; Liu, Y.; Sun, X.; Wang, B.; Ren, Y.; Zhao, Y.; Zhou, J.; Han, C.; Yin, L.; et al. Leisure-time physical activity and incident metabolic syndrome: A systematic review and dose-response meta-analysis of cohort studies. *Metabolism* **2017**, *75*, 36–44. [CrossRef] [PubMed]
15. Strasser, B. Physical activity in obesity and metabolic syndrome. *Ann. N. Y. Acad. Sci.* **2013**, *1281*, 141–159. [CrossRef] [PubMed]
16. Bull, F.; Goenka, S.; Lambert, V.; Pratt, M. Physical Activity for the Prevention of Cardiometabolic Disease. In *Cardiovascular, Respiratory, and Related Disorders*, 3rd ed.; Prabhakaran, D., Anand, S., Gaziano, T.A., Mbanya, J.C., Wu, Y., Nugent, R., Eds.; The International Bank for Reconstruction and Development/The World Bank: Washington, DC, USA, 2017; Chapter 5.
17. Myers, J. The new AHA/ACC guidelines on cardiovascular risk: When will fitness get the recognition it deserves? *Mayo Clin. Proc.* **2014**, *89*, 722–726. [CrossRef] [PubMed]
18. Franklin, B.A. physical activity to combat chronic diseases and escalating health care costs: The unfilled prescription. *Curr. Sports Med. Rep.* **2008**, *7*, 122–125. [CrossRef] [PubMed]
19. Sallis, R.E.; Matuszak, J.M.; Baggish, A.L.; Franklin, B.A.; Chodzko-Zajko, W.; Fletcher, B.J.; Gregory, A.; Joy, E.; Matheson, G.; McBride, P.; et al. Call to Action on Making Physical Activity Assessment and Prescription a Medical Standard of Care. *Curr. Sports Med. Rep.* **2016**, *15*, 207–214. [CrossRef] [PubMed]
20. Berra, K.; Rippe, J.; Manson, J.E. Making Physical Activity Counseling a Priority in Clinical Practice: The Time for Action Is Now. *JAMA* **2015**, *314*, 2617–2618. [CrossRef] [PubMed]
21. Omura, J.D.; Bellissimo, M.P.; Watson, K.B.; Loustalot, F.; Fulton, J.E.; Carlson, S.E. Primary care providers' physical activity counseling and referral practices and barriers for cardiovascular disease prevention. *Prev. Med.* **2018**, *108*, 115–122. [CrossRef]
22. U.S. Department of Health and Human Services. *Physical Activity Guidelines for Americans*, 2nd ed.; U.S. Department of Health and Human Services: Washington, DC, USA, 2018.
23. Roberts, C.K.; Hevener, A.L.; Barnard, R.J. Metabolic syndrome and insulin resistance: Underlying causes and modification by exercise training. *Compr. Physiol.* **2013**, *3*, 1–58.
24. Henriksen, E.J. Effects of acute exercise and exercise training on insulin resistance. *J. Appl. Physiol.* **2002**, *93*, 788–796. [CrossRef] [PubMed]
25. Thune, I.; Njølstad, I.; Løchen, M.L.; Førde, O.H. Physical activity improves the metabolic risk profiles in men and women: The Tromsø Study. *Arch. Intern. Med.* **1998**, *158*, 1633–1640. [CrossRef] [PubMed]
26. Laaksonen, D.E.; Lakka, H.M.; Salonen, J.T.; Niskanen, L.K.; Rauramaa, R.; Lakka, T.A. Low levels of leisure-time physical activity and cardiorespiratory fitness predict development of the metabolic syndrome. *Diabetes Care* **2002**, *25*, 1612–1618. [CrossRef] [PubMed]
27. Sisson, S.B.; Camhi, S.M.; Church, T.S.; Tudor-Locke, C.; Johnson, W.D.; Katzmarzyk, P.T. Accelerometer-determined steps/day and metabolic syndrome. *Am. J. Prev. Med.* **2010**, *38*, 575–582. [CrossRef] [PubMed]
28. Healy, G.N.; Wijndaele, K.; Dunstan, D.W.; Shaw, J.E.; Salmon, J.; Zimmet, P.Z.; Owen, N. Objectively measured sedentary time, physical activity, and metabolic risk: The Australian Diabetes, Obesity and Lifestyle Study (AusDiab). *Diabetes Care* **2008**, *31*, 369–371. [CrossRef] [PubMed]
29. Ekelund, U.; Griffin, S.J.; Wareham, N.J. Physical activity and metabolic risk in individuals with a family history of type 2 diabetes. *Diabetes Care* **2007**, *30*, 337–342. [CrossRef] [PubMed]
30. Look AHEAD Research Group. Cardiovascular effects of intensive lifestyle intervention in type 2 diabetes. *N. Engl. J. Med.* **2013**, *369*, 145–154. [CrossRef]
31. Stewart, K.J.; Bacher, A.C.; Turner, K.; Lim, J.G.; Hees, P.S.; Shapiro, E.P.; Tayback, M.; Ouyang, P. Exercise and risk factors associated with metabolic syndrome in older adults. *Am. J. Prev. Med.* **2005**, *28*, 9–18. [CrossRef]
32. Katzmarzyk, P.T.; Leon, A.S.; Wilmore, J.H.; Skinner, J.S.; Rao, D.C.; Rankinen, T.; Bouchard, C. Targeting the metabolic syndrome with exercise: Evidence from the HERITAGE Family Study. *Med. Sci. Sports Exerc.* **2003**, *35*, 1703–1709. [CrossRef]
33. Balducci, S.; Zanuso, S.; Massarini, M.; Corigliano, G.; Nicolucci, A.; Missori, S.; Cavallo, S.; Cardelli, P.; Alessi, E.; Pugliese, G.; et al. The Italian Diabetes and Exercise Study (IDES): Design and methods for a prospective Italian multicentre trial of intensive lifestyle intervention in people with type 2 diabetes and the metabolic syndrome. *Nutr. Metab. Cardiovasc. Dis.* **2008**, *18*, 585–595. [CrossRef]

34. Diabetes Prevention Program Research Group. Reduction in the Incidence of Type 2 Diabetes with Lifestyle Intervention or Metformin. *N. Engl. J. Med.* **2002**, *346*, 393–403. [CrossRef] [PubMed]
35. Tuomilehto, J.; Lindstrom, J.; Eriksson, J.G.; Valle, T.T.; Hamalainen, H.; Ilanne-Parikka, P.; Keinänen-Kiukaanniemi, S.; Laakso, M.; Louheranta, A.; Rastas, M.; et al. Prevention of type 2 diabetes mellitus by changes in lifestyle among subjects with impaired glucose tolerance. *N. Engl. J. Med.* **2001**, *344*, 1343–1350. [CrossRef] [PubMed]
36. Orchard, T.J.; Temprosa, M.; Goldberg, R.; Haffner, S.; Ratner, R.; Marcovina, S.; Fowler, S. The effect of metformin and intensive lifestyle intervention on the metabolic syndrome: The Diabetes Prevention Program randomized trial. *Ann. Intern. Med.* **2005**, *142*, 611–619. [CrossRef] [PubMed]
37. Roumen, C.; Feskens, E.J.; Corpeleijn, E.; Mensink, M.; Saris, W.H.; Blaak, E.E. Predictors of lifestyle intervention outcome and dropout: The SLIM study. *Eur. J. Clin. Nutr.* **2011**, *65*, 1141–1147. [CrossRef] [PubMed]
38. Den Boer, A.T.; Herraets, I.J.; Stegen, J.; Roumen, C.; Corpeleijn, E.; Schaper, N.C.; Feskens, E.; Blaak, E.E. Prevention of the metabolic syndrome in IGT subjects in a lifestyle intervention: Results from the SLIM study. *Nutr. Metab. Cardiovasc. Dis.* **2013**, *23*, 1147–1153. [CrossRef] [PubMed]
39. Wewege, M.A.; Thom, J.M.; Rye, K.A.; Parmenter, B.J. Aerobic, resistance or combined training: A systematic review and meta-analysis of exercise to reduce cardiovascular risk in adults with metabolic syndrome. *Atherosclerosis* **2018**, *274*, 162–171. [CrossRef] [PubMed]
40. Naci, H.; Ioannidis, J.P. Comparative effectiveness of exercise and drug interventions on mortality outcomes: Metaepidemiological study. *BMJ* **2013**, *347*, f5577. [CrossRef] [PubMed]
41. Ostman, C.; Smart, N.A.; Morcos, D.; Duller, A.; Ridley, W.; Jewiss, D. The effect of exercise training on clinical outcomes in patients with the metabolic syndrome: A systematic review and meta-analysis. *Cardiovasc. Diabetol.* **2017**, *16*, 110. [CrossRef] [PubMed]
42. Palaniappan, L.; Carnethon, M.R.; Wang, Y.; Hanley, A.J.; Fortmann, S.P.; Haffner, S.M.; Wagenknecht, L. Predictors of the incident metabolic syndrome in adults: The Insulin Resistance Atherosclerosis Study. *Diabetes Care* **2004**, *27*, 788–793. [CrossRef] [PubMed]
43. LaMonte, M.J.; Ainsworth, B.E. Quantifying energy expenditure and physical activity in the context of dose response. *Med. Sci. Sports Exerc.* **2001**, *33*, S370–S378. [CrossRef]
44. Hassinen, M.; Lakka, T.; Savonen, K.; Litmanen, H.; Kiviaho, L.; Laaksonen, D.E.; Komulainen, P.; Rauramaa, R. Cardiorespiratory Fitness as a Feature of Metabolic Syndrome in Older Men and Women. *Diabetes Care* **2008**, *31*, 1242–1247. [CrossRef] [PubMed]
45. Kelley, E.; Imboden, M.T.; Harber, M.P.; Finch, H.; Kaminsky, L.A.; Whaley, M.H. Cardiorespiratory Fitness Is Inversely Associated with Clustering of Metabolic Syndrome Risk Factors: The Ball State Adult Fitness Program Longitudinal Lifestyle Study. *Mayo Clin. Proc. Innov. Qual. Outcomes* **2018**, *2*, 155–164. [CrossRef] [PubMed]
46. LaMonte, M.J.; Barlow, C.E.; Jurca, R.; James, B.; Kampert, J.B.; Church, T.S.; Blair, S.N. Cardiorespiratory fitness is inversely associated with the incidence of metabolic syndrome: A prospective study of men and women. *Circulation* **2005**, *112*, 505–512. [CrossRef] [PubMed]
47. Adams-Campbell, L.L.; Dash, C.; Kim, B.H.; Hicks, J.C.; Makambi, K.; Hagberg, J.M. Cardiorespiratory fitness and metabolic syndrome in postmenopausal African-American women. *Int. J. Sports Med.* **2016**, *37*, 261–266. [CrossRef] [PubMed]
48. Hassinen, M.; Lakka, T.; Hakola, L.; Savonen, K.; Komulainen, P.; Litmanen, H.; Kiviniemi, V.; Kouki, R.; Heikkilä, H.; Rauramaa, R. Cardiorespiratory fitness and metabolic syndrome in older men and women. *Diabetes Care* **2010**, *33*, 1655–1657. [CrossRef] [PubMed]
49. Carnethon, M.R.; Gidding, S.S.; Nehgme, R.; Sidney, S.; Jacobs, D.R., Jr.; Liu, K. Cardiorespiratory fitness in young adulthood and the development of cardiovascular disease risk factors. *JAMA* **2003**, *290*, 3092–3100. [CrossRef]
50. Franks, P.W.; Ekelund, U.; Brage, S.; Wong, M.-Y.; Wareham, N.J. Does the association of habitual activity with the metabolic syndrome differ by level of cardiorespiratory fitness? *Diabetes Care* **2004**, *27*, 1187–1193. [CrossRef] [PubMed]
51. Earnest, C.P.; Artero, C.G.; Sui, X.; Church, T.S.; Blair, S.N. Maximal estimated cardiorespiratory fitness, cardiometabolic risk factors, metabolic syndrome in the aerobics center longitudinal study. *Mayo Clin. Proc.* **2013**, *88*, 259–270. [CrossRef]

52. Ingle, L.; Mellis, M.; Brodie, D.; Sandercock, G.R. Associations between cardiorespiratory fitness and the metabolic syndrome in British men. *Heart* **2017**, *103*, 524–528. [CrossRef]
53. Cheal, K.L.; Abbasi, F.; Lamendola, C.; McLaughlin, T.; Reaven, G.M.; Ford, E.S. Relationship to insulin resistance of the adult treatment panel III diagnostic criteria for identification of the metabolic syndrome. *Diabetes* **2004**, *53*, 1195–2000. [CrossRef]
54. Meigs, J.B.; Wilson, P.W.; Fox, C.S.; Vasan, R.S.; Nathan, D.M.; Sullivan, L.M.; D'Agostino, R.B. Body mass index, metabolic syndrome, and risk of type 2 diabetes or cardiovascular disease. *J. Clin. Endocrinol. Metab.* **2006**, *91*, 2906–2912. [CrossRef] [PubMed]
55. Despres, J.P.; Lemieux, I. Abdominal obesity and metabolic syndrome. *Nature* **2006**, *444*, 881–887. [CrossRef] [PubMed]
56. Himsworth, H.P. Diabetes mellitus: Its differentiation into insulin sensitive and insulin insensitive types. *Lancet* **1936**, *1*, 127–130. [CrossRef]
57. Yalow, R.S.; Berson, S.A. Plasma insulin concentrations in nondiabetic and early diabetic subjects. Determinations by a new sensitive immuno-assay technique. *Diabetes* **1960**, *9*, 254–260. [CrossRef] [PubMed]
58. Ginsberg, H.; Olefsky, J.M.; Reaven, G.M. Further evidence that insulin resistance exists in patients with chemical diabetes. *Diabetes* **1974**, *23*, 674–678. [CrossRef] [PubMed]
59. DeFronzo, R.A.; Tobin, J.D.; Andres, R. Glucose clamp technique: A method for quantifying insulin secretion and resistance. *Am. J. Physiol.* **1979**, *237*, E214–E223. [CrossRef] [PubMed]
60. Lillioja, S.; Mott, D.M.; Spraul, M.; Ferraro, R.; Foley, J.E.; Ravussin, E.; Knowler, W.C.; Bennett, P.H.; Bogardus, C. Insulin resistance and insulin secretory dysfunction as precursors of non-insulin-dependent diabetes mellitus. Prospective studies of Pima Indians. *N. Engl. J. Med.* **1993**, *329*, 1988–1992. [CrossRef]
61. Reaven, G.M. Banting lecture 1988. Role of insulin resistance in human disease. *Diabetes* **1988**, *37*, 1595–1607. [CrossRef]
62. Haffner, S.M.; Valdez, R.A.; Hazuda, H.P.; Mitchell, B.D.; Morales, P.A.; Stern, M.P. Prospective analysis of the insulin-resistance syndrome (syndrome X). *Diabetes* **1992**, *41*, 715–722. [CrossRef]
63. Rewers, M.; Zaccaro, D.; D'Agostino, R.; Haffner, S.; Saad, M.F.; Selby, J.V.; Bergman, R.; Savage, P. Insulin sensitivity, insulinemia, and coronary artery disease: The Insulin Resistance Atherosclerosis Study. *Diabetes Care* **2004**, *27*, 781–787. [CrossRef]
64. Solymoss, B.C.; Bourassa, M.G.; Campeau, L.; Sniderman, A.; Marcil, M.; Lespérance, J.; Lévesque, S.; Varga, S. Effect of increasing metabolic syndrome score on atherosclerotic risk profile and coronary artery disease angiographic severity. *Am. J. Cardiol.* **2004**, *93*, 159–164. [CrossRef]
65. Jones, C.N.; Pei, D.; Staris, P.; Polonsky, K.S.; Chen, Y.D.; Reaven, G.M. Alterations in the glucose-stimulated insulin secretory dose-response curve and in insulin clearance in nondiabetic insulin-resistant individuals. *J. Clin. Endocrinol. Metab.* **1997**, *82*, 1834–1838. [CrossRef]
66. Samson, S.L.; Garber, A.J. Metabolic Syndrome. *Endocrinol. Metab. Clin. N. Am.* **2014**, *43*, 1–23. [CrossRef]
67. Nolan, C.J.; Prentki, M. Insulin resistance and insulin hypersecretion in the metabolic syndrome and type 2 diabetes: Time for a conceptual framework shift. *Diabetes Vasc. Dis. Res.* **2019**, *16*, 118–127. [CrossRef]
68. Sylow, L.; Kleinert, M.; Richter, E.A.; Jensen, T.E. Exercise-stimulated glucose uptake regulation and implications for glycaemic control. *Nat. Rev. Endocrinol.* **2017**, *13*, 133–148. [CrossRef]
69. Poehlman, E.T.; Dvorak, R.V.; DeNino, W.F.; Brochu, M.; Ades, P.A. Different mechanisms leading to the stimulation of muscle glucose transport: Effects of resistance training and endurance training on insulin sensitivity in nonobese, young women: A controlled randomized trial. *J. Clin. Endocrinol. Metab.* **2000**, *85*, 2463–2468.
70. Kylin, E. Studien über das Hypertonie-Hyperglykämie- Hyperurikämiesyndrom. *Zentralblatt für Innere Medizin* **1923**, *44*, 105–127.
71. Vague, J. The degree of masculine differentiation of obesities. *Am. J. Clin. Nutr.* **1956**, *4*, 20–34. [CrossRef]
72. Kaplan, N.M. The Deadly Quartet. Upper-Body Obesity, Glucose Intolerance, Hypertriglyceridemia, and Hypertension. *Arch. Intern. Med.* **1989**, *149*, 1514–1520. [CrossRef]
73. Després, J.P.; Lemieux, I.; Bergeron, J.; Pibarot, P.; Mathiu, P.; Larose, E.; Rodés-Cabau, J.; Bertrand, O.F.; Poirier, P. Abdominal obesity and the metabolic syndrome: Contribution to global cardiometabolic risk. *Arterioscler. Thromb. Vasc. Biol.* **2008**, *28*, 1039–1049. [CrossRef]

74. McLaughlin, T.; Lamendola, C.; Liu, A.; Abbasi, F. Preferential fat deposition in subcutaneous versus visceral depots is associated with insulin sensitivity. *J. Clin. Endocrinol. Metab.* **2011**, *96*, E1756–E1760. [CrossRef]
75. Bays, H.E. Adiposopathy: Is "sick fat" a cardiovascular disease? *J. Am. Coll. Cardiol.* **2011**, *57*, 2461–2473. [CrossRef]
76. Kim, M.K.; Reaven, G.M.; Chen, Y.D.; Kim, E.; Kim, S.H. Hyperinsulinemia in individuals with obesity: Role of insulin clearance. *Obesity* **2015**, *23*, 2430–2434. [CrossRef]
77. Randle, P.J.; Garland, P.B.; Hales, C.N.; Newsholme, E.A. The glucose fatty-acid cycle. Its role in insulin sensitivity and the metabolic disturbances of diabetes mellitus. *Lancet* **1963**, *1*, 785–789. [CrossRef]
78. Cnop, M.; Ladriere, L.; Hekerman, P.; Ortis, F.; Cardozo, A.K.; Dogusan, Z.; Flamez, D.; Boyce, M.; Yuan, J.; Eizirik, D.L. Selective inhibition of eukaryotic translation initiation factor 2 alpha dephosphorylation potentiates fatty acid-induced endoplasmic reticulum stress and causes pancreatic beta-cell dysfunction and apoptosis. *J. Biol. Chem.* **2007**, *282*, 3989–3997. [CrossRef]
79. Conley, S.M.; Zhu, X.Y.; Eirin, A.; Tang, H.; Lerman, A.; van Wijnen, A.J.; Lerman, L.O. Metabolic syndrome alters expression of insulin signaling-related genes in swine mesenchymal stem cells. *Gene* **2018**, *20*, 101–106. [CrossRef]
80. Dutheil, F.; Lac, G.; Lesourd, B.; Chapier, R.; Walther, G.; Vinet, A.; Sapin, V.; Verney, J.; Ouchchane, L.; Duclos, M.; et al. Different modalities of exercise to reduce visceral fat mass and cardiovascular risk in metabolic syndrome: The RESOLVE randomized trial. *Int. J. Cardiol.* **2013**, *168*, 3634–3642. [CrossRef]
81. Kundu, N.; Domingues, C.C.; Nylen, E.S.; Paal, E.; Kokkinos, P.; Sen, S. Endothelium-derived factors influence Differentiation of Fat-Derived Stromal Cells Post-Exercise in Subjects with Prediabetes. *Metab. Syndr. Relat. Disord.* **2019**. [CrossRef]
82. Lemieux, I.; Pascot, A.; Prud'homme, D.; Almeras, N.; Bogaty, P.; Nadeau, A.; Bergeron, J.; Despres, J.P. Elevated C-reactive protein: Another component of the atherothrombotic profile of abdominal obesity. *Arterioscler. Thromb. Vasc. Biol.* **2001**, *21*, 961–967. [CrossRef]
83. Festa, A.; D'Agostino, R., Jr.; Howard, G.; Mykkanen, L.; Tracy, R.P.; Haffner, S.M. Chronic subclinical inflammation as part of the insulin resistance syndrome: The Insulin Resistance Atherosclerosis Study (IRAS). *Circulation* **2000**, *102*, 42–47. [CrossRef]
84. Lee, W.Y.; Park, J.S.; Noh, S.Y.; Rhee, E.J.; Sung, K.C.; Kim, B.S.; Kang, J.H.; Kim, S.W.; Lee, M.H.; Park, J.R. C-reactive protein concentrations are related to insulin resistance and metabolic syndrome as defined by the ATP III report. *Int. J. Cardiol.* **2004**, *97*, 101–106. [CrossRef]
85. Ridker, P.M.; Buring, J.E.; Cook, N.R.; Rifai, N. C-reactive protein, the metabolic syndrome, and risk of incident cardiovascular events: An 8-year follow-up of 14 719 initially healthy American women. *Circulation* **2003**, *107*, 391–397. [CrossRef]
86. Demidowich, A.P.; Levine, J.A.; Onyekaba, G.I.; Khan, S.M.; Chen, K.Y.; Brady, S.M.; Broadney, M.M.; Yanovski, J.A. Effects of colchicine in adults with metabolic syndrome: A pilot randomized controlled trial. *Diabetes Obes. Metab.* **2019**, *21*, 1642–1651. [CrossRef]
87. Wedell-Neergaard, A.S.; Krogh-Madsen, R.; Petersen, G.L.; Hansen, Å.M.; Pedersen, B.K.; Lund, R.; Bruunsgaard, H. Cardiorespiratory fitness and the metabolic syndrome: Roles of inflammation and abdominal obesity. *PLoS ONE* **2018**, *13*, e0194991. [CrossRef]
88. Stensvold, D.; Slørdahl, S.A.; Wisløff, U. Effect of exercise training on inflammation status among people with metabolic syndrome. *Metab. Syndr. Relat. Disord.* **2012**, *10*, 267–272. [CrossRef]
89. Povel, C.M.; Boer, J.M.; Feskens, E.J. Shared genetic variance between the features of the metabolic syndrome: Heritability studies. *Obes. Rev.* **2011**, *12*, 952–957. [CrossRef]
90. Stancakova, A.; Laakso, M. Genetics of metabolic syndrome. *Rev. Endocr. Metab. Disord.* **2014**, *15*, 243–252. [CrossRef]
91. Povel, C.M.; Boer, J.M.; Reiling, E.; Feskens, E.J. Genetic variants and the metabolic syndrome: A systematic review. *Obes. Rev.* **2011**, *12*, 952–967. [CrossRef]
92. Palizban, A.; Rezaei, M.; Khanahmad, H.; Fazilati, M. Transcription factor 7-like 2 polymorphism and context-specific risk of metabolic syndrome, type 2 diabetes, and dyslipidemia. *J. Res. Med. Sci.* **2017**, *15*, 2–24. [CrossRef]
93. Baudrand, R.; Goodarzi, M.O.; Vaidya, A.; Underwood, P.C.; Williams, J.S.; Jeunemaitre, X.; Hopkins, P.N.; Brown, N.; Raby, B.A.; Lasky-Su, J.; et al. A prevalent caveolin-1 gene variant is associated with the metabolic syndrome in Caucasians and Hispanics. *Metabolism* **2015**, *64*, 1674–1681. [CrossRef]

94. Castellano-Castillo, D.; Moreno-Indias, I.; Fernández-García, J.C.; Alcaide-Torres, J.; Moreno-Santos, I.; Ocaña, L.; Gluckman, E.; Tinahones, F.; Queipo-Ortuño, M.I.; Cardona, F. Adipose tissue LPL methylation is associated with triglyceride concentrations in the metabolic syndrome. *Clin. Chem.* **2018**, *64*, 210–218. [CrossRef]
95. Turcot, V.; Tchernof, A.; Deshaies, Y.; Pérusse, L.; Bélisle, A.; Marceau, S.; Biron, S.; Lescelleur, O.; Biertho, L.; Vohl, M.C. LINE-1 methylation in visceral adipose tissue of severely obese individuals is associated with metabolic syndrome status and related phenotypes. *Clin. Epigenetics* **2012**, *4*, 10. [CrossRef]
96. Castellano-Castillo, D.; Moreno-Indias, I.; Sanchez-Alcoholado, L.; Ramos-Molina, B.; Alcaide-Torres, J.; Morcillo, S.; Ocaña-Wilhelmi, L.; Tinahones, F.; Queipo-Ortuño, M.I.; Cardona, F. Altered adipose tissue DNA methylation status in metabolic syndrome: Relationships between global DNA methylation and specific methylation at adipogenic, lipid metabolism and inflammatory candidate genes and metabolic variables. *J. Clin. Med.* **2019**, *8*, 87. [CrossRef]
97. Gidlund, E.K. Exercise and mitochondria. In *Cardiorespiratory Fitness in Cardiometabolic Diseases Prevention and Management in Clinical Practice*; Kokkinos, P., Narayan, P., Eds.; Springer: Basel, Switzerland, 2019.
98. Alibegovic, A.C.; Sonne, M.P.; Højbjerre, L.; Bork-Jensen, J.; Jacobsen, S.; Nilsson, E.; Færch, K.; Hiscock, N.; Mortensen, B.; Friedrichsen, M.; et al. Insulin resistance induced by physical inactivity is associated with multiple transcriptional changes in skeletal muscle in young men. *Am. J. Physiol. Endocrinol. Metab.* **2010**, *299*, 752–763. [CrossRef]
99. Ling, C.; Rönn, T. Epigenetics in human obesity and type 2 diabetes. *Cell Metab.* **2019**, *29*, 1–17. [CrossRef]
100. Gomez-Abellan, P.; Hernandez-Morante, J.J.; Lujan, J.A.; Madrid, J.A.; Garaulet, M. Clock genes are implicated in the human metabolic syndrome. *Int. J. Obes.* **2008**, *32*, 121–128. [CrossRef]
101. Chaput, J.P.; McNeil, J.; Després, J.P.; Bouchard, C.; Tremblay, A. Short sleep duration is associated with an increased risk of developing features of the metabolic syndrome in adults. *Prev. Med.* **2013**, *57*, 872–877. [CrossRef]
102. Xi, B.; He, D.; Zhang, M.; Xue, J.; Zhou, D. Short sleep duration predicts risk of metabolic syndrome: A systematic review and meta-analysis. *Sleep Med. Rev.* **2014**, *18*, 293–297. [CrossRef]
103. Lian, Y.; Yuan, Q.; Wang, G.; Tang, F. Association between sleep quality and metabolic syndrome: A systematic review and meta-analysis. *Psychiatry Res.* **2019**, *274*, 66–74. [CrossRef]
104. Iftikhar, I.H.; Donley, M.A.; Mindel, J.; Pleister, A.; Soriano, S.; Magalang, U.J. Sleep duration and metabolic syndrome. An updated dose-risk meta-analysis. *Ann. Am. Thorac. Soc.* **2015**, *12*, 1364–1372. [CrossRef]
105. Chaput, J.P.; McNeil, J.; Després, J.P.; Bouchard, C.; Tremblay, A. Seven to eight hours of sleep a night is associated with a lower prevalence of the metabolic syndrome and reduced overall cardiometabolic risk in adults. *PLoS ONE* **2013**, *8*, e72832. [CrossRef]
106. Dollet, L.; Zierath, J.R. Interplay between diet, exercise and the molecular circadian clock in orchestrating metabolic adaptations of adipose tissue. *J. Physiol.* **2019**, *597*, 1439–1450. [CrossRef]
107. Gabriel, B.M.; Zierath, J.R. Circadian rhythms and exercise—Re-setting the clock in metabolic disease. *Nat. Rev. Endocrinol.* **2019**, *15*, 197–206. [CrossRef]
108. Chamarthi, B.; Gaziano, J.M.; Blonde, L.; Vinik, A.; Scranton, R.E.; Ezrokhi, M.; Rutty, D.; Cincotta, A.H. Timed Bromocriptine-QR therapy reduces progression of cardiovascular disease and dysglycemia in subjects with well-controlled type 2 diabetes mellitus. *J. Diabetes Res.* **2015**, *2015*, 157698. [CrossRef]

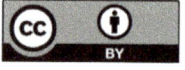

© 2019 by the authors. Licensee MDPI, Basel, Switzerland. This article is an open access article distributed under the terms and conditions of the Creative Commons Attribution (CC BY) license (http://creativecommons.org/licenses/by/4.0/).

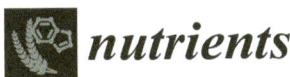

Review

Lifestyle and Metabolic Syndrome: Contribution of the Endocannabinoidome

Vincenzo Di Marzo [1,2,3,4,5,6] and Cristoforo Silvestri [3,4,5,*]

1. École de nutrition, Université Laval, Québec, QC G1V 0A6, Canada
2. Institut sur la nutrition et les aliments fonctionnels, Université Laval, Québec, QC G1V 0A6, Canada
3. Canada Excellence Research Chair on the Microbiome-Endocannabinoidome Axis in Metabolic Health, Université Laval, Québec, QC G1V 0A6, Canada
4. Centre de recherche de l'Institut universitaire de cardiologie et de pneumologie de Québec, Québec, QC G1V 4G5, Canada
5. Department de médecine, Université Laval, Québec, QC G1V 0A6, Canada
6. Institute of Biomolecular Chemistry, Consiglio Nazionale delle Ricerche, 80078 Pozzuoli, Italy
* Correspondence: cristoforo.silvestri@criucpq.ulaval.ca

Received: 16 July 2019; Accepted: 9 August 2019; Published: 20 August 2019

Abstract: Lifestyle is a well-known environmental factor that plays a major role in facilitating the development of metabolic syndrome or eventually exacerbating its consequences. Various lifestyle factors, especially changes in dietary habits, extreme temperatures, unusual light–dark cycles, substance abuse, and other stressful factors, are also established modifiers of the endocannabinoid system and its extended version, the endocannabinoidome. The endocannabinoidome is a complex lipid signaling system composed of a plethora (>100) of fatty acid-derived mediators and their receptors and anabolic and catabolic enzymes (>50 proteins) which are deeply involved in the control of energy metabolism and its pathological deviations. A strong link between the endocannabinoidome and another major player in metabolism and dysmetabolism, the gut microbiome, is also emerging. Here, we review several examples of how lifestyle modifications (westernized diets, lack or presence of certain nutritional factors, physical exercise, and the use of cannabis) can modulate the propensity to develop metabolic syndrome by modifying the crosstalk between the endocannabinoidome and the gut microbiome and, hence, how lifestyle interventions can provide new therapies against cardiometabolic risk by ensuring correct functioning of both these systems.

Keywords: endocannabinoids; endocannabinoidome; metabolic syndrome; microbiome

1. Introduction

Diets poor in essential nutritional factors (e.g., dietary fibers or vitamins) and rich in high-calorie nutrients, lack of exercise, and uncontrolled use of recreational substances or certain therapeutic drugs, together with other environmental challenges such as recently changed lifestyle habits in populations living at extreme temperatures or regarding night–day cycles, are all known to negatively affect the body's ability to regulate energy metabolism and, hence, contribute to the development of metabolic syndrome [1]. A plethora of epidemiological studies point to these aspects as major predictors of various forms of dysmetabolism, including obesity and visceral adipose tissue accumulation [2], glucose intolerance, pre-diabetes and type 2 diabetes [3], dyslipidemia [4], hypertension [5] and, eventually, the development of atherogenic inflammation [6] and the ensuing cardiovascular disorders [7]. By contrast, several other studies show how fighting bad dietary habits and the introduction of some dietary supplements and vitamins, as well as the increase of physical exercise, can successfully counteract many features of metabolic syndrome [1,8,9].

At the same time, multifaceted lifestyle aspects are emerging as having a strong impact on an endogenous system of lipid signals known as the endocannabinoid system and its more recent expansion to the endocannabinoidome (see below), which play an important role in several physiological and pathological conditions and, particularly, in the control of energy metabolism and its dysfunctions [10,11]. Endocannabinoids and endocannabinoidome mediators are ultimately derived from long-chain fatty acids, and it is therefore predictable that prolonged diets rich in some fatty acids rather than others can affect the tissue concentrations of these molecules in as much as they can change the fatty acid composition of phospholipids acting as biosynthetic precursors [12,13]. Additionally, there is evidence that pre- and probiotics can produce beneficial effects partly mediated by endocannabinoidome mediators, pointing to the possibility that at least some of the numerous physiological and pathological actions respectively displayed by a healthy or disrupted gut microbiota (known as dysbiosis) may be due to changes in this complex system of lipid chemical signals, both at the central nervous system and peripheral tissue level. This seems to be particularly true in the context of metabolic control in which the intestinal flora, like the endocannabinoidome, is known to play a major role [14–16]. This evidence is reinforced by the recent finding that some commensal bacteria produce endocannabinoid-like compounds able to activate the same receptors as their host cell counterparts [17]. Conversely, in mice, pharmacological or tissue-selective genetic manipulation of the tissue concentrations and receptor-mediated activity of endocannabinoids and endocannabinoid-like molecules was found to affect, at the same time, the relative composition in phyla, orders, genera, and species of microorganisms that populate the intestinal tract as well as the metabolic response to high-fat diets [18–21]. If one considers that gut microbiota composition is altered by the same dietary and environmental factors and unhealthy behaviors that affect the endocannabinoid system [20,22–24], then it is perhaps not so farfetched to suggest that the lifestyle–gut microbiome–endocannabinoidome triangle plays a crucial role in the development of metabolic syndrome.

In this article, we shall discuss several ways through which lifestyle-induced alterations of the endocannabinoidome—very often through direct or indirect effects on the gut microbiome (μB; that is the ensemble of genes, proteins, and metabolites provided by intestinal microorganisms)—can either worsen or ameliorate energy metabolism in mammals and, hence, influence the development of the metabolic syndrome.

2. The Endocannabinoidome

The very popular drug of abuse, marijuana, is prepared from the flowers of *Cannabis sativa* varieties containing relatively high contents of the non-psychotropic precursor of Δ^9-tetrahydrocannabinol (THC), i.e., Δ^9-tetrahydrocannabinolic acid, wherefrom the better known THC is obtained following desiccation and/or heating. However, *Cannabis sativa*—including those varieties that have been used for centuries for their fibers and employed to make ropes and paper—contains more than one hundred other THC and THC acid-like compounds in the inflorescence. These compounds have little or no psychotropic action and, together with THC and THC-acid, are known as *cannabinoids*. The euphoric, appetite-stimulating, and many other "central" actions of THC, are due to its unique capability to bind and activate a G-protein-coupled receptor (GPCR), the cannabinoid receptor type-1 (CB1), whereas another GPCR, the cannabinoid receptor type-2 (CB2), with little more than 50% homology with CB1 [1,2], is responsible for the immune-modulatory effects of this compound. So far, THC is the only plant-derived cannabinoid known to be capable of potently and efficaciously activating these receptors (which is why they should, in our opinion, be renamed "THC receptors"), although a THC congener, Δ^9-tetrahydrocannabivarine (THCV), was more recently shown to antagonize CB1 [25]. The discovery of cannabinoid receptors suggested the existence of endogenous ligands for such receptors. Two small lipids ultimately derived from arachidonic acid, *N*-arachidonoylethanolamine (AEA or anandamide) and 2-arachidonoylglycerol (2-AG), were indeed identified and shown to be capable of high-affinity binding to both CB1 and CB2 receptors, stimulating their activity with good efficacy [26,27]. These molecules were named *endocannabinoids* (eCBs) [28].

The eCBs come with their own anabolic and catabolic routes and enzymes, biosynthetic precursors, and hydrolysis products, which are inactive at cannabinoid receptors. By the turn of the last century, it was established that AEA is biosynthesized from the hydrolysis of N-arachidonoyl-phosphatidylethanolamines catalyzed by an N-acyl-phosphatidylethanolamine-specific phospholipase D-like enzyme (NAPE-PLD), whereas 2-AG is produced from the hydrolysis of 1-acyl-sn-2-arachidonoyl-glycerols (AcArGs), catalyzed by either sn-1 selective diacylglycerol lipase-α or -β (DAGLα or DAGLβ). AEA is hydrolyzed to arachidonic acid (AA) and ethanolamine by fatty acid amide hydrolase (FAAH), and 2-AG to AA and glycerol by monoacylglycerol lipase (MAGL) [29–32]. This ensemble of lipids, enzymes, and CB1 and CB2 receptors is known as the "endocannabinoid system". While the enzymes mentioned above are historically considered to be the canonical ones that regulate endocannabinoid levels, it must be noted that other pathways have also been identified (see Figure 1B, recently reviewed in [33]). For example, AEA may be synthesized by the combined action of ABDH4 and GDE1 [34] or PTPN22 [35].

It was soon realized that AEA and 2-AG, like several other lipid mediators, are quite promiscuous in their pharmacological activity in as much as they were suggested to modulate the activity of other proteins at concentrations often, but not necessarily, higher than those required to activate CB1 and CB2. These receptors were later found to often be even better targets for some of the congeners of AEA and 2-AG, i.e., the long-chain N-acylethanolamines (NAEs) and 2-monoacylglycerols (2-MAGs), respectively, and include (1) thermosensitive transient receptor potential (TRP) channels, such as the "capsaicin receptor", or TRP of vanilloid type-1 (TRPV1), the "menthol receptor", or TRP of melastatin type-8 (TRPM8), and the TRP of vanilloid type-2 (TRPV2) channels, as well as the T-type Ca^{2+} channel ($Ca_{v.3.1}$); (2) some orphan GPCRs, such as GPR55, GPR110, or GPR119; and (3) peroxisome proliferator-activated receptor-α and -γ (PPARα and PPARγ) (Figure 1A; recently reviewed in [33]. The eCB congeners, which are biosynthesized using NAPE-PLD or DAGLs from precursors similar to those of the two eCBs, and inactivated to the respective fatty acids and ethanolamine or glycerol by FAAH and MAGL, can also be produced and degraded via alternative pathways and enzymes, and, as mentioned above, this also applies to AEA and 2-AG (Figure 1B). Finally, several other long-chain fatty acid derivatives have also been identified during the last 15 years, including primary fatty acid amides and several N-acylated amino acids and neurotransmitters that often share molecular targets and/or inactivating enzymes with eCBs (Figure 1A,B). These findings led to the definition of the "expanded eCB system" or *endocannabinoidome* (eCBome), which includes a plethora of lipid mediators (including some enzymatic oxidation products of AEA and 2-AG) and tens of proteins acting as biosynthetic and inactivating enzymes, or molecular targets, for these mediators (recently reviewed in [33]).

The existence of the eCBome complicates the development of selective pharmacological and genetic tools to be used for the understanding of the several tissue-specific local functions of the eCBs, and for the exploitation of this knowledge for the development of new therapies against pathological conditions in which AEA and 2-AG are involved. On the other hand, if one looks at the eCBome as a whole and as the potential target of several physiopathological and environmental clues, and at eCBome profiles as possible personalized fingerprints of disease and responses to lifestyle, this complex signaling *hypersystem*, no matter how challenging, may open new therapeutic and diagnostic avenues. Indeed, as will be discussed below, diet and dietary components, habits, exercise, and the environment strongly impact on the eCBome—to an extent of which we have had perhaps, so far, only a partial view.

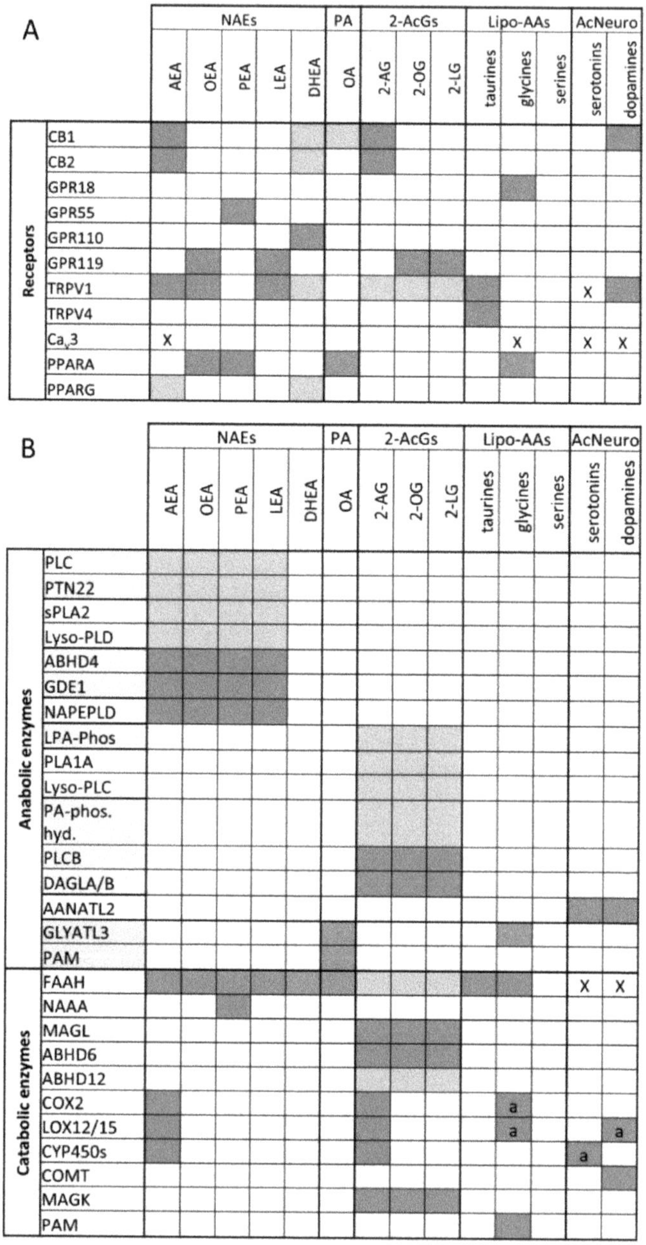

Figure 1. Endocannabinoidome mediators and their receptors (**A**) and anabolic and catabolic enzymes (**B**). Interactions are indicated by dark shaded boxes, and anabolic enzymes that function in concert are grouped together; "X" indicates inhibitory interactions; "a" indicates that enzymes only function with arachidonoyl homologs. A lighter shade of gray indicates a lower interaction with the receptors or a lesser role of the enzymes in biosynthesis or degradation.

3. Dietary Fats and the Endocannabinoidome

In the obese state, the eCB system is modulated at the level of anabolic and catabolic enzyme activity, endocannabinoid levels, and CB1 receptor expression, resulting in a generally increased eCB tone "in the wrong place and at the wrong time" [36]. BMI positively correlates with circulating AEA and 2-AG levels, especially when fat distribution is partitioned more towards intra-abdominal stores [37–39]. However, the levels of AEA are dysregulated in obesity with respect to responses to feeding or the time of day as viscerally obese men were found to have significantly lower levels of AEA in the morning than normoweights [38]. The observed increases in AEA and 2-AG levels appear to be due to changes in expression of adipose tissue-metabolizing enzymes, as the AEA-catabolizing enzyme FAAH was decreased and the 2-AG-anabolizing enzyme DAGLα was increased in the adipose tissue from obese individuals in conjunction with decreased CB1 expression, perhaps as a homeostatic compensatory response [37,39,40]. Changes in eCBome gene expression within adipose tissue appear to be depot-specific, however, since gluteal subcutaneous adipose tissue from obese subjects had decreased eCBome gene expression (including FAAH, DAGLα, and CB1) while abdominal subcutaneous adipose tissue showed the opposite trend, with visceral adipose tissue similarly having increased CB1 expression [41].

Obesogenic diets characterized by high fat content are increasingly prevalent in westernized societies. High-fat diets increase AEA and/or 2-AG levels [12,13]. While N-oleoylethanolamine (OEA), N-palmitoylethanolamine (PEA), and N-linoleoylethanolamine (LEA) levels are reduced in the jejunum and/or stomach in response to 1 week [42] or up to 8 weeks [43] of high-fat feeding, prolonged feeding (14 weeks) increased OEA levels in the stomach concomitant with increased NAPE-PLD and decreased FAAH expression [43]. In the liver, a high-fat diet increased AEA levels and CB1 signaling, which contributed to the activation of genetic programs that increase fatty acid production [13]. In a very recent study in which circulating eCBome levels were tracked over time in mice on a high-fat diet, AEA, PEA, and N-docosahexanoylethanolamine (DHEA) levels increased rapidly over the course of a week, while SEA and 2-AG increases became significant only after 4 weeks and, finally, OEA increased after 10 weeks [44]. While gene expression changes in eCBome enzymes were observed in muscle and liver tissues, they were transient; however, the expression of the 2-AG anabolic enzyme DAGLβ was constantly increased in white and brown adipose tissue (BAT) from 4 weeks, while the NAE anabolic enzyme NAPE-PLD was constantly increased only in the BAT from 3 days on [44]. This study supports the conclusions inferred from human studies, that adipose tissue is one of the main regulators of circulating 2-AG in obesity. The potential contribution of BAT (at least in mice) to the regulation of NAEs was a surprising result, though at least in the case of OEA, it cannot be ruled out that the intestinal tract is one of the major sources [43].

Changes in eCBome mediator levels in response to high-fat feeding occur very quickly in mice. Recently, Everard et al. showed that after just 4 h of initial high-fat-diet feeding, jejunal AEA and 2-AG levels decreased while OEA, 2-OG, 2-LG, and 2-PG levels increased [18], but after 5 weeks of exposure AEA, LEA increased, as did 2-OG and 2-PG.

In utero or neonatal exposure to dietary perturbations can have long-lasting effects on an individual and, indeed, the eCBome is significantly impacted by exposure to high-fat diets early on in life with long-lasting consequences. Maternal high-fat feeding resulted in sustained elevation of CB1/2, FAAH, and MAGL levels in the livers of adult male rats, with changes in redox homeostasis [45]. Maternal exposure to high-fat diet also increased CB1 in the male, and CB2 in the female hypothalamus at birth, while CB1 and FAAH expression were increased, and CB2 and MGLL were decreased in the BAT of males and females, respectively. Both sexes developed an increased adiposity and preference for high-fat diets [46].

Dietary linoleic acid (LA) is a major n-6 fatty acid component of Western diets, making up over 80% of the polyunsaturated fatty acid (PUFA) consumed in the United States [47], resulting in an imbalance the ratio of n-6/n-3 fatty acids consumed greatly in favor of the former. LA is linked to obesity and is efficiently converted to the AEA and 2-AG constituent arachidonic acid (AA), thus explaining its ability to increase AEA and 2-AG levels and to produce obesogenic effects [48,49]. Indeed, even within the context of a low-fat diet, high levels of LA increased liver AEA and 2-AG levels, promoting obesity and associated adipose tissue inflammation [50]. Inclusion of n-3 fatty acids to an LA-rich diet reverses the latter's effects on AEA and 2-AG levels [48]. Similar results have been obtained with EPA/DHA n-3 fatty acid-rich krill and, to a lesser extent, fish oil [12,51–53]. Additionally, supplementing young mice on a lard diet with flax seed oil rich in the n-3 fatty acid α-linolenic acid significantly decreased liver AEA levels and improved glucose homeostasis after a subsequent 10 weeks on a high-lard diet [54]. These effects are believed to largely be the result of decreasing the n-6/n-3 PUFA ratio, which results in AA displacement from phospholipid membranes, thus reducing the amounts of the biosynthetic precursors of AEA and 2-AG. In support of this, n-3 PUFAs provided as phospholipids, rather than free fatty acids, result in more significant decreases in eCB levels [12,52]. Correspondingly, decreasing n-3 PUFA phospholipid content increased 2-AG liver levels and promoted hepatosteatosis and insulin resistance [55].

These data suggest that some of the therapeutic properties against metabolic disorders (such as against high triglycerides) of n-3 fatty PUFA may be ascribed to a reduction of eCB overactivity, and this has also been suggested to be the case in obese humans [53]. However, the metabolic benefits of dietary n-3 PUFAs may also result from the elevation of n-3 PUFA-derived NAEs (DHEA, N-eicosapentaenoylethanolamine (EPEA)), which has been observed in several tissues and blood [52,56,57], as well as of the corresponding monoacylglycerols [58] and other monoacylamides [59], which possess anti-inflammatory and anticancer actions and potential cardiometabolic- and neuroprotective effects independent of cannabinoid receptors [60–63]. A recent study comparing DHA and EPA supplementation in diet-induced obese mice and type 2 diabetic patients found significantly increased levels of DHEA and EPEA in both circulation and adipose tissue, but decreases in AEA and 2-AG were only observed in mice [64]. Of note, this study by Rossmeisl et al. utilized n-3 PUFAs as triglycerides; however, when provided mostly as phospholipids (from krill powder) to obese men, circulating AEA levels were reduced along with triglycerides [53].

Gut microbes (collectively termed the microbiome (μB)), are not a group of commensalist microorganisms living within animals but, rather, many are mutualists, benefiting the host in a variety of ways such as aiding in energy harvesting and digestion, modulating the immune system, and influencing many aspects of metabolic health, including weight, adiposity, and lipid and glucose metabolism [65]. The μB responds quickly to dietary interventions [66], and westernized diets are linked to dysbiosis (an imbalance of microbial communities) and associated with obesity, which is generally characterized by decreased bacterial diversity with an increase in the Firmicutes/Bacteroidetes phyla ratio [67,68]. Alterations in the μB are associated with other aspects of metabolic syndrome, including dyslipidemia, hypertension, and insulin resistance (reviewed extensively in [69–72]), and their consideration for the development of targeted therapies for "precision health" plans has recently been suggested for diabetes [73,74]. Like the eCBome, the gut μB is modified by dietary fatty acids, including supplementation with n-3 fatty acids from fish oil and krill oil [22,75,76]. Although few studies have assessed the effects of α-linolenic acid, at least one clinical trial has indicated that α-linolenic acid-rich oils can modify the μB at the genera level [77].

In the study by Everard et al. discussed above, the chronic high-fat-diet-induced changes in the jejunum eCBome lipid levels were associated with significant alterations in the gut μB, with the proportions of 19 bacterial genera identified as being significantly modified [18]. The same group had previously shown that 4 weeks of high-fat-diet feeding increased 2-AG levels in the ileum which was also associated with an altered μB [78]. High-fat-diet-induced μB changes were associated with increased CB1 expression in the colon whereas FAAH was increased in the jejunum [79]. Thus, it appears that μB alterations in response to high-fat diets impacts upon the intestinal eCBome directly which, under obesity-inducing conditions, increases gut barrier permeability, subsequently resulting in increased circulating bacterially derived lipopolysaccharide (LPS) that subsequently modulates adipose tissue eCBome and functionality (reviewed in [80]).

4. Dietary Fiber and Prebiotics: Improving Gut Barrier Function through the Endocannabinoidome

The health benefits of dietary fiber have been extensively studied and reviewed, and there is little doubt that higher fiber is beneficial for cardiovascular disease, supporting prevalent recommendations that fiber intake be increased in order to maintain a healthy diet [81]. The positive effects of fiber on obesity and metabolic syndrome are believed to be intimately linked to alterations of the gut µB [23,82]. Increasing attention is being paid to "prebiotic" fiber, which is non-digestible by the host but is metabolized by gut microbiota, resulting in an alteration of the composition and/or activity of the µB, producing bioactive metabolites (such as short-chain fatty acids) that provide physiological benefits to the host [83].

One of the main positive effects of prebiotics is in regulating intestinal epithelial barrier permeability, in which short-chain fatty acids play a crucial role. The term "leaky gut" has been used to describe the phenomenon in which the tight junctions within the intestinal epithelial lining are compromised, leading to the movement of bacterially derived LPS into circulation, resulting in metabolic endotoxemia-induced inflammation that is associated with obesity [84,85]. Supplementing the diets of genetically (*ob/ob*) or diet-induced obese mice with the prebiotic oligofructose increases *Bifidobacterium* species and *Akkermansia muciniphila* in association with improved gut barrier function and decreased inflammation [79,86,87]. Similarly, women with type 2 diabetes who were given oligofructose-enriched inulin (10 g/day) for 8 weeks had significantly lower circulating levels of LPS and other inflammatory markers, along with decreased fasting glucose and glycosylated hemoglobin [88]. Finally, administration of pasteurized *A. muciniphila* improved insulin sensitivity and reduced total plasma cholesterol levels [89].

The eCBome has been found to regulate intestinal permeability. Using the same genetic model discussed above (*ob/ob* mice), Muccioli et al. showed that CB1 antagonism partially rescued tight junction integrity within the intestinal epithelium and reduced plasma LPS levels, while CB1 agonism in wild type mice increased gut permeability [79]. Further, blocking CB1 activity in mice on an obesity-inducing diet not only inhibited the development of obesity and improved glucose homeostasis, as expected, but also decreased intestinal permeability as evidenced by reduced circulating LPS levels in association with decreased adipose tissue inflammation and circulating inflammatory cytokine profile, indicating a decrease in systemic inflammation [21]. Importantly, these changes were observed in conjunction with an increase in the relative amounts of intestinal *A. muciniphila* and decreased *Lachnospiraceae*. The reduction in metabolic endotoxemia induced in *ob/ob* mice fed oligofructose correlated with decreased colonic CB1 expression and AEA levels, with the latter presumably due to increased expression of the AEA catabolic enzyme FAAH [79]. Thus, CB1 regulation of gut permeability, under the influence of the µB, is another mechanism by which CB1 regulates inflammation in addition to direct proinflammatory effects such as, for example, the stimulation of proinflammatory cytokine release from macrophages, which has developmental consequences for type 2 diabetes [90,91]. These results collectively support the notion that the cardiometabolic health effects of dietary prebiotic fiber is associated with alteration of the gut microbiota and intestinal eCBome, resulting in decreased intestinal permeability and the ensuing metabolic endotoxemia/systemic inflammation.

5. TRPV1: Linking the Endocannabinoidome to the Metabolic Benefits Attributed to Spicy Food

The consumption of spicy food has been associated with overall decreased mortality and significant reduction in hazard ratios for deaths caused by ischemic heart diseases and, in the case of the consumption of fresh chili peppers, reduced diabetes [92]. Capsaicin is the active component endowing chili peppers with their spiciness, due to activation of transient receptor potential vanilloid-1 (TRPV1) cation channels. TRPV1 channels primarily respond to noxious heat (>42 °C), but are also modulated by several eCBome members (including long-chain-saturated NAEs, monoacylglycerols, *N*-acyldopamines, and *N*-acyltaurines) [33]. Several human studies have indicated the various metabolic benefits of dietary capsaicin, which improved postprandial glucose handling in both healthy individuals and overweight individuals and women with gestational diabetes [93–95]. While a meta-analysis of capsaicin studies supported the positive effects of this dietary component on energy expenditure and appetite regulation, the overall effects were very small and more evident at high doses [96]. In rodent models, oral capsaicin is able to combat diet-induced obesity, insulin resistance, and hepatosteatosis [97]. The positive metabolic effects of capsaicin appear to be mediated by both TRPV1 and PPARα [97,98]. However, the role of TRPV1 in obesity and associated side effects—especially dysregulation of glucose homeostasis—is complex, as indicated by contrasting results from $Trpv1^{-/-}$ mice in diet-induced obesity, in which both beneficial [99] and detrimental [100] effects have been observed. These differences may be due to variations in the diets used between studies or the ages of the mice, as $Trpv1^{-/-}$ mice have been shown to have increased activity at young ages, but decreased activity at older ages, in association with increased weight gain [100,101].

Capsaicin and TRP channels have also been linked to the gut µB. The antiobesity effects of capsaicin have been associated with changes in the gut µB, including also increases in *A. muciniphila* [20,102,103]. The gut µB appears to have a causative role in mediating capsaicin antiobesity effects as gut µB transplantation from capsaicin-treated to germ-free mice replicated the capsaicin-dependent antimetabolic endotoxemia effects, which were mitigated by antibiotics in capsaicin-treated mice [104]. These changes were defined by decreases in lipopolysaccharide (LPS)-producing, gram-negative bacteria and LPS biosynthetic genes, and increases in short-chain fatty acid (SCFA)-producing bacteria, such as *Lachnospiraceae*, *Ruminococcaceae*, and *Roseburia*, as well as decreased colonic CB1 expression [104]. Accordingly, TRPV1 has been suggested to counteract increased intestinal permeability in vitro [105]. Most interestingly, in a human study, different µB enterotypes (different gut µB ecosystems) of participants were associated with the extent of capsaicin-mediated positive metabolic effects. Capsaicin increased the Firmicutes/Bacteroidetes ratio and *Faecalibacterium* abundance more prevalently in participants with the *Bacteroides* enterotype than the *Prevotella* enterotype, in combination with increased serum incretin (GIP and GLP-1) levels, which stimulate insulin production, and decreased LBP, which was assessed as a marker of inflammation [106]. As in the case of eCBs and CB1 receptors, also the communication between TRPV1 and the gut µB seems to be bi-directional. In fact, the visceral antinociceptive effects of the probiotic *Lactobacillus reuteri* has been attributed to inhibition of TRPV1 activity in mesenteric neurons [107], indicating also that the eCBome may play a significant role in mediating the activity of microbial influences on the gut–brain axis, at least with respect to pain.

6. Sunlight Effects on the Endocannabinoidome: A Role for Vitamin D?

Vitamin D deficiency represents a global health issue, with over a billion people being deficient [108], largely due to inadequate sun exposure. Yet, significant levels of deficiency still occur in populations living in areas of abundant sunlight [109]. Vitamin D is found only in a few foods and is thus a common dietary supplement recommended by health authorities, especially in winter months [110]. Several aspects of the metabolic syndrome are associated with vitamin D deficiency, including obesity, dyslipidemia, insulin resistance, hepatosteatosis, and hypertension [111]. The causal role of vitamin D in the pathophysiology of these aspects of the metabolic syndrome is not known, but the gut µB also appears to play a significant role. In a mouse model of diet-induced obesity, vitamin D deficiency aggravated high-fat-diet-induced insulin resistance and hepatosteatosis along with inflammation. These results occurred in conjunction with mucosal breakdown within the ileum, endotoxemia and dysbiosis with increased levels of pathogenic *Helicobacter hepaticus*, and decreased levels of the metabolically beneficial *A. muciniphila* [112]. Vitamin D receptor knockout mice also develop dysbiosis, exemplified by an alteration in the ratio of Bacteroidetes/Firmicutes phyla with increases in Lactobacillaceae and Lachnospiraceae families [113]. However, while the mechanisms remain to be determined, UVR has recently been found to alter the mouse gut µB independently of vitamin D [114].

Endogenous vitamin D is produced upon UV irradiation of 7-hehydrocholesterol in skin, which is then further metabolized, mostly in the liver and kidney, to produce bioactive 1,25-dihydroxyvitamin D_3 [115]. The skin contains not only 2-AG and AEA, but also several other NAEs in both the dermis and epidermis [116]. Whether the skin provides a significant source of circulating eCBome mediators remains to be determined. However, in vitro exposure of melanocytes to low doses of UVB upregulates CB1 mRNA expression and increases the levels of AEA, PEA, and 2-AG in keratinocytes [117]. Further, 6 weeks of cutaneous UV exposure increased circulating 2-AG levels in both light- and dark-skinned people, without significantly altering NAEs [118]. This finding was in apparent contrast to results obtained earlier by Magina et al., who found that in psoriasis patients, whole-body narrowband UVB therapy resulted in a decrease in AEA plasma levels without affecting 2-AG [119]. The differences in these results may have been due to a variety of factors, including the fact that the employed UV radiation regimens differed between the studies and that Madina et al. studied effects only in psoriasis patients.

Vitamin D deficiency in mice increased pain sensitization and decreased CB1, but increased CB2 and PPARα in the spinal cord along with increased AEA and DHEA [120]. In the colon, 2-AG was significantly decreased together with microbial diversity, leading to an increased Firmicutes/Bacteroidetes ratio and lower levels of *A. muciniphila*. Treatment of vitamin D-deficient mice with the PPARα agonist and AEA congener, PEA, reversed the observed pain sensitization in conjunction with an increase in the levels of several microbial genera, including *A. muciniphila* [120].

Taken together, these studies suggest that sunlight exposure, and the elevation in vitamin D levels that results from it, modify the eCBome as well as the μB. Whether there is a link between the two remains to be determined. For this reason, and given that these alterations are associated with μB changes that are believed to impact on metabolic health, such as increased Firmicutes/Bacteroidetes ratios and the presence of low *A. muciniphila* levels, it will be interesting to investigate if μB–eCBome crosstalk plays a significant role in regulating obesity and associated metabolic complications downstream of vitamin D.

7. Effects of Exercise on the Endocannabinoidome

Exercise is the second pillar, together with the diet, which maintains metabolic health. Viscerally obese men who underwent a lifestyle modification program that included the addition of regular exercise for one year had significant improvements in several metabolic parameters as well as reduced circulating 2-AG and, to a lesser extent, AEA levels [121]. These latter alterations were very likely associated with decreased adiposity. However, while physically active men have higher lymphocyte FAAH activity than sedentary controls, suggesting higher eCBome tone within these cells, basal circulating levels of AEA, PEA, and 2-AG were not found to be different from those of sedentary males [122]. By contrast, in a study of normoweight and obese women whose activity was tracked over 6 days, while 2-AG was associated with BMI, as expected, AEA and OEA levels were positively associated with moderate–vigorous physical activity [123].

In contrast to the scarcity of data on the effects of chronic physical activity on basal eCBome mediator levels, much more research has been conducted on their response to acute exercise. Many studies have shown that physical activity quickly increases circulating AEA, but not 2-AG, levels in humans ([124–126] and reviewed in [127]). However, a recent study found that 2-AG, and not AEA, increased after exercise [128], and this discrepancy with previous studies may be due to the fact that the participants fasted before exercising. Interestingly, AEA increases only appear in response to medium-intensity exercise [124]. Heyman et al. showed that similar to AEA, PEA and OEA also increase during and after exercise and, in fact, are more responsive to lower intensity exercise than AEA [126]. The source of these eCBome mediators remains to be determined. However, in rats, exercise alters the levels of many NAE metabolic enzymes within the adipose tissue [129]. It has been suggested that AEA and related NAEs exert positive metabolic effects in muscle, such as improving glucose uptake and mitochondrial activity by acting at the PPARγ and TRPV1 eCBome receptors [127]. Further, exercise may modulate AEA levels directly in muscle, as has been found in the extensor digitorum longus muscles of rats [129].

Several physiological mechanisms by which exercise affects mood have been proposed, including increasing endorphins, altered mitochondrial function, and thermogenesis, as well as modulation of the endocannabinoid system [130]. The notion that increased AEA levels may be, in part, responsible for feelings of euphoria associated with exercise is supported by the finding in mice that exercise increased AEA and OEA, but not 2-AG or PEA, levels in association with decreased GABAergic neuron CB1-dependent anxiety [131]. In fact, exercise also increases eCB tone in the brain. Mice with free access to a running wheel for 8 days had increased AEA levels and CB1 binding site density in the hippocampus [132]. Furthermore, wheel running in mice results in potentiated CB1 activity within the striatum, playing a protective role against stress [133], which does not appear to be simply due to increased CB1 expression, as chronic exercise does not alter the levels of this receptor in any part of the brain [134]. Similarly, a recent study showed that singing increased circulating AEA, PEA, and OEA levels in association with improved positive mood [135]. In the same study, the effects of 30 min of cycling were also examined, and significantly increased OEA levels were observed, while AEA and PEA only showed trends towards increases. The lack of statistical increases in AEA, commonly observed in other studies, may have been due to the intensity of the cycling or the relatively small sample size. Further, exercise addicts, which have increased negative mood in response to exercise deprivation, also have lower basal circulating AEA levels than non-addicted regular runners, and exercise withdrawal and reintroduction only decreases and increases AEA levels, respectively, in non-addicts [136]. The lack of response of AEA in exercise addicts suggests that perhaps their increased amount of exercise is a homeostatic attempt to increase eCB tone.

Recent evidence indicates that exercise and the µB interact with each other (reviewed in [24]). Germ-free mice have decreased exercise performance as compared to conventional controls, and reintroduction of a single bacterial species (*Bacteroides fragilis*) partially reversed this [137]. While the sample sizes were small, Petriz et al. found that moderate exercise differentially changes the µB in wild type Wistar, obese Zucker, and spontaneously hypertensive rats, suggesting that exercise-induced changes in the µB may be dependent on the metabolic state of the host organism [138]. Similarly, high-intensity interval training of high-fat-diet-fed mice altered the µB differentially along the gastrointestinal tract with the most significant changes found in the distal regions [139]. Interestingly, exercise reversed the high-fat-diet-induced decrease in microbial diversity and the Bacteroidetes/Firmicutes ratio, which are indicative of obesity [139]. Furthermore, fecal microbiota transplant from exercised mice to mice on a high-fat diet resulted in improved metabolic parameters, suggesting that that µB can confer, at least in part, the benefits of exercise [140]. However, a more recent study found that high- or medium-intensity training had no effect on the µB of obese Zucker rats [141]. In humans, studies on professional rugby players found that their µBs were more diverse than sedentary controls and produced more short-chain fatty acids, though these changes were also associated with dietary differences [142,143]. However, other studies have found that independent of diet or BMI, higher levels of cardiorespiratory fitness correlated with higher µB diversity and short-chain fatty acid production [144]. Similarly, independent of diet, six weeks of endurance exercise in overweight women significantly altered the µB of participants with an increase in *A. muciniphila* [145], which has been shown to increase the levels of eCBome monoacylglycerols, including 2-AG [87] and, as mentioned above, to be regulated by both CB1 and TRPV1 activity [21,103]. To date, no studies have examined the potential link between the eCBome, exercise, and the gut µB. However, given that activities of several eCBome receptors (CB1, TRPV1, PPARα) have been linked to µB changes [21,103,146], it is possible that their modulation through exercise-induced changes in eCBome mediator levels may play a role in exercise-induced changes in the µB, or vice versa.

8. Cannabis Use and Metabolic Health

The principal psychoactive component of marijuana/cannabis (THC), one of the most commonly used recreational drugs the world over, acts mainly through CB1 activation (reviewed in [25]). Given the strong association of CB1 and its ligands AEA and 2-AG with several aspects of metabolic syndrome and obesity in general [10], it is somewhat counterintuitive that cannabis use is generally associated with an improved metabolic phenotype. Analysis of the NHANES survey from 2005–2010 found that current and past cannabis use is generally associated with significantly lower odds of metabolic syndrome [147]. Combined examination of two large epidemiological studies (NESARC and NCS-R) concluded that chronic cannabis users had significantly decreased adjusted prevalence rates of obesity, from 22%–25% in non-users to 14%–17% in users [148]. A very recent prospective analysis of NESARC data supports the above, finding that cannabis use is inversely associated with BMI increases over 3 years [149]. Several large studies have also shown inverse associations between cannabis and diabetes [150–152], which were corroborated by a Swedish study involving 18,000 participants, though the observed protective effects on diabetes were attenuated when adjusted for age [153]. Interestingly, these associations, observed in large heterogeneous populations, are also observed in Inuit from the Canadian north, a relatively isolated ethnic group in which the decreased weight associated with cannabis use was found to account for an association with improved glucose metabolism [154]. Cannabis use is also associated with reduced prevalence of both alcoholic and non-alcoholic fatty liver disease [155,156]. It should be noted that cannabis use is not always associated with positive metabolic outcomes; among individuals with type 1 diabetes, it is correlated with an increased risk in ketoacidosis [157], subclinical atherosclerosis (but only among cigarette smokers) [158], and mortality in patients with myocardial infarction, despite having lower rates of diabetes and hyperlipidemia [159].

The positive metabolic effects of cannabis have been attributed to the downregulation of CB1 in response to chronic cannabis use/THC exposure. Post-mortem analysis of chronic cannabis users' brains found decreased CB1 (*CNR1*) mRNA and ligand-binding in several brain regions [160], and in vivo positron emission tomography (PET) imaging similarly showed globally decreased CB1 availability compared to controls [161]. Chronic THC administration to rats decreases 2-AG and AEA levels in the striatum, but increases AEA levels in the limbic forebrain [162], and in chronic cannabis users, AEA levels are decreased in cerebrospinal fluid while 2-AG levels are increased in the serum as compared to infrequent users [163]. The mechanism by which eCB levels were altered in these studies are unknown; however, ex vivo treatment of placental explants with THC for long (72 h) but not short (24 h) periods of time increased AEA levels, concomitant with a counterintuitive decrease in NAPE-PLD levels and a trend for increased FAAH levels [164]. In hepatocytes, THC increased both AEA and 2-AG levels, presumably by blocking the activity of fatty acid binding protein 1 (FABP1), which can act as an eCB "chaperone", allowing eCB enzymatic degradation [165]. While THC does not appear to be able to inhibit eCBome catabolic or anabolic enzymes, several other phytocannabinoids do, though at relatively high concentrations [166], suggesting that their combination within cannabis may contribute to its ability to alter eCBome mediator levels.

In agreement with epidemiological studies, chronic THC administration to mice inhibited the development of obesity in response to a high-fat diet [167]. However, other cannabis-produced phytocannabinoids are also able to elicit positive metabolic effects. Delta-9-tetrahydrocannabivarin (THCV) is a CB1 antagonist and cannabidiol (CBD) is a CB1 negative allosteric modulator,) and both are TRPV1 agonists as well as acting on other receptors (reviewed in [25]). THCV markedly improved glucose metabolism in genetically, and diet-induced obese mice [168] and as did CBD in a genetic model of type 1 diabetes [169] Similarly, a clinical study found decreased fasting glucose levels in participants treated twice per day with 5 mg of THCV [170], whereas both THCV and CBD reduced hepatic triglyceride content in genetically obese mice [168,171].

More than 25% of non-antibiotic drugs induce dysbiosis of the μB [172]. There is limited evidence that cannabis use can modulate the gut μB. To date, only two studies have investigated the effects of cannabis use on the human gut μB. Panee et al. assayed the stools of 19 lifetime cannabis users and 20 non-users for the relative abundance of only two specific genera, *Prevotella* and *Bacteroides*, given that they are main determinants of human enterotypes [173]. They found that non-users had an average 13-fold higher *Prevotella/Bacteroides* ratio than cannabis users, which has been associated with plant-based as compared to animal-based diets [174]. This raised the possibility that the observed changes were attributed to alterations in the diets of users vs non-users, consistent with observations that cannabis users consume fewer fruits and more animal products and have higher caloric intake but, paradoxically, have similar nutrient serum status and lower BMIs than non-users [175]. In a second study, archived anal swabs were used to assess the μBs of HIV-positive individuals [176]. Cannabis use in these individuals was also associated with alterations in bacterial populations, including a decreased abundance of *Prevotella* as well as *Acidaminococcus* and *Dorea*, the latter two of which have been associated with obesity [177,178], along with increased abundances of other genera. The role of the *Prevotella* genus in metabolic health is complicated, due likely to the genetic diversity between individual species and, thus, several conflicting studies exist on its association with obesity, diabetes, and NAFLD, while others report positive correlations with improvements in various metabolic parameters (recently reviewed in [179]).

Chronic treatment with THC reduced weight and fat mass gain as well as energy intake in diet-induced obese but not lean mice, in association with alterations in the gut μB, which included increased levels of *A. muciniphila* and inhibition of the obesity-induced shift in the Firmicutes/Bacteroidetes ratio [167]. In an experimental autoimmune encephalomyelitis mouse model meant to mimic multiple sclerosis, a combination of the phytocannabinoids THC and CBD attenuated the induced inflammation and disease scores and significantly modulated the μB, decreasing the levels of *A. muciniphila* [180]. Fecal material transplantation confirmed that the protective effects were mediated by changes in the μB. Further unpublished data suggest that THC-mediated effects on the μB may be due, in part, to alterations in the host immune system, which has a complex interaction with the μB throughout a host's lifespan [181].

It is still unclear if the modulation of the μB by THC is dependent on CB1 activity. However, inhibition of CB1 with the inverse agonist rimonabant alters the μB composition of diet-induced obese mice, including increasing *A. muciniphila* in conjunction with metabolic parameter improvements [21]. Further, an adipose tissue-specific knockout of a major NAE anabolic enzyme, NAPE-PLD, which reduced local OEA, PEA and SEA, but not AEA levels, inhibited adipose tissue browning, and led to increased weight gain, glucose intolerance, and dyslipidemia in addition to exacerbating diet-induced obesity [19]. These effects were associated with an alteration in the gut μB which when transferred to germ-free mice, partially reproduced the phenotype, and are therefore likely to be CB1-independent, as the affected NAEs are ligands for other eCBome receptors, including TRPV1, which, as indicated above, impacts upon metabolic health, at least in part through alteration of the μB. Taken together, the above studies indicate that cannabis use—through its psychoactive constituent, THC, and non-psychoactive phytocannabinoids—potentially impacts upon metabolic health, in part by modulating μB constituents.

9. Conclusions

In summary, we have reviewed several examples of how the lifestyle–eCBome–μB triangle, with its multifaceted aspects, is likely to play a fundamental role in both metabolic health and metabolic syndrome (Figure 2). It is likely that several healthy and "bad" lifestyle habits, in synergy with other environmental factors, independently affect both eCBome signaling and the μB, and hence help in determining their correct or defective control of energy metabolism, respectively. It is also possible, however, that eCBome and μB crosstalk—which has not yet been fully explored—directs the manner in which lifestyle cues result in virtuous or vicious circles that can respectively counteract or accelerate the development of metabolic syndrome. The molecular aspects of the lifestyle–eCBome–μB triangle, therefore, need now to be fully elucidated in order to exploit this knowledge for new lifestyle (e.g., nutritional, physical activity, etc.) and pharmacological interventions aimed at combating the appearance of one or more of the metabolic syndrome features that together contribute to the development of type 2 diabetes and cardiovascular risk factors.

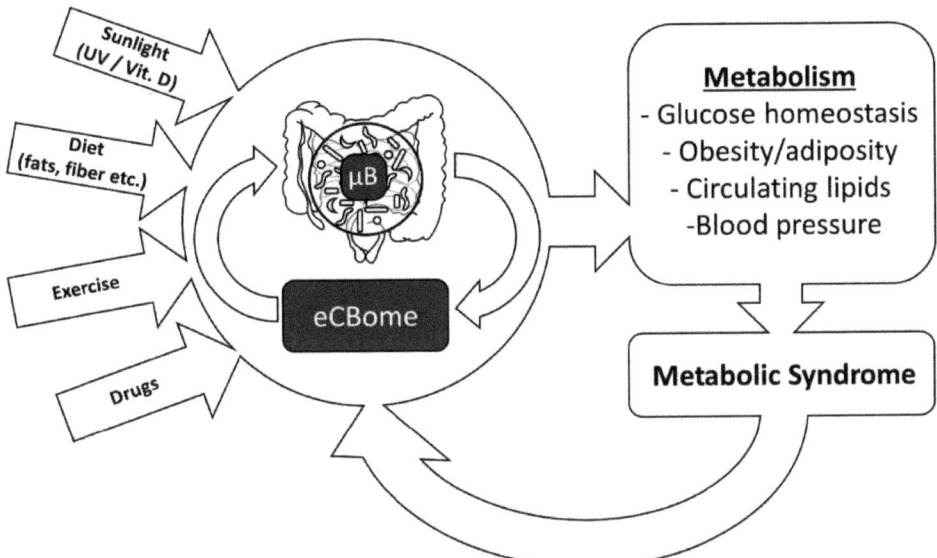

Figure 2. The endocannabinoidome–microbiome axis as a mechanism through which lifestyle choices affect various aspects of metabolism, which in turn may lead to the metabolic syndrome when dysregulated. This can, in turn, impact on both endocannabinoidome and microbiome-mediated signaling and, ultimately, also on lifestyle, thus creating potential vicious circles.

Author Contributions: C.S. and V.D.M. wrote the manuscript.

Funding: This work was performed under the scope of the Canadian Excellence Research Chair held by VD and funded by the Canadian Institute of Heath Research (CIHR), The Natural Sciences and Engineering Research Council of Canada (NSERC) and The Social Sciences and Humanities Research Council of Canada (SSHERC).

Conflicts of Interest: The authors receive research grants from GW Pharmaceuticals, not related to this work.

Abbreviations

Mediators
2-AcGs	2-acylglycerols
2-AG	2-arachidonoylglycerol
2-LG	2-linoleoyl glycerol
2-OG	2-oleoylglycerol
AcNeuro	acyl neurotransmitters
AEA	*N*-arachidonoylethanolamine
DHEA	*N*-docosahexanoylethanolamine
LEA	*N*-linoleoylethanolamine
Lipo-AAs	lipoamino acids
NAEs	*N*-acylethanolamines
OA	oleoylamide
OEA	*N*-oleoylethanolamine
PA	fatty acid primary amides
PEA	*N*-palmitoylethanolamine

Receptors

Ca_v3	T-type Ca^{2+} channel
CB1	cannabinoid receptor 1
CB2	cannabinoid receptor 2
GPR110	G protein-coupled receptor 110
GPR119	G protein-coupled receptor 119
GPR18	G protein-coupled receptor 18
GPR55	G protein-coupled receptor 55
PPARA	peroxisome proliferator-activated receptor alpha
PPARG	peroxisome proliferator-activated receptor gamma
TRPV1	transient receptor potential cation channel sub-family V member 1
TRPV4	transient receptor potential cation channel subfamily V member 4

Anabolic enzymes

AANATL2	arylalkylamine N-acyltransferase-like 2, isoform A
ABHD4	alpha/beta-hydrolase domain containing 4
DAGLA/B	diacylglycerol lipase alpha/beta
GDE1	glycerophosphodiester phosphodiesterase 1
GLYATL3	glycine N-acyltransferase-like protein 3
LPA-Phos	lysophosphatidic acid phosphatase
Lyso-PLC	lysophospholipase C Lyso-PLC, lysophospholipase D
NAPEPLD	N-acyl phosphatidylethanolamine-hydrolyzing phospholipase D
PA-phos. hyd.	phosphatidic acid phosphohydrolase
PLA1A	phospholipase A1 member A
PLC	phospholipase C
PLCB	phospholipase C beta
PTPN22	tyrosine protein phosphatase non-receptor type 22
sPLA2	soluble phospholipase A2.

Catabolic enzymes

ABHD12	alpha/beta-hydrolase domain containing 12
ABHD6	alpha/beta hydrolase domain containing 6
COMT	catechol-O-methyltransferase
COX2	cyclooxygenase 2
CYP450	cytochrome P450
FAAH	fatty acid amide hydrolase
LOX12/15	arachidonate lipoxygenase 12/15
MAGK	monoacylglycerol kinase
MGLL	monoacylglycerol lipase
NAAA	N-acylethanolamine-hydrolyzing acid amidase
PAM	peptidyl-glycine α-amidating monooxygenase

References

1. Yamaoka, K.; Tango, T. Effects of lifestyle modification on metabolic syndrome: A systematic review and meta-analysis. *BMC Med.* **2012**, *10*, 138. [CrossRef]
2. Reilly, J.J.; El-Hamdouchi, A.; Diouf, A.; Monyeki, A.; Somda, S.A. Determining the worldwide prevalence of obesity. *Lancet* **2018**, *391*, 1773–1774. [CrossRef]
3. NCD Risk Factor Collaboration (NCD-RisC). Worldwide trends in diabetes since 1980: A pooled analysis of 751 population-based studies with 4·4 million participants. *Lancet* **2016**, *387*, 1513–1530. [CrossRef]
4. Liu, H.-H.; Li, J.-J. Aging and dyslipidemia: A review of potential mechanisms. *Ageing Res. Rev.* **2015**, *19*, 43–52. [CrossRef] [PubMed]
5. Blacher, J.; Levy, B.I.; Mourad, J.-J.; Safar, M.E.; Bakris, G. From epidemiological transition to modern cardiovascular epidemiology: Hypertension in the 21st century. *Lancet* **2016**, *388*, 530–532. [CrossRef]

6. Halcox, J.P.; Banegas, J.R.; Roy, C.; Dallongeville, J.; De Backer, G.; Guallar, E.; Perk, J.; Hajage, D.; Henriksson, K.M.; Borghi, C. Prevalence and treatment of atherogenic dyslipidemia in the primary prevention of cardiovascular disease in Europe: EURIKA, a cross-sectional observational study. *BMC Cardiovasc. Disord.* **2017**, *17*, 160. [CrossRef] [PubMed]
7. Barquera, S.; Pedroza-Tobías, A.; Medina, C.; Hernández-Barrera, L.; Bibbins-Domingo, K.; Lozano, R.; Moran, A.E. Global Overview of the Epidemiology of Atherosclerotic Cardiovascular Disease. *Arch. Med. Res.* **2015**, *46*, 328–338. [CrossRef] [PubMed]
8. Saboya, P.P.; Bodanese, L.C.; Zimmermann, P.R.; da Silva Gustavo, A.; Macagnan, F.E.; Feoli, A.P.; da Silva Oliveira, M. Lifestyle Intervention on Metabolic Syndrome and its Impact on Quality of Life: A Randomized Controlled Trial. *Arq. Bras. Cardiol.* **2017**, *108*, 60–69. [CrossRef] [PubMed]
9. VanWormer, J.J.; Boucher, J.L.; Sidebottom, A.C.; Sillah, A.; Knickelbine, T. Lifestyle changes and prevention of metabolic syndrome in the Heart of New Ulm Project. *Prev. Med. Rep.* **2017**, *6*, 242–245. [CrossRef]
10. Silvestri, C.; Di Marzo, V. The Endocannabinoid System in Energy Homeostasis and the Etiopathology of Metabolic Disorders. *Cell Metab.* **2013**, *17*, 475–490. [CrossRef]
11. Cristino, L.; Becker, T.; Di Marzo, V. Endocannabinoids and energy homeostasis: An update: Regulatory Role of Endocannabinoids in Obesity. *BioFactors* **2014**, *40*, 389–397. [CrossRef] [PubMed]
12. Piscitelli, F.; Carta, G.; Bisogno, T.; Murru, E.; Cordeddu, L.; Berge, K.; Tandy, S.; Cohn, J.S.; Griinari, M.; Banni, S.; et al. Effect of dietary krill oil supplementation on the endocannabinoidome of metabolically relevant tissues from high-fat-fed mice. *Nutr. Metab. (Lond.)* **2011**, *8*, 51. [CrossRef] [PubMed]
13. Osei-Hyiaman, D.; DePetrillo, M.; Pacher, P.; Liu, J.; Radaeva, S.; Bátkai, S.; Harvey-White, J.; Mackie, K.; Offertáler, L.; Wang, L.; et al. Endocannabinoid activation at hepatic CB1 receptors stimulates fatty acid synthesis and contributes to diet-induced obesity. *J. Clin. Invest.* **2005**, *115*, 1298–1305. [CrossRef] [PubMed]
14. Bäckhed, F.; Ding, H.; Wang, T.; Hooper, L.V.; Koh, G.Y.; Nagy, A.; Semenkovich, C.F.; Gordon, J.I. The gut microbiota as an environmental factor that regulates fat storage. *Proc. Natl. Acad. Sci. USA* **2004**, *101*, 15718–15723. [CrossRef] [PubMed]
15. Esteve, E.; Ricart, W.; Fernández-Real, J.-M. Gut microbiota interactions with obesity, insulin resistance and type 2 diabetes: Did gut microbiote co-evolve with insulin resistance? *Curr. Opin. Clin. Nutr. Metab. Care* **2011**, *14*, 483–490. [CrossRef]
16. Ridaura, V.K.; Faith, J.J.; Rey, F.E.; Cheng, J.; Duncan, A.E.; Kau, A.L.; Griffin, N.W.; Lombard, V.; Henrissat, B.; Bain, J.R.; et al. Gut Microbiota from Twins Discordant for Obesity Modulate Metabolism in Mice. *Science* **2013**, *341*, 1241214. [CrossRef] [PubMed]
17. Cohen, L.J.; Esterhazy, D.; Kim, S.-H.; Lemetre, C.; Aguilar, R.R.; Gordon, E.A.; Pickard, A.J.; Cross, J.R.; Emiliano, A.B.; Han, S.M.; et al. Commensal bacteria make GPCR ligands that mimic human signalling molecules. *Nature* **2017**, *549*, 48–53. [CrossRef]
18. Everard, A.; Plovier, H.; Rastelli, M.; Van Hul, M.; de Wouters d'Oplinter, A.; Geurts, L.; Druart, C.; Robine, S.; Delzenne, N.M.; Muccioli, G.G.; et al. Intestinal epithelial N-acylphosphatidylethanolamine phospholipase D links dietary fat to metabolic adaptations in obesity and steatosis. *Nat. Commun.* **2019**, *10*, 457. [CrossRef]
19. Geurts, L.; Everard, A.; Van Hul, M.; Essaghir, A.; Duparc, T.; Matamoros, S.; Plovier, H.; Castel, J.; Denis, R.G.P.; Bergiers, M.; et al. Adipose tissue NAPE-PLD controls fat mass development by altering the browning process and gut microbiota. *Nat. Commun.* **2015**, *6*, 6495. [CrossRef]
20. Song, J.-X.; Ren, H.; Gao, Y.-F.; Lee, C.-Y.; Li, S.-F.; Zhang, F.; Li, L.; Chen, H. Dietary Capsaicin Improves Glucose Homeostasis and Alters the Gut Microbiota in Obese Diabetic ob/ob Mice. *Front. Physiol.* **2017**, *8*, 602. [CrossRef]
21. Mehrpouya-Bahrami, P.; Chitrala, K.N.; Ganewatta, M.S.; Tang, C.; Murphy, E.A.; Enos, R.T.; Velazquez, K.T.; McCellan, J.; Nagarkatti, M.; Nagarkatti, P. Blockade of CB1 cannabinoid receptor alters gut microbiota and attenuates inflammation and diet-induced obesity. *Sci. Rep.* **2017**, *7*, 15645. [CrossRef] [PubMed]
22. Costantini, L.; Molinari, R.; Farinon, B.; Merendino, N. Impact of Omega-3 Fatty Acids on the Gut Microbiota. *Int. J. Mol. Sci.* **2017**, *18*, 2645. [CrossRef] [PubMed]
23. Dahiya, D.K.; Renuka; Puniya, M.; Shandilya, U.K.; Dhewa, T.; Kumar, N.; Kumar, S.; Puniya, A.K.; Shukla, P. Gut Microbiota Modulation and Its Relationship with Obesity Using Prebiotic Fibers and Probiotics: A Review. *Front. Microbiol.* **2017**, *8*, 563. [CrossRef] [PubMed]

24. Mailing, L.J.; Allen, J.M.; Buford, T.W.; Fields, C.J.; Woods, J.A. Exercise and the Gut Microbiome: A Review of the Evidence, Potential Mechanisms, and Implications for Human Health. *Exerc. Sport Sci. Rev.* **2019**, *47*, 75–85. [CrossRef] [PubMed]
25. Pertwee, R.; Cascio, M.G. Chapter 6: Known Pharmacological Actions of Delta-9-Tetrahydrocannabinol and of Four Other Chemical Constituents of Cannabis that Activate Cannabinoid Receptors. In *Handbook of Cannabis*; Pertwee, R., Ed.; Oxford University Press: Oxford, UK, 2014; pp. 115–136. ISBN 978-0-19-178756-0.
26. Devane, W.A.; Hanus, L.; Breuer, A.; Pertwee, R.G.; Stevenson, L.A.; Griffin, G.; Gibson, D.; Mandelbaum, A.; Etinger, A.; Mechoulam, R. Isolation and structure of a brain constituent that binds to the cannabinoid receptor. *Science* **1992**, *258*, 1946–1949. [CrossRef] [PubMed]
27. Mechoulam, R.; Ben-Shabat, S.; Hanus, L.; Ligumsky, M.; Kaminski, N.E.; Schatz, A.R.; Gopher, A.; Almog, S.; Martin, B.R.; Compton, D.R. Identification of an endogenous 2-monoglyceride, present in canine gut, that binds to cannabinoid receptors. *Biochem. Pharmacol.* **1995**, *50*, 83–90. [CrossRef]
28. Di Marzo, V.; De Petrocellis, L.; Bisogno, T. The biosynthesis, fate and pharmacological properties of endocannabinoids. *Handb. Exp. Pharmacol.* **2005**, 147–185.
29. Dinh, T.P.; Carpenter, D.; Leslie, F.M.; Freund, T.F.; Katona, I.; Sensi, S.L.; Kathuria, S.; Piomelli, D. Brain monoglyceride lipase participating in endocannabinoid inactivation. *Proc. Natl. Acad. Sci. USA* **2002**, *99*, 10819–10824. [CrossRef] [PubMed]
30. Cravatt, B.F.; Giang, D.K.; Mayfield, S.P.; Boger, D.L.; Lerner, R.A.; Gilula, N.B. Molecular characterization of an enzyme that degrades neuromodulatory fatty-acid amides. *Nature* **1996**, *384*, 83–87. [CrossRef]
31. Bisogno, T.; Howlett, F.; Williams, G.; Minassi, A.; Cascio, M.G.; Ligresti, A.; Matias, I.; Schiano-Moriello, A.; Paul, P.; Williams, E.-J.; et al. Cloning of the first sn1-DAG lipases points to the spatial and temporal regulation of endocannabinoid signaling in the brain. *J. Cell Biol.* **2003**, *163*, 463–468. [CrossRef]
32. Okamoto, Y.; Morishita, J.; Tsuboi, K.; Tonai, T.; Ueda, N. Molecular Characterization of a Phospholipase D Generating Anandamide and Its Congeners. *J. Biol. Chem.* **2004**, *279*, 5298–5305. [CrossRef] [PubMed]
33. Di Marzo, V. New approaches and challenges to targeting the endocannabinoid system. *Nat. Rev. Drug Discov.* **2018**, *17*, 623–639. [CrossRef] [PubMed]
34. Simon, G.M.; Cravatt, B.F. Anandamide Biosynthesis Catalyzed by the Phosphodiesterase GDE1 and Detection of Glycerophospho-N-acyl Ethanolamine Precursors in Mouse Brain. *J. Biol. Chem.* **2008**, *283*, 9341–9349. [CrossRef] [PubMed]
35. Liu, J.; Wang, L.; Harvey-White, J.; Osei-Hyiaman, D.; Razdan, R.; Gong, Q.; Chan, A.C.; Zhou, Z.; Huang, B.X.; Kim, H.-Y.; et al. A biosynthetic pathway for anandamide. *Proc. Natl. Acad. Sci. USA* **2006**, *103*, 13345–13350. [CrossRef] [PubMed]
36. Naughton, S.S.; Mathai, M.L.; Hryciw, D.H.; McAinch, A.J. Fatty Acid modulation of the endocannabinoid system and the effect on food intake and metabolism. *Int. J. Endocrinol.* **2013**, *2013*, 361895. [CrossRef] [PubMed]
37. Bluher, M.; Engeli, S.; Kloting, N.; Berndt, J.; Fasshauer, M.; Batkai, S.; Pacher, P.; Schon, M.R.; Jordan, J.; Stumvoll, M. Dysregulation of the Peripheral and Adipose Tissue Endocannabinoid System in Human Abdominal Obesity. *Diabetes* **2006**, *55*, 3053–3060. [CrossRef] [PubMed]
38. Côté, M.; Matias, I.; Lemieux, I.; Petrosino, S.; Alméras, N.; Després, J.-P.; Di Marzo, V. Circulating endocannabinoid levels, abdominal adiposity and related cardiometabolic risk factors in obese men. *Int. J. Obes.* **2007**, *31*, 692–699. [CrossRef]
39. Engeli, S.; Böhnke, J.; Feldpausch, M.; Gorzelniak, K.; Janke, J.; Bátkai, S.; Pacher, P.; Harvey-White, J.; Luft, F.C.; Sharma, A.M.; et al. Activation of the Peripheral Endocannabinoid System in Human Obesity. *Diabetes* **2005**, *54*, 2838–2843. [CrossRef]
40. Karvela, A.; Rojas-Gil, A.P.; Samkinidou, E.; Papadaki, H.; Pappa, A.; Georgiou, G.; Spiliotis, B.E. Endocannabinoid (EC) receptor, CB1, and EC enzymes' expression in primary adipocyte cultures of lean and obese pre-pubertal children in relation to adiponectin and insulin. *J. Pediatr. Endocrinol. Metab.* **2010**, *23*, 1011–1024. [CrossRef]
41. Pagano, C.; Pilon, C.; Calcagno, A.; Urbanet, R.; Rossato, M.; Milan, G.; Bianchi, K.; Rizzuto, R.; Bernante, P.; Federspil, G.; et al. The Endogenous Cannabinoid System Stimulates Glucose Uptake in Human Fat Cells via Phosphatidylinositol 3-Kinase and Calcium-Dependent Mechanisms. *J. Clin. Endocrinol. Metab.* **2007**, *92*, 4810–4819. [CrossRef]

42. Diep, T.A.; Madsen, A.N.; Holst, B.; Kristiansen, M.M.; Wellner, N.; Hansen, S.H.; Hansen, H.S. Dietary fat decreases intestinal levels of the anorectic lipids through a fat sensor. *FASEB J.* **2011**, *25*, 765–774. [CrossRef] [PubMed]
43. Aviello, G.; Matias, I.; Capasso, R.; Petrosino, S.; Borrelli, F.; Orlando, P.; Romano, B.; Capasso, F.; Di Marzo, V.; Izzo, A.A. Inhibitory effect of the anorexic compound oleoylethanolamide on gastric emptying in control and overweight mice. *J. Mol. Med.* **2008**, *86*, 413–422. [CrossRef] [PubMed]
44. Kuipers, E.N.; Kantae, V.; Maarse, B.C.E.; van den Berg, S.M.; van Eenige, R.; Nahon, K.J.; Reifel-Miller, A.; Coskun, T.; de Winther, M.P.J.; Lutgens, E.; et al. High Fat Diet Increases Circulating Endocannabinoids Accompanied by Increased Synthesis Enzymes in Adipose Tissue. *Front. Physiol.* **2019**, *9*, 1913. [CrossRef] [PubMed]
45. Miranda, R.A.; De Almeida, M.M.; Rocha, C.P.D.D.; de Brito Fassarella, L.; De Souza, L.L.; Souza, A.F.P.D.; Andrade, C.B.V.D.; Fortunato, R.S.; Pazos-Moura, C.C.; Trevenzoli, I.H. Maternal high-fat diet consumption induces sex-dependent alterations of the endocannabinoid system and redox homeostasis in liver of adult rat offspring. *Sci. Rep.* **2018**, *8*, 14751. [CrossRef] [PubMed]
46. Dias-Rocha, C.P.; Almeida, M.M.; Santana, E.M.; Costa, J.C.B.; Franco, J.G.; Pazos-Moura, C.C.; Trevenzoli, I.H. Maternal high-fat diet induces sex-specific endocannabinoid system changes in newborn rats and programs adiposity, energy expenditure and food preference in adulthood. *J. Nutr. Biochem.* **2018**, *51*, 56–68. [CrossRef] [PubMed]
47. Kris-Etherton, P.M.; Taylor, D.S.; Yu-Poth, S.; Huth, P.; Moriarty, K.; Fishell, V.; Hargrove, R.L.; Zhao, G.; Etherton, T.D. Polyunsaturated fatty acids in the food chain in the United States. *Am. J. Clin. Nutr.* **2000**, *71*, 179S–188S. [CrossRef] [PubMed]
48. Alvheim, A.R.; Malde, M.K.; Osei-Hyiaman, D.; Lin, Y.H.; Pawlosky, R.J.; Madsen, L.; Kristiansen, K.; Frøyland, L.; Hibbeln, J.R. Dietary linoleic acid elevates endogenous 2-AG and anandamide and induces obesity. *Obesity (Silver Spring)* **2012**, *20*, 1984–1994. [CrossRef] [PubMed]
49. Matias, I.; Petrosino, S.; Racioppi, A.; Capasso, R.; Izzo, A.A.; Di Marzo, V. Dysregulation of peripheral endocannabinoid levels in hyperglycemia and obesity: Effect of high fat diets. *Mol. Cell. Endocrinol.* **2008**, *286*, S66–S78. [CrossRef]
50. Alvheim, A.R.; Torstensen, B.E.; Lin, Y.H.; Lillefosse, H.H.; Lock, E.-J.; Madsen, L.; Frøyland, L.; Hibbeln, J.R.; Malde, M.K. Dietary Linoleic Acid Elevates the Endocannabinoids 2-AG and Anandamide and Promotes Weight Gain in Mice Fed a Low Fat Diet. *Lipids* **2014**, *49*, 59–69. [CrossRef]
51. Batetta, B.; Griinari, M.; Carta, G.; Murru, E.; Ligresti, A.; Cordeddu, L.; Giordano, E.; Sanna, F.; Bisogno, T.; Uda, S.; et al. Endocannabinoids may mediate the ability of (n-3) fatty acids to reduce ectopic fat and inflammatory mediators in obese Zucker rats. *J. Nutr.* **2009**, *139*, 1495–1501. [CrossRef]
52. Rossmeisl, M.; Jilkova, Z.M.; Kuda, O.; Jelenik, T.; Medrikova, D.; Stankova, B.; Kristinsson, B.; Haraldsson, G.G.; Svensen, H.; Stoknes, I.; et al. Metabolic Effects of n-3 PUFA as Phospholipids Are Superior to Triglycerides in Mice Fed a High-Fat Diet: Possible Role of Endocannabinoids. *PLoS ONE* **2012**, *7*, e38834. [CrossRef] [PubMed]
53. Berge, K.; Piscitelli, F.; Hoem, N.; Silvestri, C.; Meyer, I.; Banni, S.; Di Marzo, V. Chronic treatment with krill powder reduces plasma triglyceride and anandamide levels in mildly obese men. *Lipids Health Dis.* **2013**, *12*, 78. [CrossRef] [PubMed]
54. Demizieux, L.; Piscitelli, F.; Troy-Fioramonti, S.; Iannotti, F.A.; Borrino, S.; Gresti, J.; Muller, T.; Bellenger, J.; Silvestri, C.; Di Marzo, V.; et al. Early Low-Fat Diet Enriched With Linolenic Acid Reduces Liver Endocannabinoid Tone and Improves Late Glycemic Control After a High-Fat Diet Challenge in Mice. *Diabetes* **2016**, *65*, 1824–1837. [CrossRef] [PubMed]
55. Pachikian, B.D.; Essaghir, A.; Demoulin, J.-B.; Neyrinck, A.M.; Catry, E.; De Backer, F.C.; Dejeans, N.; Dewulf, E.M.; Sohet, F.M.; Portois, L.; et al. Hepatic n-3 polyunsaturated fatty acid depletion promotes steatosis and insulin resistance in mice: Genomic analysis of cellular targets. *PLoS ONE* **2011**, *6*, e23365. [CrossRef] [PubMed]
56. Berger, A.; Crozier, G.; Bisogno, T.; Cavaliere, P.; Innis, S.; Marzo, V.D. Anandamide and diet: Inclusion of dietary arachidonate and docosahexaenoate leads to increased brain levels of the corresponding N-acylethanolamines in piglets. *Proc. Natl. Acad. Sci. USA* **2001**, *98*, 6402–6406. [CrossRef] [PubMed]

57. Artmann, A.; Petersen, G.; Hellgren, L.I.; Boberg, J.; Skonberg, C.; Nellemann, C.; Hansen, S.H.; Hansen, H.S. Influence of dietary fatty acids on endocannabinoid and N-acylethanolamine levels in rat brain, liver and small intestine. *Biochimica et Biophysica Acta (BBA) Mol. Cell Biol. Lipids* **2008**, *1781*, 200–212. [CrossRef] [PubMed]
58. Ramsden, C.E.; Zamora, D.; Makriyannis, A.; Wood, J.T.; Mann, J.D.; Faurot, K.R.; MacIntosh, B.A.; Majchrzak-Hong, S.F.; Gross, J.R.; Courville, A.B.; et al. Diet-Induced Changes in n-3- and n-6-Derived Endocannabinoids and Reductions in Headache Pain and Psychological Distress. *J. Pain* **2015**, *16*, 707–716. [CrossRef] [PubMed]
59. Verhoeckx, K.C.M.; Voortman, T.; Balvers, M.G.J.; Hendriks, H.F.J.; Wortelboer, H.M.; Witkamp, R.F. Presence, formation and putative biological activities of N-acyl serotonins, a novel class of fatty-acid derived mediators, in the intestinal tract. *Biochimica et Biophysica Acta (BBA) Mol. Cell Biol. Lipids* **2011**, *1811*, 578–586. [CrossRef] [PubMed]
60. Arshad, A.; Chung, W.Y.; Steward, W.; Metcalfe, M.S.; Dennison, A.R. Reduction in circulating pro-angiogenic and pro-inflammatory factors is related to improved outcomes in patients with advanced pancreatic cancer treated with gemcitabine and intravenous omega-3 fish oil. *HPB (Oxford)* **2013**, *15*, 428–432. [CrossRef]
61. Watson, J.E.; Kim, J.S.; Das, A. Emerging class of omega-3 fatty acid endocannabinoids & their derivatives. *Prostaglandins Other Lipid Mediat.* **2019**, *143*, 106337.
62. Wainwright, C.L.; Michel, L. Endocannabinoid system as a potential mechanism for n-3 long-chain polyunsaturated fatty acid mediated cardiovascular protection. *Proc. Nutr. Soc.* **2013**, *72*, 460–469. [CrossRef] [PubMed]
63. Meijerink, J.; Balvers, M.; Witkamp, R. N-Acyl amines of docosahexaenoic acid and other n-3 polyunsatured fatty acids—From fishy endocannabinoids to potential leads. *Br. J. Pharmacol.* **2013**, *169*, 772–783. [CrossRef] [PubMed]
64. Rossmeisl, M.; Pavlisova, J.; Janovska, P.; Kuda, O.; Bardova, K.; Hansikova, J.; Svobodova, M.; Oseeva, M.; Veleba, J.; Kopecky, J.; et al. Differential modulation of white adipose tissue endocannabinoid levels by n-3 fatty acids in obese mice and type 2 diabetic patients. *Biochimica et Biophysica Acta (BBA) Mol. Cell Biol. Lipids* **2018**, *1863*, 712–725. [CrossRef] [PubMed]
65. Moran, C.P.; Shanahan, F. Gut microbiota and obesity: Role in aetiology and potential therapeutic target. *Best Pract. Res. Clin. Gastroenterol.* **2014**, *28*, 585–597. [CrossRef] [PubMed]
66. David, L.A.; Maurice, C.F.; Carmody, R.N.; Gootenberg, D.B.; Button, J.E.; Wolfe, B.E.; Ling, A.V.; Devlin, A.S.; Varma, Y.; Fischbach, M.A.; et al. Diet rapidly and reproducibly alters the human gut microbiome. *Nature* **2014**, *505*, 559–563. [CrossRef]
67. Finucane, M.M.; Sharpton, T.J.; Laurent, T.J.; Pollard, K.S. A Taxonomic Signature of Obesity in the Microbiome? Getting to the Guts of the Matter. *PLoS ONE* **2014**, *9*, e84689. [CrossRef]
68. Turnbaugh, P.J.; Hamady, M.; Yatsunenko, T.; Cantarel, B.L.; Duncan, A.; Ley, R.E.; Sogin, M.L.; Jones, W.J.; Roe, B.A.; Affourtit, J.P.; et al. A core gut microbiome in obese and lean twins. *Nature* **2009**, *457*, 480–484. [CrossRef]
69. Kasselman, L.J.; Vernice, N.A.; DeLeon, J.; Reiss, A.B. The gut microbiome and elevated cardiovascular risk in obesity and autoimmunity. *Atherosclerosis* **2018**, *271*, 203–213. [CrossRef]
70. Ascher, S.; Reinhardt, C. The gut microbiota: An emerging risk factor for cardiovascular and cerebrovascular disease. *Eur. J. Immunol.* **2018**, *48*, 564–575. [CrossRef] [PubMed]
71. Ma, J.; Li, H. The Role of Gut Microbiota in Atherosclerosis and Hypertension. *Front. Pharmacol.* **2018**, *9*, 1082. [CrossRef]
72. van den Munckhof, I.C.L.; Kurilshikov, A.; ter Horst, R.; Riksen, N.P.; Joosten, L.A.B.; Zhernakova, A.; Fu, J.; Keating, S.T.; Netea, M.G.; de Graaf, J.; et al. Role of gut microbiota in chronic low-grade inflammation as potential driver for atherosclerotic cardiovascular disease: A systematic review of human studies: Impact of gut microbiota on low-grade inflammation. *Obes. Rev.* **2018**, *19*, 1719–1734. [CrossRef] [PubMed]
73. Zhou, W.; Sailani, M.R.; Contrepois, K.; Zhou, Y.; Ahadi, S.; Leopold, S.R.; Zhang, M.J.; Rao, V.; Avina, M.; Mishra, T.; et al. Longitudinal multi-omics of host–microbe dynamics in prediabetes. *Nature* **2019**, *569*, 663. [CrossRef] [PubMed]
74. Rose, S.M.S.-F.; Contrepois, K.; Moneghetti, K.J.; Zhou, W.; Mishra, T.; Mataraso, S.; Dagan-Rosenfeld, O.; Ganz, A.B.; Dunn, J.; Hornburg, D.; et al. A longitudinal big data approach for precision health. *Nat. Med.* **2019**, *25*, 792.

75. Cui, C.; Li, Y.; Gao, H.; Zhang, H.; Han, J.; Zhang, D.; Li, Y.; Zhou, J.; Lu, C.; Su, X. Modulation of the gut microbiota by the mixture of fish oil and krill oil in high-fat diet-induced obesity mice. *PLoS ONE* **2017**, *12*, e0186216. [CrossRef] [PubMed]
76. Shen, W.; Gaskins, H.R.; McIntosh, M.K. Influence of dietary fat on intestinal microbes, inflammation, barrier function and metabolic outcomes. *J. Nutr. Biochem.* **2014**, *25*, 270–280. [CrossRef]
77. Pu, S.; Khazanehei, H.; Jones, P.J.; Khafipour, E. Interactions between Obesity Status and Dietary Intake of Monounsaturated and Polyunsaturated Oils on Human Gut Microbiome Profiles in the Canola Oil Multicenter Intervention Trial (COMIT). *Front. Microbiol.* **2016**, *7*, 1612. [CrossRef] [PubMed]
78. Everard, A.; Cani, P.D. Diabetes, obesity and gut microbiota. *Best Pract. Res. Clin. Gastroenterol.* **2013**, *27*, 73–83. [CrossRef]
79. Muccioli, G.G.; Naslain, D.; Bäckhed, F.; Reigstad, C.S.; Lambert, D.M.; Delzenne, N.M.; Cani, P.D. The endocannabinoid system links gut microbiota to adipogenesis. *Mol. Syst. Biol.* **2010**, *6*, 392. [CrossRef]
80. Cani, P.D.; Plovier, H.; Van Hul, M.; Geurts, L.; Delzenne, N.M.; Druart, C.; Everard, A. Endocannabinoids—At the crossroads between the gut microbiota and host metabolism. *Nat. Rev. Endocrinol.* **2016**, *12*, 133–143. [CrossRef]
81. Veronese, N.; Solmi, M.; Caruso, M.G.; Giannelli, G.; Osella, A.R.; Evangelou, E.; Maggi, S.; Fontana, L.; Stubbs, B.; Tzoulaki, I. Dietary fiber and health outcomes: An umbrella review of systematic reviews and meta-analyses. *Am. J. Clin. Nutr.* **2018**, *107*, 436–444. [CrossRef]
82. Ahmadi, S.; Mainali, R.; Nagpal, R.; Sheikh-Zeinoddin, M.; Soleimanian-Zad, S.; Wang, S.; Deep, G.; Kumar Mishra, S.; Yadav, H. Dietary Polysaccharides in the Amelioration of Gut Microbiome Dysbiosis and Metabolic Diseases. *Obes. Control Ther.* **2017**, *4*. [CrossRef]
83. Bindels, L.B.; Delzenne, N.M.; Cani, P.D.; Walter, J. Towards a more comprehensive concept for prebiotics. *Nat. Rev. Gastroenterol. Hepatol.* **2015**, *12*, 303–310. [CrossRef] [PubMed]
84. Cani, P.D.; Amar, J.; Iglesias, M.A.; Poggi, M.; Knauf, C.; Bastelica, D.; Neyrinck, A.M.; Fava, F.; Tuohy, K.M.; Chabo, C.; et al. Metabolic endotoxemia initiates obesity and insulin resistance. *Diabetes* **2007**, *56*, 1761–1772. [CrossRef] [PubMed]
85. Cani, P.D.; Bibiloni, R.; Knauf, C.; Waget, A.; Neyrinck, A.M.; Delzenne, N.M.; Burcelin, R. Changes in gut microbiota control metabolic endotoxemia-induced inflammation in high-fat diet-induced obesity and diabetes in mice. *Diabetes* **2008**, *57*, 1470–1481. [CrossRef] [PubMed]
86. Cani, P.D.; Possemiers, S.; Van de Wiele, T.; Guiot, Y.; Everard, A.; Rottier, O.; Geurts, L.; Naslain, D.; Neyrinck, A.; Lambert, D.M.; et al. Changes in gut microbiota control inflammation in obese mice through a mechanism involving GLP-2-driven improvement of gut permeability. *Gut* **2009**, *58*, 1091–1103. [CrossRef]
87. Everard, A.; Belzer, C.; Geurts, L.; Ouwerkerk, J.P.; Druart, C.; Bindels, L.B.; Guiot, Y.; Derrien, M.; Muccioli, G.G.; Delzenne, N.M.; et al. Cross-talk between Akkermansia muciniphila and intestinal epithelium controls diet-induced obesity. *Proc. Natl. Acad. Sci. USA* **2013**, *110*, 9066–9071. [CrossRef]
88. Dehghan, P.; Pourghassem Gargari, B.; Asghari Jafar-abadi, M. Oligofructose-enriched inulin improves some inflammatory markers and metabolic endotoxemia in women with type 2 diabetes mellitus: A randomized controlled clinical trial. *Nutrition* **2014**, *30*, 418–423. [CrossRef]
89. Depommier, C.; Everard, A.; Druart, C.; Plovier, H.; Hul, M.V.; Vieira-Silva, S.; Falony, G.; Raes, J.; Maiter, D.; Delzenne, N.M.; et al. Supplementation with Akkermansia muciniphila in overweight and obese human volunteers: A proof-of-concept exploratory study. *Nat. Med.* **2019**, *25*, 1096. [CrossRef]
90. Jourdan, T.; Szanda, G.; Cinar, R.; Godlewski, G.; Holovac, D.J.; Park, J.K.; Nicoloro, S.; Shen, Y.; Liu, J.; Rosenberg, A.Z.; et al. Developmental Role of Macrophage Cannabinoid-1 Receptor Signaling in Type 2 Diabetes. *Diabetes* **2017**, *66*, 994–1007. [CrossRef]
91. Jourdan, T.; Godlewski, G.; Cinar, R.; Bertola, A.; Szanda, G.; Liu, J.; Tarn, J.; Han, T.; Mukhopadhyay, B.; Skarulis, M.C.; et al. Activation of the Nlrp3 inflammasome in infiltrating macrophages by endocannabinoids mediates beta cell loss in type 2 diabetes. *Nat. Med.* **2013**, *19*, 1132–1140. [CrossRef]
92. Lv, J.; Qi, L.; Yu, C.; Yang, L.; Guo, Y.; Chen, Y.; Bian, Z.; Sun, D.; Du, J.; Ge, P.; et al. Consumption of spicy foods and total and cause specific mortality: Population based cohort study. *BMJ* **2015**, *351*, h3942. [CrossRef] [PubMed]

93. Yuan, L.-J.; Qin, Y.; Wang, L.; Zeng, Y.; Chang, H.; Wang, J.; Wang, B.; Wan, J.; Chen, S.-H.; Zhang, Q.-Y.; et al. Capsaicin-containing chili improved postprandial hyperglycemia, hyperinsulinemia, and fasting lipid disorders in women with gestational diabetes mellitus and lowered the incidence of large-for-gestational-age newborns. *Clin. Nutr.* **2016**, *35*, 388–393. [CrossRef] [PubMed]
94. Kroff, J.; Hume, D.J.; Pienaar, P.; Tucker, R.; Lambert, E.V.; Rae, D.E. The metabolic effects of a commercially available chicken peri-peri (African bird's eye chilli) meal in overweight individuals. *Br. J. Nutr.* **2017**, *117*, 635–644. [CrossRef] [PubMed]
95. Dömötör, A.; Szolcsányi, J.; Mózsik, G. Capsaicin and glucose absorption and utilization in healthy human subjects. *Eur. J. Pharmacol.* **2006**, *534*, 280–283. [CrossRef] [PubMed]
96. Ludy, M.-J.; Moore, G.E.; Mattes, R.D. The Effects of Capsaicin and Capsiate on Energy Balance: Critical Review and Meta-analyses of Studies in Humans. *Chem. Senses* **2012**, *37*, 103–121. [CrossRef] [PubMed]
97. Kang, J.-H.; Tsuyoshi, G.; Han, I.-S.; Kawada, T.; Kim, Y.M.; Yu, R. Dietary Capsaicin Reduces Obesity-induced Insulin Resistance and Hepatic Steatosis in Obese Mice Fed a High-fat Diet. *Obesity* **2010**, *18*, 780–787. [CrossRef]
98. Zhang, L.L.; Yan Liu, D.; Ma, L.Q.; Luo, Z.D.; Cao, T.B.; Zhong, J.; Yan, Z.C.; Wang, L.J.; Zhao, Z.G.; Zhu, S.J.; et al. Activation of Transient Receptor Potential Vanilloid Type-1 Channel Prevents Adipogenesis and Obesity. *Circ. Res.* **2007**, *100*, 1063–1070. [CrossRef] [PubMed]
99. Motter, A.L.; Ahern, G.P. TRPV1-null mice are protected from diet-induced obesity. *FEBS Lett.* **2008**, *582*, 2257–2262. [CrossRef]
100. Lee, E.; Jung, D.Y.; Kim, J.H.; Patel, P.R.; Hu, X.; Lee, Y.; Azuma, Y.; Wang, H.-F.; Tsitsilianos, N.; Shafiq, U.; et al. Transient receptor potential vanilloid type-1 channel regulates diet-induced obesity, insulin resistance, and leptin resistance. *FASEB J.* **2015**, *29*, 3182–3192. [CrossRef]
101. Wanner, S.P.; Garami, A.; Romanovsky, A.A. Hyperactive when young, hypoactive and overweight when aged: Connecting the dots in the story about locomotor activity, body mass, and aging in Trpv1 knockout mice. *Aging (Albany NY)* **2011**, *3*, 450–454. [CrossRef]
102. Baboota, R.K.; Murtaza, N.; Jagtap, S.; Singh, D.P.; Karmase, A.; Kaur, J.; Bhutani, K.K.; Boparai, R.K.; Premkumar, L.S.; Kondepudi, K.K.; et al. Capsaicin-induced transcriptional changes in hypothalamus and alterations in gut microbial count in high fat diet fed mice. *J. Nutr. Biochem.* **2014**, *25*, 893–902. [CrossRef] [PubMed]
103. Shen, W.; Shen, M.; Zhao, X.; Zhu, H.; Yang, Y.; Lu, S.; Tan, Y.; Li, G.; Li, M.; Wang, J.; et al. Anti-obesity Effect of Capsaicin in Mice Fed with High-Fat Diet Is Associated with an Increase in Population of the Gut Bacterium Akkermansia muciniphila. *Front. Microbiol.* **2017**, *8*, 272. [CrossRef] [PubMed]
104. Kang, C.; Wang, B.; Kaliannan, K.; Wang, X.; Lang, H.; Hui, S.; Huang, L.; Zhang, Y.; Zhou, M.; Chen, M.; et al. Gut Microbiota Mediates the Protective Effects of Dietary Capsaicin against Chronic Low-Grade Inflammation and Associated Obesity Induced by High-Fat Diet. *mBio* **2017**, *8*, e00470-17. [CrossRef] [PubMed]
105. Karwad, M.A.; Macpherson, T.; Wang, B.; Theophilidou, E.; Sarmad, S.; Barrett, D.A.; Larvin, M.; Wright, K.L.; Lund, J.N.; O'Sullivan, S.E. Oleoylethanolamine and palmitoylethanolamine modulate intestinal permeability in vitro via TRPV1 and PPARα. *FASEB J.* **2017**, *31*, 469–481. [CrossRef] [PubMed]
106. Kang, C.; Zhang, Y.; Zhu, X.; Liu, K.; Wang, X.; Chen, M.; Wang, J.; Chen, H.; Hui, S.; Huang, L.; et al. Healthy Subjects Differentially Respond to Dietary Capsaicin Correlating with Specific Gut Enterotypes. *J. Clin. Endocrinol. Metab.* **2016**, *101*, 4681–4689. [CrossRef]
107. Perez-Burgos, A.; Wang, L.; McVey Neufeld, K.-A.; Mao, Y.-K.; Ahmadzai, M.; Janssen, L.J.; Stanisz, A.M.; Bienenstock, J.; Kunze, W.A. The TRPV1 channel in rodents is a major target for antinociceptive effect of the probiotic Lactobacillus reuteri DSM 17938. *J. Physiol.* **2015**, *593*, 3943–3957. [CrossRef]
108. Holick, M.F.; Chen, T.C. Vitamin D deficiency: A worldwide problem with health consequences. *Am. J. Clin. Nutr.* **2008**, *87*, 1080S–1086S. [CrossRef]
109. Al-Dabhani, K.; Tsilidis, K.K.; Murphy, N.; Ward, H.A.; Elliott, P.; Riboli, E.; Gunter, M.; Tzoulaki, I. Prevalence of vitamin D deficiency and association with metabolic syndrome in a Qatari population. *Nutr. Diabetes* **2017**, *7*, e263. [CrossRef]
110. Moon, R.J.; Curtis, E.M.; Cooper, C.; Davies, J.H.; Harvey, N.C. Vitamin D supplementation: Are multivitamins sufficient? *Arch. Dis. Child.* **2019**. [CrossRef]

111. Strange, R.C.; Shipman, K.E.; Ramachandran, S. Metabolic syndrome: A review of the role of vitamin D in mediating susceptibility and outcome. *World J. Diabetes* **2015**, *6*, 896–911. [CrossRef]
112. Su, D.; Nie, Y.; Zhu, A.; Chen, Z.; Wu, P.; Zhang, L.; Luo, M.; Sun, Q.; Cai, L.; Lai, Y.; et al. Vitamin D Signaling through Induction of Paneth Cell Defensins Maintains Gut Microbiota and Improves Metabolic Disorders and Hepatic Steatosis in Animal Models. *Front. Physiol.* **2016**, *7*, 498. [CrossRef] [PubMed]
113. Ooi, J.H.; Li, Y.; Rogers, C.J.; Cantorna, M.T. Vitamin D regulates the gut microbiome and protects mice from dextran sodium sulfate-induced colitis. *J. Nutr.* **2013**, *143*, 1679–1686. [CrossRef] [PubMed]
114. Ghaly, S.; Kaakoush, N.O.; Lloyd, F.; Gordon, L.; Forest, C.; Lawrance, I.C.; Hart, P.H. Ultraviolet Irradiation of Skin Alters the Faecal Microbiome Independently of Vitamin D in Mice. *Nutrients* **2018**, *10*, 1069. [CrossRef] [PubMed]
115. Bikle, D. Vitamin D: Production, Metabolism, and Mechanisms of Action. In *Endotext*; Feingold, K.R., Anawalt, B., Boyce, A., Chrousos, G., Dungan, K., Grossman, A., Hershman, J.M., Kaltsas, G., Koch, C., et al., Eds.; MDText.com, Inc.: South Dartmouth, MA, USA, 2000.
116. Kendall, A.C.; Pilkington, S.M.; Massey, K.A.; Sassano, G.; Rhodes, L.E.; Nicolaou, A. Distribution of Bioactive Lipid Mediators in Human Skin. *J. Invest. Dermatol.* **2015**, *135*, 1510–1520. [CrossRef] [PubMed]
117. Magina, S.; Esteves-Pinto, C.; Moura, E.; Serrão, M.P.; Moura, D.; Petrosino, S.; Di Marzo, V.; Vieira-Coelho, M.A. Inhibition of basal and ultraviolet B-induced melanogenesis by cannabinoid CB1 receptors: A keratinocyte-dependent effect. *Arch. Dermatol. Res.* **2011**, *303*, 201–210. [CrossRef] [PubMed]
118. Felton, S.J.; Kendall, A.C.; Almaedani, A.F.M.; Urquhart, P.; Webb, A.R.; Kift, R.; Vail, A.; Nicolaou, A.; Rhodes, L.E. Serum endocannabinoids and N-acyl ethanolamines and the influence of simulated solar UVR exposure in humans in vivo. *Photochem. Photobiol. Sci.* **2017**, *16*, 564–574. [CrossRef] [PubMed]
119. Magina, S.; Vieira-Coelho, M.A.; Moura, E.; Serrão, M.P.; Piscitelli, F.; Moura, D.; Di Marzo, V. Effect of narrowband ultraviolet B treatment on endocannabinoid plasma levels in patients with psoriasis. *Br. J. Dermatol.* **2014**, *171*, 198–201. [CrossRef] [PubMed]
120. Guida, F.; Boccella, S.; Belardo, C.; Iannotta, M.; Piscitelli, F.; De Filippis, F.; Paino, S.; Ricciardi, F.; Siniscalco, D.; Marabese, I.; et al. Altered gut microbiota and endocannabinoid system tone in vitamin D deficiency-mediated chronic pain. *Brain Behav. Immunity* **2019**. [CrossRef]
121. Di Marzo, V.; Côté, M.; Matias, I.; Lemieux, I.; Arsenault, B.J.; Cartier, A.; Piscitelli, F.; Petrosino, S.; Alméras, N.; Després, J.-P. Changes in plasma endocannabinoid levels in viscerally obese men following a 1 year lifestyle modification programme and waist circumference reduction: Associations with changes in metabolic risk factors. *Diabetologia* **2009**, *52*, 213–217. [CrossRef]
122. Gasperi, V.; Ceci, R.; Tantimonaco, M.; Talamonti, E.; Battista, N.; Parisi, A.; Florio, R.; Sabatini, S.; Rossi, A.; Maccarrone, M. The Fatty Acid Amide Hydrolase in Lymphocytes from Sedentary and Active Subjects. *Med. Sci. Sports Exerc.* **2014**, *46*, 24–32. [CrossRef]
123. Fernández-Aranda, F.; Sauchelli, S.; Pastor, A.; Gonzalez, M.L.; de la Torre, R.; Granero, R.; Jiménez-Murcia, S.; Baños, R.; Botella, C.; Fernández-Real, J.M.; et al. Moderate-Vigorous Physical Activity across Body Mass Index in Females: Moderating Effect of Endocannabinoids and Temperament. *PLoS ONE* **2014**, *9*, e104534. [CrossRef] [PubMed]
124. Raichlen, D.A.; Foster, A.D.; Seillier, A.; Giuffrida, A.; Gerdeman, G.L. Exercise-induced endocannabinoid signaling is modulated by intensity. *Eur. J. Appl. Physiol.* **2013**, *113*, 869–875. [CrossRef] [PubMed]
125. Raichlen, D.A.; Foster, A.D.; Gerdeman, G.L.; Seillier, A.; Giuffrida, A. Wired to run: Exercise-induced endocannabinoid signaling in humans and cursorial mammals with implications for the "runner's high". *J. Exp. Biol.* **2012**, *215*, 1331–1336. [CrossRef] [PubMed]
126. Heyman, E.; Gamelin, F.-X.; Goekint, M.; Piscitelli, F.; Roelands, B.; Leclair, E.; Di Marzo, V.; Meeusen, R. Intense exercise increases circulating endocannabinoid and BDNF levels in humans—Possible implications for reward and depression. *Psychoneuroendocrinology* **2012**, *37*, 844–851. [CrossRef] [PubMed]
127. Heyman, E.; Gamelin, F.-X.; Aucouturier, J.; Marzo, V.D. The role of the endocannabinoid system in skeletal muscle and metabolic adaptations to exercise: Potential implications for the treatment of obesity. *Obes. Rev.* **2012**, *13*, 1110–1124. [CrossRef] [PubMed]
128. Cedernaes, J.; Fanelli, F.; Fazzini, A.; Pagotto, U.; Broman, J.-E.; Vogel, H.; Dickson, S.L.; Schiöth, H.B.; Benedict, C. Sleep restriction alters plasma endocannabinoids concentrations before but not after exercise in humans. *Psychoneuroendocrinology* **2016**, *74*, 258–268. [CrossRef] [PubMed]

129. Gamelin, F.-X.; Aucouturier, J.; Iannotti, F.A.; Piscitelli, F.; Mazzarella, E.; Aveta, T.; Leriche, M.; Dupont, E.; Cieniewski-Bernard, C.; Montel, V.; et al. Effects of chronic exercise on the endocannabinoid system in Wistar rats with high-fat diet-induced obesity. *J. Physiol. Biochem.* **2016**, *72*, 183–199. [CrossRef] [PubMed]
130. Mikkelsen, K.; Stojanovska, L.; Polenakovic, M.; Bosevski, M.; Apostolopoulos, V. Exercise and mental health. *Maturitas* **2017**, *106*, 48–56. [CrossRef] [PubMed]
131. Fuss, J.; Steinle, J.; Bindila, L.; Auer, M.K.; Kirchherr, H.; Lutz, B.; Gass, P. A runner's high depends on cannabinoid receptors in mice. *Proc. Natl. Acad. Sci. USA* **2015**, *112*, 13105–13108. [CrossRef]
132. Hill, M.N.; Titterness, A.K.; Morrish, A.C.; Carrier, E.J.; Lee, T.T.-Y.; Gil-Mohapel, J.; Gorzalka, B.B.; Hillard, C.J.; Christie, B.R. Endogenous cannabinoid signaling is required for voluntary exercise-induced enhancement of progenitor cell proliferation in the hippocampus. *Hippocampus* **2010**, *20*, 513–523. [CrossRef] [PubMed]
133. De Chiara, V.; Errico, F.; Musella, A.; Rossi, S.; Mataluni, G.; Sacchetti, L.; Siracusano, A.; Castelli, M.; Cavasinni, F.; Bernardi, G.; et al. Voluntary exercise and sucrose consumption enhance cannabinoid CB1 receptor sensitivity in the striatum. *Neuropsychopharmacology* **2010**, *35*, 374–387. [CrossRef] [PubMed]
134. Swenson, S.; Hamilton, J.; Robison, L.; Thanos, P.K. Chronic aerobic exercise: Lack of effect on brain CB1 receptor levels in adult rats. *Life Sci.* **2019**, *230*, 84–88. [CrossRef] [PubMed]
135. Stone, N.L.; Millar, S.A.; Herrod, P.J.J.; Barrett, D.A.; Ortori, C.A.; Mellon, V.A.; O'Sullivan, S.E. An Analysis of Endocannabinoid Concentrations and Mood Following Singing and Exercise in Healthy Volunteers. *Front. Behav. Neurosci.* **2018**, *12*, 269. [CrossRef] [PubMed]
136. Antunes, H.K.M.; Leite, G.S.F.; Lee, K.S.; Barreto, A.T.; dos Santos, R.V.T.; de Sá Souza, H.; Tufik, S.; de Mello, M.T. Exercise deprivation increases negative mood in exercise-addicted subjects and modifies their biochemical markers. *Physiol. Behav.* **2016**, *156*, 182–190. [CrossRef] [PubMed]
137. Hsu, Y.J.; Chiu, C.C.; Li, Y.P.; Huang, W.C.; Huang, Y.T.; Huang, C.C.; Chuang, H.L. Effect of Intestinal Microbiota on Exercise Performance in Mice. *J. Strength Cond. Res.* **2015**, *29*, 552–558. [CrossRef] [PubMed]
138. Petriz, B.A.; Castro, A.P.; Almeida, J.A.; Gomes, C.P.; Fernandes, G.R.; Kruger, R.H.; Pereira, R.W.; Franco, O.L. Exercise induction of gut microbiota modifications in obese, non-obese and hypertensive rats. *BMC Genom.* **2014**, *15*, 511. [CrossRef] [PubMed]
139. Denou, E.; Marcinko, K.; Surette, M.G.; Steinberg, G.R.; Schertzer, J.D. High-intensity exercise training increases the diversity and metabolic capacity of the mouse distal gut microbiota during diet-induced obesity. *Am. J. Physiol.-Endocrinol. Metab.* **2016**, *310*, E982–E993. [CrossRef]
140. Lai, Z.-L.; Tseng, C.-H.; Ho, H.J.; Cheung, C.K.Y.; Lin, J.-Y.; Chen, Y.-J.; Cheng, F.-C.; Hsu, Y.-C.; Lin, J.-T.; El-Omar, E.M.; et al. Fecal microbiota transplantation confers beneficial metabolic effects of diet and exercise on diet-induced obese mice. *Sci. Rep.* **2018**, *8*, 15625. [CrossRef]
141. Maillard, F.; Vazeille, E.; Sauvanet, P.; Sirvent, P.; Combaret, L.; Sourdrille, A.; Chavanelle, V.; Bonnet, R.; Otero, Y.F.; Delcros, G.; et al. High intensity interval training promotes total and visceral fat mass loss in obese Zucker rats without modulating gut microbiota. *PLoS ONE* **2019**, *14*, e0214660. [CrossRef]
142. Barton, W.; Penney, N.C.; Cronin, O.; Garcia-Perez, I.; Molloy, M.G.; Holmes, E.; Shanahan, F.; Cotter, P.D.; O'Sullivan, O. The microbiome of professional athletes differs from that of more sedentary subjects in composition and particularly at the functional metabolic level. *Gut* **2017**. [CrossRef]
143. Clarke, S.F.; Murphy, E.F.; O'Sullivan, O.; Lucey, A.J.; Humphreys, M.; Hogan, A.; Hayes, P.; O'Reilly, M.; Jeffery, I.B.; Wood-Martin, R.; et al. Exercise and associated dietary extremes impact on gut microbial diversity. *Gut* **2014**, *63*, 1913–1920. [CrossRef] [PubMed]
144. Estaki, M.; Pither, J.; Baumeister, P.; Little, J.P.; Gill, S.K.; Ghosh, S.; Ahmadi-Vand, Z.; Marsden, K.R.; Gibson, D.L. Cardiorespiratory fitness as a predictor of intestinal microbial diversity and distinct metagenomic functions. *Microbiome* **2016**, *4*, 42. [CrossRef] [PubMed]
145. Munukka, E.; Ahtiainen, J.P.; Puigbó, P.; Jalkanen, S.; Pahkala, K.; Keskitalo, A.; Kujala, U.M.; Pietilä, S.; Hollmén, M.; Elo, L.; et al. Six-Week Endurance Exercise Alters Gut Metagenome That Is not Reflected in Systemic Metabolism in Over-weight Women. *Front. Microbiol.* **2018**, *9*, 2323. [CrossRef] [PubMed]
146. Cristiano, C.; Pirozzi, C.; Coretti, L.; Cavaliere, G.; Lama, A.; Russo, R.; Lembo, F.; Mollica, M.P.; Meli, R.; Calignano, A.; et al. Palmitoylethanolamide counteracts autistic-like behaviours in BTBR T+tf/J mice: Contribution of central and peripheral mechanisms. *Brain Behav. Immunity* **2018**, *74*, 166–175. [CrossRef] [PubMed]

147. Vidot, D.C.; Prado, G.; Hlaing, W.M.; Florez, H.J.; Arheart, K.L.; Messiah, S.E. Metabolic Syndrome among Marijuana Users in the United States: An Analysis of National Health and Nutrition Examination Survey Data. *Am. J. Med.* **2016**, *129*, 173–179. [CrossRef] [PubMed]
148. Le Strat, Y.; Le Foll, B. Obesity and Cannabis Use: Results from 2 Representative National Surveys. *Am. J. Epidemiol.* **2011**, *174*, 929–933. [CrossRef] [PubMed]
149. Alshaarawy, O.; Anthony, J.C. Are cannabis users less likely to gain weight? Results from a national 3-year prospective study. *Int. J. Epidemiol.* **2019**. [CrossRef] [PubMed]
150. Penner, E.A.; Buettner, H.; Mittleman, M.A. The Impact of Marijuana Use on Glucose, Insulin, and Insulin Resistance among US Adults. *Am. J. Med.* **2013**, *126*, 583–589. [CrossRef]
151. Alshaarawy, O.; Anthony, J.C. Cannabis Smoking and Diabetes Mellitus: Results from Meta-Analysis with Eight Independent Replication Samples. *Epidemiology* **2015**, *26*, 597–600. [CrossRef]
152. Rajavashisth, T.B.; Shaheen, M.; Norris, K.C.; Pan, D.; Sinha, S.K.; Ortega, J.; Friedman, T.C. Decreased prevalence of diabetes in marijuana users: Cross-sectional data from the National Health and Nutrition Examination Survey (NHANES) III. *BMJ Open* **2012**, *2*, e000494. [CrossRef]
153. Danielsson, A.K.; Lundin, A.; Yaregal, A.; Östenson, C.G.; Allebeck, P.; Agardh, E.E. Cannabis Use as Risk or Protection for Type 2 Diabetes: A Longitudinal Study of 18 000 Swedish Men and Women. *J. Diabetes Res.* **2016**, *2016*, 1–6. [CrossRef] [PubMed]
154. Ngueta, G.; Bélanger, R.E.; Laouan-Sidi, E.A.; Lucas, M. Cannabis use in relation to obesity and insulin resistance in the inuit population. *Obesity* **2015**, *23*, 290–295. [CrossRef] [PubMed]
155. Adejumo, A.C.; Ajayi, T.O.; Adegbala, O.M.; Adejumo, K.L.; Alliu, S.; Akinjero, A.M.; Onyeakusi, N.E.; Ojelabi, O.; Bukong, T.N. Cannabis use is associated with reduced prevalence of progressive stages of alcoholic liver disease. *Liver Int.* **2018**, *38*, 1475–1486. [CrossRef] [PubMed]
156. Adejumo, A.C.; Alliu, S.; Ajayi, T.O.; Adejumo, K.L.; Adegbala, O.M.; Onyeakusi, N.E.; Akinjero, A.M.; Durojaiye, M.; Bukong, T.N. Cannabis use is associated with reduced prevalence of non-alcoholic fatty liver disease: A cross-sectional study. *PLoS ONE* **2017**, *12*, e0176416. [CrossRef] [PubMed]
157. Akturk, H.K.; Taylor, D.D.; Camsari, U.M.; Rewers, A.; Kinney, G.L.; Shah, V.N. Association Between Cannabis Use and Risk for Diabetic Ketoacidosis in Adults With Type 1 Diabetes. *JAMA Intern. Med.* **2019**, *179*, 115. [CrossRef] [PubMed]
158. Auer, R.; Sidney, S.; Goff, D.; Vittinghoff, E.; Pletcher, M.J.; Allen, N.B.; Reis, J.P.; Lewis, C.E.; Carr, J.; Rana, J.S. Lifetime marijuana use and subclinical atherosclerosis: The Coronary Artery Risk Development in Young Adults (CARDIA) study. *Addiction* **2018**, *113*, 845–856. [CrossRef]
159. DeFilippis, E.M.; Singh, A.; Divakaran, S.; Gupta, A.; Collins, B.L.; Biery, D.; Qamar, A.; Fatima, A.; Ramsis, M.; Pipilas, D.; et al. Cocaine and Marijuana Use Among Young Adults With Myocardial Infarction. *J. Am. Coll. Cardiol.* **2018**, *71*, 2540–2551. [CrossRef] [PubMed]
160. Villares, J. Chronic use of marijuana decreases cannabinoid receptor binding and mRNA expression in the human brain. *Neuroscience* **2007**, *145*, 323–334. [CrossRef]
161. Ceccarini, J.; Kuepper, R.; Kemels, D.; van Os, J.; Henquet, C.; Laere, K.V. [18F]MK-9470 PET measurement of cannabinoid CB1 receptor availability in chronic cannabis users. *Addict. Biol.* **2015**, *20*, 357–367. [CrossRef]
162. Marzo, V.D.; Berrendero, F.; Bisogno, T.; González, S.; Cavaliere, P.; Romero, J.; Cebeira, M.; Ramos, J.A.; Fernández-Ruiz, J.J. Enhancement of Anandamide Formation in the Limbic Forebrain and Reduction of Endocannabinoid Contents in the Striatum of Δ9-Tetrahydrocannabinol-Tolerant Rats. *J. Neurochem.* **2000**, *74*, 1627–1635. [CrossRef]
163. Morgan, C.J.A.; Page, E.; Schaefer, C.; Chatten, K.; Manocha, A.; Gulati, S.; Curran, H.V.; Brandner, B.; Leweke, F.M. Cerebrospinal fluid anandamide levels, cannabis use and psychotic-like symptoms. *Br. J. Psychiatry* **2013**, *202*, 381–382. [CrossRef] [PubMed]
164. Maia, J.; Midão, L.; Cunha, S.C.; Almada, M.; Fonseca, B.M.; Braga, J.; Gonçalves, D.; Teixeira, N.; Correia-da-Silva, G. Effects of cannabis tetrahydrocannabinol on endocannabinoid homeostasis in human placenta. *Arch. Toxicol.* **2019**, *93*, 649–658. [CrossRef] [PubMed]
165. McIntosh, A.L.; Martin, G.G.; Huang, H.; Landrock, D.; Kier, A.B.; Schroeder, F. Δ^9-Tetrahydrocannabinol induces endocannabinoid accumulation in mouse hepatocytes: Antagonism by *Fabp1* gene ablation. *J. Lipid Res.* **2018**, *59*, 646–657. [CrossRef] [PubMed]

166. De Petrocellis, L.; Ligresti, A.; Moriello, A.S.; Allarà, M.; Bisogno, T.; Petrosino, S.; Stott, C.G.; Di Marzo, V. Effects of cannabinoids and cannabinoid-enriched Cannabis extracts on TRP channels and endocannabinoid metabolic enzymes. *Br. J. Pharmacol.* **2011**, *163*, 1479–1494. [CrossRef] [PubMed]
167. Cluny, N.L.; Keenan, C.M.; Reimer, R.A.; Le Foll, B.; Sharkey, K.A. Prevention of Diet-Induced Obesity Effects on Body Weight and Gut Microbiota in Mice Treated Chronically with Δ9-Tetrahydrocannabinol. *PLoS ONE* **2015**, *10*, e0144270. [CrossRef] [PubMed]
168. Wargent, E.T.; Zaibi, M.S.; Silvestri, C.; Hislop, D.C.; Stocker, C.J.; Stott, C.G.; Guy, G.W.; Duncan, M.; Di Marzo, V.; Cawthorne, M.A. The cannabinoid Δ9-tetrahydrocannabivarin (THCV) ameliorates insulin sensitivity in two mouse models of obesity. *Nutr. Diabetes* **2013**, *3*, e68. [CrossRef] [PubMed]
169. Weiss, L.; Zeira, M.; Reich, S.; Har-Noy, M.; Mechoulam, R.; Slavin, S.; Gallily, R. Cannabidiol lowers incidence of diabetes in non-obese diabetic mice. *Autoimmunity* **2006**, *39*, 143–151. [CrossRef]
170. Jadoon, K.A.; Ratcliffe, S.H.; Barrett, D.A.; Thomas, E.L.; Stott, C.; Bell, J.D.; O'Sullivan, S.E.; Tan, G.D. Efficacy and Safety of Cannabidiol and Tetrahydrocannabivarin on Glycemic and Lipid Parameters in Patients With Type 2 Diabetes: A Randomized, Double-Blind, Placebo-Controlled, Parallel Group Pilot Study. *Diabetes Care* **2016**, *39*, 1777–1786. [CrossRef]
171. Silvestri, C.; Paris, D.; Martella, A.; Melck, D.; Guadagnino, I.; Cawthorne, M.; Motta, A.; Di Marzo, V. Two non-psychoactive cannabinoids reduce intracellular lipid levels and inhibit hepatosteatosis. *J. Hepatol.* **2015**, *62*, 1382–1390. [CrossRef]
172. Le Bastard, Q.; Al-Ghalith, G.A.; Grégoire, M.; Chapelet, G.; Javaudin, F.; Dailly, E.; Batard, E.; Knights, D.; Montassier, E. Systematic review: Human gut dysbiosis induced by non-antibiotic prescription medications. *Aliment. Pharmacol. Ther.* **2018**, *47*, 332–345. [CrossRef]
173. Panee, J.; Gerschenson, M.; Chang, L. Associations between Microbiota, Mitochondrial Function, and Cognition in Chronic Marijuana Users. *J. Neuroimmune Pharmacol.* **2018**, *13*, 113–122. [CrossRef] [PubMed]
174. Wu, G.D.; Chen, J.; Hoffmann, C.; Bittinger, K.; Chen, Y.-Y.; Keilbaugh, S.A.; Bewtra, M.; Knights, D.; Walters, W.A.; Knight, R.; et al. Linking Long-Term Dietary Patterns with Gut Microbial Enterotypes. *Science* **2011**, *334*, 105–108. [CrossRef] [PubMed]
175. Smit, E.; Crespo, C.J. Dietary intake and nutritional status of US adult marijuana users: Results from the Third National Health and Nutrition Examination Survey. *Public Health Nutr.* **2001**, *4*, 781–786. [CrossRef] [PubMed]
176. Fulcher, J.A.; Hussain, S.K.; Cook, R.; Li, F.; Tobin, N.H.; Ragsdale, A.; Shoptaw, S.; Gorbach, P.M.; Aldrovandi, G.M. Effects of Substance Use and Sex Practices on the Intestinal Microbiome During HIV-1 Infection. *J. Infect. Dis.* **2018**, *218*, 1560–1570. [CrossRef] [PubMed]
177. Yun, Y.; Kim, H.-N.; Kim, S.E.; Heo, S.G.; Chang, Y.; Ryu, S.; Shin, H.; Kim, H.-L. Comparative analysis of gut microbiota associated with body mass index in a large Korean cohort. *BMC Microbiol.* **2017**, *17*, 151. [CrossRef] [PubMed]
178. Ottosson, F.; Brunkwall, L.; Ericson, U.; Nilsson, P.M.; Almgren, P.; Fernandez, C.; Melander, O.; Orho-Melander, M. Connection Between BMI-Related Plasma Metabolite Profile and Gut Microbiota. *J. Clin. Endocrinol. Metab.* **2018**, *103*, 1491–1501. [CrossRef] [PubMed]
179. Precup, G.; Vodnar, D.-C. Gut Prevotella as a possible biomarker of diet and its eubiotic versus dysbiotic roles-A comprehensive literature review. *Br. J. Nutr.* **2019**, 1–24. [CrossRef]
180. Al-Ghezi, Z.Z.; Busbee, P.B.; Alghetaa, H.; Nagarkatti, P.S.; Nagarkatti, M. Combination of cannabinoids, delta-9-tetrahydrocannabinol (THC) and cannabidiol (CBD), mitigates experimental autoimmune encephalomyelitis (EAE) by altering the gut microbiome. *Brain Behav. Immun.* **2019**. [CrossRef]
181. Becker, W.J.; Nagarkatti, M.; Nagarkatti, P.S. Δ^9-tetrahydrocannabinol (THC) activation of cannabinoid receptors induces unique changes in the murine gut microbiome and associated induction of myeloid-derived suppressor cells and Th17 cells. *J. Immunol.* **2017**, *198*, 218.11.

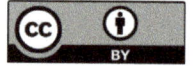

© 2019 by the authors. Licensee MDPI, Basel, Switzerland. This article is an open access article distributed under the terms and conditions of the Creative Commons Attribution (CC BY) license (http://creativecommons.org/licenses/by/4.0/).

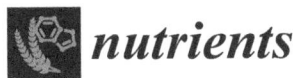

Article

Healthy Lifestyle and Incidence of Metabolic Syndrome in the SUN Cohort

Maria Garralda-Del-Villar [1], Silvia Carlos-Chillerón [2,3], Jesus Diaz-Gutierrez [2], Miguel Ruiz-Canela [2,3,4], Alfredo Gea [2,3], Miguel Angel Martínez-González [2,3,4,5], Maira Bes-Rastrollo [2,3,4], Liz Ruiz-Estigarribia [2], Stefanos N. Kales [6] and Alejandro Fernández-Montero [1,3,6,*]

1. Department of Occupational Medicine, University of Navarra, 31008 Pamplona, Navarra, Spain; mgarralda.7@alumni.unav.es
2. Department of Preventive Medicine and Public Health, University of Navarra, 31008 Pamplona, Navarra, Spain; scarlos@unav.es (S.C.-C.); jdiaz.14@alumni.unav.es (J.D.-G.); mcanela@unav.es (M.R.-C.); ageas@unav.es (A.G.); mamartinez@unav.es (M.A.M.-G.); mbes@unav.es (M.B.-R.); lruiz.29@alumni.unav.es (L.R.-E.)
3. IDISNA, Navarra Health Research Institute, 31008 Pamplona, Navarra, Spain
4. CIBER Fisiopatología de la Obesidad y Nutrición (CIBER Obn), Instituto de Salud Carlos III, 28029 Madrid, Spain
5. Department of Nutrition, Harvard T.H. Chan School of Public Health, Boston, MA 20115, USA
6. Department of Environmental Health, Harvard T.H. Chan School of Public Health, Boston, MA 20115, USA; skales@hsph.harvard.edu
* Correspondence: afmontero@unav.es; Tel.: +34-948-255-400

Received: 28 November 2018; Accepted: 24 December 2018; Published: 30 December 2018

Abstract: We assessed the relationship between a healthy lifestyle and the subsequent risk of developing metabolic syndrome. The "Seguimiento Universidad de Navarra" (SUN) Project is a prospective cohort study, focused on nutrition, lifestyle, and chronic diseases. Participants (n = 10,807, mean age 37 years, 67% women) initially free of metabolic syndrome were followed prospectively for a minimum of 6 years. To evaluate healthy lifestyle, nine habits were used to derive a Healthy Lifestyle Score (HLS): Never smoking, moderate to high physical activity (>20 MET-h/week), Mediterranean diet ($\geq$4/8 adherence points), moderate alcohol consumption (women, 0.1–5.0 g/day; men, 0.1–10.0 g/day), low television exposure (<2 h/day), no binge drinking ($\leq$5 alcoholic drinks at any time), taking a short afternoon nap (<30 min/day), meeting up with friends >1 h/day, and working at least 40 h/week. Metabolic syndrome was defined according to the harmonizing definition. The association between the baseline HLS and metabolic syndrome at follow-up was assessed with multivariable-adjusted logistic regressions. During follow-up, we observed 458 (4.24%) new cases of metabolic syndrome. Participants in the highest category of HLS adherence (7–9 points) enjoyed a significantly reduced risk of developing metabolic syndrome compared to those in the lowest category (0–3 points) (adjusted odds ratio (OR) = 0.66, 95% confidence interval (CI) = 0.47–0.93). Higher adherence to the Healthy Lifestyle Score was associated with a lower risk of developing metabolic syndrome. The HLS may be a simple metabolic health promotion tool.

Keywords: healthy lifestyle score; metabolic syndrome; SUN cohort

1. Introduction

Metabolic syndrome (MetSyn) is characterized by the clustering of several metabolic abnormalities frequently observed in clinical practice: Abdominal obesity, dyslipidemia, hyperinsulinemia, impaired fasting glucose, and high blood pressure, according to the International Diabetes Federation, the American Heart Association, and the National Heart, Lung, and Blood Institute harmonizing definition [1]. In a prospective cohort study done on middle-aged healthy men, MetSyn was associated with cardiovascular disease and mortality, and a published meta-analysis of longitudinal studies revealed an association between MetSyn and a higher risk of developing type 2 diabetes mellitus, cardiovascular disease, atherosclerosis, and higher all-cause mortality [2,3]. Due to the existence of different definitions for diagnosing this syndrome, prevalence estimates vary. However, it is accepted that the prevalence of MetSyn generally increases as body mass index and age increase [4]. In developed countries, the prevalence of MetSyn is about 25% of the adult population [5–7], and its incidence has been increasing over the last years. In Spain, MetSyn prevalence reached 10% in 2005 [8], and it increased to over 30% by 2012 [9]. Genetics cannot explain these differences alone, and environmental influences play an important role.

Several articles have shown the association between different lifestyle habits and the risk of developing MetSyn according to the harmonizing definition. In this context, eating habits are considered modifiable determinants of MetSyn. Prospective studies (that included participants who were young–middle-aged adults and that considered the harmonizing definition of MetSyn) and a systematic review (that evaluated studies with adults >18 years and that considered the ATPIII definition) analyzing nut consumption, sweet beverages, or adherence to Mediterranean diet patterns, as well as a meta-analysis on this topic (that worked with trials including adults >29 years and used the ATPIII criteria) have proven this association [10–13]. In a prospective study from the "Seguimiento Universidad de Navarra" (SUN) (that included young–middle-aged adults and used the harmonizing definition of MetSyn), physical activity was significantly associated with a lower risk of developing MetSyn [14], whereas, according to a meta-analysis (that analyzed studies whose participants were young–middle-aged adults and that used the MetSyn criteria proposed by the WHO, ATPIII, modified ATPIII, and ACE/AACE) and a longitudinal population-based study (that analyzed 43-year-old adults and used the IDF definition), active smoking and time spent viewing TV were associated with higher risks of MetSyn [15,16]. Several studies evaluating middle-aged adults and using the AHA definition, as well as studies in people who were overweight or obese, have evaluated the effect of the combination of classical healthy life factors on MetSyn (smoking, drinking, dietary habits, and physical activity) with more complex nutritional indexes and have reported them to be significantly associated with MetSyn [17,18]. These previous articles worked with middle-aged adults.

In conclusion, classic healthy lifestyle habits have proven to reduce the risk of developing MetSyn.

In a recent longitudinal study conducted in 2017 in the SUN cohort [19] (in young–middle-aged adults), a new Healthy Lifestyle Score (HLS) was associated with a significant reduction in cardiovascular disease (CVD). This HLS basically included the traditional cardiovascular healthy lifestyle factors (i.e., tobacco, alcohol, diet, and physical activity), and it also took into account other modern life habits including time spent watching television, binge drinking, napping, social life with friends, and number of hours spent working.

Therefore, since it is well known that the MetSyn is a risk factor for CVD, an important question from a public health perspective is whether a healthy lifestyle would also reduce the risk of MetSyn. Our hypothesis was that a higher adherence to the HLS would be associated with a lower risk of MetSyn.

The aim of this study was to prospectively analyze the effectiveness of this new and easy-to-apply HLS in the reduction of MetSyn risk.

2. Materials and Methods

2.1. Study Design

The "Seguimiento Universidad de Navarra" (University of Navarra Follow-Up) Project is a dynamic prospective cohort study that has been conducted in Spain since December 1999 with permanently open recruitment of university graduates. It was designed based on the model of other large cohort studies conducted at the Harvard School of Public Health (the Nurses' Health Study and the Health Professionals Follow-Up Study). Additional details on its objectives, design, and methods have been previously published [20].

Information is mainly gathered through self-reported questionnaires. Participants' information is collected biennially through mailed or electronically mailed questionnaires. Upon completion of the first questionnaire (Q_0), including a total of 554 items used as baseline information, participants receive, every other year, different follow-up questionnaires. These contain important questions to evaluate changes in lifestyle and health-related behaviors, anthropometric measures, incident diseases, and medical conditions. Participants of all ages may be included in the SUN cohort, but they must have had university studies. This inclusion criteria allows for a better control of confounding by education-related variables and by making the interpretation of results easier and therefore adding internal validity to the high-quality information derived from the questionnaires.

2.2. Participants

In our study, a subsample of the SUN cohort was selected. In order to achieve a minimum follow-up of 6 years, only participants who had at least completed the 6-year follow-up questionnaire (Q_6) were included. There were 20,622 participants eligible to be included (SUN participants who responded to the baseline questionnaire (Q_0) before March 2010). We excluded 5080 participants who had either prevalent MetSyn or any MetSyn component at baseline. We also excluded 1399 participants who had extremely low or high total energy intake [21], as well as 1411 participants lost to follow-up (retention rate = 92.7%) and 1985 subjects who did not provide all of the relevant information to diagnose metabolic syndrome at the 6-year follow-up (Figure 1). Therefore, there were 10,807 participants available for analysis.

Informed consent was obtained from all individual participants included in the study by the voluntary completion of the baseline questionnaire once participants understood the specific information needed, the methods used to deliver their data, and the future feedback from the research team. We asked their permission before any follow-up on their medical history. We informed the potential candidates of their right to refuse to participate in the SUN study or to withdraw their consent to participate at any time without reprisal, according to the principles of the Declaration of Helsinki. The Institutional Review Board of the University of Navarra approved these methods.

2.3. Exposure Assessment: Healthy Lifestyle Score Variables

We gathered information from the baseline questionnaires, which collected data on sociodemographic, clinical, anthropometric variables, and lifestyle aspects. Various studies have validated data from the self-reported questionnaires in the SUN cohort: Both anthropometric [22] and physical activity [23] data were analyzed in cohort subgroups. We used the validated 136-question semiquantitative food frequency questionnaire (FFQ) [24] for the evaluation of Mediterranean diet adherence, which was estimated with the Trichopoulou score (0–8 points) [25], (alcohol was excluded). So as to collect information on alcohol consumption, data was obtained through this questionnaire and other additional items related to alcohol consumption in the baseline questionnaire.

In order to assess adherence to a healthy lifestyle, 9 habits of the Healthy Lifestyle Score [19] were used (Table 1), excluding body mass index (BMI), as it is strongly related to MetSyn. The information for this score was gathered from the baseline questionnaire. Each participant received one point for each of the following 9 habits: Never smoking, moderate to high physical activity (>20 MET-h/week), Mediterranean diet ($\geq$4 adherence points), moderate alcohol consumption (women, 0.1–5.0 g/day; men, 0.1–10.0 g/day; abstainers excluded), low television exposure (<2 h/day), no binge drinking ($\leq$5 alcoholic drinks at any time), taking a short afternoon nap (<30 min/day), meeting up with friends >1 h/day, and working at least 40 h/week. This HLS could range from 0 (worst lifestyle) and 9 points (best lifestyle).

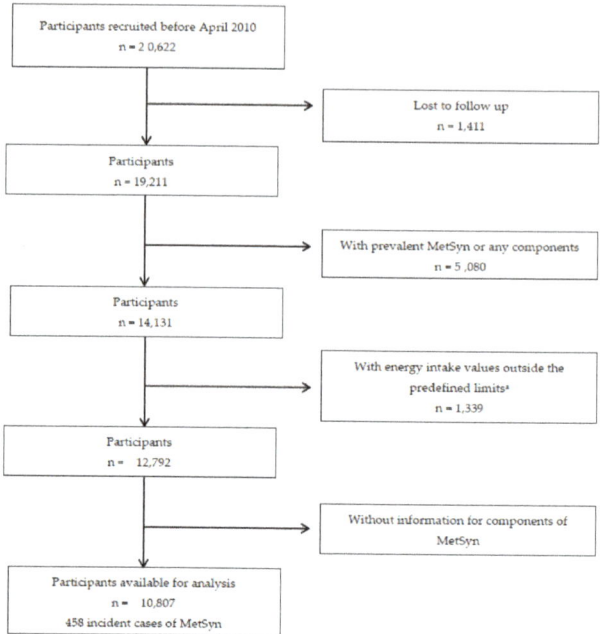

Figure 1. Flow chart depicting the selection process among participants of the Seguimiento Universidad de Navarra (SUN) cohort, 1999–2017; *n*: Number of participants; MetSyn: Metabolic Syndrome. [a] Total energy intake outside predefined limits (<800 or >4000 kcal/day for men, and<500 or >3500 kcal/day for women) [21].

2.4. Outcome Assessment: Metabolic Syndrome and Assessment of Other Variables

The study outcome was incidence of MetSyn. We followed the harmonized definition of MetSyn according to the International Diabetes Federation; the National Heart, Lung, and Blood Institute; the American Heart Association; the World Heart Federation; the International Atherosclerosis Society; and the International Association for the Study of Obesity. According to this definition, metabolic syndrome consists of at least three abnormal findings out of the following 5 criteria [1]: (i) Central adiposity ($\geq$94 cm for men and $\geq$80 cm for women, cut-off points for European populations); (ii) elevated triglycerides (TAG) ($\geq$150 mg/dL or presence of pharmacological treatment for hypertriglyceridemia); (iii) reduced high-density lipoprotein cholesterol (HDL-cholesterol) (<40 mg/dL for men and <50 mg/dL for women or presence of pharmacological treatment for reduced HDL-cholesterol); (iv) elevated blood pressure (systolic $\geq$130 mmHg or diastolic $\geq$85 mmHg or presence of pharmacological treatment for hypertension in patients with a history of this disease); and (v) fasting glucose metabolism ($\geq$100 mg/dL or pharmacological treatment for hyperglycemia).

To obtain the clinical criteria needed for the diagnosis of MetSyn, we used self-reported information provided by participants during the follow-up questionnaires. In the 6-year and 8-year follow-up questionnaires (Q_6 and Q_8), self-reported data about these specific MetSyn criteria were collected. All participants were sent a measuring tape with the Q_6 and Q_8 follow-up questionnaires, together with an explanation on how to measure their waist circumference by using the horizontal plane, midway between the inferior margin of the ribs and the superior border of the iliac crest [26]. Accuracy and validation of all self-reported data on MetSyn components had been previously analyzed in a specific subsample study from the SUN Project of 287 participants [27]. All the analytical parameters used in the validation of self-reported metabolic syndrome components were obtained from the Clinical Analyses Service of Clínica Universidad de Navarra (CUN). The analyses of glucose,

HDL-cholesterol, total cholesterol, and triglycerides were measured in blood serum with the analyzer equipment Roche/Hitachi Modular Analytics, and through spectrophotometry by the enzymatic colorimetric method with glucose oxidase and p-aminophenazone (GOD-PAP). High intraclass correlations were found for waist circumference ($r = 0.86$, 95% confidence interval (CI): 0.80–0.90) and triglycerides ($r = 0.71$, 95% CI: 0.61–0.79), whereas moderate intraclass correlations were found (between 0.46 and 0.63) for the other factors. An additional study, which compared the validity of self-reported diagnosed MetSyn and MetSyn diagnosed by the medical records of the participants, was conducted in another subsample of the SUN Project [28]. Using ATP III criteria, 91.2% of MetSyn and 92.2% (95% CI: 85.7–96.4) of non-MetSyn cases were confirmed.

An incident case of MetSyn was defined when a participant, free of this condition or any of its components at baseline, met three or more of the criteria after at least 6 years of follow-up.

Table 1. Healthy Lifestyle Score (HLS) [a].

	Score
Not smoking	
Never a smoker	1
Smoker (current and former)	0
Physical activity (MET-h/week)	
Physically active (>20 MET-h/week)	1
Not physically active (≤20 MET-h/week)	0
Mediterranean diet pattern (Trichopoulou score excluding alcohol) [b]	
High adherence (≥4)	1
Low adherence (<4)	0
Moderate alcohol consumption	
Moderate consumption (women, 0.1–5.0 g/day; men, 0.1–10.0 g/day)	1
Abstention or high consumption (women >5 g/day; men >10 g/day)	0
Low time spent watching television	
Low television watching (<2 h/day)	1
High television watching (≥2 h/day)	0
Avoidance of binge drinking	
No binge drinking (≤5 alcoholic drinks at any time)	1
Binge drinking (>5 alcoholic drinks at any time)	0
Having a short afternoon nap	
Short afternoon nap (0.1–0.5 h/day)	1
Not having an afternoon nap or having a long nap (>0.5 h/day)	0
Time with friends	
Spending time with friends (>1 h/day)	1
Not spending time with friends (≤1 h/day)	0
Time working	
Full-time work (≥40 h/week)	1
Less than full-time work (<40 h/week)	0

[a] Body mass index was excluded, as it is a component of metabolic syndrome. [b] Score from 0 to 8, because alcohol consumption was excluded.

2.5. Ascertainment of Covariates

The baseline questionnaire also collected information of potential confounding factors between HLS and MetSyn such as sociodemographic characteristics (sex, age, and education level), sleep, medical history (prevalence of cancer, cardiovascular disease, and depression), dietary factors (following a special diet and total energy intake (Kcals/day)), and anthropometric data (BMI). Our approach was to use the consideration of a priori causal knowledge to suggest which were the most relevant variables to be adjusted for. Causal diagrams were used to encode qualitative a priori subject matter knowledge. We did not use merely statistical criteria, because this statistics-only approach has been discouraged [29–31]. For instance, in reference to the prevalence of cancer, it may lead to weight loss and therefore be associated with MetSyn. Besides, it can be related to a change in diet and lifestyle, and these can influence MetSyn.

2.6. Statistical Analyses

According to their baseline HLS, participants were classified into 5 groups to ensure an appropriate sample distribution with sufficient participants and incident cases in each category. Thus, we merged extreme categories, and the distribution of these five categories was 0–3, 4, 5, 6, and 7–9 points. Logistic regression models were fit to assess the risk of metabolic syndrome (MetSyn) after a 6-year follow-up according to HLS categories. Odds ratios (ORs) and their 95% confidence intervals (95% CIs) were calculated considering the lowest category (0–3) as the reference. Linear trend tests were calculated by assigning the median score of each category to all participants in that category and treating this variable as a continuous variable.

For all the analyses, we fitted a crude model, an age- and sex-adjusted model, and a multivariable adjusted model using the following covariates as confounding factors: Age, sex, depression (yes/no), education level (technical/nongraduated, graduated, postgraduate, master's, doctorate), cardiovascular disease (yes/no), prevalent cancer (yes/no), following any special diet (yes/no), body mass index (kg/m^2), energy intake (kcal/day), hours of sleep (h/day), and year of questionnaire completion.

Additional multivariable adjusted analyses were conducted to test the association between the HLS categories and each of the individual criteria for MetSyn.

To assess the individual contribution of each specific factor of the HLS score to the risk of MetSyn, logistic regression models were fitted for each of the nine indicators of healthy life habits, adjusting for the effect of the rest of the elements that constituted the index. The reference category was the absence of the habit of healthy life (score 0 on the specific element).

We used the imputation approach because we had some missing information in important variables such as time spent watching TV, having a short afternoon nap, and time spent with friends. This statistical technique tries to overcome the problem that single imputed values are not actually observed but predicted values, and attributes the most probable value [32]. To carry out the imputation approach, we took into account potential confounding factors, each of the other components of Healthy Lifestyle Score, and each one of the components of MetSyn.

Sensitivity analyses were performed to ensure the robustness of the results in different scenarios. We repeated the analyses stratifying by age ($\geq$45) and sex and without imputation of the lost variables.

All *p*-values presented are two-tailed, and $p < 0.05$ was considered to be statistically significant. Analyses were performed using STATA/SE version 12.0.

3. Results

The main characteristics of participants according to the HLS categories are shown in Table 2. Compared to subjects who had lower HLSes (0–3 points), those who had the highest score (7–9 points) were less likely to be women, consumed less alcohol per day, had less prevalent depression, were more likely to follow a special diet, and had a slightly higher total energy intake per day. There were no differences in age, baseline BMI, and the prevalence of CVD and cancer.

Of the participants, 458 (4.24%) (272 men, 186 women) initially free of metabolic syndrome (MetSyn) were newly diagnosed as incident cases during the 6-year follow-up. Those who had high HLSes (7 to 9 points) had a significant 34% lower risk of developing MetSyn than those who had lower HLSes (0 to 3), after adjusting for other factors related to MetSyn (Table 3).

Table 4 shows the multivariable-adjusted ORs for each component of MetSyn across HLS categories after the 6-year follow-up. With the exception of HDL-cholesterol, all point estimates of ORs for the upper versus lower category of the HLS suggested inverse associations. However, only the associations with waist circumference and elevated blood pressure showed statistically significant associations (*p* for trend < 0.05).

Table 2. Baseline characteristics of participants according to the number of Healthy Lifestyle Factors (HLFs) (the SUN cohort).

Number of Healthy Lifestyle Factors	0–3	4	5	6	7–9	p-Value
Participants, n	1468	1993	2599	2525	2222	
Sex, women (%)	69.8	68.0	68.3	66.3	63.7	<0.001
Age, years	35.8 ± 10.6	36.5 ± 11	35.9 ± 10.7	35.9 ± 10.8	34.2 ± 10	<0.001
Body mass index in men	24.9 ± 2.5	24.6 ± 2.3	24.6 ± 2.3	24.6 ± 2.2	24.3 ± 2.3	<0.001
Body mass index in women	22.0 ± 2.5	21.9 ± 2.5	21.9 ± 2.5	21.6 ± 2.4	21.6 ± 2.4	<0.001
Smoking, packs per year	8.8 ± 10.2	7.1 ± 9.4	5.4 ± 8.1	4.21 ± 7.8	1.9 ± 5.8	<0.001
Physical activity, MET-h/week	16.1 ± 15.2	21.4 ± 19.3	25.1 ± 21.8	30.3 ± 25	36.7 ± 26	<0.001
Mediterranean diet pattern [a]	3.04 ± 1.54	3.56 ± 1.7	3.89 ± 1.73	4.24 ± 1.69	4.71 ± 1.49	<0.001
Alcohol consumption, g/day	8.0 ± 11.1	6.9 ± 9.4	6.2 ± 8.7	5.1 ± 7.1	3.9 ± 5.1	<0.001
Watching television, h/day	2.27 ± 1.51	1.81 ± 1.4	1.58 ± 1.31	1.33 ± 1.11	1.09 ± 0.83	<0.001
No binge drinking (%) [b]	44.3	60.7	71	77.2	86.6	<0.001
Afternoon nap, min/day	0.3 ± 0.45	0.27 ± 0.39	0.25 ± 0.34	0.22 ± 0.29	0.22 ± 0.22	<0.001
Meeting up with friends, h/day	1.11 ± 1	1.24 ± 1.05	1.34 ± 1.09	1.39 ± 1	1.54 ± 1.03	<0.001
Working ≥40 h/week (%)	25.4	37.7	49.2	60.6	76.3	<0.001
Sleeping, h/day	7.5 ± 1.1	7.4 ± 1	7.4 ± 1	7.4 ± 0.9	7.4 ± 0.9	0.011
Depression disease (%)	12.7	11.2	10.7	9.2	9.3	0.001
Prevalent cardiovascular disease (%) [c]	1.43	2.06	1.89	1.43	1.53	0.512
Prevalent cancer (%)	3.07	3.21	2.89	3.05	2.43	0.826
Education level						<0.001
No college (%)	8.86	9.13	8.96	10.18	10.26	
College (%)	26.6	22.9	25.2	23.1	21.1	
Postgraduate (%)	51.2	51.9	49.5	47.9	49.1	
Master's (%)	5.93	7.02	7.7	8.08	8.51	
Doctorate (%)	7.43	9.03	8.66	10.73	10.98	
On any special diet (%)	4.36	6.77	5.73	6.81	7.25	0.003
Caloric consumption	2282 ± 607	2302 ± 594	2359 ± 603	2392 ± 606	2428 ± 593	<0.001

[a] Trichopoulou score (from 0 to 8, with alcohol consumption excluded). [b] Less than 5 alcoholic drinks at any time. [c] Atrial fibrillation, paroxysmal tachycardia, coronFary artery bypass surgery or another revascularization procedure, heart failure, aortic aneurysm, pulmonary embolism, or peripheral venous thrombosis.

Table 3. Incidence of metabolic syndrome at 6-year follow-up, according to the number of Healthy Lifestyle Score factors (the SUN cohort). OR: Odds ratio; CI: Confidence interval.

	Number of Healthy Lifestyle Factors					
	0–3	4	5	6	7–9	p for Trend
Participants, n	1468	1993	2599	2525	2222	
Incident cases	80	92	109	103	74	
Crude OR (95% CI)	1 (ref.)	0.86 (0.64–1.17)	0.73 (0.54–0.98)	0.75 (0.56–1.01)	0.57 (0.42–0.80)	0.002
OR adjusted for age and sex (95% CI)	1 (ref.)	0.77 (0.56–1.05)	0.68 (0.50–0.93)	0.69 (0.51–0.94)	0.60 (0.43–0.83)	0.003
Multivariable adjusted OR [a]	1 (ref.)	0.82 (0.59–1.13)	0.72 (0.52–0.98)	0.76 (0.77–1.05)	0.66 (0.47–0.93)	0.027

ref: reference category. [a] Adjusted for age, sex, depression, education level, cardiovascular disease, prevalent cancer, following any special diet, body mass index, energy intake, hours of sleep, year of questionnaire completion.

Figure 2 shows the multivariable-adjusted ORs across the 9 habits of the HLS and the risk of MetSyn. Only low television exposure (<2 h/day) and a short afternoon nap (<30 min/day) were significantly related to the incidence of MetSyn.

In the stratified analysis, we found a significant inverse association between HLS and MetSyn in men and in those older than 55 years, but we did not find any significant interaction (Figure 3).

When we performed the analyses without imputation, the results did not change in magnitude, but they were no longer significant (OR = 0.67, 95% CI = 0.44–1.02).

Table 4. Odds ratios and 95% confidence intervals for each component of metabolic syndrome at the 6-year follow-up, according to the number of HLFs (the SUN Cohort).

	Number of Healthy Lifestyle Factors					
	0–3	4	5	6	7–9	p for Trend
Waist Circumference (>94 cm men, 80 cm women) [a]	1 (ref.)	0.88 (0.75–1.02)	0.74 (0.64–0.86)	0.74 (0.64–0.86)	0.68 (0.58–0.79)	<0.001
Elevated triglycerides (>150 mg/dL) [a]	1 (ref.)	0.84 (0.64–1.12)	0.80 (0.62–1.07)	0.72 (0.54–0.95)	0.87 (0.66–1.16)	0.213
Reduced HDL-cholesterol (<40 mg/dL) [a]	1 (ref.)	1.00 (0.73–1.38)	1.27 (0.95–1.70)	1.10 (0.81–1.49)	1.10 (0.80–1.51)	0.483
Elevated blood pressure (systolic >130 or diastolic >85 mmHg) [a]	1 (ref.)	1.02 (0.85–1.24)	0.93 (0.78–1.12)	0.89 (0.74–1.07)	0.86 (0.71–1.05)	0.033
Elevated glucose (>100 mg/dL) [a]	1 (ref.)	0.82 (0.64–1.05)	0.86 (0.68–1.09)	0.93 (0.74–1.17)	0.73 (0.57–0.94)	0.127

ref: reference category. [a] Adjusted for age, sex, depression, education level, cardiovascular disease, prevalent cancer, following any special diet, body mass index, energy intake, hours of sleep, year of questionnaire completion. HDL-cholesterol: High-density lipoprotein cholesterol.

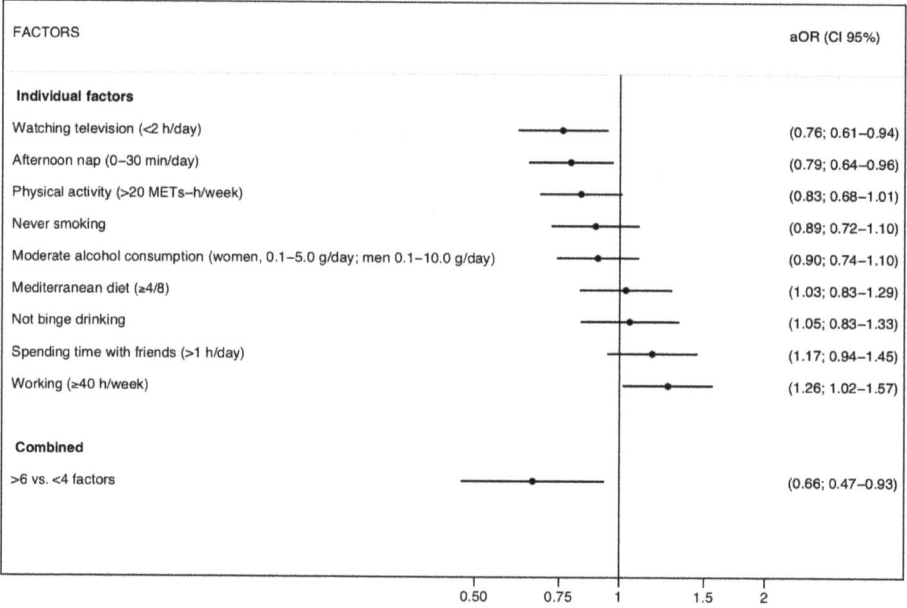

Figure 2. Risk of metabolic syndrome for each factor of the Healthy Lifestyle Score (the SUN cohort); aOR: Adjusted odds ratio; CI: Confidence interval.

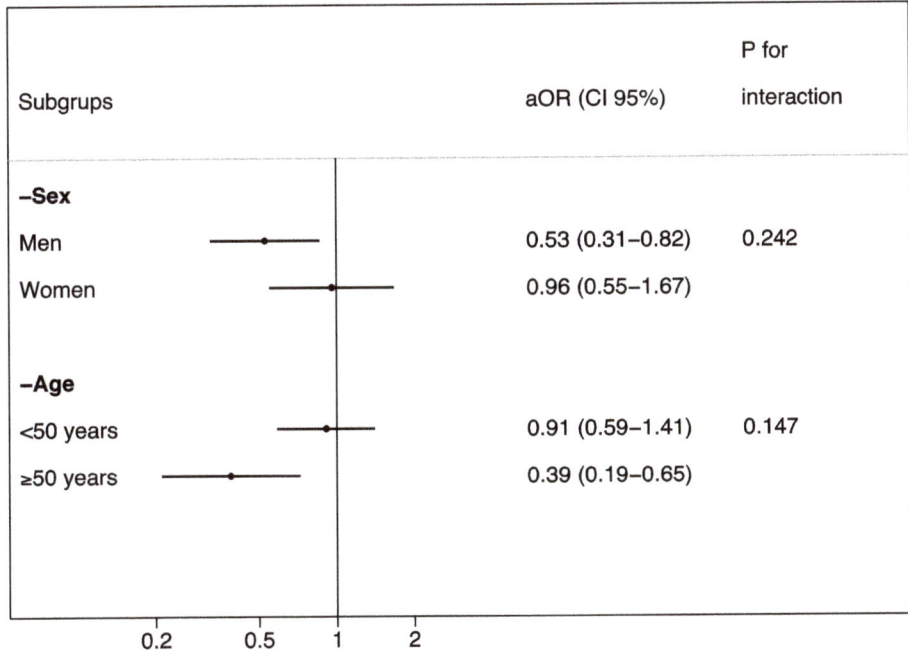

Figure 3. Risk of metabolic syndrome in the highest category compared to the lowest category of the Healthy Lifestyle Score. Stratified analyses (the SUN cohort); aOR: Adjusted odds ratio; CI: Confidence interval.

4. Discussion

This prospective study of initially healthy young–middle-aged Mediterranean university graduates showed that a high adherence to a Healthy Lifestyle Score (7 to 9 points) was associated with a lower risk of incident MetSyn after 6 years of follow-up compared to participants with the lowest number of healthy lifestyle factors (0 to 3). Regarding the components of MetSyn, the highest inverse association of this HLS was observed for a high waist circumference and blood pressure. Although we observed a strong and consistent association, only two healthy lifestyle factors, reduced time watching TV and napping less than 30 min, were significantly associated with a risk reduction of MetSyn. This finding suggests that the synergistic effect of the combination of several lifestyle factors is probably more important than the individual effect of each one of them when considered individually.

The HLS has already been shown to present a strong inverse association with cardiovascular disease in this same cohort [19]. Our study is of interest given that MetSyn is not only a risk factor for cardiovascular diseases, but also for type 2 diabetes, atherosclerosis, and all-cause mortality [17,18], among others.

Our findings were consistent with several previous studies supporting the beneficial impact of combinations of healthy lifestyle behaviors on the primary prevention of MetSyn. These studies demonstrated that the risk of MetSyn decreased as the number of lifestyle factors increased, suggesting that a constellation of factors rather than a single factor is more associated with decreased risks of MetSyn [17,18,33,34].

Our findings were also consistent with previous studies demonstrating an association between lifestyle scores and health-related outcomes, such as mortality [35] and cardiovascular diseases [19]. A recent prospective cohort study conducted in the United States showed that five healthy lifestyle-related factors—physical activity (>30 min/day of moderate or vigorous activities), a healthy diet, moderate alcohol consumption, never smoking, and a normal BMI (18.5 to 24.9 kg/m^2)—are associated with lower risk of all-cause mortality (hazard ratio (HR) 0.26 (95% CI, 0.22–0.31)), cancer mortality (HR 0.35 (95% CI, 0.27–0.45)), and CVD mortality (HR 0.18 (95% CI, 0.12–0.26)) compared to participants with zero low-risk factors [36]. Similar findings of reduced mortality were demonstrated in another prospective cohort study of Spanish older adults, investigating the combined impact between three traditional (diet, physical activity, and smoking) and three nontraditional health behaviors (social interaction, sedentary time, and sleep duration) on mortality [37].

Our HLS combined indicators of lifestyle habits (never smoking, physical activity, Mediterranean diet, and moderate alcohol consumption) with other factors not typically included in risk scores (television exposure <2 h/day, no binge drinking, taking a short afternoon nap (<30 min), meeting up with friends for more than 1 h/day, and working at least 40 h/week).

According to the literature, and consistent with our results, smoking is associated with a higher risk of developing MetSyn [15,38,39]. Physical activity is also associated with a reduction in the risk of MetSyn [14,40–42]: However, we did not find a significant association between physical activity and MetSyn, only a trend.

Many studies have shown, in agreement with our results, the association between the Mediterranean dietary pattern and the risk of MetSyn [43–46]. However, this finding did not reach statistical significance. A potential explanation for these results may rely on the fact that our population was composed of healthy young–middle-aged Mediterranean university graduates, as shown in Table 2. In addition, the Mediterranean diet score proposed by Trichopoulou et al. [25,47] included alcohol intake: Nevertheless, in our study this was considered a separate lifestyle element because the literature suggests that excessive consumption is related to an increased risk of MetSyn [48,49]. Inconsistent with the literature, our results showed that avoidance of "binge drinking" was not associated with a lower risk of MetSyn. However, this could be explained by the fact that we defined avoidance of binge drinking as never having had more than five alcoholic drinks in a single occasion. Therefore, since the prevalence of binge drinking in Spain has been found to be moderately high [50,51], people with healthy lifestyle habits were included in the unhealthy allocation, potentially leading to a non-differential misclassification bias.

Consistent with our results, some studies have reported the relation between TV viewing and MetSyn [52], as TV viewing may displace physical activity. A meta-analysis [53] demonstrated a J-curve relation between nap time and the risk of MetSyn. This study proved that longer than 40 min/day napping was associated with an increased risk of MetSyn.

Social relationships have been suggested as a protective factor, as they are positively related to minutes of physical activity per week and days of physical activity per week. However, they have been positively associated with number of servings of wine per week and increased high-density lipoprotein cholesterol [54], which may explain why our results showed no protection related to social relationships (variable: Spending time with friends) and MetSyn.

Finally, even if O'Reilly and Rosato found that professionals or managers who worked more than 40 h/week had a lower risk of death [55], which may be explained by maintaining a healthy lifestyle [56], other articles have not found a significant association [57]. In our study, working ≥40 h/week was associated with a higher risk of metabolic syndrome (OR 1.26; 95% CI 1.02–1.57): However, the results should be examined carefully, since our population consisted of university graduates whose work may be related to sedentary, seated jobs.

As expected, and consistent with the literature, adherence to various lifestyle habits showed a greater synergistic effect than a single habit in particular. Therefore, if individuals are concerned about their health, the total number of healthy habits should be increased [58].

It is important when interpreting our results to emphasize that the variables that made up this HLS were categorized in a dichotomous way. Most studies divide these variables into more categories to find greater differences between the extremes. This may be the reason why the differences found between healthy lifestyle factors analyzed individually (regarding the risk of MetSyn (Figure 2)) were more modest than in other investigations [38,44].

Therefore, healthy lifestyle scores can potentially be used as health promotion tools, which help people make health-conscious decisions regarding their behaviors. Future research should be conducted in different scenarios to better analyze the potential effects of HLSes on healthy behaviors and health outcomes.

The present study had several limitations. We observed an incidence of 4.24% of MetSyn. This incidence was lower than that described in the general population [8], but expected in a cohort of young adults with low baseline body mass index, a high educational level and, especially, after selecting only participants without any criteria for MetSyn at the baseline. As is the case in most cohort studies, the sample was not representative of the total population, and generalizing the results should be interpreted carefully. Another potential limitation was the self-reported data collection. Nevertheless, previously published validation studies were carried out in the SUN study, which evaluated the validity of our methods and the quality of the self-reported data by our highly trained volunteers. In any case, this would be expected to be nondifferential and would make the bias more likely to tend to null. Moreover, our analyses assumed that baseline habits remained stable throughout the 6-year follow-up, yet there might have been some changes, which would probably have led to underestimating the protective effects of the HLS. On top of this, as participants were young–middle-aged graduates and had few risk factors, there were few incidence cases. This could be associated with a lower statistical power. However, despite missing values of lifestyle behaviors being imputed, the magnitude of the results hardly changed.

The strengths of the present study included its dynamic participation, prospective design, long follow-up period, and high retention rate. As it is an open cohort, the number of participants is large and constantly increasing, which leads to more powerful results. Finally, validation studies were available for some variables, the outcomes were confirmed using medical records, and the findings were adjusted for a large number of covariables, therefore reducing the existence of potential confounding bias, although we cannot rule out the existence of residual confounding.

5. Conclusions

In summary, in this prospective cohort study of healthy young–middle-aged Mediterranean university graduates, a significant association was found between higher Healthy Lifestyle Scores and a reduction in the risk of incident metabolic syndrome. These results suggest the importance of promoting a comprehensive HLS to maintain metabolic health and allow for rapid evaluation in clinical practice. Further longitudinal and intervention studies in the general population should be conducted to confirm this relationship and to enable extrapolation.

Author Contributions: Each participated sufficiently in the conception and design of the work, in the analysis of the data, writing, and editing of the manuscript. M.G.-D.-V. contributed to data research, extracted data, performed data analysis, and drafted the manuscript. S.C.-C., S.N.K., and J.D.-G. reviewed the data analysis and contributed to the discussion and revision of the manuscript and intellectual revision of the manuscript. A.G., L.R.-E., M.B.-R., M.A.M.-G., and M.R.-C. reviewed the data analysis and contributed to the discussion and revision of the manuscript. A.F.-M. contributed to the design, the generation of the database, the data analysis, and the intellectual revision of the manuscript. This article's contents have not been previously presented elsewhere.

Funding: European Research Council (Advanced Research Grant 2013–2018; 340918) granted to MAM-G. The SUN Project has received funding from the Spanish Government-Instituto de Salud Carlos III and the European Regional Development Fund (FEDER) (RD 06/0045, CIBER-OBN, Grants PI10/02658, PI10/02293, PI13/00615, PI14/01668, PI14/01798, PI14/01764 PI17/01795, and G03/140), the Navarra Regional Government (45/2011, 122/2014), and the University of Navarra. The funding sources had no involvement in the study design; in data collection, analysis, or interpretation of data; in the writing of the report; or in the decision to submit the paper for publication.

Acknowledgments: We thank the collaboration of other members of the SUN Group: Alvarez-Alvarez, I.; Alonso, A.; Balaguer, A.; Barrio López, M.T.; Basterra-Gortari, F.J.; Benito Corchón, S.; Beunza, J.J.; Carmona, L.; Cervantes, S.; de Irala Estévez, J.; de la Fuente-Arrillaga, C.; de la Rosa, P.A.; Delgado Rodríguez, M.; Donat Vargas, C.L.; Galbete Ciáurriz, C.; García López, M.; Gómez-Donoso, C.; Goñi Ochandorena, E.; Guillén Grima, F.; Hernández, A.; Lahortiga, F.; Llorca, J.; López del Burgo, C.; Marí Sanchís, A.; Martí del Moral, A.; Martín-Calvo, N.; Martínez, J.A.; Núñez-Córdoba, J.M.; Pérez de Ciriza, P.; Pimenta, A.M.; Razquin C, Rico-Campà, A., Romanos, A.; Ruiz Zambrana, A.; Sánchez Adán, D.; Sánchez-Villegas, A.; Sayón-Orea, C.; Toledo, E.; Vázquez Ruiz, Z.; and Zazpe, I. All of them contributed to the building of this cohort and to the validation of the questionnaires used in this study.

Conflicts of Interest: The authors declare no conflicts of interest.

References

1. Alberti, K.G.M.M.; Eckel, R.H.; Grundy, S.M.; Zimmet, P.Z.; Cleeman, J.I.; Donato, K.A.; Fruchart, J.-C.; James, W.P.T.; Loria, C.M.; Smith, S.C. Harmonizing the Metabolic Syndrome. *Circulation* **2009**, *120*, 1640–1645. [CrossRef] [PubMed]
2. Lakka, H. The Metabolic Syndrome and Total and Cardiovascular Disease Mortality in Middle-aged Men. *JAMA* **2002**, *288*, 2709. [CrossRef] [PubMed]
3. Gami, A.S.; Witt, B.J.; Howard, D.E.; Erwin, P.J.; Gami, L.A.; Somers, V.K.; Montori, V.M. Metabolic Syndrome and Risk of Incident Cardiovascular Events and Death. *J. Am. Coll. Cardiol.* **2007**, *49*, 403–414. [CrossRef] [PubMed]
4. Ervin, R.B. Prevalence of metabolic syndrome among adults 20 years of age and over, by sex, age, race and ethnicity, and body mass index: United States, 2003–2006. *Natl. Health Stat. Rep.* **2009**, 1–7.
5. Ford, E.S.; Giles, W.H.; Dietz, W.H. Prevalence of the Metabolic Syndrome Among US Adults. *JAMA* **2002**, *287*, 356. [CrossRef] [PubMed]
6. Lim, S.; Shin, H.; Song, J.H.; Kwak, S.H.; Kang, S.M.; Won Yoon, J.; Choi, S.H.; Cho, S.I.; Park, K.S.; Lee, H.K.; et al. Increasing Prevalence of Metabolic Syndrome in Korea: The Korean National Health and Nutrition Examination Survey for 1998–2007. *Diabetes Care* **2011**, *34*, 1323–1328. [CrossRef] [PubMed]
7. Delavari, A.; Forouzanfar, M.H.; Alikhani, S.; Sharifian, A.; Kelishadi, R. First Nationwide Study of the Prevalence of the Metabolic Syndrome and Optimal Cutoff Points of Waist Circumference in the Middle East: The National Survey of Risk Factors for Noncommunicable Diseases of Iran. *Diabetes Care* **2009**, *32*, 1092–1097. [CrossRef] [PubMed]
8. Laclaustra, M.; Ordoñez, B.; Leon, M.; Andres, E.M.; Cordero, A.; Pascual-Calleja, I.; Grima, A.; Luengo, E.; Alegria, E.; Pocovi, M.; et al. Metabolic syndrome and coronary heart disease among Spanish male workers: A case-control study of MESYAS. *Nutr. Metab. Cardiovasc. Dis.* **2012**, *22*, 510–516. [CrossRef]
9. Fernández-Bergés, D.; Cabrera de León, A.; Sanz, H.; Elosua, R.; Guembe, M.J.; Alzamora, M.; Vega-Alonso, T.; Félix-Redondo, F.J.; Ortiz-Marrón, H.; Rigo, F.; et al. Metabolic Syndrome in Spain: Prevalence and Coronary Risk Associated With Harmonized Definition and WHO Proposal. DARIOS Study. *Rev. Esp. Cardiol.* **2012**, *65*, 241–248. [CrossRef]
10. Yamaoka, K.; Tango, T. Effects of lifestyle modification on metabolic syndrome: A systematic review and meta-analysis. *BMC Med.* **2012**, *10*, 138. [CrossRef]
11. Fernández-Montero, A.; Bes-Rastrollo, M.; Beunza, J.J.; Barrio-Lopez, M.T.; De La Fuente-Arrillaga, C.; Moreno-Galarraga, L.; Martínez-González, M.A. Nut consumption and incidence of metabolic syndrome after 6-year follow-up: The SUN (Seguimiento Universidad de Navarra, University of Navarra Follow-up) cohort. *Public Health Nutr.* **2013**, *16*, 2064–2072. [CrossRef] [PubMed]
12. Barrio-Lopez, M.T.; Martinez-Gonzalez, M.A.; Fernandez-Montero, A.; Beunza, J.J.; Zazpe, I.; Bes-Rastrollo, M. Prospective study of changes in sugar-sweetened beverage consumption and the incidence of the metabolic syndrome and its components: The SUN cohort. *Br. J. Nutr.* **2013**, *110*, 1722–1731. [CrossRef] [PubMed]
13. Esposito, K.; Kastorini, C.-M.; Panagiotakos, D.B.; Giugliano, D. Mediterranean diet and metabolic syndrome: An updated systematic review. *Rev. Endocr. Metab. Disord.* **2013**, *14*, 255–263. [CrossRef] [PubMed]
14. Hidalgo-Santamaria, M.; Fernandez-Montero, A.; Martinez-Gonzalez, M.A.; Moreno-Galarraga, L.; Sanchez-Villegas, A.; Barrio-Lopez, M.T.; Bes-Rastrollo, M. Exercise Intensity and Incidence of Metabolic Syndrome: The SUN Project. *Am. J. Prev. Med.* **2017**, *52*, e95–e101. [CrossRef] [PubMed]
15. Sun, K.; Liu, J.; Ning, G. Active Smoking and Risk of Metabolic Syndrome: A Meta-Analysis of Prospective Studies. *PLoS ONE* **2012**, *7*, e47791. [CrossRef] [PubMed]
16. Wennberg, P.; Gustafsson, P.E.; Howard, B.; Wennberg, M.; Hammarström, A. Television viewing over the life course and the metabolic syndrome in mid-adulthood: A longitudinal population-based study. *J. Epidemiol. Community Health* **2014**, *68*, 928–933. [CrossRef] [PubMed]
17. Chang, S.-H.; Chen, M.-C.; Chien, N.-H.; Wu, L.-Y. CE: Original Research: Examining the Links between Lifestyle Factors and Metabolic Syndrome. *Am. J. Nurs.* **2016**, *116*, 26–36. [CrossRef] [PubMed]

18. Sotos-Prieto, M.; Bhupathiraju, S.N.; Falcón, L.M.; Gao, X.; Tucker, K.L.; Mattei, J. A Healthy Lifestyle Score Is Associated with Cardiometabolic and Neuroendocrine Risk Factors among Puerto Rican Adults. *J. Nutr.* **2015**, *145*, 1531–1540. [CrossRef]
19. Díaz-Gutiérrez, J.; Ruiz-Canela, M.; Gea, A.; Fernández-Montero, A.; Martínez-González, M.Á. Association between a Healthy Lifestyle Score and the Risk of Cardiovascular Disease in the SUN Cohort. *Rev. Esp. Cardiol.* **2018**, *71*, 1001–1009. [CrossRef]
20. Carlos, S.; De La Fuente-Arrillaga, C.; Bes-Rastrollo, M.; Razquin, C.; Rico-Campà, A.; Martínez-González, M.A.; Ruiz-Canela, M. Mediterranean Diet and Health Outcomes in the SUN Cohort. *Nutrients* **2018**, *10*, 439. [CrossRef]
21. Willett, W. *Nutritional Epidemiology (pp. 74–100)*, 3rd ed.; Oxford University Press: New York, NY, USA, 2013.
22. Bes-Rastrollo, M.; Pérez-Valdivieso, J.R.; Sánchez-Villegas, A.; Alonso, A.; Martínez-González, M.Á. Validación del peso e índice de masa corporal auto-declarados de los participantes de una cohorte de graduados universitarios. *Rev. Esp. Obes.* **2005**, *3*, 352–358.
23. Martínez-González, M.A.; López-Fontana, C.; Varo, J.J.; Sánchez-Villegas, A.; Martinez, J.A. Validation of the Spanish version of the physical activity questionnaire used in the Nurses' Health Study and the Health Professionals' Follow-up Study. *Public Health Nutr.* **2005**, *8*, 920–927. [CrossRef] [PubMed]
24. De la Fuente-Arrillaga, C.; Vázquez Ruiz, Z.; Bes-Rastrollo, M.; Sampson, L.; Martinez-González, M.A. Reproducibility of an FFQ validated in Spain. *Public Health Nutr.* **2010**, *13*, 1364–1372. [CrossRef] [PubMed]
25. Trichopoulou, A.; Costacou, T.; Bamia, C.; Trichopoulos, D. Adherence to a Mediterranean Diet and Survival in a Greek Population. *N. Engl. J. Med.* **2003**, *348*, 2599–2608. [CrossRef] [PubMed]
26. Klein, S.; Allison, D.B.; Heymsfield, S.B.; Kelley, D.E.; Leibel, R.L.; Nonas, C.; Kahn, R. Waist Circumference and Cardiometabolic Risk: A Consensus Statement from Shaping America's Health: Association for Weight Management and Obesity Prevention; NAASO, The Obesity Society; the American Society for Nutrition; and the American Diabetes Associat. *Diabetes Care* **2007**, *30*, 1647–1652. [CrossRef] [PubMed]
27. Fernández-Montero, A.; Beunza, J.J.; Bes-Rastrollo, M.; Barrio, M.T.; de la Fuente-Arrillaga, C.; Moreno-Galarraga, L.; Martínez-González, M.A. Validity of self-reported metabolic syndrome components in a cohort study. *Gac. Sanit.* **2011**, *25*, 303–307. [CrossRef] [PubMed]
28. Barrio-Lopez, M.T.; Bes-Rastrollo, M.; Beunza, J.J.; Fernandez-Montero, A.; Garcia-Lopez, M.; Martinez-Gonzalez, M.A. Validation of metabolic syndrome using medical records in the SUN cohort. *BMC Public Health* **2011**, *11*, 867. [CrossRef]
29. Williamson, E.J.; Aitken, Z.; Lawrie, J.; Dharmage, S.C.; Burgess, J.A.; Forbes, A.B. Introduction to causal diagrams for confounder selection. *Respirology* **2014**, *19*, 303–311. [CrossRef]
30. Flanders, W.D.; Eldridge, R.C. Summary of relationships between exchangeability, biasing paths and bias. *Eur. J. Epidemiol.* **2015**, *30*, 1089–1099. [CrossRef]
31. Hernan, M.A. Causal Knowledge as a Prerequisite for Confounding Evaluation: An Application to Birth Defects Epidemiology. *Am. J. Epidemiol.* **2002**, *155*, 176–184. [CrossRef]
32. Groenwold, R.H.H.; Donders, A.R.T.; Roes, K.C.B.; Harrell, F.E.; Moons, K.G.M. Dealing with Missing Outcome Data in Randomized Trials and Observational Studies. *Am. J. Epidemiol.* **2012**, *175*, 210–217. [CrossRef] [PubMed]
33. Lee, J.A.; Cha, Y.H.; Kim, S.H.; Park, H.S. Impact of combined lifestyle factors on metabolic syndrome in Korean men. *J. Public Health* **2016**, *39*, 82–89. [CrossRef] [PubMed]
34. Mitchell, B.L.; Smith, A.E.; Rowlands, A.V.; Parfitt, G.; Dollman, J. Associations of physical activity and sedentary behaviour with metabolic syndrome in rural Australian adults. *J. Sci. Med. Sport* **2018**, *21*, 1232–1237. [CrossRef] [PubMed]
35. Khaw, K.-T.; Wareham, N.; Bingham, S.; Welch, A.; Luben, R.; Day, N. Combined Impact of Health Behaviours and Mortality in Men and Women: The EPIC-Norfolk Prospective Population Study. *PLoS Med.* **2008**, *5*, e12. [CrossRef]
36. Li, Y.; Pan, A.; Wang, D.D.; Liu, X.; Dhana, K.; Franco, O.H.; Kaptoge, S.; Di Angelantonio, E.; Stampfer, M.; Willett, W.C.; et al. Impact of Healthy Lifestyle Factors on Life Expectancies in the US Population. *Circulation* **2018**, *138*, 345–355. [CrossRef] [PubMed]

37. Martínez-Gómez, D.; Guallar-Castillón, P.; León-Muñoz, L.M.; López-García, E.; Rodríguez-Artalejo, F. Combined impact of traditional and non-traditional health behaviors on mortality: A national prospective cohort study in Spanish older adults. *BMC Med.* **2013**, *11*, 47. [CrossRef] [PubMed]
38. Kim, B.J.; Kim, B.S.; Sung, K.C.; Kang, J.H.; Lee, M.H.; Park, J.R. Association of Smoking Status, Weight Change, and Incident Metabolic Syndrome in Men: A 3-Year Follow-Up Study. *Diabetes Care* **2009**, *32*, 1314–1316. [CrossRef]
39. Nakanishi, N.; Takatorige, T.; Suzuki, K. Cigarette smoking and the risk of the metabolic syndrome in middle-aged Japanese male office workers. *Ind. Health* **2005**, *43*, 295–301. [CrossRef]
40. Pattyn, N.; Cornelissen, V.A.; Eshghi, S.R.T.; Vanhees, L. The Effect of Exercise on the Cardiovascular Risk Factors Constituting the Metabolic Syndrome. *Sports Med.* **2013**, *43*, 121–133. [CrossRef]
41. Strasser, B. Physical activity in obesity and metabolic syndrome. *Ann. N. Y. Acad. Sci.* **2013**, *1281*, 141–159. [CrossRef]
42. Zhang, D.; Liu, X.; Liu, Y.; Sun, X.; Wang, B.; Ren, Y.; Zhao, Y.; Zhou, J.; Han, C.; Yin, L.; et al. Leisure-time physical activity and incident metabolic syndrome: A systematic review and dose-response meta-analysis of cohort studies. *Metabolism* **2017**, *75*, 36–44. [CrossRef] [PubMed]
43. Ahluwalia, N.; Andreeva, V.A.; Kesse-Guyot, E.; Hercberg, S. Dietary patterns, inflammation and the metabolic syndrome. *Diabetes Metab.* **2013**, *39*, 99–110. [CrossRef] [PubMed]
44. Kastorini, C.M.; Milionis, H.J.; Esposito, K.; Giugliano, D.; Goudevenos, J.A.; Panagiotakos, D.B. The effect of mediterranean diet on metabolic syndrome and its components: A meta-analysis of 50 studies and 534,906 individuals. *J. Am. Coll. Cardiol.* **2011**, *57*, 1299–1313. [CrossRef] [PubMed]
45. Kesse-Guyot, E.; Ahluwalia, N.; Lassale, C.; Hercberg, S.; Fezeu, L.; Lairon, D. Adherence to Mediterranean diet reduces the risk of metabolic syndrome: A 6-year prospective study. *Nutr. Metab. Cardiovasc. Dis.* **2013**, *23*, 677–683. [CrossRef] [PubMed]
46. Grosso, G.; Mistretta, A.; Marventano, S.; Purrello, A.; Vitaglione, P.; Calabrese, G.; Drago, F.; Galvano, F. Beneficial Effects of the Mediterranean Diet on Metabolic Syndrome. *Curr. Pharm. Des.* **2014**, *20*, 5039–5044. [CrossRef] [PubMed]
47. Martínez-González, M.A.; Hershey, M.S.; Zazpe, I.; Trichopoulou, A. Transferability of the Mediterranean Diet to Non-Mediterranean Countries. What Is and What Is Not the Mediterranean Diet. *Nutrients* **2018**, *9*, 1226. [CrossRef]
48. Sun, K.; Ren, M.; Liu, D.; Wang, C.; Yang, C.; Yan, L. Alcohol consumption and risk of metabolic syndrome: A meta-analysis of prospective studies. *Clin. Nutr.* **2014**, *33*, 596–602. [CrossRef]
49. Im, H.-J.; Park, S.-M.; Choi, J.-H.; Choi, E.-J. Binge Drinking and Its Relation to Metabolic Syndrome in Korean Adult Men. *Korean J. Fam. Med.* **2014**, *35*, 173. [CrossRef]
50. Valencia-Martín, J.L.; Galán, I.; Rodríguez-Artalejo, F. Binge Drinking in Madrid, Spain. *Alcohol. Clin. Exp. Res.* **2007**, *31*, 1723–1730. [CrossRef]
51. Soler-Vila, H.; Galán, I.; Valencia-Martín, J.L.; León-Muñoz, L.M.; Guallar-Castillón, P.; Rodríguez-Artalejo, F. Binge Drinking in Spain, 2008–2010. *Alcohol. Clin. Exp. Res.* **2014**, *38*, 810–819. [CrossRef]
52. Tremblay, M.S.; LeBlanc, A.G.; Kho, M.E.; Saunders, T.J.; Larouche, R.; Colley, R.C.; Goldfield, G.; Gorber, S.C. Systematic review of sedentary behaviour and health indicators in school-aged children and youth. *Int. J. Behav. Nutr. Phys. Act.* **2011**, *8*, 98. [CrossRef] [PubMed]
53. Yamada, T.; Shojima, N.; Yamauchi, T.; Kadowaki, T. J-curve relation between daytime nap duration and type 2 diabetes or metabolic syndrome: A dose-response meta-analysis. *Sci. Rep.* **2016**, *6*, 38075. [CrossRef] [PubMed]
54. Fischer Aggarwal, B.A.; Liao, M.; Mosca, L. Physical Activity as a Potential Mechanism through Which Social Support May Reduce Cardiovascular Disease Risk. *J. Cardiovasc. Nurs.* **2008**, *23*, 90–96. [CrossRef] [PubMed]
55. O'Reilly, D.; Rosato, M. Worked to death? A census-based longitudinal study of the relationship between the numbers of hours spent working and mortality risk. *Int. J. Epidemiol.* **2013**, *42*, 1820–1830. [CrossRef] [PubMed]
56. Kivimaki, M.; Nyberg, S.T.; Fransson, E.I.; Heikkila, K.; Alfredsson, L.; Casini, A.; Clays, E.; De Bacquer, D.; Dragano, N.; Ferrie, J.E.; et al. Associations of job strain and lifestyle risk factors with risk of coronary artery disease: A meta-analysis of individual participant data. *Can. Med. Assoc. J.* **2013**, *185*, 763–769. [CrossRef] [PubMed]

57. Pimenta, A.M.; Bes-Rastrollo, M.; Sayon-Orea, C.; Gea, A.; Aguinaga-Ontoso, E.; Lopez-Iracheta, R.; Martinez-Gonzalez, M.A. Working hours and incidence of metabolic syndrome and its components in a Mediterranean cohort: The SUN project. *Eur. J. Public Health* **2015**, *25*, 683–688. [CrossRef]
58. Spring, B.; Moller, A.C.; Coons, M.J. Multiple health behaviours: Overview and implications. *J. Public Health* **2012**, *34*, i3–i10. [CrossRef]

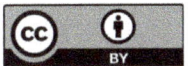

© 2018 by the authors. Licensee MDPI, Basel, Switzerland. This article is an open access article distributed under the terms and conditions of the Creative Commons Attribution (CC BY) license (http://creativecommons.org/licenses/by/4.0/).

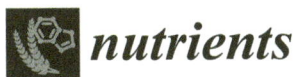

Communication

Population Approaches Targeting Metabolic Syndrome Focusing on Japanese Trials

Hitoshi Nishizawa * and Iichiro Shimomura

Department of Metabolic Medicine, Graduate School of Medicine, Osaka University, 2-2-B5, Yamada-oka, Suita, Osaka 565-0871, Japan; ichi@endmet.med.osaka-u.ac.jp
* Correspondence: hitoshin1127@endmet.med.osaka-u.ac.jp; Tel.: +81-6-6879-3732; Fax: +81-6-6879-3739

Received: 17 April 2019; Accepted: 23 June 2019; Published: 25 June 2019

Abstract: The clinical importance of assessment of metabolic syndrome lies in the selection of individuals with multiple risk factors based on visceral fat accumulation, and helping them to reduce visceral fat. Behavioral modification by population approach is important, which adds support to the personal approach. The complexity of visceral fat accumulation requires multicomponent and multilevel intervention. Preparation of food and physical environments could be useful strategies for city planners. Furthermore, actions on various frameworks, including organizational, community, and policy levels, have been recently reported. There are universal public health screening programs and post-screening health educational systems in Japan, and diseases management programs in Germany. Understanding one's own health status is important for motivation for lifestyle modification. The U.S. Preventive Services Task Force recommends that primary care practitioners screen all adults for obesity and offer behavioral interventions and intensive counseling. Established evidence-based guidelines for behavioral counseling are needed within the primary care setting.

Keywords: atherosclerotic cardiovascular disease; visceral fat accumulation; universal public health screening program; health check-up; health guidance; city planning

---

1. Introduction

Visceral fat accumulation is associated with glucose intolerance, dyslipidemia, hypertension, and atherosclerotic cardiovascular diseases (ACVD), conceptualized as metabolic syndrome (Figure 1). Several definitions of metabolic syndrome have been used worldwide. Abdominal obesity is one of the risk factors in the harmonized criteria by AHA (American Heart Association), IDF (International Diabetes Federation), NHLBI (National Heart, Lung, and Blood Institute), and other organizations (2009) [1], while in the original criteria of IDF (2005) [2] and the Japanese criteria [3,4], abdominal obesity or visceral fat accumulation is an essential component of metabolic syndrome. The latter criteria consider visceral fat accumulation as the basal pathogenic component of metabolic syndrome. An important aspect of the diagnosis of visceral fat-based metabolic syndrome is to select subjects with multiple risk factors based on visceral fat accumulation, and enroll them in health educational programs conducted at health check-up and medical facilities. The cornerstone of effective improvement of multiple risk factors for ACVD is the reduction of visceral fat (Figure 2).

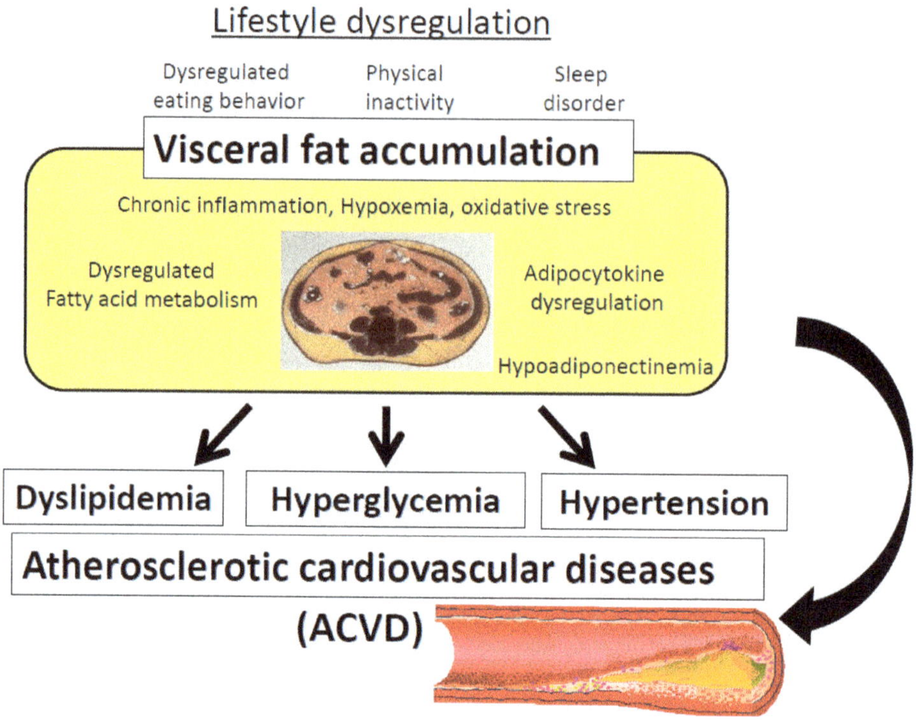

Figure 1. Concept of metabolic syndrome.

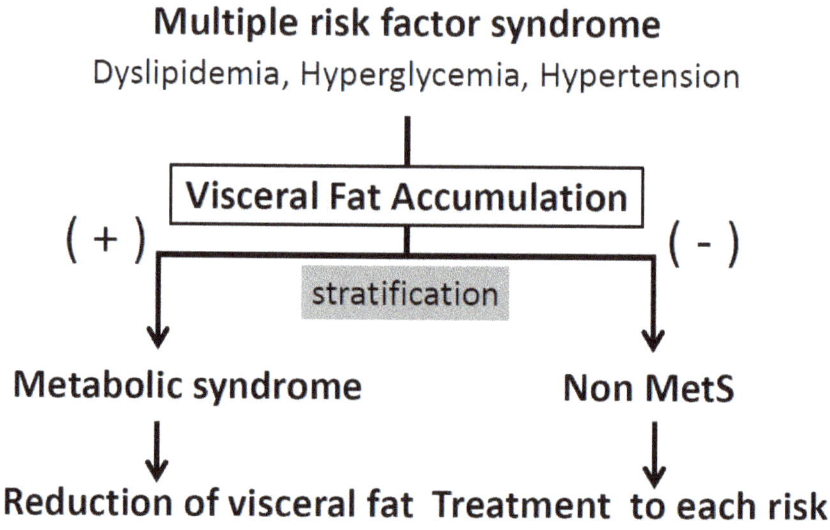

Figure 2. Management of multiple risk factor syndrome for prevention of atherosclerotic cardiovascular diseases (ACVD); "Metabolic syndrome (Mets)-oriented approach".

The cause of worldwide obesity and visceral fat accumulation is multifactorial at multiple levels, including food environment, physical activity levels, and policies. One of the important approaches to reduce visceral fat involves behavioral modification of individuals (personal approach), such as modifications to dietary and physical habits. Another is the population approach, which provides support to the personal approach, and could be even more important.

2. Obesity and Obesity Disease

Obesity is a state of excess body fat accumulation in individuals, and body mass index (BMI) is used as an index of obesity. Obesity is defined as BMI ≥ 30 kg/m^2 in Europe and the United States, and ≥ 25 kg/m^2 in Japan, where there are fewer obese individuals [5–7]. Obesity, per se, is not always clinically necessary to be subjected to aggressive medical intervention. On the other hand, "obesity disease" is defined in Japan as visceral fat obesity (BMI ≥ 25 kg/m^2 plus visceral fat area ≥ 100 cm^2), or obesity (BMI ≥ 25 kg/m^2) with obesity-related complications, such as metabolic or orthopedic disorders that require weight reduction for their improvement [7]. Therefore, "Obesity disease" should be dealt with as a clinical condition requiring medical intervention.

3. Visceral Fat and Subcutaneous Fat

It is well known that obesity is accompanied by glucose intolerance, dyslipidemia, and hypertension. Following the spread of the Western diet and motor vehicles, the prevalence of obesity and type 2 diabetes has increased worldwide [5,6]. East Asians, including Japanese, are more easily affected by metabolic disorders even with a mild degree of obesity, compared with Europeans and Americans. On the other hand, such disorders are not always accompanied by massive obesity. These disorders cannot be explained by the absolute value of BMI, and therefore understanding of body fat distribution is considerably important [8]. Analysis of body fat distribution using abdominal computed tomography (CT) has demonstrated that visceral fat obesity poses a higher risk for metabolic disorders and ACVD than subcutaneous obesity [9]. A recent Japanese study involving subjects who underwent health checks concluded that visceral fat area (VFA), but not subcutaneous fat area (SFA), correlated positively with the number of cardiovascular risk factors [10]. The same study also demonstrated that the mean number of risk factors exceeded one at 100 cm^2 of VFA, both in males and females. Therefore, the cutoff value of visceral fat accumulation was set to 100 cm^2 in Japan [10].

4. BMI and Visceral Fat Area

The BMI and VFA vary considerably among individuals, especially in males. In a study of Japanese male employees (mean age 48.0 ± 10.5 years, ±SD), 26.8% (n = 401/1497) of normal weight subjects (BMI < 25 kg/m^2) had visceral fat accumulation (VFA ≥10 0cm^2) (Figure 3) [11]. Irrespective of BMI, the mean number of metabolic risk factors in the subjects with visceral fat accumulation was significantly higher than those without (solid bars in Figure 3). Also, a study from the United Kingdom reported a relatively high mortality rate for individuals with central obesity, despite having normal weight (BMI <25 kg/m^2) [12]. Interestingly, reduction of body weight and VFA is closely associated with improvement of metabolic risk factors, such as diabetes, dyslipidemia, and hypertension [11,13]. These data suggest that assessment of visceral fat accumulation is important for selection of individuals who should avoid over-nutrition.

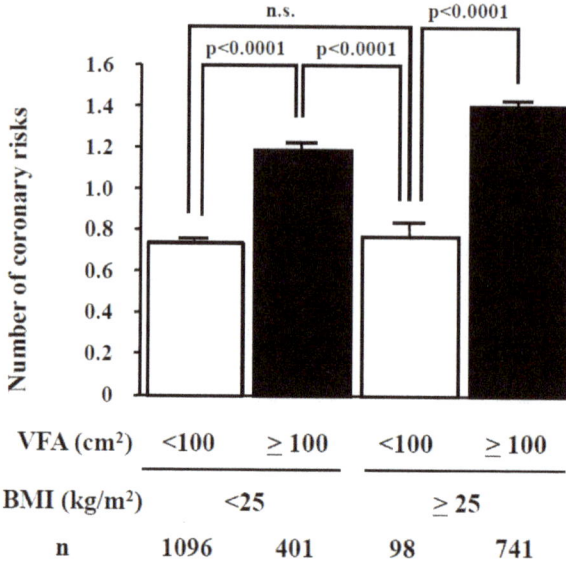

Figure 3. Relationship between number of metabolic risk factors and body fat distribution. Subjects were divided according to their BMI (cutoff value 25 kg/m^2) and VFA (cutoff value 100 cm^2). Data are mean ± SEM. BMI = body mass index; VFA = visceral fat area;. Data from Diabetes Care 2007; 30: 2392-94 [11], by permission of American Diabetes Association.

5. Clinical Significance of Metabolic Syndrome in Atherosclerotic Cardiovascular Diseases

It is important to take measures against individual risk factors, such as hypertension, smoking, and hypercholesterolemia, to prevent atherosclerotic cardiovascular diseases (ACVD). Since the 1990s, multiple risk factor syndrome and metabolic syndrome have been the focus of attention as residual risks, in which dysregulation of glucose and lipid metabolism, hypertension, and obesity coexisted in each individual [1,14,15]. Among them, the concept of metabolic syndrome was selected in the original criteria of IDF (2005) along with in Japan, stating that visceral fat accumulation is the basis of the pathogenesis of atherosclerosis complicated with dysregulation of glucose and lipid metabolism and elevated blood pressure (Figure 1). There are two types of arteriosclerosis—atherosclerosis that affects relatively large vessels, such as coronary arteries and middle cerebral arteries, and arteriosclerosis that affects relatively small vessels, such as cerebral perforating arteries. Atherosclerosis is the pathological process underlying myocardial infarction and cerebral thrombosis, whereas arteriosclerosis is that of cerebral hemorrhage and lacunar infarction. In Europe and the United States, atherosclerosis based on dyslipidemia and metabolic syndrome is more frequent due to over-intake of dietary fat. On the other hand, in East Asia, arteriosclerosis based on hypertension has been the predominant type due to over-intake of dietary salt [16]. Recently, even in East Asia and Japan, visceral fat based-metabolic syndrome has been increasing. However, hypertension and hypercholesterolemia should be important therapeutic targets in any clinical management program designed to prevent ACVD independent of the metabolic syndrome.

6. Pathogenesis of Visceral Fat Accumulation

Visceral fat is the adipose tissue that adheres and accumulates in the mesenterium and omentum, and acts as transient energy reservoir from gut to liver through the portal vein. In fasting and starvation, lipolysis efficiently occurs in visceral fat resulting in supply of free fatty acids and glycerol to hepatocytes. However, through excessive lipolysis in the accumulated visceral fat, large amounts of free fatty acids and glycerol overflow into the liver, resulting in the dysregulation of lipid metabolism and gluconeogenesis [17]. Although the weight of adipose tissue accounts for about 15–20% of total body weight, that of obese subjects reaches up to 30–50%. Therefore, the massive adipose tissue considerably affects the pathogenic condition of individuals.

Adipocyte precursor cells in visceral adipose tissue are relatively difficult to differentiate or proliferate compared to those in the subcutaneous adipose tissue [18]. Thus, visceral adipose cells, in parallel to over-nutrition, are considered hypertrophic adipocytes. Since the number of adipocytes can increase only during childhood and adolescence [19], over-nutrition in adulthood induces hypertrophy of visceral adipose cells, which are affected by hypoxia and inflammation, complicating the production of oxidative stress and dysregulation of adipocytokines and adipokines, such as hypoadiponectinemia. This is the pathogenic basis of visceral fat accumulation associated with metabolic syndrome (Figure 1) [20,21].

Fat distribution varies considerably between males and females and also among different ethnic groups. In Asian individuals, VFA is relatively larger than SFA [22,23]. This is probably related to genetic (ethnic) differences in the proliferative potential of subcutaneous adipose precursor cells, as well as differences in the duration of over-nutrition. Therefore, the susceptibility of Asian individuals to the metabolic syndrome could be higher, with visceral fat accumulation even in lower BMI relative to Europeans and Americans.

7. Population Approaches Targeting the Metabolic Syndrome

There is a need to reduce accumulated visceral fat in subjects with metabolic syndrome, rather than treat each metabolic risk factor with medications. To achieve this aim, it is important to provide health education about healthy diet and physical exercise to these individuals (personal approach). Next, improvement of various metabolic risk factors can be achieved through reduction of accumulated visceral fat [11,13]. Therefore, for assessment of the metabolic syndrome, it is clinically important to identify individuals with large amounts of visceral fat during medical or health check-ups, who are affected, or are supposed to be, by multiple metabolic disorders, even if each disorder is mild. Moreover, it is important to enroll the subjects with metabolic syndrome into the health education system. We will focus here on population approaches to combat metabolic syndrome (Figure 4), as individual programs on lifestyles, such as diet and physical exercise, are discussed in other chapters of this review and have also been described previously [24].

1. Strategies addressing lifestyle behavior and policies targeting the environment (diet, physical activity, sleep, and mental health)

a. Health education at school and for parents
b. Calorie labels on menus, taxation for "harmful" food
c. City planning (e.g. walking and cycling lane, sports facilities and training gym, green area, and TV program)

2. Screening and intervention program against the metabolic syndrome

a. Community or organization-based prevention
Multicomponent and multilevel intervention (e.g. city planning)

b. Healthcare program by public system
Health checkup and intervention program using public health insurance system (e.g. Japan)
Disease management program conducted on national level (e.g. German)

c. Behavioral approach including motivational interviewing

Figure 4. Population Approaches targeting the metabolic syndrome.

8. Strategies Addressing Lifestyle Behavior and Policies Targeting the Environment (Diet, Physical Activity, Sleep, and Mental Health)

For lifestyle modification, it is first important to have a clinical understanding of one's own health status. For this aim, health check-ups followed by health guidance is a good approach. Recent studies have provided evidence for the role of pictorial presentation of silent atherosclerosis in the prevention of cardiovascular diseases and its usefulness in reducing the low adherence to medications and lifestyle modification [25]. Therefore, scientific understanding of one's own health is the most important factor for motivation towards lifestyle modification. Once subjects are motivated to improve their lifestyle to reduce accumulated visceral fat, health promotion strategies, which address lifestyle behavior and policies targeting the environment, are potentially effective in the prevention of visceral fat accumulation.

Since dieting and disordered eating behaviors during childhood and adolescence are considered to continue to be present among young adults [26], some strategies were found to be useful, such as health education on nutrition for students and their parents in school and provision of healthy food at school (Figure 4) [27,28]. At the population level, public policies and economic strategies are important to improve food and physical environments. For example, calorie and nutritional information on food menus and packaging are useful for individuals who care about dietary modification and also to avoid harmful food components, such as saturated fatty acids and excess salt. In some countries, higher taxes have been enforced on harmful foods, such as fast foods, unhealthy fats, and sugar-sweetened drinks (Figure 4) [29].

High physical activity is reported to be associated with low risk of mortality and cardiovascular disease [30], and diet-plus-exercise was more effective in weight loss than diet-only interventions [31]. Strategies that encourage individuals to exercise are important. Walking and cycling can serve for both transportation and recreational purposes, and both can reduce motor vehicle dependency. Therefore, it should be important to support lifestyle choices through city planning, such as preparation for walking, running, and cycling lanes (Figure 4) [32]. In general, aerobic exercise several days per week (total: 150 min/week) has been recommended in physical activity guidelines [33]. However, it was recently reported that there was no significant difference in the likelihood of metabolic syndrome in the general population between frequently active participants (≥5 days per week) and infrequently active participants (1–4 days per week) after adjustment for total weekly moderate-to-vigorous physical activity [34], suggesting that only weekend exercise could be effective in preventing metabolic syndrome if sufficient weekly physical activity was performed. Preparation of sports gymnasiums, playing fields, and parks that are easily accessed by citizens are useful strategies that should be instituted in city planning.

Sleep is considerably associated with eating behaviors and physical activity. Insufficient sleep has been reported to be associated with dysregulation of leptin and ghrelin [35], resulting in hyperphagia and physical inactivity due to sleepiness. Moreover, a late bedtime with shorter sleep time were reported to be closely associated with weight gain and visceral fat accumulation [36,37]. To facilitate more sleeping hours, many communities have attempted to change TV programming [32]. Since control of psychological status is important to continue lifestyle modification, green areas in communities are useful for stress management (Figure 4) [28,32].

9. Screening and Intervention Program Against the Metabolic Syndrome

9.1. Community or Organization-Based Prevention

The complexity of visceral fat accumulation requires multicomponent and multilevel intervention [28]. Multicomponent intervention is effective in weight loss programs, which consist of changes that combine food choices, physical environments, sleep, and stress management, as described above (Figure 4). Furthermore, multilevel approaches focus on changing health behaviors by acting on multiple frameworks, including individual, interpersonal, organizational, community, and policy levels. Many intervention programs at the community level have been used to combat metabolic syndrome [28,38,39]. For instance, the healthy living program delivered by community coaching staff for overweight and obese me, who were football fans of the Scottish Premier League football clubs proved effective for weight loss of 4.94 kg (95% CI 3.95–5.94) after 12 months [39].

Step1 : Abdominal obesity and/or overweight
    Waist circumference Male ≥ 85cm. Female ≥ 90 cm → Group (1)
    Waist circumference Male < 85cm. Female < 90 cm, but Body Mass Index ≥ 25 → Group (2)
Step2 : Additional risk factors
    1) Fasting Plasma glucose   FPG ≥ 100 mg/dl and/or HbA1c ≥ 5.6%
    2) TG and HDL-cholesterol   TG ≥ 150 mg/dl and/or HDL-cholesterol < 40mg/dl
    3) Blood pressure   SBP ≥ 130 mmHg and/or DPB ≥85 mmHg
    4) Smoking   (counted only for those who have 1 risk or more from 1-3)
Step3 : Classification for Health guidance Program
    Group (1) Additional risks at Step2
        ≥ 2   Intensive Health Guidance program
        2   Motivational Health Guidance program
    Group (2) Additional risks at Step2
        ≥ 3   Intensive Health Guidance program
        1 or 2 Motivational Health Guidance program
Step4 :
People taking medication for diabetes, hypertension, or high cholesterol are excluded
People aged 65-74 who are eligible for health guidance are allocated to
Motivational Health Guidance program regardless of risk profile

Figure 5. Participant classification for the Health Guidance program by the Ministry of Health, Labor, and Welfare in Japan [40].

9.2. Healthcare Program by the Public System

Atherosclerotic cardiovascular diseases (ACVD) are life-threatening. Development of ACVD is often followed by serious complications. Therefore, it is important to detect asymptomatic cardiovascular risk factors and provide counter measures. For this purpose, a health check-up is a good opportunity to assess one's own health status and assess the risk for cardiovascular diseases. In many countries, individuals are left on their own to decide whether to receive health check-ups or not. However, in the case of Japan, there is a universal public health screening program and a post-screening health educational system in place at the nation level to deal with metabolic syndrome, as described below [4,40]. There is also a disease management program (DMP) nationally in Germany. The Japanese intervention program aims at primary disease prevention, while the German DMP aims at secondary disease prevention (Figure 4) [41].

The Japanese criteria for metabolic syndrome were established in 2005 [3,4], in which visceral fat accumulation was an essential component. In 2008, the Japanese government started a new screening and educational system for metabolic syndrome, focusing on visceral fat accumulation [40]. This new public health care system has the following features: (1) medical insurers are obliged to perform free health check-ups followed by health guidance to their subscribers aged 40 to 74 years; (2) methods of health check-ups and health guidance are standardized and health data are collected and assessed electronically; (3) subjects who need health guidance are stratified based on visceral fat accumulation and smoking habits (Figure 5). Participants who are thought to be "downstream" of metabolic syndrome are subjected to an intensive health guidance program with intermittent support over three months after the first interview followed by assessment six months later [40,42]. Recently, descriptive analysis in Japan has shown greater improvement in metabolic syndrome profiles in those individuals that participated in specific health guidance programs for three years than nonparticipants, although selection bias may be present [42]. Since it is difficult to set control conditions, there are only a few population-level or policy-level studies on health behaviors [42,43]. Further randomized control trials of health guidance programs are theoretically needed, which are now being undertaken in Japan [44].

9.3. Behavioral Approach Including Motivational Interviewing

In 2003, the U.S. Preventive Services Task Force recommended that primary care practitioners screen all adults for obesity and offer behavioral interventions and intensive counseling (Figure 4) [38]. Although a meta-analysis demonstrated that behavioral intervention resulted in a mean weight loss of 3.01 kg (95% CI: 4.02–2.01) [38], there are no established evidence-based guidelines for behavioral weight loss counseling in a primary care setting [28,38,45].

To encourage improvement of unhealthy lifestyles in health check-ups followed by health guidance, the following are important points: (1) individuals free of symptoms can assess their health status with regard to visceral fat accumulation to metabolic syndrome through what is called the "Where am I? chart" [46], for example using health data and pictorial presentation of carotid artery echograms; (2) individuals can go back to review their past and their own lifestyle using past health data, and understand the significance of reduction of accumulated visceral fat; (3) individuals can find out how to improve their lifestyle; and finally (4) individuals can appreciate improvement of health data, such as changes in blood glucose, lipid, and blood pressure, as well as weight loss and reduction of visceral fat in health check-ups to be conducted in subsequent years [42,46]. Behavioral modification in lifestyle by face-to-face individual counseling is important in reduction of visceral fat [40,42,46]. One recent innovation in improvement of face-to-face counseling is the implementation of online tools, including e-mail counseling and internet treatment programs (telemedicine) [47].

Health education (Figure 4) and preparation of food and physical environments (Figure 4) should be useful in facilitating behavioral modifications and practicing lifestyle improvements.

Since healthy living programs were reported to be effective for weight loss [39], recreational exercise might be useful as exercise therapy to combat metabolic syndrome. Recreational exercise and sports could be more feasible than the exercise therapy-based FITT (frequency, Intensity, time, type) principle, because recreation and sports are fun and encouraging for individuals. Therefore, recreational exercise and sports are suitable community-based strategies for physical activity and city planning [32].

It has been reported that on average, visceral fat accumulation is increasing in 20 to 30 year-old Japanese males, and exceeded 100 cm^2 in 40-year old individuals [10]. Therefore, for prevention of metabolic syndrome, it is important to approach younger individuals. One of the targets of management of metabolic syndrome should be prevention of ACVD in the community. In the community, health education on lifestyle modification is important, and health guidance for acceleration of referral to physicians is also important for high-risk individuals [44]. In the medical field, medical intervention by focusing on visceral fat accumulation should be more efficient, since the etiology of metabolic diseases is diverse (Figure 2). Diabetic patients with visceral fat accumulation have dysregulated eating or sleeping behavior and progression of atherosclerosis [37,48]. Therefore, it is important to improve multiple metabolic diseases comprehensively by persistent lifestyle modification targeting reduction of visceral fat (Figure 1) [11,13,42]. On the other hand, an individual approach to each metabolic disease is needed for individuals with multiple risks without visceral fat accumulation (Figure 1; Figure 2) [49]. Programs against smoking, hypertension, and hypercholesterolemia are also quite important for individuals with or without visceral fat accumulation.

10. Conclusions

Taken together, the clinical significance of assessment of the metabolic syndrome is to link individuals with visceral fat–related multiple risk factors to follow health guidance, and to prevent atherosclerotic cardiovascular diseases by reducing visceral fat. To achieve this aim, in addition to personal approaches, population approaches are important to combat metabolic syndrome. Established evidence-based guidelines and programs are needed within primary care setting.

Author Contributions: H.N. wrote the manuscript. I.S. reviewed the manuscript. The authors approved the final manuscript.

Acknowledgments: We thank Norikazu Maeda, Ken Kishida, Midori Noguchi, Tohru Funahashi (Osaka University), and Yuji Matsuzawa (Sumitomo Hospital) for the helpful discussion and direction.

Conflicts of Interest: The authors declare no conflict of interest.

Abbreviations

ACVD	atherosclerotic cardiovascular disease
BMI	body mass index
Mets	metabolic syndrome
SFA	subcutaneous fat area
VFA	visceral fat area

References

1. Alberti, K.G.; Eckel, R.H.; Grundy, S.M.; Zimmet, P.Z.; Cleeman, J.I.; Donato, K.A.; Fruchart, J.C.; James, W.P.; Loria, C.M.; Smith, S.C., Jr. Harmonizing the metabolic syndrome: A joint interim statement of the International Diabetes Federation Task Force on Epidemiology and Prevention; National Heart, Lung, and Blood Institute; American Heart Association; World Heart Federation; International Atherosclerosis Society; and International Association for the Study of Obesity. *Circulation* **2009**, *120*, 1640–1645. [PubMed]
2. Alberti, K.G.; Zimmet, P.; Shaw, J.; IDF Epidemiology Task Force Consensus Group. The metabolic syndrome—a new worldwide definition. *Lancet* **2005**, *366*, 1059–1062. [CrossRef]
3. Matsuzawa, Y. Metabolic syndrome–definition and diagnostic criteria in Japan. *J. Atheroscler. Thromb.* **2005**, *12*, 301. [CrossRef] [PubMed]
4. Yamagishi, K.; Iso, H. The criteria for metabolic syndrome and the national health screening and education system in Japan. *Epidemiol. Health* **2017**, *39*, e2017003. [CrossRef] [PubMed]
5. Malik, V.S.; Willett, W.C.; Hu, F.B. Global obesity: Trends, risk factors and policy implications. *Nat. Rev. Endocrinol.* **2013**, *9*, 13–27. [CrossRef] [PubMed]
6. González-Muniesa, P.; Mártinez-González, M.A.; Hu, F.B.; Després, J.P.; Matsuzawa, Y.; Loos, R.J.F.; Moreno, L.A.; Bray, G.A.; Martinez, J.A. Obesity. *Nat. Rev. Dis. Primers* **2017**, *3*, 17034. [CrossRef] [PubMed]
7. Examination Committee of Criteria for 'Obesity Disease' in Japan; Japan Society for the Study of Obesity. New criteria for 'obesity disease' in Japan. *Circ. J.* **2002**, *66*, 987–992. [CrossRef]
8. Neeland, I.J.; Poirier, P.; Després, J.P. Cardiovascular and metabolic heterogeneity of obesity: Clinical challenges and implications for management. *Circulation* **2018**, *137*, 1391–1406. [CrossRef]
9. Fujioka, S.; Matsuzawa, Y.; Tokunaga, K.; Tarui, S. Contribution of intra-abdominal fat accumulation to the impairment of glucose and lipid metabolism in human obesity. *Metabolism* **1987**, *36*, 54–59. [CrossRef]
10. Hiuge-Shimizu, A.; Kishida, K.; Funahashi, T.; Ishizaka, Y.; Oka, R.; Okada, M.; Suzuki, S.; Takaya, N.; Nakagawa, T.; Fukui, T.; et al. Absolute value of visceral fat area measured on computed tomography scans and obesity-related cardiovascular risk factors in large-scale Japanese general population (The VACATION-J study). *Ann. Med.* **2012**, *44*, 82–92. [CrossRef]
11. Okauchi, Y.; Nishizawa, H.; Funahashi, T.; Ogawa, T.; Noguchi, M.; Ryo, M.; Kihara, S.; Iwahashi, H.; Yamagata, K.; Nakamura, T.; et al. Reduction of visceral fat is associated with decrease in the number of metabolic risk factors in Japanese men. *Diabetes Care* **2007**, *30*, 2392–2394. [CrossRef] [PubMed]
12. Hamer, M.; O'Donovan, G.; Stensel, D.; Stamatakis, E. Normal-weight central obesity and risk for mortality. *Ann. Intern. Med.* **2017**, *166*, 917–918. [CrossRef] [PubMed]
13. Pi-Sunyer, X.; Blackburn, G.; Brancati, F.L.; Bray, G.A.; Bright, R.; Clark, J.M.; Curtis, J.M.; Espeland, M.A.; Foreyt, J.P.; Graves, K.; et al. Look AHEAD Research Group. Reduction in weight and cardiovascular disease risk factors in individuals with type 2 diabetes. *Diabetes Care* **2007**, *30*, 1374–1383. [PubMed]

14. Alberti, K.G.; Zimmet, P.Z. Definition, diagnosis and classification of diabetes mellitus and its complications. Part 1: Diagnosis and classification of diabetes mellitus provisional report of a WHO consultation. *Diabet. Med.* **1998**, *15*, 539–553. [CrossRef]
15. National Cholesterol Education Program (NCEP) Expert Panel on Detection, Evaluation, and Treatment of High Blood Cholesterol in Adults (Adult Treatment Panel III). Third Report of the National Cholesterol Education Program (NCEP)Expert Panel on Detection, Evaluation, and Treatment of High Blood Cholesterol in Adults (Adult Treatment Panel III) final report. *Circulation* **2002**, *106*, 3143–3421.
16. Iso, H. A Japanese health success story: Trends in cardiovascular diseases, their risk factors, and the contribution of public health and personalized approaches. *EPMA J.* **2011**, *2*, 49–57. [CrossRef] [PubMed]
17. Kuriyama, H.; Shimomura, I.; Kishida, K.; Kondo, H.; Furuyama, N.; Nishizawa, H.; Maeda, N.; Matsuda, M.; Nagaretani, H.; Kihara, S.; et al. Coordinated regulation of fat-specific and liver-specific glycerol channels, aquaporin adipose and aquaporin 9. *Diabetes* **2002**, *51*, 2915–2921. [CrossRef]
18. Tchkonia, T.; Thomou, T.; Zhu, Y.; Karagiannides, I.; Pothoulakis, C.; Jensen, M.D.; Kirkland, J.L. Mechanisms and metabolic implications of regional differences among fat depots. *Cell Metab.* **2013**, *17*, 644–656. [CrossRef]
19. Spalding, K.L.; Arner, E.; Westermark, P.O.; Bernard, S.; Buchholz, B.A.; Bergmann, O.; Blomqvist, L.; Hoffstedt, J.; Näslund, E.; Britton, T.; et al. Dynamics of fat cell turnover in humans. *Nature* **2008**, *453*, 783–787. [CrossRef]
20. Kusminski, C.M.; Bickel, P.E.; Scherer, P.E. Targeting adipose tissue in the treatment of obesity-associated diabetes. *Nat. Rev. Drug Discov.* **2016**, *15*, 639–660. [CrossRef]
21. Maeda, K.; Okubo, K.; Shimomura, I.; Mizuno, K.; Matsuzawa, Y.; Matsubara, K. Analysis of an expression profile of genes in the human adipose tissue. *Gene* **1997**, *190*, 227–235. [CrossRef]
22. Nyamdorj, R.; Pitkäniemi, J.; Tuomilehto, J.; Hammar, N.; Stehouwer, C.D.; Lam, T.H.; Ramachandran, A.; Janus, E.D.; Mohan, V.; Söderberg, S.; et al. Ethnic comparison of the association of undiagnosed diabetes with obesity. *Int. J. Obes.* **2010**, *34*, 332–339. [CrossRef]
23. Kadowaki, T.; Sekikawa, A.; Murata, K.; Maegawa, H.; Takamiya, T.; Okamura, T.; El-Saed, A.; Miyamatsu, N.; Edmundowicz, D.; Kita, Y.; et al. Japanese men have larger areas of visceral adipose tissue than Caucasian men in the same levels of waist circumference in a population-based study. *Int. J. Obes. (Lond)* **2006**, *30*, 1163–1165. [CrossRef] [PubMed]
24. De Toro-Martín, J.; Arsenault, B.J.; Després, J.P.; Vohl, M.C. Precision nutrition: A review of personalized nutritional approaches for the prevention and management of metabolic syndrome. *Nutrients* **2017**, *9*, E913. [CrossRef] [PubMed]
25. Näslund, U.; Ng, N.; Lundgren, A.; Fhärm, E.; Grönlund, C.; Johansson, H.; Lindahl, B.; Lindahl, B.; Lindvall, K.; Nilsson, S.K.; et al. VIPVIZA trial group. Visualization of asymptomatic atherosclerotic disease for optimum cardiovascular prevention (VIPVIZA): A pragmatic, open-label, randomised controlled trial. *Lancet* **2019**, *393*, 133–142.
26. Neumark-Sztainer, D.; Wall, M.; Larson, N.I.; Eisenberg, M.E.; Loth, K. Dieting and disordered eating behaviors from adolescence to young adulthood: Findings from a 10-year longitudinal study. *J. Am. Diet. Assoc.* **2011**, *111*, 1004–1011. [CrossRef]
27. Shah, R.; Kennedy, S.; Clark, M.D.; Bauer, S.C.; Schwartz, A. Primary care-based interventions to promote positive parenting behaviors: A meta-analysis. *Pediatrics* **2016**, *137*, e20153393. [CrossRef]
28. Ewart-Pierce, E.; Mejía Ruiz, M.J.; Gittelsohn, J. "Whole-of-Community" Obesity Prevention: A review of challenges and opportunities in multilevel, multicomponent interventions. *Curr. Obes. Rep.* **2016**, *5*, 361–374. [CrossRef]
29. Cornelsen, L.; Green, R.; Dangour, A.; Smith, R. Why fat taxes won't make us thin. *J. Public Health (Oxford)* **2015**, *37*, 18–23. [CrossRef]
30. Lear, S.A.; Hu, W.; Rangarajan, S.; Gasevic, D.; Leong, D.; Iqbal, R.; Casanova, A.; Swaminathan, S.; Anjana, R.M.; Kumar, R.; et al. The effect of physical activity on mortality and cardiovascular disease in 130,000 people from 17 high-income, middle-income, and low-income countries: The PURE study. *Lancet* **2017**, *390*, 2643–2654. [CrossRef]
31. Wu, T.; Gao, X.; Chen, M.; van Dam, R.M. Long-term effectiveness of diet-plus-exercise interventions vs. diet-only interventions for weight loss: A meta-analysis. *Obes. Rev.* **2009**, *10*, 313–323. [CrossRef] [PubMed]

32. Giles-Corti, B.; Vernez-Moudon, A.; Reis, R.; Turrell, G.; Dannenberg, A.L.; Badland, H.; Foster, S.; Lowe, M.; Sallis, J.F.; Stevenson, M.; et al. City planning and population health: A global challenge. *Lancet* **2016**, *388*, 2912–2924. [CrossRef]
33. World Health Organization. *Global Recommendations on Physical Activity for Health*; World Health Organization: Geneva, Switzerland, 2010.
34. Clarke, J.; Janssen, I. Is the frequency of weekly moderate-to-vigorous physical activity associated with the metabolic syndrome in Canadian adults? *Appl. Physiol. Nutr. Metab.* **2013**, *38*, 773–778. [CrossRef] [PubMed]
35. Taheri, S.; Lin, L.; Austin, D.; Young, T.; Mignot, E. Short sleep duration is associated with reduced leptin, elevated ghrelin, and increased body mass index. *PLoS Med.* **2004**, *1*, e62. [CrossRef] [PubMed]
36. Knutson, K.L. Sleep duration and cardiometabolic risk: A review of the epidemiologic evidence. *Best Pract. Res. Endcrinol. Metab.* **2010**, *24*, 731–743. [CrossRef] [PubMed]
37. Fukuda, S.; Hirata, A.; Nishizawa, H.; Nagao, H.; Kimura, T.; Fujishima, Y.; Yamaoka, M.; Kozawa, J.; Imagawa, A.; Funahashi, T.; et al. Characteristics of sleep-wake cycle and sleep duration in Japanese type 2 diabetes patients with visceral fat accumulation. *J. Diabetes Invest.* **2018**, *9*, 63–68. [CrossRef] [PubMed]
38. Leblanc, E.S.; O'Connor, E.; Whitlock, E.P.; Patnode, C.D.; Kapka, T. Effectiveness of primary care-relevant treatments for obesity in adults: A systematic evidence review for the U.S. Preventive Services Task Force. *Ann. Intern. Med.* **2011**, *155*, 434–447. [CrossRef] [PubMed]
39. Hunt, K.; Wyke, S.; Gray, C.M.; Anderson, A.S.; Brady, A.; Bunn, C.; Donnan, P.T.; Fenwick, E.; Grieve, E.; Leishman, J.; et al. A gender-sensitised weight loss and healthy living programme for overweight and obese men delivered by Scottish Premier League football clubs (FFIT): A pragmatic randomised controlled trial. *Lancet* **2014**, *383*, 1211–1221. [CrossRef]
40. Kohro, T.; Furui, Y.; Mitsutake, N.; Fujii, R.; Morita, H.; Oku, S.; Ohe, K.; Nagai, R. The Japanese national health screening and intervention program aimed at preventing worsening of the metabolic syndrome. *Int. Heart J.* **2008**, *49*, 193–203. [CrossRef] [PubMed]
41. Stock, S.A.; Redaelli, M.; Lauterbach, K.W. Disease management and health care reforms in Germany - does more competition lead to less solidarity? *Health Policy* **2007**, *80*, 86–96. [CrossRef] [PubMed]
42. Tsushita, K.; Hosler, A.S.; Miura, K.; Ito, Y.; Fukuda, T.; Kitamura, A.; Tatara, K. Rationale and descriptive analysis of specific health guidance: The nationwide lifestyle intervention program targeting metabolic syndrome in Japan. *J. Atheroscler. Thromb.* **2018**, *25*, 308–322. [CrossRef]
43. Gregg, E.W.; Ali, M.K.; Moore, B.A.; Pavkov, M.; Devlin, H.M.; Garfield, S.; Mangione, C.M. The importance of natural experiments in diabetes prevention and control and the need for better health policy research. *Prev. Chronic Dis.* **2013**, *10*, E14. [CrossRef] [PubMed]
44. Noguchi, M.; Kojima, S.; Sairenchi, T.; Kinuta, M.; Yamakawa, M.; Nishizawa, H.; Takahara, M.; Imano, H.; Kitamura, A.; Yoshida, T.; et al. Study Profile: Japan Trial in High-risk Individuals to Accelerate their Referral to Physicians (J-HARP)—A Nurse-led, Community-based Prevention Program of Lifestyle-related Disease. *J. Epidemiol.* in press.
45. Kelley, C.P.; Sbrocco, G.; Sbrocco, T. Behavioral modification for the management of obesity. *Prim. Care* **2016**, *43*, 159–175. [CrossRef]
46. Ryo, M.; Nakamura, T.; Funahashi, T.; Noguchi, M.; Kishida, K.; Okauchi, Y.; Nishizawa, H.; Ogawa, T.; Kojima, S.; Ohira, T.; et al. Health education "Hokenshido" program reduced metabolic syndrome in the Amagasaki visceral fat study. Three-year follow-up study of 3,174 Japanese employees. *Intern. Med.* **2011**, *50*, 1643–1648. [CrossRef] [PubMed]
47. Tate, D.F. A series of studies examining internet treatment of obesity to inform Internet interventions for substance use and misuse. *Subst. Use Misuse* **2011**, *46*, 57–65. [CrossRef] [PubMed]
48. Fukuda, S.; Hirata, A.; Nishizawa, H.; Nagao, H.; Kashine, S.; Kimura, T.; Inoue, K.; Fujishima, Y.; Yamaoka, M.; Kozawa, J.; et al. Systemic arteriosclerosis and eating behavior in Japanese type 2 diabetic patients with visceral fat accumulation. *Cardiovasc. Diabetol.* **2015**, *14*, 8. [CrossRef] [PubMed]
49. Kishida, K.; Funahashi, T.; Matsuzawa, Y.; Shimomura, I. Visceral adiposity as a target for the metabolic syndrome. *Ann. Med.* **2012**, *44*, 233–241. [CrossRef] [PubMed]

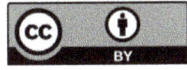

© 2019 by the authors. Licensee MDPI, Basel, Switzerland. This article is an open access article distributed under the terms and conditions of the Creative Commons Attribution (CC BY) license (http://creativecommons.org/licenses/by/4.0/).

MDPI
St. Alban-Anlage 66
4052 Basel
Switzerland
Tel. +41 61 683 77 34
Fax +41 61 302 89 18
www.mdpi.com

Nutrients Editorial Office
E-mail: nutrients@mdpi.com
www.mdpi.com/journal/nutrients

www.ingramcontent.com/pod-product-compliance
Lightning Source LLC
LaVergne TN
LVHW070224100526
838202LV00015B/2086